KU-460-204

Introduction to
PHARMACOLOGY

Third Edition

Mannfred A. Hollinger, Ph.D.

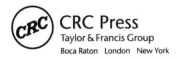

CRC Press
Taylor & Francis Group
Boca Raton   London   New York

CRC Press is an imprint of the
Taylor & Francis Group, an informa business

CRC Press
Taylor & Francis Group
6000 Broken Sound Parkway NW, Suite 300
Boca Raton, FL 33487-2742

© 2008 by Taylor & Francis Group, LLC
CRC Press is an imprint of Taylor & Francis Group, an Informa business

No claim to original U.S. Government works
Printed in the United States of America on acid-free paper
10 9 8 7 6 5 4 3 2 1

International Standard Book Number-13: 978-1-4200-4741-7 (Softcover)

This book contains information obtained from authentic and highly regarded sources. Reprinted material is quoted with permission, and sources are indicated. A wide variety of references are listed. Reasonable efforts have been made to publish reliable data and information, but the author and the publisher cannot assume responsibility for the validity of all materials or for the consequences of their use.

No part of this book may be reprinted, reproduced, transmitted, or utilized in any form by any electronic, mechanical, or other means, now known or hereafter invented, including photocopying, microfilming, and recording, or in any information storage or retrieval system, without written permission from the publishers.

For permission to photocopy or use material electronically from this work, please access www.copyright.com (http://www.copyright.com/) or contact the Copyright Clearance Center, Inc. (CCC) 222 Rosewood Drive, Danvers, MA 01923, 978-750-8400. CCC is a not-for-profit organization that provides licenses and registration for a variety of users. For organizations that have been granted a photocopy license by the CCC, a separate system of payment has been arranged.

Trademark Notice: Product or corporate names may be trademarks or registered trademarks, and are used only for identification and explanation without intent to infringe.

Library of Congress Cataloging-in-Publication Data

Hollinger, Mannfred A.
    Introduction to pharmacology / by Mannfred A. Hollinger. -- 3rd ed.
        p. ; cm.
    "A CRC title."
    Includes bibliographical references and index.
    ISBN-13: 978-1-4200-4741-7 (hardcover : alk. paper)
    ISBN-10: 1-4200-4741-8 (hardcover : alk. paper)
    1. Pharmacology. I. Title.
    [DNLM: 1. Pharmacology. 2. Pharmaceutical Preparations. QV 4 H741i 2008]

RM300.H65 2008
615'.1--dc22   2007017046

Visit the Taylor & Francis Web site at
http://www.taylorandfrancis.com

and the CRC Press Web site at
http://www.crcpress.com

Introduction to
PHARMACOLOGY

Third Edition

LIVERPOOL
JOHN MOORES UNIVERSITY
AVRIL ROBARTS LRC
TEL. 0151 231 4022

LIVERPOOL JMU LIBRARY

3 1111 01260 3922

Contents

"In the ocean depths off Madagascar, obsolete fish keep their laggard appointments. In the depths of the human mind, obsolete assumptions go their daily rounds. And there is little difference between the two, except that the fish do no harm."

Robert Ardrey
African Genesis

"That which in the beginning may be just like poison, but at the end is like nectar, and which awakens one to self-realization, is said to be happiness in the mode of goodness."

Bhagavad Gita

"Nothing in life is to be feared, it is only to be understood."

Marie Curie

"As thinking beings with the capacity for rational thought it is our responsibility to utilize our brains to wrestle with seemingly imponderable questions such as 'the meaning of life.' Simply put, there is no reason. Only what we make of it. We are not guided by some whimsical celestial force but are, fortunately, the product and manager of consistent, unalterable physical laws."

Anonymous

… "the pharmacologist has been a 'jack of all trades' borrowing from physiology, biochemistry, pathology, microbiology and statistics."

Gaddum

Preface to the First Edition

The topic of pharmacology usually escapes the attention of many college students by virtue of the fact that pharmacology itself is rarely taught at the undergraduate level. It is generally reserved for post-baccalaureate students enrolled in the health professions associated with medicine, dentistry, nursing, and the veterinary sciences. However, certain upper division undergraduates are interested in the subject. This book is the product of teaching undergraduates the principles of pharmacology over 20 years. During that period of time the author continually searched for an appropriate textbook for students who normally had some background in biochemistry and physiology. Medical school texts were of no use since their coverage is far too extensive and clinically oriented. On the other hand, "softer" texts tended to overemphasize certain areas, such as drug abuse, which was often the driving force behind their creation. While both types of texts were good, in their own right, they just did not "hit the mark." Students frequently expressed a desire for more "hard" science while not becoming inundated by "boiler plate" text. It is because of my agreement with their sentiment that the present book was constructed. The goal of this book is not to be a mini-medical school pharmacology text. Rather, it is intended to address a wider audience of advanced undergraduate students who have an interest in learning about the diverse aspects of pharmacology in society, not simply about the curative aspects of drugs. It is hoped that not only students in the biological sciences but also those in the social sciences will find some, if not all, of the book's contents informative and useful.

The underlying strategy in the organization of this book is to provide a logical continuum of information relating to drugs, beginning with the historical discovery of the pharmacological properties of certain foods. With this background, important pharmacological principles will be considered relating to drug absorption, distribution, metabolism, and elimination. This material will form the *corpus* of the chapters comprising Section 1. In essence, the emphasis will be placed on pharmacokinetic aspects of drug action. Having gained access to the body, how do drugs produce an effect and how can the effect be quantified for comparative purposes? In Section 2, the student is exposed to the concepts of drug–receptor interaction and the transduction of drug binding into pharmacodynamic or toxicodynamic responses. Factors influencing drug toxicity, as well as underlying principles of managing drug overdose, will also be presented as the inevitable "other side of the coin." Section 3 reiterates, in more detail, the concept introduced in Section 1 that drugs can be classified into three broad categories: (1) drugs that replace physiological inadequacies; (2) drugs that cure; and (3) drugs that treat symptoms. In this regard, hormones, antibiotics, and neuroactive agents will provide examples, respectively, in their own chapters. In addition, the pharmacology of substance abuse as well as the evolution of drug abuse laws and the use of drugs in sports will also be discussed. In Section 4, the final four chapters deal with the development of drugs by the pharmaceutical industry and the challenges they face in new drug discovery as well as dealing with the FDA. In addition, this section will include a discussion of the controversial use of experimental animals in research, an area often neglected in the study of pharmacology.

Preface to the Second Edition

Since the publication of the first edition the author has reevaluated the content of the book as well as its purpose. It became clear over the years that certain important areas that had been omitted in the first edition needed to be included in a revision, if a revision was to be meaningful. Therefore, additional areas added to the second edition include cardiovascular drugs, anticancer drugs, neuroleptics, designer drugs, bioterrorism, placebos, recombinant DNA technology, apoptosis, gaseous anesthetics, local anesthetics, vitamins, and the cigarette industry Master Settlement Agreement. In addition, in the intervening period since the publication of the first edition, the issue of alternative medicine has become very topical. For that reason, a new chapter on this subject has been added.

While identifying areas of omission was relatively straightforward, the question of how to make the book more attractive to the author's intended audience was more illusive. It has always been the author's goal to reach upper division, undergraduate students beyond those in the traditional "hard" science paths. Surely, there must be students and faculty in the humanities, in fields such as sociology and psychology, for example, who would find certain aspects of the study of drugs interesting and, perhaps, even provocative. Areas such as animal experimentation, the development of drug laws, drugs in sports, the drug-discovery process, and bioterrorism are not typical subjects expanded on in graduate-level texts. These are stand-alone subjects that do not require mastery of pharmacokinetics and pharmacodynamics, which essentially comprise the introductory Chapters 2–7.

In order to assist the student in evaluating his or her progress in dealing with the subject matter, the author has included a set of ten self-assessment questions at the end of each chapter (answers are provided at the back of the book). Hopefully, these questions will emphasize the important facts, principles, and personalities that the student should become familiar within the field of pharmacology. To further enhance the teaching power of the book, the new edition contains 41 new tables and 31 new figures.

Preface to the Third Edition

The roles of pharmacology in Western societies have greatly changed since its initial development in the late-nineteenth century. For example, the discovery of new drugs has permitted scientists to consider pharmacotherapy as one of the milestones of medicine in the past century. The direct consequence of the success of drug discovery has been a prodigious increase of scientific information exemplified by the development of pharmacogenomics and proteomics.

The introduction of recombinant DNA technology during the past 20 years has altered radically our approach to drug discovery and has had a fundamental impact on how drug targets are selected. Witness the power of molecular biology and the impact that such a discipline brings to modern-day pharmacology. Within a decade of the cloning of constitutive and inducible cyclooxygenase isoenzymes (Cox-1 and COX-2), selective COX-2 inhibitors were launched. Thus, these powerful cloning techniques have revolutionized how existing therapies are refined.

One of the challenges of teaching pharmacology is to define a core of knowledge. Examples of formal efforts to achieve this goal include (1) the formulation of a core curriculum for *Honours BSc in Pharmacology* by The Education Committee of the British Pharmacological Society and (2) the *Erasmus Program* and *Bologna Declaration* to develop comparable studies across universities in European higher education.

Whereas pharmacology was once only taught to health professionals, it is increasingly found that students with a biological or technological background are receiving instruction in this discipline. In addition, students from journalism, economic sciences, and lawyers are more and more interested in pharmacology.

How to integrate these new areas with the "old" pharmacology will be a challenge in the new millennium. Given the development of molecular biology, immunology, and genomics, modern pharmacologists will have to develop expertise in these disciplines if they plan to be robust participants in the pharmacology of the twenty-first century. Conversely, principles derived from past experience can still be applied to new drug development even if they are derived from proteomics or from biotechnology. It has been suggested that it may be easier for a pharmacologist to understand the principles of molecular biology than for a molecular biologist to grasp all the knowledge of pharmacology needed to correctly evaluate new drugs. Pharmaceutical industries are, in fact, increasingly searching for young researchers with pharmaceutical background rather than those with only molecular biology skills.

Knowledge and competence of pharmacologists will always be recognized as essential to develop drugs in the present century, regardless of the method from which they are obtained. Simply put, drugs are drugs, regardless of their origin, and students should be trained in the principles of pharmacology to understand how they treat a disease, how they can harm a patient, and how they are developed.

Pharmacology is a living discipline. It is subject to a constant evolution of changes. All these changes are not as exciting as molecular biology but, in their own ways, illustrate the diversity of the impact of drugs on society. For example, the beginning of the new century has seen the appearance of unprecedented counterfeiting of some of the most important drugs on the market (e.g., Viagra), while drugs such as OxyContin and some AIDS drugs are popular targets for thieves. These drugs will be among the first to carry *radio chip tracking devices* under a new FDA initiative. Although the FDA has said that less than 1% of prescription drugs sold in the United States are fake, they believe that counterfeiting is becoming more common and criminals are using more sophisticated techniques.

Another interesting development that may be edging forward in the future is an expanding liberal attitude to drug use. In 2004, the Drug Enforcement Agency (DEA) agreed to let a South Carolina physician treat 12 trauma victims with the illegal street drug *ecstasy* in what will be the first U.S.-approved study of the recreational drug's therapeutic potential. The goal is to help people with debilitating posttraumatic stress disorder. The DEA's move marks an historic turn for a drug that has long been both venerated and vilified.

One of the greatest developments in information transfer of the last century is, of course, the Internet. It offers a large number of pharmacological resources that can help students find information regarding all drug topics. A recent study has shown that >80% of European pharmacologists rate Internet information as good to excellent; their American colleagues are at least as enthusiastic.

Whenever possible, the author has taken advantage of new information that has become available since publication of the second edition. This is particularly true of knowledge that has been gained at the molecular level. In almost all areas, we know so much more than 5 years ago about intimate details about mechanistic aspects of drugs and toxins. While not all this information is appropriate for the introductory student, much of it will be helpful in appreciating the interrelationship between physiology, biochemistry, and pharmacology. In this regard, each individual instructor should feel free to pick and choose from the contents of this book in a manner that best reflects the background and interest of his students. Toward this end, a number of new tables and figures have been added.

Mannfred A. Hollinger, PhD
Oro Valley, Arizona

Acknowledgments

The author would like to express his sincere thanks for the continuing support of his wife Georgia throughout the three iterations of this book project. In addition, the kind comments of former students have been greatly appreciated. The author is fortunate to have sons Randy and Chris who have developed mature intellects and insights into some of the thornier issues of contemporary drug use. The author appreciates their input. The author would also like to acknowledge the excellent graphic design provided in much of this book by Tsunami Graphics, Sacramento, California. (Thanks Randy.)

Appendix I has been reproduced with kind permission from PJD Publications Limited, Westbury, New York, and from M.A. Hollinger, *Res. Commun. Alc. Sbst. Abuse,* Vol. 16, pp. 1–23, 1995. Copyright 1995 by PJD Publications Ltd.

Author

Mannfred A. Hollinger, PhD, was a professor in the Department of Medical Pharmacology and Toxicology, School of Medicine, University of California, Davis. He was chair of the department from 1991 to 2001. Dr Hollinger was the former editor of *Current Topics in Pulmonary Pharmacology and Toxicology*, *Focus on Pulmonary Pharmacology and Toxicology*, and *Yearbook of Pharmacology*, and assistant editor of *The Journal of Pharmacology and Experimental Therapeutics*. He served on the editorial advisory board of *The Journal of Pharmacology and Experimental Therapeutics*, *Research Communications in Chemical Pathology and Pharmacology*, and *The Journal of the American College of Toxicology*. He was the series editor of *Pharmacology and Toxicology: Basic and Clinical Aspects* published by CRC Press. He was a member of the American Society of Pharmacology and Experimental Therapeutics and the Society of Toxicology.

Born in Chicago, he earned his BS from North Park College in 1961 and his MS (1965) and PhD (1967) from Loyola University. He was employed by Baxter Laboratories from 1961 to 1963. From 1967 to 1969, Dr Hollinger was a postdoctoral research fellow in the Department of Pharmacology, Stanford University Medical School. On moving to the UC Davis in 1969, Dr Hollinger participated in several team-taught courses for undergraduate, graduate, and medical students.

While at Davis, Dr Hollinger published numerous research papers as well as a monograph on respiratory pharmacology and toxicology. He served as a referee for many of the principal pharmacology and toxicology journals. Dr Hollinger was the recipient of a Burroughs–Wellcome Visiting Scientist Fellowship to Southampton, England, in 1986 as well as a National Institutes of Health Fogarty Senior International Fellowship to Heidelberg, Germany, in 1988. Dr Hollinger resided in Oro Valley, Arizona.

Part I

Fundamentals of Pharmacokinetics

1 Introduction

HISTORY

Pharmacology is one of the pillars of the drug discovery process. While the medicinal/organic chemist may create the candidate compound (sometimes referred to as a new chemical entity [NCE], an acronym that will recur later in this book), it is the pharmacologist who is responsible for testing it for pharmacological activity. A NCE is eventually investigated by several other groups of scientists (e.g., toxicologists, microbiologists, and clinicians), if it has demonstrated a potential therapeutic effect.

Pharmacology studies the effects of drugs and how they exert their effects. For example, penicillin cures certain bacterial infections and acetylsalicylic acid (ASA) can reduce inflammation. How do they accomplish these respective effects? Through research we now know that penicillin can disrupt the synthesis of cell walls in susceptible bacterial strains by inhibiting a key enzyme while ASA can inhibit the action of a cell membrane enzyme known as cyclooxygenase that is responsible for the synthesis of a number of inflammatory mediators.

Modern pharmacology owes part of its development to Friedrich Wörler, who inaugurated the field of synthetic organic chemistry in 1828 with the synthesis of *urea*. This achievement catalyzed the formation of an entire industry (German-dye) that ultimately led to the synthesis of NCEs; many of which were subsequently introduced as possible therapeutic agents. Prior to this achievement, physiological pharmacologists had been restricted to the study of crude preparations of natural substances such as strychnine (*Francois Magendie* showed that its convulsant action was produced at the spinal cord level) and curare (*Claude Bernard* demonstrated that it produces paralysis of skeletal muscle by blocking the neuromuscular junction).

Medical research in mid-nineteenth-century Europe was localized in Germany. In distinction to the relatively undeveloped state of laboratory-based research in Britain and France, experimental science blossomed in German university laboratories. However, things were about to change in the twentieth century, particularly in the field of physiology in France, thanks to one of the greatest scientists of his era. His name was *Claude Bernard*.

Unlike Germany, France had few bastions of laboratory medical research in the nineteenth century. Medical research in France was closely linked with the observation of hospital patients. Critics of this practice claimed that instead of the hospital, the laboratory was the ideal setting for experimentation. Laboratory medicine dated back to the seventeenth century, but the nineteenth century created a unique culture in which microscopy, vivisection, and chemical investigation were used in a controlled environment conducive to experimentation.

New research traditions emerged from the European laboratories of the mid-nineteenth century. Physiology, histology, cytology, pharmacology, and other fields grew to maturity on German university campuses. French medicine did not take to laboratory research as quickly. The French national universities emphasized teaching and accreditation of doctors and did not incorporate German ideas quickly. Medicine in France was bureaucratic and was centralized in Paris. The long-standing French tradition of hospital-based observation led to an almost complete repudiation of the new university-centered laboratories.

Despite the poor research environment in France, there were some notable researchers in those years. I have mentioned two above. *François Magendie*, a surgeon and anatomist, was professor at the Collège de France and was notorious for his willingness to perform vivisections. Yet, even more famous would be his protégé, the physiologist *Claude Bernard*.

Born on July 12, 1813, Claude Bernard's earliest interests were literature and drama, not science. In what turned out to be a fortuitous event for medical science, a Parisian literary critic read one of Bernard's plays and convinced the young man that his future was *not* in the theater. The critic encouraged Bernard to take up a more stable profession in order to make a living, leading to his enrollment in the University of Paris to study medicine.

Bernard proved to be a poor student, finishing 26th out of 29 total students. Eventually, he took a post as an assistant physician, where his skills at dissection caught the attention of Magendie. While working under the tutelage of Magendie, Bernard discovered his true calling. His first publication dealt with a branch of the facial nerve, the *chorda tympani,* while his medical dissertation focused on the function of gastric juice in nutrition.

As time passed, his research interests expanded to include further work digestion and a collaborative study of the South American poison curare. Bernard's studies of curare led him to reject long-standing concepts that all drugs have generalized, nonspecific effects in the body. Alternatively, he postulated that certain drugs act at localized sites. For example, curare causes paralysis by preventing a nerve impulse from making a muscle contract at a specific location. These precise locations were later determined for other drugs and the concept of "receptors" became central to the development of pharmacology.

One of Bernard's most important discoveries was the handling of sugar by the liver. He discovered glycogen in the liver and theorized that the liver was making sugar independently. Bernard concluded that the body not only broke down complex molecules in digestion but made its own chemicals in normal functioning. He suggested that the body created glycogen as a storage reserve of glucose. Bernard called the glycogenic process "internal secretion," a term that would become fundamental to endocrinology.

Another critical explanation of a physiological process was his description of the regulation of the blood supply by the vasomotor nerves. He discovered that the vasomotor nerves control the dilation and constriction of blood vessels in response to environmental temperature changes. For example, in cold weather the blood vessels of the skin constrict to conserve heat, and in hot weather they dilate to dissipate excess heat.

Bernard's discovery of this control mechanism, in concert with his knowledge of the glycogenic function of the liver, led Bernard to theorize about how an organism regulates its *"internal environment"* in the midst of changing external conditions. He emphasized the importance of this concept: *"The stability of the internal environment is the prime requirement for free, independent existence."* The regulatory measures and control systems that Bernard described were eventually termed "homeostasis," a concept central to modern physiology and pharmacology.

A key figure in the development of pharmacology, as a discipline, was *Oswald Schmiedeberg* (1838–1921). He obtained his medical doctorate in 1866, with a thesis on the measurement of chloroform in blood. He worked at the University of Dorpat in Hungary under *Rudolph Buchheim* (see Chapter 5), in what is generally considered to be the first department of pharmacology, and ultimately succeeded him in 1869. Only 3 years later, he was a professor at the University of Strasbourg and head of an institute of pharmacology. In 1878, he published the classic text *Outline of Pharmacology.*

In his 46 years at Strasbourg, he trained a list of preeminent scientists who populated the great centers of scientific learning throughout many countries. One of which was *John Jacob Abel.* Abel became the first chairman of pharmacology in the United States at the University of Michigan. Abel was an excellent scientist and is credited with the isolation of both epinephrine and histamine, as well as the preparation of crystalline insulin. Additional important individuals in the history of pharmacology are shown in Table 1.1.

Clinical pharmacology owes much of its foundation to the work of *William Withering.* Born in Shropshire, England, Withering was interested in various aspects of science, eventually graduating with an MD from the University of Edinburgh. Withering became interested in the disorder known as "dropsy" and eventually learned about an herbal treatment for this disorder from an old woman herbalist in Shropshire. However, her herbal recipe contained more than 20 plants. Fortunately, because of his interest and knowledge of botany, he identified the active ingredient as coming from

TABLE 1.1

Important Figures in the Development of Pharmacology

- *Dioscorides* (57 AD), Greek, one of the first materia medica of approximately 500 plants and remedies
- *Paracelsus* (1493–1541), Swiss scholar and alchemist, often considered the "grandfather of Pharmacology"
- *William Withering* (1741–1799), English, published *An Account of the Foxglove* in 1785
- *Sertürner*, isolated morphine the first *pure* drug in 1805
- *Paul Ehrlich*, German pathologist and Nobel prize winner, who is credited with developing the concept of chemotherapy
- *Gerhard Domagk*, German pathologist and Nobel Prize winner, observed the antibacterial property of a prototypical sulfonamide (Prontosil); considered to be the first selective antimicrobial agent
- *Horace Wells and William T.G. Morton*, introduced volatile anesthetics in the 1840s
- *Henri Bequerel* (1896), *Pierre and Marie Curie* (1898), discovery and awareness of radioactive principles
- *William Fleming*, discoverer of Penicillin
- *J. Watson* and *F. Crick* (1953) Structure of DNA
- *Rosalyn Yalow* (1921–), development of the radioimmunoassay, Nobel Prize in 1977
- *Stanley Cohen* and *Herbert Boyer*, genetic engineering in the 1980s
- *Sune K. Bergström, Bengt I. Samuelsson, and John R. Vane*, for their discoveries concerning prostaglandins and related biologically active substances (1982)
- Kary Mullis, inventor of polymerase chain reaction (1983)
- *Alfred G. Gilman and Martin Rodbell*, for their discovery of G-proteins and the role of these proteins in signal transduction in cells (1994)
- *Robert F. Furchgott, Louis J. Ignarro, and Ferid Murad*, for their discoveries concerning nitric oxide as a signalling molecule in the cardiovascular system (1998)

the plant *Digitalis purpurea*. With publication of his book *An Account of the Foxglove*, published in 1785, Withering introduced *Digitalis* for the therapy of congestive heart failure, or dropsy, as he knew the condition.

Withering was unaware that dropsy was caused by cardiac insufficiency. In common with his time, he believed that the kidney was responsible for dropsy (peripheral fluid accumulation) and, therefore, was the site of action of *Digitalis* in the condition. Nevertheless, his clinical observations were precise: "Let the medicine therefore be given in doses, and at the intervals mentioned above; let it be continued until it either acts on the kidneys, the stomach, the pulse or the bowels; let it be stopped upon the first appearance of any one of these effects, and I will maintain that the patient will not suffer from its exhibition, nor the practitioner be disappointed in any reasonable expectation."

In the process of observing the pharmacological effects of *Digitalis*, Withering identified desired endpoints to include increased urine production (now believed to be the result of increased cardiac output and increased blood flow through the kidneys) and a decreased pulse rate. Withering also noted the toxic central and cardiac effects of *Digitalis*. Withering's major contribution was not so much a discovery as the construction of a way of rationally approaching a therapeutic problem. Withering replaced the anecdotal (testimonial) basis of medicine with evidence-based medicine, derived from careful observation, uncontaminated with prejudice.

DEFINITIONS

Pharmacology is the science of drugs (Greek *pharmakos*, medicine or drug; and *logos*, study). Pharmacology has been defined as an experimental science that studies changes brought about *in vivo* and *in vitro* by chemically acting substances, whether used for therapeutic purposes or not. In the broadest sense, pharmacology is the science of studying the effect of drugs on living organisms. It attempts to describe the biological responses produced by drugs and define the underlying

TABLE 1.2
Pharmacology Definitions

- *Pharmacodynamics* is the study of how drugs act; an emphasis on mechanisms
- *Pharmacokinetics* is the study of how the body absorbs, distributes, metabolizes, and excretes drugs; the calculation of various rates brings a quantitative component to assessing drug action
- *Pharmacotherapeutics* is the use of drugs to treat disorders; the emphasis is on clinical management
- *Pharmacoepidemiology* is the study of the effect of drugs on populations; questions dealing with the influence of genetics are particularly important
- *Pharmacoeconomics* is the study of the cost-effectiveness of drug treatments; this is particularly important since the cost of medications is a world-wide concern, particularly among certain groups such as the elderly and AIDS patients

mechanisms by which the responses are generated. Because of this, pharmacology is an integrative discipline involving other fields of study such as physiology, biochemistry, microbiology, and immunology, for example. Pharmacology should be distinguished from the profession of pharmacy whose responsibilities include the identification, verification, standardization, compounding, and dispensing of drugs and dosage forms of drugs. Additional useful definitions relative to pharmacology are shown in Table 1.2.

Associating the word science with pharmacology implies a systematic investigation of observable phenomena that can be quantified and controlled for, a state that reflects much of modern pharmacology. However, as we shall see, this has not always been the case. As mentioned above, pharmacology involves the study of drugs. However, what is a drug?

The word drug is believed to have been derived from the French word "*drogue*," which refers to a dry substance and probably reflects the use of herbs in early therapy. Broadly defined, a drug is a chemical substance that can alter or influence the responsiveness of a biological system. The action of a drug is mediated by a naturally occurring process of the body. A drug either mimics, facilitates, or antagonizes a normally occurring phenomenon. Although people can, and do, argue about what a drug is to them, perhaps it may be helpful, at this point, to present several "official" views as to what a drug is. To begin with, let's examine how the governmental agency most concerned with drugs defines a drug. According to the *Food and Drug Administration* (FDA)

A. All drugs are chemicals, but, all chemicals are not drugs
  1. All drugs are poisons, but, all poisons are not drugs
B. Definitions
  1. Chemical: a substance composed of a combination of elements (electrons, protons, and neutrons)
  2. Drug: a chemical which is utilized for the diagnosis, prevention, cure, or amelioration of an unwanted health condition
    a. F.D. & C. Sec. 201. [321] (g) (1)—The term "drug" means (A) articles recognized in the official United States Pharmacopeia, official Homeopathic Pharmacopoeia of the United States, or official National Formulary, or any supplement to any of them; and (B) articles intended for use in the diagnosis, cure, mitigation, treatment, or prevention of disease in man or other animals; and (C) articles (other than food) intended to affect the structure or any function of the body of man or other animals; and (D) articles intended for use as a component of any articles specified in clause (A), (B), or (C);...
      (1) "Food" (201). [321] (a) (f) means (1) articles used for food or drink for man or other animals, (2) chewing gum, and (3) articles used for components of any other such article

Furthermore, according to the Federal Food, Drug, and Cosmetic Act, the term "drug" means (1) articles recognized in the official United States Pharmacopoeia (USP) (see end of chapter), official Homeopathic Pharmacopoeia of the United States, or official National Formulary, or any supplement to any of them; (2) articles intended for use in the diagnosis, cure, mitigation, treatment, or prevention of disease in man or other animals; (3) articles (other than food) intended to affect the structure or any function of the body of man or other animals; and (4) articles intended for use as a component of any article specified in clause (1), (2), or (3); but does not include devices or their component parts or accessories.

As one can appreciate, deciding what a drug is, or is not, can become an exercise as complicated as one wishes. For example, are salt water, sugar water, synthetic saliva (there is such a product [Salivart®]), artificial tears, placebos, or tetrodotoxin drugs? We will not debate this question at this time; however, with these official guidelines behind us, we may now proceed to investigate the world(s) of drugs and their diverse influences on the human experience.

BACKGROUND

The roots of pharmacology extend backward in time to our earliest Pleistocene hominid ancestors on the African savanna, approximately 5–10 million years ago. These primitive forebearers grubbed for existence in the brush, where berries, shoots, leaves, tubers, flowers, seeds, nuts, and roots were plentiful. Our predecessors became specialized vegetarians who, only later, acquired an appetite for meat. It was their vegetarian diet that served to join gastronomic needs with pharmacological discovery.

As our species evolved, we developed the higher reasoning centers of the brain. One of the manifestations of this increased capacity for thought was the ability to recognize *cause-and-effect* relationships between our environment and us. One specific relationship that our ancestors learned was that the dietary ingestion of certain plants (regardless of which part) produced significant, corresponding physiological changes in their bodies, in addition to providing essential minerals and calories. Thus began our long-standing relationship with plants, which continues to the present time.

HISTORY—ROLE OF PLANTS

Since time immemorial, plants have been used for treating diseases in humans and animals, as well as for spiritual needs in humans. Their role in early religion can be seen in friezes (carvings) from eighth century BC in Mesopotamia. These carvings clearly depict mandrake flowers and poppy heads. Early belief in the curative powers of plants and certain substances rested exclusively on traditional knowledge, that is, empirical information not subjected to critical examination (i.e., ethnopharmacology).

The use of natural products has been the single most important strategy in the discovery of novel medicines. Not only have most medical breakthroughs been based on compounds of natural origin, such compounds also represent a large share of the market. In 1999, half of the top 20 best-selling drugs were natural products, and their total sales amounted to $16 billion. Of the ~500 NCEs approved by regulatory authorities around the world in the past decade, nearly half are from natural sources. Thus, it is likely that newly identified compounds will continue to reach the market.

What are the reasons why natural compounds will continue to be successful as leads in the future? Most of the currently available classes of drugs either contain natural products or have these as original leads. This applies not only to relatively old drugs, but also to newer drugs. For many of these drugs, synthetic counterparts have not yet been developed.

The number of different natural plant species is estimated at over a quarter of a million, but only a small fraction of these has been studied. Together with even less-investigated sources, such as microorganisms and marine organisms, these have resulted in the identification of >160,000 natural compounds, a number that grows at a rate of >10,000 per year.

The question has been asked: "How over time, have we been 'shaped' by the shifting alliances that we have formed and broken with various members of the vegetable world as we have made our way through the maze of history?" The answer, in part, is that plants have always played a significant role in mediating human cultural experiences in the world at large; be that role dietary, medicinal, or to alter consciousness. These are roles that they still play today, whether in the realm of medicine, religion, or jurisprudence.

One of the most provocative theories relating to our relationship with plants is the suggestion that their consumption may have contributed to the relatively rapid organization of the human brain's information processing capacity. This is a process that occurred over a relatively short anthropological time frame. Specifically, this proposal suggests that hallucinogenic compounds such as psilocybin, dimethyltryptamine, and harmaline were present in the protohuman diet and that their psychopharmacological effects catalyzed the emergence of human self-reflection.

The theory boldly suggests that the tripling of human brain size from *Homo hablis* was facilitated by mutagenic, psychoactive plants that functioned as a chemical "missing link." While this proposal certainly does not represent a mainstream scientific view, it illustrates, nevertheless, the impact that plants, particularly psychoactive ones, continue to have in our attempts to define ourselves.

We can only speculate as to the actual sequence of events in the genesis of our relationship with plants. However, the knowledge of plant effects undoubtedly began with individual experiences. It was only after the epigenetic (i.e., learned rather than genetically based) development of language (i.e., communication) that members of a familial or tribal group could receive "instruction" based on the experience of senior members. This view is based, of course, on the premise that language, of any kind, is the primary fulcrum of teaching and/or learning.

Verbal communication does not appear to be an absolute prerequisite, however. For example, mother chimps routinely offer choice tidbits of food to their infants and will snatch unusual, possibly dangerous, foods from their mouths. Primatologists in Tanzania have observed that chimpanzees periodically include leaves of the *Aspilia* plant in their diet. Despite its bitter taste, it's consumed by both sexes, all ages, the healthy as well as the sick. The chimps eat these leaves regularly, but consume very few of them at one time, indicating that their nutritional value is in doubt. In the rainy season, though, when intestinal worms and other illnesses plague apes, ingestion increases dramatically. Analysis of these leaves has shown them to contain the chemical *thiarubrine-A*, which has antibacterial properties.

Leaves from the same plant are also used by natives of the area to treat wounds and stomachaches. How is "chimpanzee ethnomedicine" possible? Could it be based on some kind of hereditary information? Or, more probably, is this *cultural* information passed on—by emulation or instruction—from generation to generation, and subject to rapid change if the available medicinal plants change, or if new diseases arise, or if new ethnobotanical discoveries are made? With the exception of the lack of professional herbalists, chimpanzee folk medicine does not seem so different from human folk medicine etiology. While the *Aspilia* story is particularly instructive, chimps are also known to eat plants other than Aspilia to treat intestinal disorders, as well as soil from particular cliff faces, presumably to provide mineral nutrients such as salt.

It has been said that until experience can be summarized by symbols—whether words or manual gestures—and the symbols grouped, filed, isolated, and selected to perform the thinking process, then experience is no more than a silent film. Symbols allow us to store information outside the physical brain for retrieval and transmission across space and time. The capacity to relate past experiences to future possibilities and deal in symbols, particularly language, is an inheritance from our Pliocene past, which has evolved from warning cries in the *Oldavi gorge* to *Senate filibusters* and "*Rap music.*"

In this way, knowledge of the effect of plants on bodily functions probably became part of our collective memory. Before the advent of writing, this collective memory had to be communicated verbally and became the responsibility of certain members of the group, a practice that continued into the middle ages in the form of lyrical song or verse, in order to make the information easier to remember.

There are many examples of plants that played significant roles in the lives of ancient man. Perhaps one of the more interesting examples deals with a parasitic shrub that we still use in our own traditional Christmas celebrations. *Mistletoe* (*Viscum album*) was celebrated for its mysterious powers by the ancient Celts (fourth century BC). Celtic priests (the *Druids*) were fascinated by the haphazard growing and blooming of the shrub and considered it the most sacred plant of all. Interestingly, the presence of mistletoe pollen in the peat moss "grave" of the 1500-year-old "*Lindow Man*," unearthed in 1984 near Manchester, England, contributed to the theory that this individual had, in fact, been a Druid prince.

Druids harvested the mistletoe berry yearly and used it in their winter celebrations, known as *samain* and *imbolc*, which were centered on the winter solstice. For this celebration, the Druids concocted a strong potion of the berries, which researchers have subsequently discovered to contain a female-like steroid that may have stimulated the libido (presumably structurally related to either estrogen or progesterone). Mistletoe has, of course, become a contemporary symbol to Yuletide merrymakers as a license to kiss.

The Celts, and others, also used mistletoe for medical purposes. The Roman historian Pliny the Younger wrote that mistletoe was "deemed a cure for epilepsy; carried about by women it assisted them to conceive, and it healed ulcers most effectually (sic) if only the sufferer chewed a piece of the plant and laid another piece on the sore." Modern herbalists continue to recommend mistletoe for the treatment of epilepsy, hypertension, and hormone imbalances. However, it should be appreciated that homemade brews made from the berries and leaves of the North American species (Phoradendron flavescens) are poisonous and should be avoided.

In the New World, specialists similar to the Druids existed in "primitive" societies and functioned as *Shamans*. The Shaman is a priest-doctor who uses "magic" to cure the sick, to divine the hidden, and to control events that affect the welfare of the people. The Shaman seeks to achieve "ecstasy" often by the use of plants containing psychedelic drugs. The central role that drugs played in fourteenth-century life in Columbia, for example, is clearly illustrated by much of their artwork. Sculptures clearly depict the use of *coca leaves* as well as the veneration of the *mushroom*. The writings of *Carlos Castaneda* and others have popularized the *Shaman* and the use of hallucinogenic drugs in contemporary literature.

While Shamans were inculcating the role of drugs in the New World, the Middle Ages were not a particularly good time for plants and drugs. For example, the medieval church actively suppressed knowledge of plants suspected of playing a role in the nocturnal activities of the practitioners of *witchcraft*. Specifically, use of extracts from the *thorn apple* (*Datura*) was prohibited, since the application of ointments containing this substance was believed to confer the gift of flight.

Throughout medieval Europe witches routinely rubbed their bodies with hallucinogenic ointments made from belladonna, mandrake, and henbane; all structurally related to Datura. In fact, much of the behavior associated with witches was attributed to these drugs. Their journey was not through space, however, but across the hallucinatory landscape of their minds. A particularly efficient means of self-administering the drug for women is through the moist tissues of the vagina; the witches' broomstick or staff was considered a most effective applicator.

Fortunately, a Swiss named *Phillippus Theophrastus von Hohenheim* (1493–1541) began to question doctrines handed down from antiquity. In 1516, he assumed the name *Paracelsus* (Para: beside, beyond, and Celsus: a famous Roman physician). He encouraged development of knowledge of the active ingredient(s) in prescribed remedies, while rejecting the irrational concoctions and mixtures of medieval medicine. Paracelsus discounted the humoral theory of *Galen*, whose rediscovered works became the foundation of medicine at the time. Galen postulated that there were *four humors* in the body (*blood, phlegm, and yellow and black bile*); when these were in balance, one enjoyed health, and when there was imbalance, sickness ensued. Paracelsus was a free thinker and an iconoclast. His disenchantment with the teaching of medicine at the University of Basle reached its climax on July 24, 1527, when he publicly burned the standard medical textbooks of the day (e.g., Galen's). All this behavior was deemed heresy, and not acceptable to the medical community of his time.

Paracelsus prescribed chemically defined substances with such success that enemies within the profession had him prosecuted as a poisoner. This was primarily based on his use of inorganic

TABLE 1.3
**Examples of Plant Compounds and
Their Therapeutic Uses**

- *Atropine*—Anticholinergic (mydriatic)
- *Caffeine*—CNS stimulant
- *Cocaine*—Local anesthetic
- *Colchicine*—Antigout
- *Digoxin*—Cardiotonic
- *Ephedrine*—Bronchodilator
- *Morphine*—Analgesic
- *Oubain*—Cardiotonic
- *Physostigmine*—Cholinergic
- *Quinine*—Antimalarial
- *Scopolamine*—Anticholinergic
- *Theophylline*—Bronchodilator
- *D-Tubocurarine*—Skeletal muscle relaxant
- *Vincristine*—Antineoplastic

substances in medicine, because his critics claimed that they were too toxic to be used as therapeutic agents. He defended himself with the thesis that has become axiomatic in pharmacology/toxicology: "*If you want to explain any poison properly, what then isn't a poison? All things are poisons, nothing is without poison; the dose alone causes a thing not to be poison.*"

Plants, and natural products, continue to play a vital role in modern society both as the source of conventional therapeutic agents as well as herbal preparations in "health" food stores. In 1994, half of the top 25 drugs on the market in terms of sales were either natural products or based on natural products, now made synthetically or semisynthetically. Examples of active plant compounds with therapeutic uses are shown in Table 1.3.

It is estimated that 80% of people in developing countries are almost totally dependent on traditional healers for their health care, and that plants are the major source of drugs for their traditional medical practitioners. In theory, in as much as 80% of the world's population live in developing countries; approximately 64% of the world's population depends, therefore, almost entirely on plants for medication.

The anti-ovarian cancer compound *Taxol* is a classic case of how supply can be critical for drugs based on natural products. In the late 1980s, the only known source of this drug was the bark of the relatively rare Pacific yew tree *Taxus brevifolia*. Unfortunately, in the Pacific Northwest, nearly 90% of the yew's native habitat has been destroyed in the last century. The decline in yew population had serious implications for patients with ovarian cancer.

It has been estimated that 6-inch diameter trees would have to be sacrificed for enough Taxol to treat one woman suffering from ovarian cancer. Considering that the number of potential patients in the late 1980s numbered approximately 12,000, an eventual limitation of Taxol was possible. Fortunately, the problem was solved in the early 1990s by the partial synthesis of Taxol from a precursor produced in needles and twigs from the more renewable *Taxus baccata*. This has secured the supply of Taxol for its current therapies and made it the best-selling anticancer agent ever, with sales exceeding $1 billion annually.

The approval of Taxol for marketing in December of 1992 was the culmination of 35 years of work. During this period of time, the *National Cancer Institute (NCI)* and the *U.S. Department of Agriculture* (USDA) collaborated to collect, identify, and screen U.S. native plant material for antitumor activity. The year 1992 also marked, coincidentally, the discovery of the "*Ice Man*" in the Italian Alps. This Bronze Age man, who died 5300 years ago, was found in possession of a pure copper axe set in a yew wood handle and an unfinished 6-ft yew bow. Obviously, the yew tree has played a number of important roles for humans throughout history.

Taxol is a potent inhibitor of eukaryotic cell replication, blocking cells in the late G2, or mitotic phase of the cell cycle. Interaction of Taxol with cells results in the formation of discrete bundles of *stable microtubules* as a consequence of reorganization of the microtubule cytoskeleton. Microtubules are normally not static organelles but rather are in a state of dynamic equilibrium with their components (i.e., soluble tubulin dimers). Taxol alters this normal equilibrium, shifting it in favor of the stable, nonfunctional microtubule polymer. At present, the number of different classes of natural compounds that cause microtubule stabilization has risen to eight.

In addition to being an essential component of the mitotic spindle, and required for the maintenance of cell shape, microtubules are involved in a wide variety of cellular activities, such as cell motility and communication between organelles within the cell. Any disruption of the equilibrium within the microtubule system would be expected to disrupt cell division and normal cellular activities in which microtubules are involved.

As indicated above, plant products can be useful as starting material for the semisynthetic preparation of other drugs. An important example in this regard is the Mexican yam, which produces a steroid precursor (*diosgenin*) that serves as a vital precursor in the synthesis of steroidal hormones used in oral contraceptives (i.e., progesterone). The availability of diosgenin eliminates numerous expensive steps in the organic synthesis of the basic steroid molecule. It was this discovery that contributed to the development of the pharmaceutical company Syntex (now a subsidiary of Hoffman LaRoche) and the development of the first birth control pill.

CONTEMPORARY ISSUES REGARDING PLANTS

It is our historical relationship with plants that has led contemporary *ethnobotanists* to attempt to raise our consciousness regarding the disappearance of rain forests; and their indigenous richness in discovered and undiscovered drug sources. For example, it has been estimated that between 2,000 and 40,000 plant species are lost annually through destruction of tropical rainforests. This is significant since less than 1% of the world's flowering plants have been tested for their effectiveness against disease. In an attempt to counteract this scenario, several drug companies have committed financial resources to support increased acquisition and evaluation of remaining plant material. In addition, royalties have been guaranteed to South American tribes whose Shamans provide successful drug leads.

There are estimated to be at least 250,000 species of higher plants and 30 million botanical species remaining, most of which have not been tested for biological activity. To this end, a drug company was formed in the early 1990s to specifically deal with this challenge (appropriately named Shaman Pharmaceuticals). By forming consortiums with larger drug companies (e.g., Lilly), they hope to accelerate the rate of discovery of new drug entities discovered from botanical sources.

Major technological advances in screening processes (see Chapter 14) have promoted the belief that the drug discovery process may become abbreviated. Pharmacologists have traditionally had to analyze in the approximate neighborhood of 15,000 NCEs, before one could qualify for testing in humans. This normally requires many years and hundreds of millions of dollars. Until relatively recent, animal testing was the only way to go. However, initial screening can often be done in a matter of days without using animals. This can be achieved by using isolated enzymes or receptors to determine if the drug has any binding affinity (see Chapter 14) at all.

However, not everyone agrees that this renewed drug company enthusiasm for going out in the field to seek plant-based drugs will be particularly widespread or particularly effective in the long-term. Nonenthusiasts contend that labor-intensive plant collection methods are being supplanted by newer, laboratory-based chemistry techniques (see Chapter 15) that are more efficient in creating new drug leads. For every proven anticancer drug like Taxol, there are hundreds of plant compounds that demonstrate initial promise in the test tube only to prove a disappointment later.

In the final analysis, will rational drug design, chemical synthesis, or combinatorial chemistry prove to be enough? Or, will the abundant natural diversity of chemical structures found in nature provide new scaffolds and new chemical space for even greater advancement in NCEs.

In the Western hemisphere, there are more than 40 species of plants that are used for hallucinogenic purposes alone. Although the structures of hallucinogenic substances varies significantly, most plants owe their hallucinogenic properties to alkaloids, which are cyclic structures containing nitrogen. At least 5000 higher plants contain alkaloids. Despite their wide distribution among plants, our knowledge of their pharmacology is still largely incomplete.

One of the challenges facing early, as well as contemporary, chemists is how to extract the pharmacologically active principle (such as an alkaloid) from a plant. This is desirable because it allows identification, assessment of pharmacological effects, constant dosage, and the opportunity to create liquid forms of the extract. For example, soaking plants in alcohol (ethanol) creates a *tincture*, which is, undoubtedly, one of the first organic extractions performed by man.

In the process of preparing a tincture, some pharmacologically active constituents of the plant are extracted by the alcohol. Although not all substances are soluble in alcohol, those that are include the alkaloids. In the case of a tincture of raw opium, the soluble alkaloids include morphine, codeine, noscapine, papavarine, and others. Such tinctures of opium were the infamous laudanum preparations of the late 1800s (see Appendix I).

In addition to providing drugs, plants have also been recently utilized for ecological purposes via the process of *phytoremediation*. Phytoremediation refers to the ability of some plants to remove toxic compounds from the soil, concentrate them in their own tissues, and, therefore, achieve a certain degree of detoxification. Current interest has specifically focused on removing metals from poisoned sites. Among the poisoned sites are abandoned mines containing zinc and lead; military bases contaminated with lead and cadmium; municipal waste containing copper, mercury, and lead; and sewage sludge where numerous metals can be a problem. Agricultural applications are also being researched (e.g., selenium removal by the mustard plant). The process of metal scavenging appears to be mediated by phytochelatins, small peptides that bind metals in forms that are less toxic to the plant.

MICROORGANISMS

Plants are not the only natural products used as a source for drugs. Microorganisms have, of course, been extensively screened for antibiotics since Alexander Fleming's discovery of the antibacterial activity of *Penicillin notatum* in the 1920s. Numerous useful antibiotics are also produced by bacteria of the Streptomyces genus (including streptomycin, neomycin, tetracycline, and chloramphenicol) as well as fungi (griseofulvin and cyclosporin C). Antibiotics will be discussed in more detail in Part III, Chapter 10.

MARINE SOURCES

Drugs and other products from the sea have been a steadily growing area of research interest for the past 20 years. In 1992, the U.S. government spent approximately $44 million in the area of marine biotechnology research. U.S. industrial investment in marine biotechnology was approximately $60 million in 1994 (both small and large companies are involved). By collecting, growing, or synthesizing natural compounds made by an array of marine creatures (e.g., microbes, sponges, corals, sea slugs, and others), investigators are screening compounds in hopes of adding to the medical armamentarium against cancer, AIDS, inflammation, and other conditions.

Marine species comprise approximately one-half of total global diversity (estimates range from 3 to 500 million different species). Therefore, the marine world would appear to offer significant potential resources for novel pharmacological compounds. Unfortunately, much of the literature on marine natural products is characterized by compounds with demonstrable cytotoxicity rather than pharmacological efficacy.

However, toxicological properties can conceivably be utilized therapeutically. For example, one current therapeutic candidate, based on its cytotoxicity, is bryostatin 1; Bryostatin, from the bryozoan *Bugula neritina*. Development is currently underway to develop aquaculture techniques for the harvesting of the bryozoan source. Because of the relatively large number of possible drug candidates from marine sources, pharmaceutical companies are forced to utilize their high-throughput screening technologies with extensive arrays of drug-target specific assays (see Part IV, Chapter 15 for more details) to test marine extracts.

An example of a natural product from a marine organism that has been commercialized is an extract from sea whips (*Pseudopterogoogia elisabethae*). This extract is used in the manufacture of certain cosmetic products. The active ingredient is believed to be a class of diterpine glycosides (pseudopterosins), which apparently has some anti-inflammatory activity.

Another marine product undergoing development is docosahexaenoic acid (DHA), developed via fermentation of a microalgae. DHA is a major component in human gray matter and is important for normal healthy development in infants. Various groups, such as the World Health Organization, have recommended DHA's inclusion in infant formulas at levels similar to those found in human milk. DHA is presently used in Belgium and Holland, and is expected to gain approval in the United States.

ANIMAL SOURCES

Today, animal products such as insulin (extracted from the pancreas of cows and pigs) are being used less frequently for the treatment of diabetes mellitus because of the introduction of synthetic recombinant human derivatives (e.g., Lantus®). However, it should be appreciated that less attractive members of the animal world can still provide therapeutic features. For example, *maggots*, which are the larval form of approximately one-half of the more than 85,000 species of flies, have and still are occasionally used to treat open wounds (a procedure known as maggot debridement therapy [MDT] or, more commonly, maggot therapy). MDT is practiced in more than 150 hospitals in the United States and 1000 centers worldwide.

The use of maggots to treat wounds dates back to ancient times; in fact, the 2000 Academy Award film *Gladiator* portrayed the hero's shoulder being healed by maggot therapy. The modern father of MDT was William S. Baer, who developed the strategy based on his observation during World War I that wounded soldiers, whose wounds harbored living maggots, did not develop gangrene. The maggots had the lovely habit of selectively debriding the necrotic tissue in the wounds, but left the healthy tissue unmolested. This is particularly true for the popular *Lucilia sericata* (greenbottle blowfly larvae) that actually starves on healthy tissue, making them ideal for medicinal use. Another of Baer's contributions to the field involved a method to sterilize the maggots. Today, commercial and research laboratories produce sterile larvae.

The ability of maggots to promote healing of lacerations on skin wounds is apparently the result of their secretion of the chemical *allantoin*. A less offensive source of allantoin is the synthetic form. Synthetic allantoin is available today to accelerate wound healing and is used in skin ulcer therapy when applied topically (similar uses exist in veterinary medicine). An alternative theory to explain the maggot's "mechanism of action" is that they secrete antimicrobial waste products such as ammonium, calcium, or other bicarbonates that break down only the necrotic tissue in wounds; these secretions also change the alkalinity of the wound to help it heal.

The soft-bodied, legless larvae were widely used to clean wounds until the 1940s, when antibiotics supplanted them. However, interest in this "biosurgery" using specially bred, germ-free maggots is currently increasing within certain clinical specialties (e.g., plastic surgery), particularly in the United Kingdom. Three-day-old maggots from the greenbottle fly have been used in the treatment of open wounds such as ulcers. Apparently, 100 maggots can eat 10–15 g of dead tissue a day, leaving wounds clean and healthy (today, the scientific standard of 10 larvae/cm^2 is used). In one case, an 83-year-old man with severe leg ulcers was saved the trauma of an amputation due to successful treatment with maggots.

In a similar context, a recombinant version of a protein from a blood-feeding *hookworm* is currently being investigated for its use in preventing blood clots. A protein, designated NAP-5, is a member of a family of anticoagulant proteins. Apparently, the protein acts by inhibiting Factor Xa in the initial step of the blood-clotting cascade, leading to fibrin formation. If successful, this protein may replace an entire class of 40-year-old "blood-thinning" drugs, called heparins, which are widely used to protect against clot formation in heart-attack patients.

Another natural anticoagulant is *hirudin*, derived from the saliva of the *leech* (*hirudo* is the Latin word for leech). Medicinal-leech mania swept through Europe and North America in the mid-1800s. Records from that time show that while practicing so-called hirudotherapy, French physicians used more than a billion medicinal leeches each year. The demand for fresh European medicinal leeches was so great that a leech "express" operated from Moscow to Paris. Because collecting wild leeches for pharmaceutical suppliers was so easy, wild leeches were over collected and nearly disappeared from ponds and wet lands. (Today, several nations have crafted conservation plans for protecting the wild species.)

The red-and-white striped barber pole originates from the days of bloodletting, which was often performed in barbershops. Bloodied bandages were hung on a pole outside the shops and became a symbol of the service rendered by the proprietor. By the 1850s, most physicians had come to recognize that bloodletting, with or without medicinal leeches, was weakening and sometimes even killing their patients. Soon after, medicinal leeches joined the unemployed.

Leeches are still occasionally used therapeutically for certain topical applications. In the United States, Dr. Joseph Upton made headlines in 1985, when he applied two dozed medicinal leeches to the head of a five-year-old boy during a successful ear reattachment. As others subsequently discovered, medicinal leeches are particularly helpful in restoring blood circulation to grafted tissues and to reattached fingers and toes. While feeding, the leeches can remove any congested blood at the site of reattachment, allowing normal circulation to return to the tissues and facilitating fast healing.

Another possible drug to be used for the dissolution of blood clots is derived from *bat saliva* and acts as a plasminogen activator. It appears as though saliva is a good place to look for possible drugs affecting the blood clotting system since *sand fly* saliva is also being examined for this property. Bat and sand fly saliva are not the only salivary source for an exciting new drug. The Southwest's reclusive Gila monster is the source for salivary proteins used in the treatment of type 2 diabetes (see Chapter 9). Numerous patients taking this drug (Byetta, exenatide) have reported reductions in their blood sugar as well as body weight. In a 2-year study presented in June 2006, at an *American Diabetes Association* meeting, 283 patients who added *Byetta* to their current diabetes treatment lost an average of 10 pounds and reduced their fasting blood glucose 25 milligrams per deciliter.

Byetta was approved by the FDA in April 2005, for use as an additional treatment for patients unable to control their type 2 diabetes with a sulfonylurea drug or Metformin. Pharmaceutical companies Amylin and Eli Lilly launched Byetta in June 2005; it is now fifth (October, 2006) among branded diabetes drugs for number of "new" prescriptions written. Net sales in its first year exceeded $242 million.

Snake venoms have also been found to possess ingredients with important pharmacological properties. Perhaps the best-known example is the drug captopril, which is used in the management of hypertension. This drug is a dipeptide analogue of bradykinin-potentiating peptides (BPPs), originally identified in the venom of the pit viper *Bothrops jararaca*. The drug acts by inhibiting angiotensin-converting enzyme (ACE), whose normal function is to catalyze the formation of a vasoconstrictor peptide (angiotensin II). When the snake injects its venom, the BPPs inhibit ACE thus ensuring circulation of the venom by inhibiting vasoconstriction in the same manner.

DEVELOPMENT OF FORMULARIES

Archeological evidence confirms our assumption that drug taking is an extremely old human characteristic. Human use of alcohol in the form of fermented grains, fruits, and plants is particularly ancient.

For example, fragmentary evidence exists that beer and hackle berry wine were used as early as 6400 BC. However, it was not for several more millennia before organized, written compendia (i.e., a brief compilation of a whole field of knowledge) were developed.

The Egyptian Ebers papyrus (ca. 1550 BC) contains the description of several active medicinal ingredients that are still used today. In India, an extensive list of the therapeutic uses of plant material was developed by approximately 1000 BC. To put Western knowledge of drugs into perspective, the modern era of pharmacology did not begin until the work of Francois Magendie (1783–1855), who prepared a medical formulary of "purified drugs." His book contained a list of medicinal substances and formulas for making medicines.

The earliest Chinese records indicate the use of natural products after approximately 500 BC. It was also during this period that the Chinese might have been the first to distill alcohol; thus making it the first drug to be isolated and purified.

The Chinese have one of the most extensive herbal traditions. The earliest known written work on Chinese herbs is *The Herbal Classic of the Devine Plowman* written anonymously in approximately 100 BC. This treatise recommended the therapeutic use of 365 drugs (252 from plants, 67 from animals, and 46 from minerals).

PHARMACOPOEIAS

A pharmacopoeia is simply a compendium of drugs, along with information about their preparation. Historically, they have ranged from herbals—lists of plants with medicinal properties (real or imagined)—to lists and recipes used by apothecaries, to the modern formularies used by health care plans and recognized by governments. Along the way, pharmacopoeias have helped those who prepare drugs to separate themselves as a distinct discipline among the healing professions, culminating in modern pharmacy in the nineteenth and twentieth centuries.

It is claimed that the world's first pharmacopoeia is the *De Materia Medica* (ca. AD 79) by the Greco-Roman military physician Dioscorides. This publication described hundreds of pharmaceutical preparations made from vegetable, animal, and mineral sources.

Later, Galen (AD 131–201), who wrote widely about many aspects of medical practice, influenced pharmaceutical practice for centuries to come. Not only did he have a robust medical practice that served gladiators and emperors, but Galen maintained a well-stocked pharmacy. Although Galen influenced medieval medicine significantly, medieval pharmacy was largely a matter of local remedies. One of these was Hildegard of Bingen (1098–1179). As Abbess of the Benedictine convent in Rupertsburg, she compiled and organized information about the pharmaceutical uses of plants and kept records of plant combinations she deemed efficacious.

One of the largest sources of European pharmaceutical information was the mid-thirteenth-century *Compendium of Medicine* of *Gilbertus Anglicus*. Gilbertus's manuscript contained instructions for making numerous preparations, as well as guides to diagnosis and prognosis. It contained some 400 ingredients. The *Compendium* was translated into English in the early fifteenth century, indicating perhaps that apothecaries were increasingly distinguishing themselves from others who sought to govern health.

The word *apothecary* is derived from the Latin *apotheca*, a place where herbs, spices, and wine were sold. During the Middle Ages in England, it came to describe a person who sold these commodities from a shop or stall. London apothecaries were originally members of the Grocer's Guild, which was derived from the *Guild of Pepperers* formed in 1180.

Among other sundries, some of these grocers sold herbs and drugs (which they compounded and sold to the public); this group achieved separate status on December 6, 1617, when James I granted a royal charter for their incorporation. They were the forerunners of the first truly national pharmacopoeia (*London Pharmacopoeia)* in 1618.

Perhaps the most significant written work on Chinese herbs was the *Ben Cao Kong Mu*, published in 1596 and, subsequently, translated into English, French, German, Russian, and Japanese.

Following the 1911 Revolution, The Ministry of Health of the Nationalist government sought to curtail or eliminate traditional Chinese medicine. However, after the communist revolution of 1949, the new government reversed the ban on traditional medicine, establishing a number of traditional medical colleges and institutes, whose role is to train physicians and further investigate the uses of herbs. Even in Western hospitals in China, apothecaries are available to dispense herbs on request.

SOURCES OF DRUG INFORMATION IN AMERICA

Today, in the United States, there are numerous sources of drug information including the *Physicians Desk Reference* (PDR), which is an industry-supported reference. The PDR contains information identical to that contained in package inserts. No comparative information on efficacy, safety, or cost is included. PDR versions covering both trade name protected as well as generic preparations are available.

The USP, founded in 1820, originally contained "recipes" (formulas) for the preparation of drugs and drug products. The evolution of the USP actually began in 1817, when a New York physician, Lyman Spalding, recognized the need for *drug standardization*. At that time, medicine names and formulations differed from one region to another.

Spalding organized a meeting with ten other physicians in January of 1820 in the U.S. Capitol's Senate Chamber. Following the 1-week meeting, the groundwork was laid for the compilation of the first *Pharmacopoeia of the United States of America*. The book was designed to standardize 217 of the most fully recognized and best understood medicines of that era.

USP standards first became legislatively mandated in 1848, when Congress enacted the *Drug Import Act*. The USP gained further recognition in the *1906 Food and Drugs Act* and the *1938 Federal Food, Drug, and Cosmetic Act* (see Appendix I), in which its standards of strength, quality, purity, packaging, and labeling are recognized. These acts also recognized the standards of the USP's sister publication, the *National Formulary* (NF).

From the beginning, the NF sought to list those "unofficial" medicines and local remedies excluded from the USP. The NF was intended to detail and standardize preparations made of many ingredients, whereas the USP focused on those drugs containing a few ingredients. In essence, the USP set the standard for those drugs that were generally the first used therapeutically, whereas the NF detailed those whose drugs in the general public justified inclusion.

Today, the USP contains standards of identity, strength, quality, purity, packaging, and labeling for more than 3200 drug substances and products. With the incorporation of the NF in 1975, the standards for approximately 250 excipients (inert additives) are also now included.

Manufacturer compliance with the combined USP–NF standards ensures that drug products (dosage forms) and their ingredients are of appropriate strength, quality, and purity; are properly packaged; and that the product labeling includes the names and amounts of active ingredients, expiration dates, and storage conditions.

Over the centuries, pharmacopoeias have served not only as standard references for drugs and other pharmaceuticals but also as a means for pharmacists to distinguish themselves among the medical professions. With these standards, pharmacists transformed themselves from mere vendors of herbs and potions to highly trained professionals, charged with ensuring that patients receive the appropriate medicine for their ailment.

ALTERNATIVE SOURCES

In addition to the publications listed above dealing with ingredients, there are also publications dealing with nomenclature (e.g., USAN and USP Dictionary of Drug Names), information indexing (e.g., *PubMed, National Library of Medicine*), and information retrieval (e.g., computer-based Medical Literature Analysis and Retrieval System; *MEDLARS and MEDLINE, National Library of Medicine*).

There are also over 1500 medical journals and books published in the United States that comprise the primary (research publications), secondary (review articles), and tertiary (textbooks) literature. The pharmaceutical industry also supplies promotional material, often via "detail" persons. With the development of the Internet, vast amounts of drug-related information have become readily available to the general public. Governmental (e.g., NIH), commercial (e.g., Pharminfo; WebMD), and individual's web sites provide hard-data as well as controversial platforms for alternative viewpoints regarding drugs.

Reasons for the proliferation of this resource material include the major role that drugs play in modern therapeutics, the considerable profitability associated with their sale, and problems associated with drug abuse. Millions of prescriptions are written every year for more than 700 active ingredients available in several thousand different pharmaceutical preparations. In addition, there are many additional thousands of OTC preparations.

CLASSIFICATION

In reading any of the above-described drug information sources, you will find that drugs can be classified in many different ways, ranging from their chemical structure to the principle effect they produce, or the disease that they treat. Which method of classification used is usually dependent on one's point of view. For example, the drug amphetamine could be classified in at least five different ways depending on who was doing the classification:

1. Physician: appetite suppressing agent (anorexigenic)
2. Pharmacologist: sympathomimetic
3. Chemist: 2-amino-1-phenylpropane
4. Lawyer: drug of abuse falling in schedule II of the 1970 federal drug law
5. Psychologist: stimulant

By analyzing the method of classification imposed on a drug, we can gain some insight into which of its characteristics is being emphasized by the classifier. However, there is an alternative classification system to those described above, which can also be instructive. This system seeks to put drugs into *four functionally distinct categories* that divulge important distinctions about therapeutic and nontherapeutic principles. The four categories are listed below. More in-depth coverage will be presented in Part III.

1. *Drugs used to combat infection*—drugs in this category are based on the concepts of selective toxicity and chemotherapy developed by *Paul Ehrlich* in the late nineteenth and early twentieth centuries. Ehrlich made the observation that the dye methylene blue specifically stained neural tissue but not any other. From this *specific* observation he *generalized* that some molecular characteristic of neural tissue conferred selectivity on the dye and that a similar situation might exist in foreign organisms, which could form the basis for selective chemotherapy.

Unfortunately, there are few pure examples of true selective toxicity. Perhaps the best is *penicillin*. The therapeutic specificity of this antibiotic is based on the *qualitative* difference between bacterial cell wall synthesis and mammalian cell membrane synthesis. Synthesis of the former can be inhibited by penicillin while the latter is unaffected. Thus, penicillin is one of the few examples of a drug that can actually "*cure*" an illness. A similar example involves the sulfa drugs, which interfere with the synthesis of folic acid, used in nucleic acid formation, in bacteria. While bacteria must synthesize their own folic acid, mammalian cells utilize dietary, preformed folic acid and are not susceptible to interference with its formation.

1. *Drugs used to replace inadequacies of naturally occurring substances*—in an ideal sense, this class of drugs represents the "purest" form of drug used in that they are not "foreign" to the body. Examples include the use of hormones, such as insulin, in

replacement therapy. Insulin is obviously an endogenous hormone and, if the *human recombinant preparation* is used, is exactly the same in all of us. The therapeutic goal in treating *Diabetes Mellitus* is to replace normal, physiological levels of insulin. The neurogenic chemical L-dopa can also be thought of in a similar manner since it is used to treat inadequate brain levels of dopamine in certain cases of Parkinsonism. It must be understood, however, that if hormones are given in supraphysiological amounts they have the capacity to produce undesirable affects just as any xenobiotic.

2. *Drugs that change regulation*—this group contains the largest total number of drugs used, since they deal with the treatment of *symptoms*. Drugs used in this category do not cure, or replace, but can effectively manage acute or chronic disorders, often involving regulatory changes in the cardiovascular or nervous system, for example. Drugs in this category include antihypertensives, antianginals, diuretics, anticoagulants, analgesic and antipyretics, sedatives, anticonvulsants, and birth control pills.

3. *Drugs that alter mood or behavior*—this class includes relatively widely used licit, as well as illicit, drugs such as tranquilizers, alcohol, and tetrahydrocannabinol (the active ingredient in marijuana). In addition, "hard" drugs such as cocaine, opiates, methamphetamine, and hallucinogens are also included. This class of drugs is usually taken to *change our perceptions* of our environment and ourselves. They are often taken to relieve anxiety or to facilitate our involvement in certain social or "recreational" settings.

In addition to the variety of drug classification systems described above, a similar diversity, and somewhat bewildering array of systems are used to name drugs during their development. This is due to the fact that in the course of a drug's development it usually acquires more than one identifying name. Below is an example using the common drug aspirin.

1. *Chemical name*—a systematized and standardized nomenclature that encodes within the name descriptive information about the molecular constitution of the drug (e.g., 2-Acetoxybenzoic acid).

2. *Trivial name*—a coined name in general use. It is a common name by which the drug is identified, although it may not be intrinsically descriptive. There may be more than one trivial name (e.g., ASA).

3. *Generic or established name*—a similarly or contrived or coined name in general use. It usually refers to the U.S. name adopted by nomenclature groups known as the United States Approved Name (USAN) and USP Committees. The generic or established names are trivial names, but they have a somewhat more official status (e.g., Aspirin).

4. *Trade name*—a brand or proprietary name, a legally registered trademark of a drug or dosage form of a drug. This name is the property of the registrant. There may be more than one trade name for a drug (e.g., Empirin™).

Before considering the pharmacology of any particular class of drugs, it is important to understand the basic underlying principles of drug action. The following two chapters in this section will deal with an important subject traditionally covered in the area of pharmacology, known as *pharmacokinetics* (i.e., time related factors such as absorption, distribution, metabolism, and excretion). Pharmacokinetics is the branch of pharmacology that is concerned with both the *rates* with which drug uptake and elimination proceed as well as those processes that influence the time course of drug movement between one biological compartment and another.

The rates of absorption and distribution govern the time of onset of the drug's action; the rates of metabolism and excretion govern its duration, while the size of the dose, in combination with these effects, governs the intensity.

In addition to these fundamental aspects of drug action, the important area of *drug interactions* will be considered in the fourth chapter. Although this subject does not require exhaustive coverage, it is important to appreciate its ramifications early in the study of pharmacotherapeutics, since the coincidental administration of drugs can affect their respective pharmacokinetics, pharmacodynamics, and toxicity. In some cases, their interaction can be clinically significant.

THE PLACEBO EFFECT

Before we move on to the first "serious" topic of pharmacology, it is necessary for at least a cursory consideration of the placebo. To the average pharmacologist this is really not an issue. However, for those of you who go on to be clinicians or, more specifically, clinical pharmacologists (involved with human clinical trials), the issue of a placebo effect will often have to be dealt with.

The word placebo comes from the Latin word meaning "I shall please." A placebo is any treatment (including drugs, psychotherapy, quack therapy, and surgery) that achieves an ameliorative effect on a symptom or disease but that is actually ineffective or is not specifically effective for the condition being treated. The good news is that this phenomenon can be taken advantage of in relieving the symptoms of certain patients. What type of patients? Many effective antianxiety drugs have been prescribed both knowingly and unknowingly at placebo dosages, for example. But how effective can this effect really be? Hundreds of studies have demonstrated the *effectiveness of antidepressant drugs* for the treatment of depression in a range of 45–80% of patients. Pretty impressive until we realize that *placebo effectiveness in depression* is also high, ranging from 30 to 50%.

Placebos are effective for a variety of conditions. Their efficacy in dealing with depression is not particularly surprising since people may vary in their mood normally from day-to-day. However, it is more difficult to explain the fact that some patients with *angina pectoris* (chest pain produced by insufficient blood flow to the heart) respond to placebo surgery in which surgeons made only an incision in the chest. And in a study of the drug propranolol, which is used after heart attacks to prevent further damage, investigators noticed that patients who took placebo pills regularly had a lower death rate than patients who took placebos sporadically. Therefore, the placebo effect is not unique to psychiatric illness.

There was a time when doctors would prescribe phony medication, so-called "sugar pills" to their patients who they regarded as *hypochondriacs*. When they reported positive results the idea of the placebo effect was born.

As mentioned above, placebo pills are used in clinical trials to assess the true effect of a drug or supplement. Ideally, they are made of an inert substance that resembles the real drug in every respect so that neither the patient nor the doctor can detect the active preparation and, thus, be biased in reporting their experience. Before conducting human trials for drugs, pharmaceutical companies are often aware of many side effects of the products they are testing. For example, if a drug is known to cause dizziness and hypertension, the drug company running the test wants the placebo to have the same side effects. They rightly believe that, ideally, the placebo should mimic the drug being tested … warts and all … so that the control group (placebo) of the experiment will have side effects similar to their candidate drug. Without taking this precaution, the results of a blind study would be compromised. These preparations are known as "active placebos."

What types of patients are not really amenable to a placebo effect? If you are a type I (insulin-dependent) diabetic (Chapter 9) who goes into hypoglycemic shock, a placebo effect will not help you. No matter how much you believe in whatever you are, or are not, taking, nothing will change the physiological dynamics between your circulating blood glucose level and your brain's extremely high need for this energy substrate *Period*.

Ideally, in clinical trials, the placebo effect should be controlled for. If not, how can the investigator know if it is his company's NCE effectiveness or the patient's belief system? On the surface this seems rather straightforward, right? Simply give a "sugar-pill" and your problems are solved. Not. As mentioned above, simply having an inert control may not be adequate because it can often be detected by the patient. Color, shape, texture, dissolution rate, and taste are but a few of the parameters that can be discerned by humans and constitute a very real problem in the formulation of placebos.

ZOMBIES

Throughout this first chapter the author has tried to emphasize the extremely wide diversity of drugs and their impact on the human scene. Sometimes such examples can be truly dramatic and bizarre. One of these is the putative role of drugs/poisons in the creation of *zombies*. Article 240 of the *Haitian penal code* deals with zombie poison and prohibits the use of any substance that induces a *lethargic coma* "*indistinguishable from death*." Haitians do not fear zombies; they fear being turned into one.

According to one theory of zombiism, victims are "converted" into a zombie in a two-step process. Initially, the intended victim is treated with the paralytic *nerve toxin tetrodotoxin*, applied surreptitiously to an open wound. This nerve toxin is readily available in the Caribbean area. As the toxin does its work, the victim presents with all the symptoms of death (see below). Often, not realizing this error in diagnosis, the victim is placed in a coffin and buried. Within a day or two, a priest (bokor) resurrects the highly traumatized victim, who is then forced to eat a strong dose of a plant called the zombie's cucumber (*Datura stramonium*) that brings on a state of disorientation and *amnesia*.

Tetrodotoxin is present in the *puffer fish* and is one of the most potent poisons known. It has been estimated to be more than 500 times more potent than cyanide. This fact makes the voluntary consumption of puffer fish all the more remarkable. In Japan, for example, puffer fish (fugu) is considered a culinary delicacy that requires preparation by specialized fugu chefs. Their job is to reduce the level of the toxin, so the meal is not fatal but still retains enough of the toxin to produce some of its effects. These include a mild numbing or tingling of the tongue and lips, sensations of warmth, a flushing of the skin, and a general feeling of euphoria. If the dose is too high, difficulty in breathing occurs and a coma-like state develops. In some cases, people have appeared to have died, been declared clinically dead only to rise from the examining table.

SELECTED BIBLIOGRAPHY

Bowman, W.C. (1979) Drugs ancient and modern, *Scot. Med. J.* 24: 131–140.
Brown, W.A. (1998) The placebo effect, *Sci. Amer.* January: 90–95.
Cowen, D.L. and Helfand, W.H. (1990) *Pharmacy: An Illustrated History*, New York: Harry N. Abrams.
Davis, W. (1997) *The Serpent and the Rainbow*, Carmichael: Touchstone Books.
Harvey, A.L. (Ed.) (1993) *Drugs from Natural Products*, Chichester: Ellis Horwood Ltd.
Huang, K.C. (1993) *The Pharmacology of Chinese Herbs*, Boca Raton: CRC Press.
Mann, J. (1992) *Murder, Magic, and Medicine*, New York: Oxford University Press.
McKenna, T. (1992) *Food of the Gods*, New York: Bantam Books.
Midgley, J.M. (1988) Drug development: From sorcery to science, *Pharm. J.* 241: 358–365.
Moore, M. (1979) *Medicinal Plants of the Moutain West*, Santa Fe: The Museum of New Mexico Press.
Mowrey, D.B. (1986) *The Scientific Validation of Herbal Medicine*, New Canaan, CO: Keats Publishing, Inc.
One Hundred Years of the National Formulary: A Symposium; American Institute of the History of Pharmacy: Madison, WI
Rouli, A. Maureen (1997) Seeking drugs in natural products, *Chem. Eng. News*, April, p. 14.
Ross, A and Robins, D. (1989) *The Life and Death of a Druid Prince*, New York: Touchstone.
Shapiro, A.K. and Shapiro, E. (1997) *The Powerful Placebo*, Baltimore: The Johns Hopkins University Press.
Suffness, M. (Ed.) (1995) *Taxol® Science and Applications*, Boca Raton: CRC Press.
Wallace, S. (1999) *Mostly Medieval: Exploring the Middle Ages*; www.skell.org.

SAMPLE QUESTIONS

1. Which of the following individuals is credited with the first synthesis of an organic compound (urea)?
    a. John Jacob Abel
    b. Oswald Schmiedeberg

    c. Friedrich Worler

    d. Francois Magendie

    e. Claude Bernard

2. Which of the following is credited with isolating the first pure drug (morphine)?

    a. Friedrich Wörler

    b. Sertürner

    c. Paul Ehrlich

    d. Paracelsus

    e. William Withering

3. Man's first experience with pharmacology was the result of which of the following?

    a. Dreams

    b. Word of mouth

    c. Ancient material medica

    d. Food

    e. Observing animals

4. Which of the following statements is/are true regarding pharmacology?

    a. It is an integrative discipline

    b. Pharmacological effects can be studied *in vitro* and *in vivo*

    c. The word pharmacology is believed to be derived from the French word drogue

    d. Drug effects are mediated by naturally occurring processes in the body

    e. All of the above

5. Drugs play a role in which of the following?

    a. Sports

    b. Religion

    c. Politics

    d. The judicial system

    e. All of the above

6. A Shaman is which of the following?

    a. A fraud

    b. A priest-doctor

    c. Can employ hallucinogenic drugs

    d. Generally works for Western drug companies

    e. b and c above*

7. The first department of pharmacology in the world is generally associated with which of the following universities?

    a. University of Michigan

    b. Cambridge University

    c. Montpelier University

    d. University of Dorpat

    e. Oxford University

8. Which of the following is concerned with the study of drug absorption, distribution, metabolism, and excretion?

    a. Pharmacodynamics

    b. Pharmacokinetics

    c. Pharmacotherapeutics

    d. Pharmacoepidemiology

    e. Pharmacoeconomics

9. Extracts from which of the following were believed to confer the gift of flight?
    a. Mistletoe
    b. Tobacco
    c. Tomatoes
    d. Thorn apple
    e. Cannabis

10. Which of the following produces a steroid precursor that was used in the synthesis of progesterone?
    a. Mistletoe
    b. Coca plant
    c. North American potatoes
    d. Southwestern mushrooms
    e. Mexican yam

2 Absorption and Distribution

ABSORPTION

BACKGROUND

As mentioned in Chapter 1, our human species' earliest experiences with "drug effects" occurred *unintentionally*, as a result of *intentionally* eating plants for nourishment. Obviously, these effects would have to be classified as "side-effects," of sorts, since obtaining nutritive value was, of course, the real goal. Nevertheless, this paradigm illustrates an important principle in pharmacology—that drugs are usually substances that are chemically foreign to the human body (i.e., *xenobiotics*). Therefore, because they are produced in plants (be they botanical or pharmaceutical), they usually have to gain entrance *into* the body in order to produce an effect; the exception being those that produce a topical (skin) effect.

Today, there are a number of methods that can be used to introduce a drug into the body. Because of its convenience, the most common delivery system is the oral route. However, sometimes the oral route is not the most appropriate. In addition to the oral route, some of the alternative routes of drug administration with the oldest history include, not surprisingly, inhalation, and, surprisingly, rectal and vaginal, as illustrated by the following examples.

On landing in the New World, members of Columbus's crew described natives on the island of present-day Cuba, who inserted burning roles of leaves (called tobaccos) into their nostrils and "drank the smoke." The crew quickly took up this practice and the custom was subsequently introduced into Europe on their return. Nicotine is the addictive alkaloid constituent of tobacco (it was named after the French diplomat Jean Nicot [1530–1600], who brought tobacco to Europe). Tobacco proved to be a runaway success in Europe for many reasons, not the least of which was the belief that it would increase libido. Nicotine was not the first drug taken for this reason and will not be the last. Inhalation proved an extremely efficient method for conveying nicotine into the human body, in order to obtain its alleged aphrodisiac effect.

Today, the advantage of inhalation as a therapeutic route of drug administration is utilized for the concentrated localization of certain drugs within the tracheobronchioler region of the airway. For example, ipratropium and cromolyn are drugs used in the treatment of *asthma*. However, they are poorly absorbed from the intestine when they are taken orally. Therefore, they are essentially devoid of therapeutic effectiveness when taken by this route. Fortunately, when these drugs are given by inhalers for the treatment of asthma, they are effective in many patients. The large surface area of the terminal alveoli permits rapid absorption of drugs other than antiasthmatics, such as "crack" cocaine and gaseous anesthetics.

Drug companies around the world are now exploring the possibility of having patients inhale more of their medicines. The hope is that tiny particles inhaled deeply into the lung will cross through the thin epithelial cells lining the alveoli into the bloodstream and then make their way to their intended destination in the body. Clinical trials are already underway with inhaled formulations of currently marketed drugs including insulin, morphine, and drugs to fight osteoporosis. As mentioned above, asthmatics have long used inhalers to deliver bronchodilators such as albuterol. In 1994, Genentech began marketing the first aerosol-delivered protein, a recombinant form of the natural human enzyme *deoxyribonuclease* that degrades excess DNA that accumulates in the lungs of patients suffering from *cystic fibrosis*.

Unfortunately, the current devices for delivering drugs to the lungs, used primarily for asthma medications, are too inefficient at delivering their cargo to make them economically viable for more than a handful of products. These devices, called nebulizers (which deliver drugs in a water-based mist) and metered-dose inhalers (in which the drug is suspended in a propellant) only manage to get approximately 5–10% of the drug from the inhaler into the lungs; the nature of the propellant system as well as particle size are prime determinants. For example, particles <1 μm in diameter favor coalescence while those >5 μm tend to be physically trapped due to the architecture of the airway.

The utility of alternate routes for drug administration is not a new phenomenon. The ancient Maya and Peruvians, for example, employed *enemas* (AD 600–800) for drug delivery. The exact nature of the drugs used is unknown, but may have included tobacco and a fermented beverage called *balche*, as well as morning glory seeds. In Europe, the Danish physician Thomas Bartholin recommended, in 1661, the use of tobacco-juice and tobacco-smoke enemas as purgatives (i.e., to induce vomiting). Delivery of smoke was via pipes specifically designed for this purpose.

Ancient Egyptians used *vaginal inserts containing honey mixed with lint* as contraceptive devices, while an eighteenth-century French physician named Buc'hoz advocated the use of intra-vaginal insufflation of tobacco smoke to cure hysteria. The above examples illustrate the degree to which our species will go to introduce drugs into the body. In this regard, nicotine has probably been delivered into the body by more routes than any other drug (e.g., oral, nasal, inhalation, vaginal, rectal, and topical).

Since the oral route is basically passive and relatively time consuming, more direct routes now allow us to inject directly (i.e., intravenously) or indirectly (i.e., intramuscularly or subcutaneously) into the circulatory system. Administration via these *parenteral* routes was facilitated by the invention of the hypodermic syringe credited to the Scotsman Alexander Wood, in 1853 (Figure 2.1). Traditionally, the principle routes of administration have been divided into two major classes: *enteral*, which refers to the gastrointestinal tract, and *parenteral*, which indicates other than the gastrointestinal tract.

Wood's may not have been the original inventor, however, since archeological research during the eighteenth century uncovered medical items that look remarkably similar. In any event, before this invention, physicians had used creative devices such as the hollow stems of the lilac plant to introduce drugs into the body. Today, more subtle technologies have been developed for facilitating the movement of drugs across the skin (e.g., transdermal patches and iontophoresis).

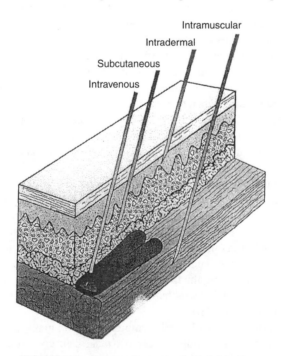

FIGURE 2.1   Routes of parenteral administration.

In certain situations, drugs can be given by continuous infusion. The drug is added to a large volume of parenteral fluid (up to 1000 mL), and the solution is then slowly and continuously administered into a vein. This is why an indwelling venous catheter is often implanted in the upper wrist on admission to the hospital so that drugs can be readily administered without the disadvantage of continuous injections (Figure 2.2)

This method allows fluid and drug therapy to be administered simultaneously. It provides an excellent control of drug plasma levels over a prolonged period of time. Drug plasma levels can be easily controlled by adjusting the infusion flow rate.

Considerable research in recent years has successfully yielded drug preparations that can also be given intranasally (e.g., calcitonin for osteoporosis) or by inhalation (e.g., bronchodilators for asthmatics). A more complete list of possible routes of drug administration is presented in Table 2.1. However, we will concern ourselves only with the principle routes of administration. An important point to remember is that all these routes vary in terms of influencing a drug's onset of action. ·

THE ORAL ROUTE

The human body can be basically thought of as a container of water (a polar medium) within which various aqueous compartments are separated by lipid membranes that contain both polar and non-polar components. The oral route is, for most drugs, the most desirable route for administration into the body because of the ease of self-administration. However, oral agents must be able to withstand

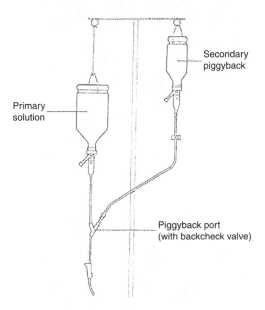

FIGURE 2.2   Primary IV with piggyback.

TABLE 2.1
Possible Routes of Drug Administration

Oral	Sublingual
Intravenous	Rectal
Intramuscular	Topical
Subcutaneous	Intravaginal
Inhalation	Intranasal
Intra-arterial	Subarachnoid

the acidic environment of the stomach and must permeate the gut lining (a mucousal membrane) before entering the blood stream.

In general, drugs must traverse biological membranes in order to (1) gain access to the circulatory system and, hence, distribution throughout the body and (2) entry into cells. The facility with which a chemical crosses these membranes is a major determinant in estimating rates of absorption and subsequent distribution as well as the eventual pharmacological effect of the drug. This is particularly important for drugs that must cross the mucousal lining of the gastrointestinal (GI) tract, since this will, in all probability, be the first of many. In order to gain some insight into the factors that affect the passage of xenobiotics, such as drugs, across biological membranes in the body, we should have some appreciation of important membrane characteristics that can influence drug absorption, particularly in the GI tract.

The conventional model developed to explain cell membrane characteristics influencing drug permeability is routinely referred to as the *fluid-mosaic model*. In this model, the main components, for our purposes, are a phospholipid (e.g., sphingomyelin and phosphatidylcholine) bilayer (8 nm), with polar moieties at both the external and internal surfaces, with proteins periodically traversing the phospholipid plane perpendicularly (Figures 2.3 and 2.4).

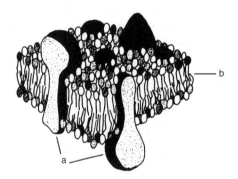

FIGURE 2.3   The three-dimensional structure of the animal cell membrane. Proteins (a) are interspersed in the phospholipid bilayer (b). (From J. A. Timbrell (1995), *Introduction to Toxicology.* With permission.)

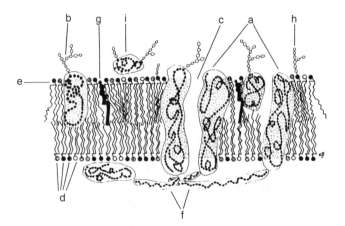

FIGURE 2.4   The molecular arrangement of the cell membrane: a, integral proteins; b, glycoprotein; c, pore formed from integral protein; d, various phospholipids with saturated fatty acid chains; e, phospholipid with unsaturated fatty acid chains; f, network proteins; g, cholesterol; h, glycolipid; i, peripheral protein. There are four different phospholipids: phosphatidyl serine; phosphatidyl choline; phosphatidyl ethanolamine; sphingomyelin represented respectively as. The stippled area of the protein represents the hydrophobic portion. (From J.A. Timbrell (1995), *Introduction to Toxicology.* With permission.)

The bilayer forms because of the physicochemical properties of the phospholipid constituents and their interaction with water. The round "head" regions depicted in the figure are *polar* because they contain *charged* phosphate, choline, and ethanolamine groups. However, the tail regions are the predominant components and consist of *nonpolar* fatty acyl chains. Because orientation of polar groups is favored toward other polar groups, such as water, the bilayer is oriented both inwards and outwards toward extracellular and intracellular water, respectively. This architecture forms a diffusion barrier that is virtually impermeable to charged (polar) molecules and ions attempting to move in either direction.

The lipid layer favors uptake of *nonpolar* compounds (lipophilic; having an affinity for fat) while certain globular proteins embedded in the membrane form aqueous pores or channels, which allow penetration of small polar substances (hydrophilic; having an affinity for water) such as ethanol or ions such as sodium chloride. However, the ordered structure of the phospholipid membrane is not highly conducive to the presence of numerous pores. Therefore, *high lipid solubility* is a predominant characteristic that favors membrane absorption of a chemical. It is an important feature for oral absorption into the body as well as distribution within the body, since, as mentioned above, the body is basically a series of polar, aqueous media chambers separated by phospholipid barriers containing polar groups.

Molecules that do *not* contain electrical charges (uncharged) or whose electron distribution is *not* distorted (nonpolar) are compatible with the nonpolar region of cell membranes. For charged or polar molecules, the aqueous pores that do exist within the protein channels can provide an alternate route. These pores do allow the passage of *some* poorly lipid soluble nonelectrolytes, as well as *some* charged molecules. However, they must be *low* in molecular weight.

Transmission of extracellular signals to the cell interior is based on receptor-induced recruitment and assembly of proteins into signaling complexes at the inner leaflet of the plasma membrane. Protein–protein, as well as protein–lipid, interactions play a crucial role in the process in which molecular proximity in specially formed membrane subdomains provides the special and temporal constraints that are required for proper signaling. The phospholipid bilayer is *not* merely a passive hydrophobic medium for this assembly process, but a site where the lipid, as well as the protein components, are enriched by a dynamic process (see Chapter 5).

TRANSMEMBRANE PROCESSES

Transmembrane movement of a chemical can occur by several processes including (1) *passive diffusion* through the membrane phospholipid according to *Fick's Law* (rate of passage is *directly* proportional to the concentration gradient, surface area of the membrane, and partition coefficient of the chemical and *inversely* proportional to membrane thickness). Therefore, a concentration gradient must exist and the xenobiotic must be lipid soluble and nonionized; (2) *filtration* of small molecules may occur through pores in membrane protein, also down a concentration gradient; (3) *active transport* of a select group of molecules can occur but requires a specific membrane carrier and the expenditure of metabolic energy. Because of these requirements, the process can be inhibited by metabolic poisons, is saturable, and the carrier sites subject to competition from other chemicals. However, active transport can occur against a concentration gradient; (4) *facilitated diffusion* also utilizes a specific membrane carrier (saturable) and requires a concentration gradient but *no* energy expenditure is required; and (5) *phagocytosis and pinocytosis* are processes that involve the invagination of part of the membrane to enclose a particle or droplet, respectively, that might contain a drug.

PARTITION COEFFICIENT

Because lipid solubility is so important for transmembrane movement of a drug, attempts have been made over the years to assess this characteristic as a predictor of drug activity. Perhaps the most useful method employs a simple relationship referred to as the oil/water partition coefficient. The coefficient may be obtained relatively easily by adding the drug to a mixture of equal volumes of a nonpolar medium (e.g., an organic aliphatic alcohol such as octanol) and a polar medium (water). The mixture is then agitated (usually with a mechanical shaking device) until equilibrium is reached, whereupon the phases are separated and assayed for the drug; the greater the partition coefficient of a drug (i.e., the greater the concentration in the organic phase) the more lipid soluble the drug. This principle is illustrated in Table 2.2 for a number of structurally related barbiturates.

Comparing the lipophilicity of the barbiturates above with their uptake across the GI tract (colon) demonstrates that the membrane permeability of each member of the series is proportional to its partition coefficient. Apparently, there can be some differential effect on partitioning, depending on which organic solvent is used in making the determination. For example, the gastrointestinal membrane is believed to behave more like an octanol/water pairing, while drug uptake into the brain is more closely mimicked by a heptane/water combination.

ADDITIONAL MAJOR FACTORS AFFECTING ABSORPTION

Within the GI tract, the major anatomical absorption site is the upper small intestine because of its huge *surface area* (e.g., 500–1000 times that of the stomach; Figure 2.5 and Table 2.3). In addition to

TABLE 2.2
The Effects of Partition Coefficient on Absorption of Drugs

	Partition Coefficient	% Absorbed
Barbital	0.7	12
Aprobarbital	4.9	17
Phenobarbital	4.8	20
Cyclobarbital	11.7	24
Pentobarbital	28.0	30
Secobarbital	50.7	40

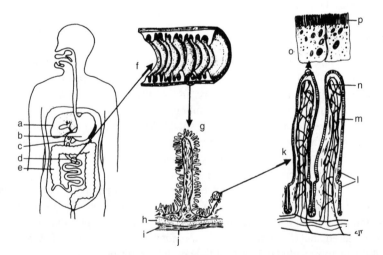

FIGURE 2.5   The mammalian gastrointestinal tract showing important features of the small intestine, the major site of absorption for orally administered compounds: a, liver; b, stomach; c, duodenum; d, ileum; e, colon; f, longitudinal section of the ileum showing folding that increases surface area; g, detail of fold showing villi with circular and longitudinal muscles, h and i respectively, bounded by the serosal membrane, j; k, detail of villi showing network of capillaries, m, lacteals, n, and epithelial cells, I; o, detail of epithelial cells showing brush border or microvilli, p. The folding, vascularization, and microvilli all facilitate absorption of substances from the lumen. (From J.A. Timbrell (1995), *Introduction to Toxicology*. With permission.)

TABLE 2.3
Comparison of the Size of the Absorptive Surface of the Various Parts of the Gastrointestinal Tract

Oral cavity	0.02
Stomach	0.1–0.2
Small intestine	100
Large intestine	0.5–1.0
Rectum	0.04–0.07

surface area, other important factors include drug solubility (drugs must dissolve before absorption), particle size, and contact time with the absorption surface, membrane integrity, and pH. Materials that are quite insoluble in both polar and nonpolar media are pharmacologically inert. For example, barium sulfate is a highly toxic material if absorbed into the body. However, because of its poor solubility in the GI tract, it can be swallowed and used as a contrast medium for radiography in this region without toxicological hazard.

The Effect of pH

Hydrogen ion concentration (pH) has particular relevance to drug absorption since approximately 75% of all clinically utilized drugs can behave as either weak acids or bases (i.e., they can take up or release a hydrogen ion and become charged, polar entities). As mentioned above, uncharged molecules are compatible with the lipid environment of cellular membranes. Therefore, acidic and basic drugs are preferentially absorbed in their *nonionized* form, the proportion of which exists at any moment being pH dependent.

Calculations regarding the influence of pH on the ionization of weak acids and bases may be solved by applying the *Henderson–Hasselbalch* equation (pH – pKa = log [base/acid]), which may be familiar to you from taking a class in biochemistry. This equation essentially describes the relationship between pH and the degree of ionization of weak acids and bases. When applied to drugs, the equation tells us that when pH equals the apparent equilibrium dissociation constant of the drug (pK), 50% of the drug will be in the unionized form and 50% will be in the ionized form (i.e., log [base/acid] = 0 and antilog of 0 = 1, or unity). Application of the *Henderson–Hasselbalch* equation can, therefore, allow one to mathematically determine the exact proportion of ionized and nonionized species of a drug in a particular body compartment, if the pK of the drug and the pH of the local environment are known.

A practical method for determining the general effect of pH on the degree of ionization of a drug can be determined in a straightforward manner by applying the *principle of LeChatelier*. This principle states that if the conditions of a system, originally in equilibrium, are changed; the new equilibrium shifts in such a direction as to restore the original conditions. When applying this principle to the effect of pH on drug ionization, the following relationships occur. For a weak acid, the dissociation equilibrium can be expressed as follows:

$$AH \leftrightarrow A^- + H^+$$

In this situation, if the hydrogen ion concentration increases (pH becomes lower) the reaction will be driven to the left by mass action, the original condition, and the proportion of the drug in the *nonionized* form will increase and, hence, the number of lipid soluble molecules. For example, if the pK_a of a weak acid is 5.0 and is placed in a medium of pH 4.0, 90% will be in the unionized form. Therefore, weak acids are preferentially absorbed in a relatively acidic environment. For a weak base, the equilibrium dissociation constant can be expressed as follows:

$$BH^+ \leftrightarrow B + H^+$$

TABLE 2.4
Comparison of pH Values in Some Human Body Compartments

Blood	7.35–7.45
Oral cavity	6.2–7.2
Stomach (at rest)	1.0–3.0
Duodenum	4.8–8.2
Jejunum	6.3–7.3
Ileum	7.6
Colon	7.8–8.0
Rectum	7.8
Cerebral fluid	7.3–7.4
Vagina	3.4–4.2
Urine	4.8–7.5
Sweat	4.0–6.8
Milk	6.6–7.0

In this situation, if the hydrogen ion concentration increases, the proportion of drug in the *ionized* form, the original condition, increases. Therefore, consequences of a shift in pH away from equilibrium conditions are opposite for weak acids and weak bases. For example, a solution of the weak base dextromethorphan (a drug present in cough preparations with a pK_a of 9.2) in the stomach (pH 1) will have approximately 1 of every 160,000,000 molecules in the unionized form. Obviously, gastric absorption will be significantly curtailed.

As important as this pH effect is it can be subordinated by other factors, however. For example, as indicated above, the absorptive area that a drug is exposed to can be a predominating factor. In this context, even though the acidic environment of the stomach favors the absorption of weak acids (e.g., acetylsalicylic acid), aspirin is still absorbed to a greater extent, in totality, in the small intestine. A partial list of the pH of several body compartments is shown in Table 2.4. The fact that there are some variations suggests that the disposition of some drugs may be differentially affected.

The oral route is, of course, the principle enteral route of drug administration. However, two other examples are worthy of note. First, the sublingual route (beneath the tongue) provides relatively good absorption because of its rich capillary bed; it is routinely used for the administration of nitroglycerin tablets in the treatment of angina pectoris. Because the stomach is bypassed, acid lability and gut permeability need not be considered. Secondly, the rectal route can be found useful for unconscious or vomiting patients or small children.

Although the oral route is certainly the most convenient mode of drug delivery, it is not appropriate for all drugs or all situations. For example, administration of insulin by the oral route results in destruction of the hormone's physiological activity. This is due to the fact that the proteinaceous nature of insulin renders it susceptible to degradation within the stomach owing to the acidic environment as well as the presence of proteases. Therefore, insulin must be given by injection (note: attempts are being made to develop new insulin preparations that can be given by other routes (e.g., intranasally), thus avoiding the necessity of repeated injections). Absorption from the GI tract is also relatively slow and may not be appropriate for an emergency situation. For these and other reasons, alternative routes of drug administration are often utilized.

INJECTION

As indicated in Table 2.1, drugs may be injected into veins, muscles, subcutaneous tissue, arteries, or into the subarachnoid space of the spinal canal (intrathecal). For obvious reasons, intra-arterial and intrathecal injections are reserved for specialized drug administration requirements, such as regional perfusion of a tumor with a toxic drug or induction of spinal anesthesia, respectively.

Therefore, the more routine injection routes are intravenous (IV), intramuscular (IM), and subcutaneous (SC). Because these three modalities involve skin puncture, they carry the risks of infection, pain, and local irritation.

Intravenous administration of a drug achieves rapid onset of drug action. For this reason IV lines are routinely established in many emergency rooms and inpatient situations (e.g., unconsciousness), in order to establish a "permanent" portal for drug injection (Figure 2.2).

While IV injection achieves rapid action it also must be used with discretion for several reasons: (1) administration is irreversible; (2) if the rate of injection is too rapid, the drug is delivered in more of a bolus form, thus presenting the heart and vascular system with a more concentrated "hit"; (3) severe allergic reactions may be particularly severe for the same reason; (4) accidental injection of air can form air emboli in the circulatory system; and (5) mixing certain drugs may cause a chemical interaction between them such as precipitation (e.g., precipitation of sulfonamides by tetracyclines).

In addition to the factors listed above, IV drugs must also be delivered in a sterile medium and be free of insoluble material. Failure to respect these requirements can produce serious consequences. For example, it is well recognized that IV drug abusers are a population at particular risk for bacterial endocarditis, viral hepatitis, and AIDS. Fortunately, free-needle programs can significantly reduce the likelihood of cross-infections when implemented.

Drug abuse often involves attempts to "solubilize" oral medication for IV injection. This practice, with drugs such as amphetamine or cocaine for example, can result in severe pulmonary injury. This is due to the inadvertent coadministration of insoluble talc (hydrous magnesium silicate) that is routinely present as a filler material in the original preparation manufactured for oral use. Because of their size, the insoluble talc particles (particularly in the 10–17 μm range) can become trapped in small blood vessels in the lung and serve as "foreign body" loci for connective tissue accumulation. Depending on the quantity of talc deposited, patients will experience varying degrees of compromised lung function ranging from dyspnea (difficulty in breathing) to death.

Fortunately, not all drugs need to be injected IV. Common alternatives include IM and SC injections that can provide depot sites for more prolonged entrance of drug into the circulatory system (see new table for principles). If a drug is given either IM (directly into muscle) or SC (beneath the skin), it passes through *capillary* walls to enter the bloodstream. Rate of absorption is influenced by several factors including the drug's formulation (oil-based preparations are absorbed slowly, aqueous preparations are absorbed rapidly) and regional blood flow.

For drugs deposited in the proximity of the peripheral capillary beds of muscle and subcutaneous tissue, lipid solubility is considerably less important than the oral route, since even ionized forms of drugs are absorbed with relative ease. The capillary wall in these areas is of sufficient porosity that even drugs with molecular weights as great as 60,000 Da may be absorbed by passive diffusion. This fact explains why a protein, such as insulin (5808 Da), can be given SC and is absorbed into the blood stream.

The rate and efficiency of drug absorption following IM or SC injection may be greater than, equal to, or less than that following oral administration, depending on the drug under consideration. In addition, blood flow in the area of drug injection is a major determinant in the rate of drug absorption from both IM and SC sites. This fact can be utilized in altering the absorption of certain drugs. For example, local anesthetics are usually injected in combination with a vasoconstricting agent such as epinephrine. Epinephrine serves to elicit contraction of the vascular smooth muscle, achieving a reduction in both the absorptive surface area of the vessel as well as blood flow through the area. The cumulative effect is that the local anesthetic remains in the proximity of the injection site (sensory nerve) for a longer period of time.

TOPICAL ABSORPTION

Increasingly today, more and more drugs are prepared in patch form to be applied directly to the surface of the skin; this is known as *topical* application. One of the earliest examples of this strategy was the creation of the nicotine patch. These patches contain a known quantity of nicotine that was dissolved in a matrix that permitted a predictable amount of the drug embedded in the patch to dissolve and pass through the layers of the skin via four transport pathways: (1) intercellular (between cells), (2) transcellular (through cells), (3) follicular (via follicle openings), and (4) via eccrine routes. Ideally, in this fashion, blood level of nicotine could be managed ... helping the patient to gradually withdraw from the drug and minimize withdrawal symptoms. Examples of drugs given via topical patches other than nicotine include sex steroids and antidepressants; others in the pipeline are analgesics, as well as drugs for Alzheimer's and attention deficit hyperactivity disorder.

BIOAVAILABILITY

An important consequence of administering drugs by different routes is that there can be a difference in their bioavailability. Bioavailability refers to that fraction of an administered drug that gains access to the systemic circulation in an unchanged form. The standard of comparison in determining bioavailability, against which all other routes are compared, is the IV dose. In practice, drug serum or plasma levels are monitored at different time points following various routes of administration, such as oral, and the respective ratios of the *area under the curve* (AUC) are calculated:

$$\text{Bioavailability} = AUC_{oral}/AUC_{iv}$$

In Figure 2.6, the serum concentrations of three tablet forms of a drug are compared with its IV form. As you can see, tablets A and B have approximately the same bioavailability (AUC). Tablet C, on the other hand, has significantly less. Poor oral bioavailability can obviously influence a drug's ideal mode of delivery. It is because of poor oral bioavailability (approximately 25%) of heavily charged weak bases, such as the opiates (pK's in the range of 8.0–9.0), that heroin and morphine abusers resort to injection of the drugs in order to maximize their effects.

If drugs have the same bioavailability (i.e., the same AUC), they are said to be *bioequivalent*. This is a particularly important aspect in the development of generic drugs (see below). However, it should be appreciated that bioavailability refers ultimately to plasma concentration per se. It does not tell us anything about *therapeutic equivalence*, which deals with comparable efficacy and safety (issues to be addressed in subsequent chapters).

Generic products tested by the FDA and determined to be therapeutic equivalents are listed by the FDA in their publication *Approved Drug Products with Therapeutic Equivalence Evaluations*.

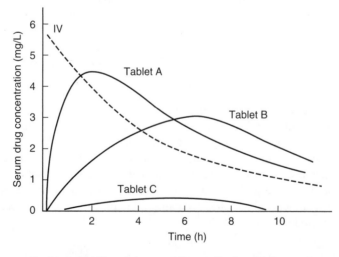

FIGURE 2.6 Comparative bioavailability of three oral forms of a drug. Reference is serum level of the drug administered in its intravenous (IV) form. (From Pharmacia and Upjohn, *Pharmacokinetics Applied to the Treatment of Asthma*. With permission.)

These products contain the same active ingredients as their brand-name counterparts and also meet bioequivalence standards. The FDA recommends substitution only among products listed as therapeutically equivalent.

Factors that can affect bioavailability include metabolism (to be discussed in more detail in Chapter 3), lipid solubility of the drug, chemical stability of the drug (e.g., penicillin G is unstable at gastric pH), and the nature of the drug formulation (i.e., particle size, salt form, presence of inert binders, etc.).

GENE THERAPY

After nearly 30 years of speculation, one of the most provocative avenues of "drug" administration currently receiving substantial interest and financial resources is the area of gene therapy—an area of continuing evolution. There are at least two different kinds of gene therapy. Which one is employed depends on an assessment of the disease and the needs of the patient. In "traditional" *replacement-gene therapy*, a functional copy of the gene in question is administered to replace the faulty activity of the defective gene in question. *Pharmacological-gene therapy* transmits a gene not for replacement but for the production of a novel therapeutic product, essentially turning the patient's own cells into pharmaceutical manufacturing plants. To date, clinical research has focused on gene-replacement therapy.

One of the first patients to be treated with gene replacement was a 4-year-old girl, in 1990. She was born with a defective gene for making the essential enzyme *adenosine deaminase* (ADA), which is vital for the function of the immune system. Since that time, hundreds of clinical trials (mostly phase I safety trials—see Part IV) have been started, dealing with single gene disorders such as *cystic fibrosis*, as well as acquired disorders such as cancer and AIDS. Clinical progress, with acquired disorders, appears to be occurring at a faster rate using gene addition, since a greater diversity of approaches is possible.

This diversity of approaches in treating acquired illnesses is illustrated in the gene therapy strategies that have been proposed for treating AIDS and various cancers. Treatment of HIV infection could conceivably be based on the interruption of viral processes that directly contribute to the pathogenesis of AIDS. This could be achieved by several potential mechanisms, including inserting a gene that produces antisense mRNA or ribozymes (see Chapter 15 for more information), or a dominant negative mutant protein.

There are many reasons why gene therapy has not proven to be straightforward. Challenges to be dealt with are as follows: Is it the right form of the gene to solve the specific disease problem? Is the gene product stable enough to act as a replacement for the missing or aberrant "natural product"? What is the most effective promoter to get the new gene to express properly (in time, space, and amount)? Finally, how does one get the introduced gene to breach the numerous membrane barriers and other defense mechanisms that have evolved to keep out foreign genetic material?

VECTORS

Although all of the notoriety of gene therapy rests in finding prospective genetic solutions to various diseases, the pedestrian issue of safe and effective transport and delivery of genetic "magic bullets" can make or break a therapeutic protocol. Therefore, creating an efficacious gene or gene product depends on the development of a corresponding carrier, that is, the appropriate vector.

A major challenge in gene therapy is to find safe vectors capable of transporting genes efficiently into target cells and getting these target cells to express the genes once inserted. In fact, most researchers blame current problems on difficulties with the vectors for lack of progress in the field. The messengers intended to deliver healthy genes into patients have instead betrayed the goals of therapy, causing allergic reactions and cancers, or simply failing to perform. This should not be surprising since the vectors chosen have been adapted from viruses known to cause human disease.

Gene therapy has been conducted using three main virus vectors: *retroviruses, adenoviruses,* and *adenovirus-associated viruses* (AAVs). Retroviruses infect the cell naturally and incorporate the gene of interest directly into the human chromosome. Adenoviruses are modified from a variety of human and animal pathogens. AAVs are nonpathogenic to humans and cause a lower immune response, providing a transient burst of therapeutic protein on infection. The most commonly used retrovirus vectors are based on *murine leukemia virus* (MLV) that can infect mouse and human cells. Inactivated versions of this retrovirus have been loaded with genes and used in approximately 30–40% of human trials to date.

Although this murine retrovirus is relatively easy to make and use, retroviruses insert genes only into cells that are actively dividing and growing and possess, therefore, some theoretical danger of eliciting tumor formation—so-called *insertional oncogenesis*. Such "toxicity" is believed to have occurred in a French study in which 1 of 11 children developed a leukemia-like cancer that the researchers determined was attributed to the insertion of the vector into a well-known oncogenic site.

For the reasons mentioned above, retroviruses have been used in *ex vivo* procedures such as ADA deficiency. For example, in the case of the 4-year-old girl mentioned above, a sample of her blood was removed, T lymphocytes were isolated from it, the gene for ADA was inserted into the cells via a retrovirus, and the cells reinfused into her body.

Attempts to obviate the limitations of retrovirus vectors include the use of alternative virus vectors such as adeno-associated viruses (now used in approximately 20% of clinical trials) and lentiviruses, as well as nonviral vectors such as plasmid-based vectors, alone, in combination with liposomes, or linked to a ligand. Other, more theoretical, strategies proposed involve the creation of a "human artificial chromosome." In this case, a 25th chromosome containing "suites" of genes would, hopefully, be introduced into the nucleus of a target cell.

In the final analysis, it is likely that no universal vector will be found to be appropriate for all situations.

The Future

Although the potential therapeutic benefits of gene therapy appear to be great, it remains to be seen how successful attempts will be to overcome present problems. These problems include the need to develop improved gene-transfer methodology, reduced vector antigenicity, as well as the appreciation of new pharmacokinetic paradigms. For example, with *in vivo* gene transfer, it will be necessary to account for the fate of the DNA vector itself (e.g., volume of distribution, clearance rate, etc.), as well as determining the consequences of altered gene expression and protein function.

In addition to the challenges of gene transfer and expression noted above, there are also potential adverse consequences that could conceivably occur as a result of gene transfer. These include immunological responses to both the newly transcribed protein as well as to the vector itself. The 1999 *death* of an 18-year-old boy (the first reported death from gene therapy) being treated for a deficiency of *ornithine transcarbamylase*, as well as others developing nonlethal leukemia-like conditions in 2002 have been ascribed to an immunological response to the massive doses of an adenovirus vector that are needed in clinical trials. The latter event led to the FDA's decision in January 2003 to halt trials using retroviral vectors in blood stem cells. Furthermore, a state of replication-defectiveness must be maintained in the vector in order to protect against the potential inherent pathogenicity of the carrier.

To date, clinical trials of gene therapy have shown little evidence of positive therapeutic effects. An NIH report in 1995 indicated that all the "vectors" used so far to transfer genes into target cells are inefficient, with a "very low" rate of gene transfer. In addition, the same report concluded that gene therapists and their sponsors are "overselling" the technology and that there should be less hype and more emphasis on good biology.

To develop improved viral alternatives, researchers are investigating DNA sequences from bacteriophages to provide them with an "ideal" method for insertion. Despite these disappointing results and the increasing awareness of gene therapy's limitations, pharmaceutical companies have invested nearly $1 billion in gene biotechnology companies, since the summer of 1995. Research firms estimate that the market for gene therapy treatments will generate between $2 and $3 billion in worldwide revenues in the new millennium. In addition, current NIH funding for gene therapy will remain at approximately $200 million per year.

There have been some encouraging results, however, including the results of two phase 1 studies reported in 2000. In a phase 1 gene transfer trial for Hemophilia B "significant reduction in whole blood clotting times was observed in patients for several months after receiving intramuscular administration of the lowest dose of a recombinant adeno-associated virus expressing the human coagulation factor IX gene." In another study, patients who received autologous transplants of bone marrow stem cells transformed *in vitro* using an MLV retrovirus-derived vector containing the complement to the normal gene for X-linked SCID (bubble-boy syndrome) have "reconstituted their immune systems for up to one year and the children are now living normally with their families."

Perhaps the most significant cause for renewed enthusiasm for gene therapy is the first commercial milestone with the licensing and marketing in China of a new cancer treatment. Unexpected by many, the first commercialized gene therapy is the result of Chinese entrepreneurship, expanded for production with the use of technology developed in the West. The product, called *Gendicine* (projected to cost $360/injection), *is a new treatment for head and neck squamous cell carcinoma*—a highly lethal cancer that strikes some 300,000 people yearly in China.

Whether or not the product will be an unqualified success, it is not a radical approach remains to be seen. The therapy relies on the use of an adenovirus vector delivery system expressing the *p53* tumor suppressing gene. In humans, the *p53* gene product is a phosphorylated protein that acts as a transcriptional activator important in regulating cell growth. Its tumor suppression activity is due to its ability to trigger apoptosis (see Chapter 7) by signaling cytotoxic T cells to destroy aberrant cells. Many cancers contain defective *p53* genes or insufficient *p53* gene product, to induce an apoptotic response. Gene therapies based on *p53* have been and are currently the subject of numerous clinical trials in the United States and Europe. Many believe that if there is to be a "magic bullet" against multiple forms of cancer, *p53*-based therapies are the most promising approach.

Gene therapy is not just about cancer, however. Gene therapy is also under investigation for a wide variety of conditions, including hemophilia, Gaucher's and Fabry diseases, cystic fibrosis, Alzheimer's disease, leukocyte adherence deficiency disease, bedsores, and others.

Despite its checkered past, the story of genes as drugs is only just beginning; it is a technology in transition.

DISTRIBUTION

After a drug is administered to the body, it goes through various phases of distribution. If we were to make periodic plasma measurements of a drug following its administration, its plasma profile would be a composite of various simultaneous dynamic processes, serving to increase or decrease its concentration. The processes of distribution can be considered in terms of movement of a drug through various *compartments*.

Absorption of a drug into the theoretical central or main compartment may be followed by distribution into one or more peripheral compartments, or the drug may undergo excretion or metabolism from the central compartment. While compartmental analysis of drug distribution can be quite informative, it is beyond the scope of this book. For more details on the effect of multicompartmental distribution of a drug on pharmacokinetics, see references in the Bibliography.

With the exception of the more complicated aspects of gene delivery methodologies described above, after a drug is absorbed into the systemic circulation via a conventional route of administration, it is basically transported throughout the body either free or bound to plasma proteins.

TABLE 2.5
Tissue Perfusion (% of Cardiac Output in the Human)

Brain	14.0
Heart	3.3
Kidney	22.0
Liver	26.5
Viscera	30.0
Adipose tissue	4.7

Source: Data derived from U.S. Environmental Protection Agency, Reference Physiological Parameters in Pharmacokinetic Modeling, Arms, A.D. and Travis, C.C. *Office of Risk Analysis*, EPA No., 600/6–88/004, 1988.

In order for a drug to reach its site of action, it must usually leave the blood stream. Drug permeability occurs largely in the capillary bed, where both surface area and contact time are maximal, owing to extensive vascular branching and low velocity of flow. However, capillary beds in different organs vary in their penetrability (i.e., pore size between adjacent endothelial cells). For example, the liver capillary bed is "leaky" while brain is not.

Before *steady state* is reached (when the concentrations of drug in all body compartments are in equilibrium), distribution is principally dependent on *blood flow*. In fact, the fraction of drug that can diffuse into a specific organ is proportional to the blood flow into that organ. A comparison of organ perfusion is shown in Table 2.5.

Tissues that are highly perfused, such as kidneys, liver, heart, and brain, therefore, are promptly exposed to a drug. A useful concept in drug distribution is referred to as the *apparent volume of distribution* (V_d) of a drug. It is defined as:

$$V_d = \text{Total drug dose (mg)/plasma concentration } at \text{ } equilibrium \text{ (mg/ml)}$$

Therefore, V_d is the apparent fluid volume, usually expressed in ml or liters, in which the drug appears to be dissolved. Values of V_d compatible with the known volume of a body compartment may suggest that the drug is confined to that compartment. Values of V_d greater than the total body volume of water indicate that the drug is concentrated in a tissue compartment.

Many lipid-soluble drugs are stored in body fat, for example, which can range from 10% to 50% of body weight. Therefore, fat can serve as an important reservoir for highly lipid soluble drugs. This can have important implications for the distribution and time course of drug action. It has been shown, for example, that 3 h after the IV administration of the short-acting barbiturate thiopental, 70% of the dose can be found in the fatty tissues, thus contributing to the rapid termination of its initial action.

Another example of the effect of fat storage on a drug is tetrahydrocannabinol (THC). THC is the psychoactive component in *Cannabis sativa* and is quite lipid soluble (hence its ability to affect the brain and be stored in adipose tissue). THC is released very slowly from fat cells, which explains why it can have a lingering effect and be detected in the urine many days following a single exposure. The potential liability of this pharmacokinetic fact is obvious in this era of workplace drug testing. A person could test positive for urinary THC, as it slowly equilibrates out of adipose tissue, without being under its influence. Conversely, rapid weight loss (i.e., fat reduction by exercise at a health club) could also conceivably result in accelerated release of THC from adipose tissue that is breaking down.

TABLE 2.6
Comparison of Apparent Volumes
of Distribution (Liters)

- Acetylsalicylic acid-11
- Amoxicillin-29
- Captopril-40
- Chloroquine-13,000

Some relevant volumes of body compartments are (in liters) plasma water (3), erythrocyte water (3), extracellular water excluding blood (11), and intracellular water (24); the total body water is approximately 41 L. A comparison of selected drugs with apparent volumes of distribution (L), approximating various body compartments, is shown in Table 2.6.

In certain cases of drug distribution there can be advantageous cellular selectivity. For example, tetracyclines, organic arsenicals, griseofulvin, and cyanocobalamin (vitamin B_{12}) concentrate in bacteria, trypanosomes, fungi, and bone marrow, respectively. The antimalarial drug chloroquine also concentrates outside the plasma, localizing in parasitic protozoans. This aspect of chloroquine's pharmacokinetics explains its therapeutic usefulness as well as an apparent volume of distribution in *excess* of 10,000 L. This value is obviously a physiological impossibility and, therefore, represents only a mathematical concept, and hence the term apparent is applied. Many drugs have very large distribution volumes because they are highly bound to tissue proteins. However, the site of concentration within the body is not necessarily a drug's target organ.

It should also be pointed out that the % body water varies between infants and adults. Infants possess approximately 77% body water while adults approximately 58%. Conversely, the elderly have lower percent body water. This can have significant implications in terms of drug clearance (see Chapter 3).

If a drug passes through cell membranes, but is not taken up into any particular cells, it will be evenly distributed throughout total body water when equilibrium is reached. It will therefore have an apparent volume of distribution of about 41 L. A prime example of such a drug is ethanol.

After arriving at a particular organ, it is the free, unbound form of the drug that is able to cross first the endothelial cells of the capillaries into the interstitial space and, subsequently, the cellular membrane of the tissue. Capillary permeability is largely determined by: (1) capillary structure and (2) the chemical nature of the drug. The membrane-related factors influencing distribution of drugs between blood plasma and tissues are essentially the same as those described previously between the gastrointestinal tract and blood plasma.

CHIRALITY

To this point, various physicochemical properties of drugs such as lipophilicity, ionization, and partition coefficient have been discussed. While these are certainly major factors, there is an additional factor that can influence drug distribution, namely *chirality*. Chirality is a relatively unique structural characteristic of certain molecules that can exist in two asymmetric, nonsuperimposable isomers (enantiomers), owing to the presence of a chiral center (a carbon atom that is attached to four different functional groups (see Chapters 5 and 16).

Chirality does not really become a significant factor unless enantioselectivity exists in processes such as active transport. The distribution of a drug can be markedly affected by its ability to bind to plasma proteins, since only free drug is able to cross cell membranes and the blood-brain barrier. The plasma proteins to which drugs bind are enantioselective and the fraction of the free, active drug can be widely different between the enantiomers of highly protein bound drugs such as ibuprofen and warfarin (50% in each case).

BLOOD-BRAIN BARRIER

In the periphery, capillary walls are generally quite porous, depending on the area (e.g., liver>kidney> muscle>brain). Most drugs, whether ionized or not, are able to pass through gaps (fenestrations) between endothelial cells and within the basement membrane. An important *exception* to this, however, is the central nervous system (*CNS, brain,* and *spinal cord*), where capillary endothelial cells are tightly packed adjacent to each other, precluding the existence of gaps, and are closely associated with a covering of astrocytes. Therefore, in the CNS, like the gastrointestinal tract, drug absorption is also significantly influenced by its lipophilicity (i.e., its state of ionization and polarity).

The result of this anatomical characteristic of endothelial cells in the CNS is an increased resistance to water soluble and ionized drugs entering the brain, and cerebral spinal fluid (CSF), from capillary blood. However, in a few areas of the brain, the barrier is absent. These areas include the lateral nuclei of the hypothalamus, the area postrema of the fourth ventricle, the pineal body, and the posterior lobe of the hypophysis. Highly lipophilic compounds can cross the barrier. Tranquilizers such as diazepam and its analogs are known to rapidly gain access to the CSF with a half-life ($t^{1/2}$) entry time of less than 1 min.

In addition to the more tightly packed endothelial cells in CNS capillaries, the capillaries are also surrounded by glial cells (astrocytes), mentioned above, that form an *additional* sheath surrounding the capillary network. The CNS, therefore, has two protective barriers between free drug and brain tissue. This membrane complex is referred to as the *blood-brain barrier* or the blood-CSF barrier. Under normal circumstances it is quite effective. However, if the barrier membranes become inflamed, a wider range of substances can pass through because of the development of "leaky" pores. In addition, this barrier is incompletely developed at birth, so neonates are less protected against drugs gaining access to the CNS.

PLACENTAL TRANSFER

A relatively unique but particularly significant aspect of drug distribution is the placental transfer of drugs from the maternal circulation into that of the fetus. Any xenobiotic that gains access to the maternal circulation should be considered capable of crossing the placenta, unless demonstrated to the contrary. In general, lipophilic, unionized, low molecular weight drugs in their unbound form tend to cross the placenta. Although the human placenta contains some detoxification enzymes (see Chapter 3) responsible for oxidation, reduction, hydrolysis, and conjugation, their capacity is extremely limited and they do not significantly contribute to drug clearance.

A number of drugs are known to have adverse or teratogenic effects on the developing fetus. The most infamous, of course, is thalidomide (a sedative used during the early 1960s). Thalidomide was manufactured in West Germany and was used by millions of people in 46 nations, before it was discovered that it caused birth defects during the first trimester of pregnancy. This is the period of gestation when the developing fetus is most susceptible to teratogenic effects, and a single dose of thalidomide at the right/wrong time is sufficient to produce its effect.

Specifically, thalidomide produced a characteristic stunting of limb bud tissue, apparently owing to interference with normal vascularization. The result was the development of a relatively unique syndrome known as *phocomelia*. At least 10,000 children, most of them German, were born with "flippers" instead of arms or legs. Unfortunately, some thalidomide babies are apparently still being born in South America, where the drug continues to be manufactured and many people are unaware of its proper uses (it is used fairly extensively for treating certain skin lesions in leprosy patients).

Despite thalidomide's embryo toxicity, it is relatively nontoxic in other contexts. Therefore, research projects are currently underway, or proposed, to investigate thalidomide's possible use in cancer patients, because of its presumed antiangiogenesis and immune-modulating effects. In addition, some AIDS patients have also reported that thalidomide seems to provide some relief for their rapid weight loss and possibly provide relief for mouth ulcers.

ETHANOL

At the present time there are several contemporary, widely used drugs that pose particular dangers to the developing fetus because of the relative prevalence of their use and their distribution across the placenta. These include alcohol, tobacco, and cocaine.

As mentioned above, ethanol distributes within total body water. This includes the body water of a developing fetus. Maternal consumption of ethanol is, therefore, a major cause of birth defects today, with its maximal expression being the *fetal alcohol syndrome* (FAS). FAS is characterized by: (1) growth retardation, (2) CNS abnormalities, and (3) a particular pattern of craniofacial abnormalities. The minimal amount of maternally consumed ethanol needed to elicit the syndrome is controversial. However, consumption of at least 165 g/week or 1 ounce per day is generally accepted as sufficient to generate abnormalities. Not surprisingly, the fetus appears to be particularly sensitive to binge drinking where blood levels can reach devastating amounts and exceed the mother's capacity to inactivate it (see Chapter 3). The fetotoxic effects of ethanol are probably mutifactorial. However, restricted placental blood supply is a possible cause mediated by the release of prostaglandins resulting in fetal hypoxia.

TOBACCO

Obvious concern regarding the exposure of pregnant women to tobacco dust and smoke has existed since at least the middle of the nineteenth century. During the subsequent years, many studies have reported the association of cigarette smoking with numerous problems of pregnancy. One of the most important observations in experimental animals was reported in 1940. In this study, it was found that the young of nicotine-treated as well as tobacco-smoke-exposed rats were *underweight* compared to those of control rats. This observation was confirmed in 1957. *In general, babies of pregnant women who smoke are 200 g lighter than babies born to comparable pregnant women who are nonsmokers.* In addition to lower birth weight, smoking increases prematurity, spontaneous abortion, and prenatal mortality.

The fetotoxic causative agent(s) in tobacco is (are) not known with certainty. One of the reasons for this is that a lit cigarette generates more than 2000 known compounds. These can be divided into five groups: (1) tobacco alkaloids and their metabolites; (2) nitrosamines; (3) tobacco gases; (4) metals; and (5) toxic hydrocarbons. The three components in the highest concentration per cigarette are carbon dioxide (68.1 mg), carbon monoxide (16.2 mg), and nicotine (0.1–2.5 mg). Proposed mechanisms for tobacco fetotoxicity include decreased utilization of amino acids (negative nitrogen balance) and hypoxia due to the displacement of oxygen from hemoglobin (e.g., the affinity of hemoglobin for carbon monoxide is approximately 300 times that for oxygen).

COCAINE

One of the most significant contemporary pediatric problems is cocaine abuse in pregnant women ("crack" cocaine being a particularly prevalent form). Surveys indicate that women of childbearing age (18–34 years) constitute 15% of all regular users of cocaine. It is estimated that 2–3% of pregnant women use cocaine in the United States. The use of cocaine by pregnant women has caught the attention of the courts. In some U.S. jurisdictions, mothers have been sentenced to jail time for causing the addiction of their baby.

The hazards of cocaine specific to pregnant women include premature rupture of placental membranes, spontaneous abortion, abnormal labor, and several general medical risks (e.g., hypertension). Their babies typically have growth retardation with consequent lowered birth weight. Cocaine use is also related to *sudden infant death syndrome* characterized by abnormal respiratory control, particularly during sleep.

It is not clearly understood to what extent cocaine and/or its metabolites contribute to fetotoxicity. However, the end result appears to be a reduction in uterine blood flow possibly via blockade of neuronal amine reuptake (see CNS section for more details). Cocaine may also decrease placental transport of amino acids, as well as hypertension.

SELECTED BIBLIOGRAPHY

Albert, A. (1979) *Selective Toxicity*, London: Chapman & Hall.

Brody, T.M., Larner, J., Minneman, K.P., and Neu, H.C. (Eds.) (1994) *Human Pharmacology: Molecular to Clinical*, 2nd ed., St. Louis: Mosby.

First commercial gene therapy; www.nbsc.com/files/press/pr20031105.pdf.

Goldstein, A., Aronow, L., and Kalman, S. (1974) *Principles of Drug Action: The Basis of Pharmacolgy*, 2nd ed., New York: John Wiley & Sons.

Hardman, J.G. and Limbird, L.E. (Eds.) (2001) *Goodman and Gillman's The Pharmacological Basis of Therapeutics*, 10th ed., New York: McGraw-Hill.

Mutschler, E. and Derendorf, H. (Eds.) (1995) *Drug Actions: Basic Principles and Therapeutic Aspects*, Boca Raton: CRC Press.

Niesink, R.J.M., de Vries, J., and Hollinger, M. (Eds.) (1995) *Toxicology: Principles and Applications*, Boca Raton: CRC Press.

Rama Sastry, B.V. (1995) *Placental Toxicology*, Boca Raton, CRC Press

Smith, C.M. and Reynard, A.M. (Eds.) (1995) *Essentials of Pharmacology*, Philadelphia: W.B. Saunders.

Timbrell, J.A. (1995) *Introduction to Toxicology*, 2nd ed., London: Taylor & Francis.

QUESTIONS

1. Following oral administration of a drug, the first major organ the drug would reach would be which of the following?
   a. Heart
   b. Lung
   c. Brain
   d. Liver
   e. Kidney

2. Following IV administration of a drug, the first major organ the drug would reach would be which of the following?
   a. Heart
   b. Lung
   c. Brain
   d. Liver
   e. Kidney

3. A drug that is highly lipid soluble:
   a. Is absorbed slowly from the GI tract
   b. Is rapidly excreted by the kidneys
   c. Is probably active in the CNS
   d. Requires an active transport system
   e. None of the above

4. Administering a drug by way of inhalation:
   a. Can be a slow way to get the drug in the bloodstream
   b. Can be an ideal route for certain drugs
   c. Is a good route to ensure a long duration of drug action
   d. Is the fastest way to get a drug into the blood stream
   e. Is the ideal route for all drugs

5. You have overheard a physician talking about the parenteral administration of a drug. Which route would he/she <u>not</u> have been referring to?
    a. Sublingual
    b. Topical
    c. Intradermal
    d. Inhalation
    e. Intramuscular

6. An advantage of the IV route is/are which of the following?
    a. Once injected IV the drug can be easily removed
    b. Rapid injections can be made free of acute toxic effects
    c. Large volumes of drug solution can be introduced over a long period of time
    d. Ideal route to deliver drugs to the liver
    e. Both b and c

7. The blood-brain barrier is believed to be:
    a. Fully developed at birth
    b. Impermeable to lipid soluble drugs
    c. Believed to be a specialized lining of blood vessels in the brain and adjacent astrocytes
    d. A means of keeping drugs out of the peripheral nervous system
    e. All of the above

8. Which of the following is/are <u>not</u> true regarding Fick's law?
    a. Rate of passage directly proportional to concentration gradient
    b. Rate of passage directly proportional to surface area of membrane
    c. Rate of passage directly proportional to partition coefficient
    d. Rate of passage directly proportional to membrane thickness
    e. None of the above

9. Which of the following is/are true regarding the affect of pH on drug absorption?
    a. Weak acids are preferentially absorbed in relatively acidic environments
    b. Weak bases are preferentially absorbed in relatively acidic environments
    c. Weak acids are preferentially absorbed in relatively basic environments
    d. b and c above
    e. None of the above

10. The fetus is most susceptible to <u>teratogenic</u> effects of drugs during which period(s) of gestation?
    a. First trimester
    b. Second trimester
    c. Third trimester
    d. Fourth trimester
    e. Equally throughout

3 Metabolism and Elimination

GENERAL PRINCIPLES

After a drug or any xenobiotic gains access to the body and distributes within it, there must be some mechanism(s) whereby the molecule has its bioactivity terminated; otherwise, drug effects could last the lifetime of the recipient. For most drugs, their duration of action is inversely proportional to the rate at which they are metabolically inactivated. For example, if *hexobarbital* (a sedative/hypnotic drug that can produce sleep) is given to mice and dogs, dogs will sleep, on average, 26 times longer than mice, even if they receive *half* the dose on a per weight basis. This increased sleeping time in dogs correlates reasonably well with the elevated half-life (time required for the blood level to decrease by one-half) of hexobarbital in that species.

In view of the fact that we have evolved in a manner in which we obtain our energy primarily by way of the GI system, this route also became the most likely portal for the inadvertent introduction of toxic substances. Therefore, as a survival necessity, the body had to evolve a strategy for the early interception and processing of potentially toxic xenobiotic substances. Anatomically, this is primarily accomplished by the *hepatic portal venous system*, which delivers substrates absorbed from the gut directly to a succession of chemical-transforming enzyme systems located in the liver.

An important consequence of the hepatic-portal system is that before a drug can reach the heart and from there the rest of the body, it has to initially pass through the liver. This is referred to as the *first-pass effect* and can result in nearly complete metabolism (>90%) of certain substances. It is for this reason that some drugs are not given orally (e.g., nitroglycerin) but by an alternative route (e.g., transdermally across the skin or sublingually across the mucous membrane beneath the tongue), because they are so completely inactivated. Xenobiotics introduced into the body via alternative routes will, of course, ultimately find their way to the liver via the general circulation (i.e., *hepatic artery*).

The chemical modification of xenobiotics in the body is called *biotransformation, metabolism*, or *metabolic clearance*. Enzymes involved in metabolism are either membrane bound (e.g., *endoplasmic reticulum* and *mitochondria*) or freely soluble within the *cytosol*. Because these metabolic enzymes are not particularly substrate specific, they can metabolize compounds with fairly diverse chemical structures, including some endogenous compounds such as steroids, bile acids, and heme.

In general, all biotransformation reactions can be assigned to one of two major categories called Phase I and II reactions (Table 3.1); these terms are frequently used interchangeably with Phase 1 and 2. *Richard Tecwyn Williams* (1909–1979) was one of the founders of the study of drug

---

TABLE 3.1
Examples of Metabolic Phase 1 and Phase 2 Reactions

Phase 1	Phase 2
Oxidation	Glucuronidation
Reduction	Methylation
Hydrolysis	Acetylation
	Amino acid conjugation
	Glutathione conjugation

---

metabolism at the molecular level. Williams is perhaps best remembered for introducing the idea of various phases of drug metabolism; a classification that has greatly influenced subsequent thinking in pharmacology and toxicology.

William's influential textbook *Detoxication Mechanisms: The Metabolism of Drugs and Allied Organic Compounds* was published in 1947; a second edition appeared in 1959. In the second edition of his book, William's distinguished between the two classes of *drug metabolism*, which he called "Phase 1" and "Phase 2." "Phase 1" included *oxidation*, *reduction*, and *hydrolysis* reactions. "Phase 2"encompassed *conjugation* reactions, such as glucuronidation and sulfation, which typically yield *water-soluble* urinary metabolites. Williams also recognized that metabolism could result in either detoxication or increased toxicity.

Using William's designations, Phase 1 reactions *are nonsynthetic* biotransformation reactions. Phase 2 reactions, on the other hand, *are synthetic* reactions and involve conjugation of the drug with a new moiety. Often, a drug may undergo sequential biotransformation through both Phase 1 and 2 pathways. The usual net effect of these reactions is to produce metabolites that are *more polar* (i.e., *more* water soluble and *less* lipophilic at cellular membranes). Therefore, the metabolites are partitioned into the aqueous media, being less likely to cross subsequent cellular membranes than the parent molecule and, conversely, more likely to be excreted by the kidneys.

PHASE 1 REACTIONS

Enzymatic mediated oxidation in the liver is the predominant metabolic process responsible for the transformation of xenobiotics in many species, including humans. This process is often the *rate-limiting step* in the elimination of a compound from the body. Large differences can exist between different species, as illustrated above by hexobarbital sleeping time in the mouse and dog, as well as between different individuals within a species, as well as gender, in their capacity to metabolize xenobiotics. The reason that mice sleep significantly less following two times as much hexobarbital as dogs is that they have nearly a 17-fold higher liver *hydroxylase* activity (which is the enzyme that inactivates hexobarbital). Although the liver is the most important xenobiotic metabolizing organ, other tissues can have varying activity (Table 3.2).

Interspecies and interindividual variability in drug metabolism is influenced by both genetic and environmental factors. The basal rate of drug metabolism in a particular individual is determined *primarily by genetic constitution*, but also varies with age, gender, and environmental factors such as diet, disease states, and concurrent use of other drugs.

For most drugs, oxidative biotransformation is performed primarily by a class of P450 enzymes, discovered during the early 1960s. These enzymes are all cytochromes that when treated appropriately (complexing with carbon monoxide) show a strong spectrophotometric absorption peak at $\lambda_{max} = 450$ nm. In 1962, Tsuneo Omura and Ryo Sato, in Osaka, purified the protein responsible for the 450 chromophore. They found that the absorption was due to a previously unknown class of heme proteins.

TABLE 3.2
Tissue Localization of Xenobiotic-Metabolizing Enzymes

Relative Amount	Tissue
High	Liver
Medium	Lung, kidney, intestine
Low	Skin, testes, placenta, adrenals
Very low	Nervous system tissues

P450 enzymes are often identified by their catalytic activities. The common feature to P450 catalysis is insertion of a single oxygen atom into an organic substrate, hence the name "mono-oxygenase," which has replaced the more archaic term *"mixed-function oxidase enzyme system."*

P450 ENZYMES

P450s are actually a super family of heme-containing enzymes found throughout the animal and plant kingdoms, and in yeast and bacteria. Mammalian P450 enzymes are membrane bound and present in very large amounts. In the liver, for example, P450 enzymes are the predominant proteins of the endoplasmic reticulum. The prevailing view is that microsomal P450s are exposed on the cytosolic side of the endoplasmic reticulum and anchored into the endoplasmic membrane by a hydrophobic "tail."

These proteins are classified into families and subfamilies on the basis of their amino acid similarities. Human genes encode about 66 functional P450 proteins. P450 enzymes involved in the oxidation of drugs and xenobiotics are widely distributed in the body, with highest concentrations in the *endoplasmic reticulum* of liver, kidney, lung, nasal passages, gut, and skin—organs that must cope with exposure to diverse foreign compounds.

A dozen or so P450 enzymes dominate the metabolism of drugs and xenobiotics. The mammalian P450s involved in the oxidation of foreign compounds are designated CYP1, CYP2, CYP3, and CYP4. The human gene encoding P450 1A2 is approximately 8 kbp in length and comprises seven exons/six introns; among its substrates include acetaminophen, aflatoxin B_1, caffeine, clozapine, ethoxyresorufin, and phenacetin. Other isoforms interact with coumarin, nicotine, cyclophosphamide, diazepam tamoxifen, hexobarbital, and tolbutamide, for example. Many other P450s catalyze specific steps in secondary metabolism, particularly *steroid synthesis*.

Human hepatic P450 content can be accounted for by enzymes 1A2, the 2C subfamily, 2E1, and the most abundant P450 enzyme, 3A4; the student should be aware that even a P450 expressed at a low level may control the metabolism of a substance for which it has high specificity. For example, P450 2A6 is probably not one of the highly expressed hepatic forms, but it accounts for most of the nicotine detoxication activity and is a major determinant of smoking behavior. Individuals with high activity metabolize nicotine quickly, and smoke more frequently.

P450 INDUCTION

All three enzymes of the P450 1 family are *induced* by compounds such as 3 methylcholanthrene. Increased activity of an enzyme following exposure to an environmental factor (such as a dietary factor, drug, or toxicant) is referred to as *induction*. The rise in enzyme activities, following administration of an inducing agent, usually takes several days to reach a maximum. Sustained elevation depends on the continued presence of the inducing agent; if the inducing agent is withdrawn, enzyme activities slowly return to baseline, due to normal messenger RNA and protein degradation and turnover.

As the sciences of molecular pharmacology and toxicology developed, induction (discovered in the late 1950s) became an increasingly important field of research. For a long time, however, studies remained theoretical rather than mechanistic. The principle roadblock to progress was the difficulty of identifying and characterizing the protein receptors that mediate the induction response and to which xenobiotics bind. These impediments were overcome in the early 1990s with the cloning of the aryl hydrocarbon (AH) receptor. P450 induction is a phenomenon with significant implications for clinical pharmacology. Humans are typically exposed to complex mixtures of chemicals in the environment and multiple drugs are often prescribed simultaneously ("polypharmacy"). The P450 induction effect of one agent may alter the actions of another. Induction can significantly

- Change the rate of elimination of a xenobiotic from the body
- Alter the fraction of an oral dose of a drug that reaches a target organ
- Shift the proportions of the various metabolites formed from a xenobiotic

---

TABLE 3.3
Examples of Inducing Agents

- 3-Methylcholanthrene
- 2,3,7,8-Tetrachlorodibenzodioxin
- β-Naphthoflavone
- Phenobarbital
- Benzo[a]-pyrene
- Barbital
- Dimethylaminoazobenzene
- Aminopyrene
- Phenylbutazone
- Clofibrate
- Pregnenolone-16α-carbonnitrile
- "Arachlor" (mixture of PCB isomers)
- TCPOBOP (1, 4-bis[2-(3,5-dichloropyridyloxy)]benzene)

The increased metabolic activities following induction reflect an increase in the amounts of specific forms of P450 present in the tissue. *The amount of a specific P450 can be increased by up to two orders of magnitude* by exposure to xenobiotics, although there is usually no more than a two- to threefold increase in the *total* content of P450 protein in the tissue. Significant elevations in conjugating enzymes, such as *glucuronosyl transferases* and *glutathione transferases*, also occur in response to xenobiotic exposures (Table 3.3).

GENETICS OF P450

Sequence-based analysis of P450 evolution indicates that the number of animal P450 genes increased suddenly about 400 million years ago, at about the time when animals *evolved* from the sea to the land. It has been speculated that the selective pressure resulting from fierce molecular struggles between plants (evolving biosynthetic pathways for elaboration of natural product toxins, to deter foraging animals) and animals (evolving detoxication enzymes to metabolize these toxins, thereby allowing the animals to eat the plants) drove the expansion of the P450 superfamily.

An early but erroneous idea was that each P450 substrate would induce the P450 activity responsible for its metabolism. While this may occur, it is not a fixed rule. Similarly, another theory was that the P450 enzymes are themselves the receptors that mediate the induction process. It is now appreciated that the induction process is complex and may involve regulation at the *transcriptional*, *translational*, and *posttranslational* levels. However, the most important mechanism of P450 induction is *enhanced transcription*.

More than 20 different human CYP isoforms have been characterized. It has been estimated that over 50% of the most commonly used prescribed drugs are metabolically cleared primarily by CYPs. Pharmacogenetics today, to a great extent, deals with genes encoding drug transporters, drug-metabolizing enzymes, and drug targets. It is clear that the polymorphism of metabolizing enzymes, and in particular that of P450s, has the greatest effect on interindividual variability of drug response. These polymorphisms affect the response of individuals to drugs used in the treatment of depression, psychosis, cancer, cardiovascular disorders, ulcers and gastrointestinal disorders, and pain and epilepsy, among others.

Codeine intoxication can occur in individuals who are ultrarapid CYP2D6 metabolizers because of CYP2D6 gene duplication. In Switzerland, a 62-year-old man developed life-threatening opioid intoxication in 2004, after ingesting "small doses" of codeine (25 mg three times a day) to relieve cough associated with pneumonia. Codeine is normally metabolized by CYP2D6 into *morphine,* and genotyping showed that the patient had *three or more functional CYP2D6 alleles*, a finding consistent with ultrarapid metabolism of codeine to morphine. The total amount of morphine and metabolites in this patient corresponded to 75% of the total amount of codeine present in his body. Normally, the usual amount of morphine that is produced after administration of multiple doses of codeine rarely reaches 10% of the total amount of codeine in a person.

P450 OXIDATION

The mechanism of oxidation by CYPs within the monooxygenase system has been determined in quite detail, but is beyond the scope of this book. The interested reader may consult any major medical pharmacology text for in-depth coverage; the mini-review by Snyder cited at the end of the chapter is also a good start. However, we now recognize the stoichiometry of the general formulation of a P450-dependent drug oxidation as summarized below:

$$NADPH + H^+ + O_2 + RH \rightarrow NADP^+ + ROH + H_2O$$

Examples of oxidative reactions are shown in Table 3.4. *Generally, reduction and hydrolysis reactions play subordinate roles in xenobiotic metabolism compared to oxidation reactions.* Examples of reduction and hydrolysis reactions are shown in Tables 3.5 and 3.6, respectively. To reiterate: the net result of Phase 1 reactions is the formation of *more polar, less lipid soluble* metabolites that will have a greater tendency to remain within the circulatory system, until they are eliminated via the kidneys.

TABLE 3.4
Examples of Oxidative Reactions

Reaction Class	Structural Change		Drug Example
Hydroxylation	RCH_2CH_3	$\rightarrow RCH_2CH_2OH$	Phenobarbital
Dealkylation	RNHCH3	$\rightarrow RNH_2 + CH_2O$	Morphine
Desulfuration	R_1CSR_2	$\rightarrow R_1COR_2$	Thiopental
Deamination	$RC(NH_2)HCH_3$	$\rightarrow RCOCH_3 + NH_3$	Amphetamine
Sulfoxide formation	R_1SR_2	$\rightarrow R_1SOR_2$	Cimetidine

TABLE 3.5
Examples of Reduction Reactions

Reaction Class	Structural Change		Drug Example
Aldehyde reduction	RCHO	$\rightarrow RCH_2OH$	Chloral hydrate
Azo reduction	$R_1-N=N-R_2$	$\rightarrow R_1- NH_2 + R_2 - NH_2$	Sulfachrysoldine
Nitroreduction	O_2N-R	$\rightarrow H_2N - R$	Chloramphenicol

Note: Tend to occur when oxygen tension is low.

TABLE 3.6
Examples of Hydrolysis Reactions

Reaction Class	Structural Change		Drug Example
Ester hydrolysis	R_1COOR_2	$\rightarrow R_1 - COOH + HOR_2$	Acetylsalicylic acid
Amide hydrolysis	R_1CONHR_2	$\rightarrow R_1 COOH + H_2N - R_2$	Procaineamide

Note: Esters and amides are hydrolyzed by the same enzymes, however, esters are hydrolyzed much faster.

PHASE 2 REACTIONS

Phase 2 reactions involve a different type of mechanism whereby either the parent drug or oxidized metabolite becomes *conjugated to a new moiety*. The resulting conjugate is, once again, *more* polar and *less* lipid soluble. Conjugation of weak acids is particularly important because they tend to be unionized at the relatively *low pH of urine and, therefore, subject to reabsorption* (remember the principle of LeChatelier). There are a number of drugs that are primarily cleared metabolically by Phase 2 reactions, including tricyclic antidepressants, β_2-agonists, and some anti-AIDS drugs.

There are a variety of Phase 2 conjugating enzyme systems that react with functional groups such as –OH, –COOH, –NH2, and –SH, which are either present originally on the target xenobiotic or have been generated by Phase 1 reactions.

Glucuronide conjugation and *sulfate* conjugation are the major Phase 2 conjugation pathways and are enzymatically mediated by uridine diphosphoglucuronosyltransferase and sulfotransferase, respectively. In addition to the transferase enzymes, these two conjugation reactions require coenzymes and ATP. In both cases, the conjugated moiety is provided by an *activated donor source* (e.g., uridine diphosphate-glucuronic acid [UDPGA] and 3′-phosphoadenosine 5′-phosphosulfate, respectively). Other important conjugating substances include glutathione and amino acids such as glycine.

An example of glucuronide conjugation is shown in Figure 3.1. In general, both glucuronide and sulfate conjugation result in the formation of a biologically inert metabolite that is more readily excreted. In relatively rare situations, however, exceptions can occur.

Glucuronic acid conjugation is one of the most important pathways for biotransformation of many foreign substances, including natural products (e.g., morphine), pollutants (e.g., aromatic amines, hydroxylated metabolites of polycyclic aromatic hydrocarbons), and drugs (e.g., acetaminophen). This pathway accounts for more than one-third of all conjugation reactions involved in drug metabolism. In addition, several endogenous lipophilic compounds (bilirubin, bile salts. steroid hormones, etc.) are metabolized by conjugation to glucuronic acid.

Glucuronides are recognized by the biliary and renal organic anion transport systems, which enable their secretion into the bile or urine. Addition of glucuronic acid to a xenobiotic radically changes the structure of the molecule and alters its biological activity. Usually, the activity of the *aglycone* (without sugar) is reduced or abolished, due to reduction in affinity for the biological target (and facilitation of excretion). Therefore, glucuronide formation is mainly (but not exclusively) a detoxication process leading to inactive metabolites. For example, morphine-6-glucuronide may

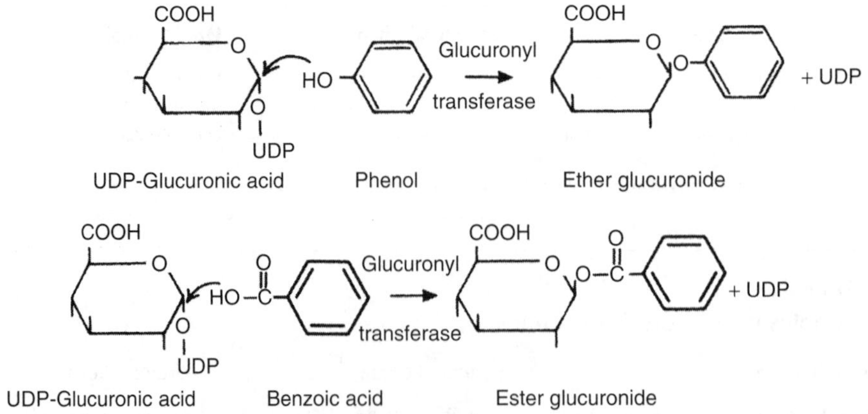

FIGURE 3.1   Conjugation of a phenol and a carboxylic acid with glucuronic acid. (From J.A. Timbrell (1991), *Principles of Biochemical Toxicology*. With permission.)

possess superior analgesic effect compared to its parent aglycone, morphine (see bioactivation below for a broader discussion).

Feline species have a very poor capacity for glucuronidation of phenolic compounds (e.g., acetaminophen), although they can glucuronidate bilirubin satisfactorily. Consequently, cats tend to excrete drugs as sulfate conjugates rather than glucuronides. This peculiarity of drug biotransformation has to be particularly considered in veterinary pharmacological practice.

GLUTATHIONE

Glutathione (GSH) is one of the most important molecules in the body's defense against toxic compounds, including drugs. This protective function is largely the result of its ability to undergo conjugation reactions with electrophiles, catalyzed by *S-transferases*. Reduced glutathione (its active form) is a tripeptide composed of glutamic acid, cysteine, and glycine.

GSH is the most abundant low-molecular-mass thiol in all mammalian cells. It is found in most cells but is particularly abundant in mammalian liver, where it reaches a concentration of 5–10 mM. The production of GSH in the adult human body has been estimated at about 10 g per day. Extracellular media, such as blood plasma and cerebrospinal fluid, contain lower (micromolar) but still significant concentrations.

The presence of *cysteine* is the key component of GSH since its sulphydryl group is *nucleophilic* and will tend to attract highly reactive, toxic *electrophiles* (see Chapter 7). The cellular balance between reduced GSH and its disulfide is maintained largely in favor of the reduced form (normally >98%).

Electrophiles may be chemically reactive products of Phase 1 reactions or they may be somewhat more stable xenobiotics that have been ingested. Therefore, reduced glutathione can protect cells by removing reactive metabolites (see below) via conjugation. Unlike glucuronic acid conjugation, however, reduced glutathione is not part of an activated donor source utilizing ATP. Instead, it provides a *direct target* for electron seeking electrophiles.

BIOACTIVATION AND BIOTOXIFICATION

While the term biotransformation generally implies inactivation and detoxification, there are exceptional cases where a metabolite is actually more chemically active or more toxic than the parent compound. In these situations, the processes of *bioactivation* and *biotoxification* are said to have occurred, respectively. An example of bioactivation is the formation of the commonly used drug acetaminophen from phenacetin in the liver (Figure 3.2). The latter drug was once widely used as an analgesic agent but, because of kidney toxicity, has been replaced by other more potent, less toxic substitutes including, of course, acetaminophen itself. In this particular bioactivation pathway, the process occurs via normal oxidative dealkylation.

In the context described above, phenacetin can be thought of as a *prodrug*, that is, an inactive or less active precursor of a more active drug form. The classic example of a prodrug is *Prontosil*. Prontosil was the first antibacterial sulphonamide introduced in 1935 by Gerhard Domagk; as such, it has historical significance. However, within a year of its introduction, it was discovered that Prontosil itself was inactive. The actual active substance was found to be *sulphanilamide*, which was formed from prontosil by bacterially mediated *fission of the parent compound* in the gut (see Chapter 10 for additional coverage).

Aspirin, one of the most widely used drugs in the United States (estimated annual consumption of 10–20 thousand tons), also has a prodrug background. The antifebrile property of *willow bark* (*Salix alba*) has been known by many cultures for centuries and is due to the presence of a glucoside called *salicin*. In humans, salicin is hydrolyzed in the GI tract to glucose and salicyl alcohol. The latter substance subsequently undergoes cytoplasmic oxidation to *salicylic acid, the true active ingredient*.

However, because of the irritating effect of sodium salicylate when administered orally, the molecule was subsequently modified to acetylsalicylic acid and became commercially available in 1899. Today, considerable research is being devoted to the development of prodrugs that can be activated in target tissues other than the liver or gut.

An example of *biotoxification* is the formation of paraoxon from the insecticide parathion via sulfoxidation. The simple substitution of an oxygen atom for a sulfur atom in the molecule results in a cholinesterase inhibitor with several-fold more potency. Similarly, the toxic action of methanol in producing blindness is the result of its metabolism to formaldehyde. Examples of bioactivation and biotoxification reactions are shown in Figure 3.2.

It should also be pointed out that there are reports in the literature relating to the *paradoxical toxicity* of glutathione conjugates (Table 3.7). Glutathione conjugates of drugs such as menadione and *p*-aminophenol have both been reported to produce nephrotoxicity in rodents. Ethylene dibromide, a compound used as a fumigant and insecticide, is converted by GSH conjugation into a reactive conjugate that cyclizes to form an alkylating agent. Therefore, although thiols such as reduced

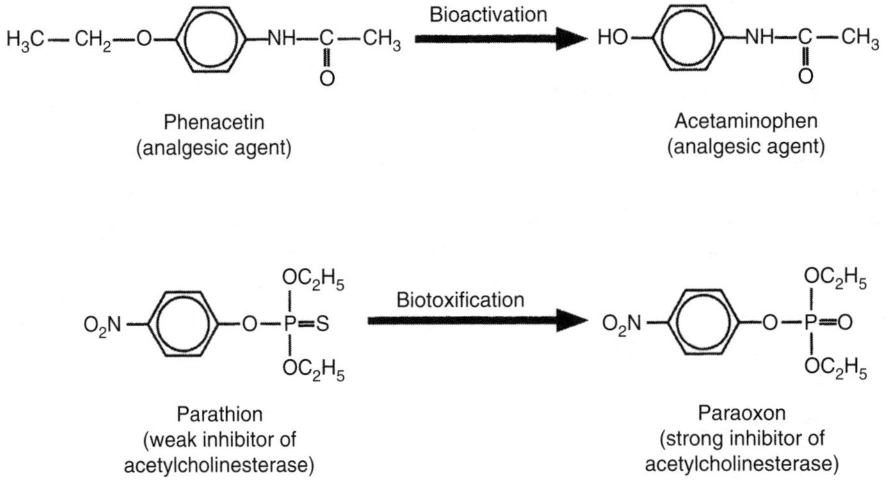

FIGURE 3.2   Comparison of metabolic bioactivation and biotoxification processes.

TABLE 3.7
Examples of Drugs that can Form GSH-Reactive Conjugates

Compound

Acetaminophen
Amodiaquine
Carbamazepine
Clozapine
Diclofenac
Felbamate
Imipramine
Indomethacin
Pioglitazone
Rosiglitazone
Sulfamethoxazole
Valproic acid

glutathione are generally considered to be antioxidants, the redox cycling (see Chapter 7) of thiols may lead, themselves, to the formation of reactive oxygen species.

ENZYME INDUCTION

One of the more interesting and clinically relevant aspects of the drug metabolizing capacity of the liver is that it is subject to *fluctuations* in activity. As mentioned previously, the basal rate of many liver enzymes can be modified by a number of factors including xenobiotics (e.g., drugs, environmental pollutants, natural products, and pesticides). Enzyme activity can be either increased or decreased. When enzyme activity is increased, the process is referred to as hepatic *enzyme induction*.

The induction of liver enzymes has been demonstrated in many species, including humans, and probably represents a homeostatic, defense mechanism. Induction usually requires multiple exposures to the inducing agent over a period of several days, the time required for the synthesis of new protein. Enzymes induced include cytochrome P450 monooxygenase system, glucuronyltransferase, microsomal ethanol-oxidative system, and steroid-metabolizing system.

There are basically three types of cytochrome P450 inducers: (1) phenobarbital-like (the major class), (2) methylcholanthrene-like (which actually increases a P448 isozyme), and (3) anabolic steroids. The former two have been the most frequently studied. Research over the last 40–50 years indicates that their mechanism of action involves genetic interaction, possibly via derepression of a "repressor" gene, and the subsequent synthesis of mRNA for the specific enzyme proteins. Examples of phenobarbital-like inducers, the most common, are shown in Table 3.8.

There are a number of clinical consequences of liver drug metabolizing enzyme induction by phenobarbital-like drugs. For example, a drug can increase its own rate of metabolism. If the non-steroidal anti-inflammatory drug phenylbutazone is administered for 5 days to a dog, the drug's blood level will decrease by 85%, even though the dose administered remains constant. The decline in blood level is the result of enzyme *self-induction*. Similarly, phenobarbital can increase its own rate of metabolism by inducing cytochrome P450, thus requiring the need for a higher dose. This type of tolerance is referred to as *pharmacokinetic* tolerance.

In addition to self-induction, the metabolism of other drugs and endogenous compounds can also be increased (i.e., *cross-induction*). In one classic case, a hospitalized heart patient was treated with an anticlotting drug (e.g., coumarin) to prevent additional heart attacks. In order to assist the patient in sleeping, the sedative/hypnotic phenobarbital was administered. After several days, the effectiveness of coumarin began to wane and its dose was *increased*. Following release from the hospital, the use of phenobarbital was discontinued, but the elevated dose of coumarin was continued. The result was a severe bleeding episode because the inducing effect of phenobarbital is *reversible*, and the higher, compensatory dose of coumarin was being metabolized at a *reduced* rate.

TABLE 3.8
Examples of Phenobarbital-Like Enzyme Inducers

Drug Group	Example	Strength of Induction
Antibiotic	Rifampin	4
Anticonvulsant	Diphenylhydantoin	3
Antihistamine	Chlorcyclizine	2
Antipsychotic	Chlorpromazine	2
Muscle relaxant	Carisoprodol	1
Nonsteroidal anti-inflammatory	Phenylbutazone	3
Oral hypoglycemic	Tolbutamide	3
Sedative	Phenaborbital	4

A similar type of situation has been reported in female epilepsy patients who were participants in a program studying the effectiveness of birth control pills. In this case, users of the antiepilepsy medication diphenylhydantoin (see Table 3.8) were found to have a higher incidence of pregnancy. This was subsequently shown to be due to the induction of liver enzymes metabolizing the steroids in their birth control pills. Obviously, the simultaneous use of enzyme inducing drugs in women taking birth control pills has potentially significant complications and must be monitored carefully.

Rifampin, a semisynthetic antibiotic effective in the treatment of tuberculosis, is a well-characterized inducer of the CYP3A4 isoform in man and is known to result in significant drug interactions with a relatively diverse range of drugs. The capacity for metabolic clearance of drugs by CYP3A4 can increase between 5- and 8-fold following treatment with rifampin, which translates into a 20- to 40-fold reduction in plasma concentration of subsequently administered drugs such as *oral contraceptives*, cyclosporin, verapamil, and nifedipine.

ENZYME INHIBITION

Drug metabolism in the liver can also be inhibited by certain xenobiotics. Enzyme inhibition can occur by decreased synthesis of drug metabolizing enzymes, increased degradation of the enzyme, or competition of two or more drugs for the same binding site. In general, inhibition of the capacity of the liver for detoxification is the result of pathological changes in the organ. For example, cirrhosis of the liver has been reported to diminish the glucuronidation of several drugs, including morphine and acetaminophen. In addition, hepatotoxicants such as carbon tetrachloride and toluene can also produce an inhibitory effect.

Apparently, relatively innocuous factors can also sometimes influence liver enzyme activity. For example, the metabolic elimination of the bronchodilator theophylline (see Chapter 13) has been reported to be prolonged in patients with influenza A or adenovirus infections. In 1990, an influenza epidemic in Seattle resulted in the admission of 11 children with high serum levels of theophylline and confirmed drug toxicity. These effects appear to be confined to cytochrome P450-based drug biotransformation. They may be related to the generation of interferons as a result of these infections, which, presumably, are causally related to the inhibitory effect on hydroxylases and demethylases.

In addition, something seemingly as innocent as grapefruit juice has also been shown to inhibit the metabolism of certain calcium channel blockers (e.g., nifedipine; taken to treat hypertension [see Chapters 4 and 12]). This effect is caused by the presence of relatively high concentrations of specific flavenoids in grapefruit juice. Patients taking calcium channel blockers should be warned of the food–drug interaction since blood levels of the drug can increase by 100–150%, resulting in rapid decrease in blood pressure.

RENAL ELIMINATION

In order for a drug or its metabolite(s) to be completely eliminated from the body, it must undergo excretion as well as metabolism. Excretion represents the final common pathway for the elimination of drugs. The kidneys are the most significant of the excretory sites. Extrarenal sites include biliary, pulmonary, sweat, salivary, and mammary glands in order of decreasing importance. For the purposes of our discussion, the renal pathway will be emphasized. The *renal processes* operating to modify the blood level of a drug include (1) *glomerular filtration*, (2) *tubular secretion*, and (3) *tubular reabsorption*.

The fundamental functional unit of the kidney is the *nephron*, of which approximately 1.2 million are present in each human being (Figure 3.3). If placed end to end, one person's nephrons would stretch approximately 50 miles. Structurally, each nephron consists of a porous tube within a nonporous tube, and is U-shaped. At the beginning of each nephron is a small tuft of blood capillaries called the *glomerulus*. Blood flows unidirectionally into this tuft, which has a porous

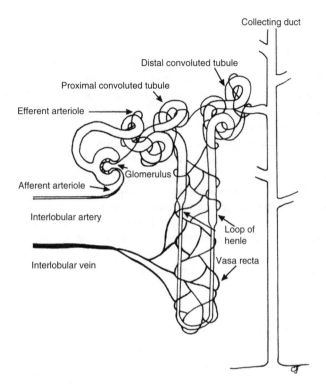

Collecting duct

Distal convoluted tubule

Proximal convoluted tubule

Efferent arteriole

Glomerulus

Afferent arteriole

Interlobular artery

Loop of henle

Vasa recta

Interlobular vein

FIGURE 3.3 Structure of the mammalian kidney. (From J.A. Timbrell (1991), *Principles of Biochemical Toxicology*. With permission.)

membrane that retains large blood components (e.g., erythrocytes) and most of the plasma protein (e.g., albumin; the presence of excess protein in the urine is suggestive of kidney damage) but allows passage of low molecular weight compounds (<500 Da). Therefore, drugs that are bound to plasma proteins will not be filtered and their clearance will be directly related to the free fraction.

After traversing the proximal and distal regions of the nephron, the filtrate eventually exits into the ureter that leads to the urinary bladder. Molecules and ions that the body needs are reabsorbed back across the epithelial layer of the tubules into the blood. The human kidneys produce approximately 180 L of glomerular filtrate per day, with the tubules reabsorbing all but 1.5 L of water and many dissolved endogenous and exogenous substances.

GLOMERULAR FILTRATION

The kidneys receive approximately one-fifth of the cardiac output (i.e., 1200 mL/min of blood). Therefore, each minute they are exposed to approximately 650 mL of plasma. However, the actual normal rate of plasma filtration in the *specific region* of the glomeruli is 125 mL/min (i.e., the glomerular filtration rate). The *volume* of plasma filtered by the glomeruli per unit time is *independent* of the plasma concentration of the drug. In individuals, the actual glomerular filtration capacity of the kidneys can be quantified. This is accomplished by measuring the *urinary excretion* of a substance that is *unbound* and *does not undergo appreciable tubular secretion or reabsorption* (e.g., *creatinine*, which is only processed by glomerular filtration).

At the early stage of the elimination process in the glomerulus, lipophilic drugs are filtered just as readily as hydrophilic. If a drug is excreted solely by glomerular filtration, its excretion rate (mg/min) will be the product of its glomerular filtration rate (mL/min) times its plasma concentration (mg/mL). However, if drug disappearance studies show that the renal clearance is either significantly greater or lower than 125 mL/min, some other factor(s) must be involved.

TUBULAR SECRETION

In the case of certain drugs, such as the penicillin class, there are *energy-dependent* active secretory processes that take place in the proximal tubule cells. These secretory processes selectively *facilitate the excretion* of certain acids (anions) and bases (cations) from the plasma over and above that provided by glomerular filtration. Therefore, in these cases, renal clearance is the sum of glomerular filtration and tubular secretion.

Because carrier systems are involved, the secretory process has a limited carrying capacity and can be saturated. Therefore, in distinction with glomerular filtration, tubular secretion is *dependent* on the plasma concentration of the drug. Like all active transport processes, secretion of a drug into the tubular fluid can be competitively inhibited by other drugs that are transported by the same carrier.

For example, coadministration of the drug probenecid reduces the tubular secretion of penicillin G because both are organic acids that are transported by a common carrier. The oral administration of probenecid in conjunction with penicillin G results in higher and more prolonged concentrations of the antibiotic in plasma than with penicillin alone. The elevation in plasma penicillin level can be at least twofold and sometimes much greater. The ability to reduce the dose of the antibiotic required is particularly important in the treatment of resistant infections.

REABSORPTION

The renal clearance of many drugs is low because they are significantly reabsorbed passively from the distal portion of the tubules. This is because of the large concentration gradient that exists between the free drug in the tubular lumen and that in plasma. Reabsorption depends on two separate routes: a transcellular pathway (through cell cytoplasm via selective pumps and cotransporters on epithelial cell plasma membranes) and a paracellular pathway (through the intercellular space between cells). For most drugs reabsorption is a passive process that is influenced by the lipid solubility of the drug, the pK of the drug, and pH of the urine. Lipophilic drugs, which are well absorbed in the GI tract, are also generally reabsorbed across the tubule epithelium. Conversely, hydrophilic drugs, which are poorly absorbed orally, are also reabsorbed poorly and, therefore, more readily excreted in the urine.

If urine flow increases, the time that a drug is exposed to the reabsorbtive surface of the kidney is decreased. This principle forms the basis for the treatment of certain extreme cases of acute drug overdose. In these situations patients undergo forced diuresis with large volumes of fluid in order to accelerate drug clearance (e.g., meprobamate poisoning).

The effect of urinary pH on drug ionization also has toxicological implications. For example, in cases of phenobarbital (a weak acid barbiturate) overdose, the urine can be alkalinized (elevate the pH) by administering sodium bicarbonate to the patient. The resultant increase in pH shifts the dissociation equilibrium for this weak acid to the right producing an increase in the proportion of the ionized form (as one would predict), less reabsorption in the kidneys, and more rapid elimination. Conversely, acidifying the urine with ammonium chloride will increase the excretion rate of drugs that are weak bases, since they will be more protonated (ionized) and less reabsorbed (more polar, less lipophilic).

CLEARANCE, ELIMINATION RATE CONSTANT, AND HALF-LIFE

In this chapter, we have seen that drugs are distributed in the body and subsequently metabolized and eliminated. All these factors contribute to regulating the ultimate duration of the drug's presence in the body. In concluding this section, there are some basic kinetic relationships between volume of distribution of a drug (discussed in Chapter 2), circulating drug concentration, and duration of drug in the body that the introductory student should be familiar with. If you go to a professional school (medical, pharmacy, etc.), you will run into them again. These relationships allow us to *quantify* important drug parameters that have significant pharmacological and toxicological implications.

An important concept relating to the ability of the body to eliminate a drug is *total body clearance* (CL_t). Total body clearance is a term that indicates the rate at which a drug is cleared from the body. It is defined as the volume of plasma from which all drug is removed in a given time (i.e., mL/min) by *all* routes, as expressed in the following equation:

$$CL_t = \frac{\text{Rate of drug removal (mg/min)}}{\text{Plasma concentration of drug (mg/mL)}}$$

Since drug elimination mechanisms in humans generally follow *first-order kinetics* (nonsaturated), an *elimination rate constant* (K_e) can be determined according to the following formula (assuming a one compartment model): The important feature of first-order kinetics in this context is that *they are not saturated*. In other words, the reactions are not operating maximally. This has important toxicological implications:

$$K_e = \frac{\text{Total body clearance (mL/min)}}{V_d \text{ (mL)}}$$

For example, if a drug has a total body clearance rate of 100 mL/min and its V_d is 2000 mL, the corresponding K_e would be 0.05 min^{-1}. This value indicates that approximately 5% of the *remaining* drug is eliminated per minute. In a first-order process, the concentration of the remaining chemical is rate limiting.

It should be understood that the total body elimination rate constant is a composite parameter. It encompasses *all* rate constants for all routes of elimination including excretion in the urine and feces, biotransformation, as well as sequestration in tissues.

Determination of clearance rate (for first-order reactions) also allows us to calculate another very important drug characteristic, namely its *half-life* ($t^{1/2}$), according to the following formula:

$$t^{1/2} = 0.693/k_e,$$

Therefore

$$t^{1/2} = 0.693 \times \frac{V_d \text{(mL)}}{\text{Clearance (mL/min)}}$$

In this equation, 0.693 is a constant obtained during the derivation of the formula (log 0.5). If we substitute our hypothetical values as used above, we would obtain a $t^{1/2}$ of approximately 14 min; *this is an important value to know since the time required to reach a steady-state plateau, and maintain it for first-order metabolism,* is dependent on the drug's half-life. In our case, therefore, it would take approximately 70 min (i.e., 5 half-lives) to reach approximately 97% of steady state. *In first-order reactions, $t^{1/2}$ is independent of dose*, because, under normal circumstances, that is, therapeutic, the system is not saturated since dosage is in the subgram amount.

In the example above, the drug has a very short half-life. In fact, it would really not be practical for a therapeutic agent, particularly if given orally. While this relationship between half-life and duration holds true for most drugs, there are exceptions. Adrenal glucocorticosteroids, for example, produce many of their anti-inflammatory effects after gaining access to intracellular receptors that transport the steroid into the nucleus. The steroid then induces gene expression of specific protein. As with all protein synthesis, this process takes time (i.e., a latent period). It continues after blood levels of the steroid have become diminished, but the effect lingers on.

When possible, a "once a day oral dose" represents an ideal regimen for drug administration. In view of the fact that approximately 90% of a dose is eliminated within three plasma half-lives of a compound, this would indicate that a half-life of approximately 8 h would be ideal. Compounds that have half-lives in humans in excess of 12 h will likely demonstrate systemic accumulation with daily

LIVERPOOL JOHN MOORES UNIVERSITY
LEARNING SERVICES

dosing in that all of the previous day's dosage will not be 100% eliminated before the successive dose is administered. Obviously, this has significant toxicological implications.

It should be pointed out at this point that although *most* drug elimination is via first-order kinetics, there can be some important exceptions. Drugs that *saturate* routes of elimination will disappear from plasma in a *nonconcentration-dependent manner*, which is *zero-order* kinetics. The most common example of a drug that has zero-order kinetics is ethanol. The reason that ethanol displays zero-order kinetics is that it is usually consumed in 5–10 g quantities that overwhelm (saturate) *alcohol dehydrogenase* in the liver.

Important characteristics of zero-order reactions are (1) a *constant amount* of drug is eliminated per unit time, since the system is saturated (maximized); (2) the *half-life is not constant* for zero-order reactions, but depends on the concentration; the higher the concentration, the longer the half-life. Therefore, the term zero-order half-life has little practical significance, since it can change; and (3) zero-order kinetics is also known as nonlinear or dose-dependent. For example, if the body can metabolize ethanol at a rate of 10 mL/h, then if one consumes 60 mL, it will take 3 h to metabolize half of it (the half-life under these circumstances). However, if 80 mL is consumed, the half-life will now become 4 h. This is particularly significant regarding ethanol toxicity.

Blood Alcohol Level

The amount of alcohol (ethanol) in your blood stream is referred to as blood alcohol level (BAL). It is recorded in milligrams of alcohol per 100 mL of blood, or mg%. For example, a BAL of 0.10 means that 1/10 of 1% (or 1/1000) of your total blood content is alcohol. When you drink alcohol, it goes directly from the stomach into the bloodstream and distributes evenly throughout the body. BAL is primarily influenced by weight, gender, genetic factors, and rate of consumption. On average, it takes the liver approximately an hour to metabolize the amount of alcohol found in 12 oz of beer, 4 oz of wine, or 1 oz of 50 proof (25%) hard liquor.

The *National Highway Traffic Safety Administration* in the United States estimates that it takes a 170-pound male 4–5 drinks (5 ounce glasses of 11% wine) within an hour on an empty stomach to reach a BAL of 0.08% (the legal limit in California and most states, for example). Conversely, it is estimated that a 137-pound female requires only three drinks over the same time frame to reach the same BAL. Therefore, the difference between 0.08 and 0.10% could be one drink in an hour for a large man, or half a drink for a petite woman. The significance of BAL in terms of behavior and toxicity are shown in Table 3.9.

The reason for the significant increase in severity of effects from elevated BAL is that from the first drink onwards, liver enzymes are saturated and that continued drinking will only elevate BAL. This fact is little appreciated by *binge drinkers*; defined as four drinks within an hour for females and five for males. Binge drinking has become an unfortunate aspect of college life. Unfortunately, surveys indicate that college students are not dissuaded by drinking-related deaths. To illustrate: one student died celebrating his 21st birthday by consuming 20 shots within 10 min and another 15 shots

---

TABLE 3.9
Relationship of BAL (mg%) to Human Behavior and Toxicity

- 0.02—Mellow feeling, slight body warmth, less inhibited
- 0.05—Noticeable relaxation, less alert. Less self-focused, impairment of coordination begins
- 0.08—Drunk driving limit in many states, definite impairment in coordination and judgment
- 0.10—Noisy, possible embarrassing behavior, mood swings, reduction in reaction time
- 0.15—Impaired balance and movement, clearly drunk
- 0.30—Many lose consciousness
- 0.40—Most lose consciousness, some die
- 0.50—Breathing stops, many die

---

within 15 min. Another student died with a BAL of 0.588, a level that would require 20–25 drinks in an hour. This is equivalent to unintentional suicide. Each new school year brings the inevitable addition of new names to this death list. Binge drinking can no longer be viewed as a rite of passage; it is a major health threat.

Those dying from alcohol poisoning experience no pain because the central nervous system becomes severely compromised. Initially, blood glucose begins to drop, signaling *hypoglycemia.* This is critical because blood glucose is the principle metabolic substrate for the brain to function. Following hypoglycemia, *hypothermia* sets in. The body's temperature drops, and because the central mechanism that regulates the body's temperature is impaired, natural responses to a cold environment, such as shivering, do not occur. Veins dilate and allow heat to escape at the skin level, causing the body's exterior to actually feel hot even as its core temperature is dropping.

The next phase of intoxication involves the development of *acidosis,* in which the body's pH level begins to fall. In an acid environment, the body's many vital systems go awry and start trying to compensate for the imbalance. Breathing may speed up and then slow down. The kidneys may attempt to excrete more acids. Blood pressure rises. All these conditions—hypoglycemia, hypothermia, and acidosis—begin in most people when BAL reaches 0.15–0.20% and higher.

Driving is a daily activity for most people in developed countries. Unfortunately, however, traffic accidents are one of the major causes of death. In the European Union (EU) in 2000, >40,000 people were killed and approximately 1.7 million suffered some kind of injury on the roads. The EU is aiming to reduce the accident mortality rate to 50% by the year 2010. To achieve this reduction, the EU has compiled an action program "to combat the scourge of drink-driving and find solutions to the issue of the use of drugs and medicines."

Although traffic accidents have many different causes, the most common is driving under the influence of alcohol. Were this not enough, it has been estimated that approximately 10% of all people killed or injured in road-traffic accidents were also taking *psychotropic medication*—clearly indicating a potential for interacting with alcohol. Several studies have provided evidence, in fact, that drivers taking benzodiazepines and tricyclic antidepressant drugs are at greater risk of having accidents than those not taking the medication.

EXTRARENAL CLEARANCE OF DRUGS

In addition to metabolism, the liver contributes to clearance by secreting approximately 0.5–1.0 L of *bile* daily (Figure 3.4). Important constituents of bile include conjugated bile salts, cholesterol, phospholipid, bilirubin diglucuronide, electrolytes, and drugs. Biliary excretion is primarily important for compounds with a molecular weight >500, while compounds with a molecular weight <300 (most drugs) are preferentially excreted into the urine.

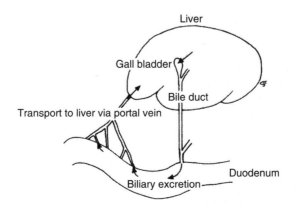

FIGURE 3.4 Biliary excretion route for foreign compounds. (From J.A. Timbrell (1991), *Principles of Biochemical Toxicology.* With permission.)

Bile is initially concentrated in the gall bladder and subsequently transported to the small intestine (duodenum) via the bile ducts. Drugs entering the duodenum may be eliminated in the feces or recycled back into the general circulation (i.e., enterohepatic circulation). Therefore, biliary excretion is truly a route of elimination only to the extent that the excreted drug fails to be reabsorbed. A mechanism facilitating the reabsorption of certain drugs is the hydrolysis of glucuronide conjugates via β-glucuronidase present in intestinal flora.

The *lungs* are the primary site of elimination for gaseous anesthetics and any other compounds that are volatile. For example, certain aromatic hydrocarbons are largely eliminated in the expired air. The major pathway for the elimination of ethanol, of course, is metabolism by the liver. However, approximately 2% is eliminated via the lungs. The equilibrium partition coefficient for ethanol between blood and alveolar air in humans is approximately 2100:1. Therefore, the ethanol concentration in end-expiratory air can be measured and multiplied by 2100 (e.g., by the *Breathalyzer* machine) to provide a fairly accurate estimate of ethanol concentration in the blood.

A number of drugs are eliminated partially by transport into *milk* during lactation. For most drugs, their concentration in milk is similar to that in the mother's circulation. The usual percentage of maternal dose transferred to the infant is in the range of 0.05–2%. In some cases, a significant pharmacological effect can be produced in babies who are breast-feeding. Among the drugs that are specifically contraindicated during breast-feeding are cocaine, lithium, and methotrexate. In addition, a number of drugs should be used with caution, including aspirin and phenobarbital.

SELECTED BIBLIOGRAPHY

Albert, A. (1979) *Selective Toxicity*, London: Chapman & Hall.

Brody, T.M., Larner, J., Minneman, K.P. and Neu, H.C. (Eds.) (1994) *Human Pharmacology: Molecular to Clinical*, 2nd ed., St. Louis: Mosby.

Goldstein, A., Aronow, L., and Kalman, S. (Eds.) (1974) *Principles of Drug Action: The Basis of Pharmacolgy*, 2nd ed., New York: John Wiley & Sons.

Hardman, J.G. and Limbird, L.E. (Eds.) (2001) *Goodman and Gillman's The Pharmacological Basis of Therapeutics*, 10th ed., New York: McGraw-Hill.

Mutschler, E. and Derendorf, H. (Eds.) (1995) *Drug Actions: Basic Principles and Therapeutic Aspects*, Boca Raton: CRC Press.

Rowland, M. and Tozer, T.N. (1980) *Clinical Pharmacokinetics: Concepts and Applications*, Philadelphia: Lea & Febiger.

Smith, C.M. and Reynard, A.M. (Eds.) (1995) *Essentials of Pharmacology*, Philadelphia: W.B. Saunders.

Snyder, R. (2000) Profiles in toxicology: Microsomal enzyme induction, *Toxicol. Sci.*, 55: 233–234.

Timbrell, J.A. (1995) *Introduction to Toxicology*, 2nd ed., London: Taylor & Francis.

QUESTIONS

1. In the process of drug action, the primary function of the liver is
   a. To initiate the deactivation process
   b. To aid in the transportation of the drug to the site of action
   c. To excrete the drug
   d. To speed up the absorption of the drug into the bloodstream
   e. To initiate the activation process

2. During the metabolism of a drug, most chemical changes of the drug's molecular structure result in products that are
   a. Less ionized
   b. Less rapidly excreted by the kidneys

    c. More lipid soluble

    d. More active pharmacologically

    e. More water soluble

3. Mechanisms for metabolizing certain drugs in the body may be impaired by
    a. Illness or damage to the liver
    b. Inadequate diet
    c. Advanced age
    d. Grapefruit juice
    e. All of the above

4. A drug may be excreted through the
    a. Lungs
    b. Urine
    c. Skin
    d. Kidneys
    e. All of the above

5. The primary enzymes responsible for the oxidation of drugs are located in the:
    a. Cytoplasm
    b. Mitochondria
    c. Smooth endoplasmic reticulum
    d. Nucleus
    e. Cell membrane

6. Which of the following is/are a Phase II reaction?
    a. Reduction
    b. Oxidation
    c. Hydrolysis
    d. Conjugation
    e. a, b, and c above

7. The consequences of stimulation of the smooth endoplasmic reticulum is/are more likely with regard to which of the following?
    a. Acute administration of a drug
    b. Chronic administration of a drug
    c. Phenobarbital
    d. Rifampin
    e. b, c, and d above

8. The mixed-function oxidase system is/are composed of which of the following?
    a. A superfamily of heme-containing proteins
    b. Cytochrome P450s
    c. Cytochrome P450 reductase
    d. b and c above
    e. a, b, and c above

9. Which of the following is/are true regarding "prodrugs"?
    a. They are an inactive or less active precursor of a more active metabolite
    b. They have only been developed during the past 10 years
    c. Their "activation" occurs primarily in the gastric mucosa
    d. They are far more potent than drugs considered "amateurs"
    e. a and b above

10. Which of the following drugs is/are most likely to be eliminated by zero-order kinetics?
    a. Birth control pills
    b. Penicillin
    c. Digoxin
    d. Alcohol (ethanol)
    e. b and d above

4 Drug Interactions

There are currently approximately 13,000 prescription drugs available in the United States and 3,000 in the United Kingdom. A new entity is approved for human use approximately every 2–3 weeks and two-thirds of all physician visits culminate in a drug being prescribed. No other risk factor compares with *polypharmacy* as a cause of adverse drug reactions and interactions, particularly in the *geriatric* population. A number of British and American studies have indicated that persons over 65 years of age living independently take an average of 2.8 drugs per day. In skilled nursing homes, the number increases to an average of 3.4 while approximately 9 drugs per day are prescribed for the hospitalized elderly.

It has been reported that there is a ninefold increased risk of having an adverse drug reaction when four or more drugs are taken simultaneously. In addition, 3–5% of all hospital admissions are related to adverse drug reactions and, of all the admissions for the elderly, 15–25% are complicated by an adverse drug reaction. Some of these reactions are life threatening, and it is estimated that fatal adverse drug reactions in the United States may run in the thousands each year.

Results obtained by counting the number of interactions of major clinical significance indicate substantial variation among different drug classes. For example, oral anticoagulants appear to have the greatest tendency followed by oral antidiabetics, monoamine oxidase inhibitors, phenothiazines, and anticonvulsants. The former two are not surprising since they are among the most frequently prescribed in the elderly.

When it comes to *drug–drug interactions* (DDIs), there is a spectrum of pharmacological issues that should be considered. For example, some drug interactions are very common such as the lipid-elevating effect of combining thiazide diuretics and beta-blockers, but the clinical consequences are usually not life threatening, produce few symptoms, are easily managed, transient, and well tolerated. However, in other situations, the statistical risk of incurring a drug interaction may be very low but the drug-related consequences may be life threatening (e.g., cardiac arrhythmias produced by the combination of erythromycin and terfenadine [the latter subsequently withdrawn from the market]).

To minimize an inadvertent drug–drug interaction, numerous pharmacies maintain records of prescription drugs currently used by individuals. Compendia of possible drug interactions are also available in both written and computer-based formats. Community pharmacists rely on their knowledge of interactions and dispensing software to identify potential DDIs. Interestingly, a study in 2004 of 1377 patients (>30 years of age) with hypertension—taking four or more oral medications—suggested that "higher-intensity pharmacies (the busiest) may have been more successful in minimizing the risk for clinically significant drug–drug interactions when compared with lower-intensity pharmacies."

As the number of drugs continue to proliferate and the population ages, the likelihood of drug interactions will undoubtedly continue to increase. Of all prescription drugs, 25% are taken by people over 65 years of age, although this group presently comprises approximately 12% of the population. The average older person fills more than twice as many prescriptions as those under age 65. Polypharmacy, variable compliance, and multiple diseases, combined with altered physiological response, make the elderly especially prone to adverse drug reactions.

The 1999 Institute of Medicines (IOM) report suggested that between 44,000 and 98,000 persons die annually from *medical errors* within hospitals. The IOM identified medication errors as a major subcategory of all medical errors. In 2000, an analysis of drug-related morbidity and mortality totaled $177.4 billion.

Up to 10% of adverse drug events involve drug–drug interactions. One case report involving an interaction of two antidepressants (fluoxetine and selegiline) illustrates the potential seriousness of the problem. In this situation, their concurrent use required a 15-day hospitalization, emergency room visits, ambulance services, magnetic resonance imaging, electrocardiogram, laboratory tests, and consultations to the extent of $17,213.

In addition to the elderly, patients with AIDS have a higher incidence of toxic reactions to medications than other subgroups treated with similar drugs. These individuals frequently consume 5–10 different medications daily, including antiretroviral drugs, as well as a number of antibiotic or antifungal agents that are used for prophylaxis against opportunistic infections. Often, nonapproved drugs are also used. Although the exact reasons for this increased sensitivity to drug-related side effects are not fully understood, it is possible that HIV-infected individuals tend to take multiple medications for long periods and also have multiorgan system compromise.

INTERACTIONS WITH HERBAL MEDICATIONS

At least 16% of people using prescription medication in the United States concurrently take herbal supplements. An estimated 15 million Americans are at risk of herb–drug interactions. Ginseng is one of the most commonly used herbals. Human case reports and animal studies indicate that ginseng may reduce the anticoagulant effect of warfarin (coumarin), a commonly used drug in the elderly. Ginseng may also promote bleeding in surgical patients.

INTERACTIONS DURING DISTRIBUTION AND METABOLISM

As mentioned previously, it is the free, unbound form of a drug that is able to be absorbed across cellular membranes. However, many drugs are reversibly bound to red blood cells and plasma proteins (particularly albumin, which represents 50–65% of the total). In humans, the blood concentration of albumin is normally 4% and each molecule possesses 109 cationic and 120 anionic groups at physiological pH. Albumin is referred to as *"high capacity, low affinity."* Acidic drugs tend to bind to albumin while basic drugs tend to bind to α1 acid glycoprotein (AAG), which is present in plasma at approximately 1% the concentration of albumin. Plasma levels of AAG are more subject to change than albumins. AAG is often referred to as *"low capacity, high affinity,"* in terms of binding sites.

The drug fraction bound to plasma protein cannot diffuse, cannot be metabolized, and cannot be excreted, because the molecular weight of the drug–protein complex exceeds 65,000 Da. The bound fraction represents, therefore, a storage form that is released when the concentration of free drug decreases and a new equilibrium is established. The normal therapeutic dose of a drug is determined taking this into account.

One of the potentially significant ramifications of plasma protein binding of drugs is in the area of drug interactions. The binding sites that exist on albumin, the principle plasma protein for drug binding, are designated as two forms, type I (warfarin site) and type II (benzodiazepine site). They are nonspecific and are finite in number. Therefore, whenever two different drugs (that are normally significantly albumin bound, i.e., >80%) are in the blood stream together, competition for binding sites can occur. Binding is usually expressed in percentage terms that describe the fraction of the concentration of drug in plasma that is bound to plasma proteins.

The drug with the higher affinity constant will successfully *displace* the drug with the lower. The result is an increase in the free-drug concentration of the latter. For example, tolbutamide (an oral hypoglycemic agent used in maturity-onset *Diabetes Mellitus*) is approximately 95% bound and 5% free (see Table 4.1). In the presence of the anti-inflammatory drug phenylbutazone (which is nearly 100% bound), essentially all of the bound tolbutamide can be displaced (i.e., a 20-fold increase from 5 to 100%), leading to potential toxicity (e.g., severe lowering of blood sugar).

Whether or not a drug interaction of this type is clinically significant depends on the distribution and elimination properties of the drug affected. Competition between two drugs for the same plasma protein-binding site is fairly common. However, it is only clinically relevant if the drugs have high protein binding, a low therapeutic index (see Part II), and a relatively small volume of distribution.

TABLE 4.1
Comparison of Drug Plasma Protein Binding

Drug	Percent Bound
Caffeine	0
Alcohol	0
Procainamide	10–20
Digoxin	30–40
Gentamicin	40–50
Penicillin G	50–60
Theophylline	60
Phenobarbital	70
Carbamazepine	70–80
Quinidine	85
Phenytoin	90
Tolbutamide	92–95
Propranolol	92–95
Diazepam	92–95
Digitoxin	97
Warfarin	99.5
Phenylbutazone	99.5
Dicumarol	99.9

In the case of tolbutamide, second-generation derivatives (e.g., gliburide) have been developed with less protein binding affinity and, hence, less probability for this type of interaction. It should also be remembered that even if the unbound fraction of a drug becomes elevated, vis-à-vis a receptor site, it is also presented to the eliminating organs, resulting in more rapid clearance. Consequently, with the exception of the criteria mentioned above, the principle effects of a protein binding displacement are to decrease total concentration and increase % unbound. Therefore, a new equilibrium between drug effect and drug elimination is achieved, which tends to dampen any consequences of this type of interaction.

In addition to displacement of plasma protein-bound drug, another major example of drug interactions includes acceleration or inhibition of drug metabolism (discussed previously in Chapter 3). Among the drugs that are known to increase the metabolism of selected drugs are ethanol, antihistamines, phenytoin, barbiturates, and glutethimide. For more specific examples, the reader is referred to more advanced medical pharmacology texts. Similarly, drugs such as phenylbutazone, chloramphenical, allopurinal, cimetidine, desipramine, and methylphenidate inhibit the metabolism of certain drugs.

In addition to displacement of protein-bound drug and alteration of drug metabolism, there are other types of drug interactions. These include impaired uptake of drug from the GI tract and altered renal clearance, for example. A summary of mechanisms by which nutrients and drugs can influence each other is shown in Table 4.2.

INTERACTION IN THE GASTROINTESTINAL TRACT

Because drugs are often taken orally at the same time, the gastrointestinal tract is a relatively common site for drug interactions to occur. Possible interactions during absorption include changes in local pH (e.g., antacids), altered gastric emptying and intestinal motility, and the formation of complexes.

TABLE 4.2

Mechanisms by Which Nutrients and Drugs Can Influence Each Other

Process	Mechanism
Ingestion	Both drugs and disease can cause changes in appetite and nutrient intake; resultant malnutrition can impact on drug efficacy
Absorption	Drugs and foods can have mechanical effect, via binding or adsorption, that can influence the absorptive processes, resulting in $\uparrow$ or $\downarrow$ drug and nutrient absorption. Some drugs can affect GI motility, thereby $\downarrow$ or $\uparrow$ absorption of nutrients. Chemical factors, in particular pH of the stomach contents and the influence of foods therein, can affect the subsequent absorption of drugs
Transluminal transport	The ability of drugs and nutrients to be transported can depend on such factors as lipid solubility and competition for amino acid transport systems
Metabolism	The effectiveness of the mixed function oxidase (MFO) and conjugase systems in the liver and elsewhere for converting drugs and nutrients into their active and, ultimately, excretory forms is dependent on the availability of specific nutrient cofactors. In addition, certain drugs can increase the activity of the MFO systems required to convent nutrient precursors into their active forms. Nonnutritive components in foods can induce MFO activity, thereby affecting drug metabolism
Distribution	The utilization of both drugs and nutrients depends on body composition, the availability and functional integrity of transport proteins, receptor integrity, and intracellular metabolic machinery
Elimination	Drugs and nutrients can synergistically and competitively interact to cause increased or decreased excretion. Systemic factors such as pH and physiological state (e.g., sweating) can dictate whether a drug or nutrient is excreted or reabsorbed

Source: From E. Massaro, (Ed.) (1997), *Handbook of Human Toxicology*, Boca Raton, FL: CRC Press. Reprinted with permission.

With regard to complex formation, tetracyclines and cholestyramine are common examples—although their mechanisms are different. In the case of tetracyclines, complexes of the antibiotic can be formed with a number of positive, polyvalent mineral ions such as Al^{+3}, Ca^{++}, and Mg^{++}. Such minerals are commonly present in antacids and milk. The result of such complex formation is diminished absorption of tetracycline. This is the reason why patients taking tetracyclines are directed to avoid taking milk with their medication.

Complexes can also be formed with compounds that act as *ion-exchange resins*. The cholesterol-lowering drug cholestyramine acts in this manner and can complex with acidic (anionic) compounds such as the oral anticoagulant drug coumadin. Similar interactions have been reported for thyroid hormone, tetracyclines, bile acids, and iron compounds. In each case, the result is interference with absorption.

INTERACTIONS DURING EXCRETION

A number of drugs are known to inhibit the renal secretion of certain other drugs, resulting in decreased clearance of the latter. Examples of drugs decreasing the renal clearance of other drugs include probenecid, salicylates, sulfinpyrazone, phenylbutazone, and thiazide diuretics. As previously mentioned, the inhibition of penicillin secretion by probenecid due to competition between the two for renal tubule "carriers" is used therapeutically to increase penicillin blood levels.

DRUG–FOOD INTERACTIONS

For many drugs, it is not known how food intake affects their pharmacokinetic profile (other than the obvious physical effect). However, as a generalization, it can be said that such interactions do

TABLE 4.3
Some Selected Drug–Food Interactions

Drug	Food	Adverse Interaction
Calcium antagonists (felodipine, nifedipine, nitrendipine); terfenadine; caffeine	Grapefruit juice	Increased bioavailability; inhibition of first-pass metabolism; Increased toxicity
MAO inhibitors	Foods containing tyramine (liver, pickled herring, cheese, bananas, avocados, soup, beer, wine, yogurt, sour cream, yeast, nuts)	Palpitations, headache, hyper-tensive crises
Digitalis	Licorice	Digitalis toxicity
Griseofulvin	Fatty foods	Increased blood levels of griseofulvin
Timed-release drug preparations	Alcoholic beverages	Increased rate of release for some
Lithium	Decreased sodium intake	Lithium toxicity
Quinidine	Antacids and alkaline diet (alkaline urine)	Quinidine toxicity
Thiazide diuretics	Carbohydrates	Elevated blood sugar
Tetracyclines	Dairy products high in calcium; ferrous sulfate or antacids	Impaired absorption of tetracycline
Vitamin B_{12} (cyanocobalamin)	Vitamin C—large doses	Precipitate B_{12} deficiency
Fenfluramine	Vitamin C addition	Antagonism of antiobesity effect of Fenfluramine
Thiamine	Blueberries, fish alcohol	Decreased intake, absorption, utilization
Benzodiazepines	Caffeine	Antagonism of antianxiety action

MAO = monoamine oxidase.

Source: From *Essentials of Pharmacology*, C. Smith and Reynard (Eds.), W.B. Saunders Company, Philadelphia, 1995 (with permission).

occur and that they can be clinically significant. A selected list of some drug–food interactions is shown in Table 4.3.

In addition, although there can be disagreement regarding classifying alcoholic beverages as food or drug, alcohol consumption can potentially have a number of important interactions with drugs (Table 4.4).

An important example of a food–drug interaction involves a drug used in the treatment of AIDS. *Sanquinavir*, a protease inhibitor, has very low bioavailability—only about 4% of the drug taken orally reaches the general circulation. This is partly because the drug is poorly absorbed, and partly because it is rapidly destroyed by the cytochrome P450 system (cytochrome P450 3A4, also called CYP3A4) that is present in the liver and also the intestinal wall. Some foods inhibit this enzyme, thus increasing the bioavailability (AUC) of Saquinavir. One such food is *grapefruit juice*. Human studies indicate that when a 150 mL glass of ordinary reconstituted frozen grapefruit juice is taken with the Saquinavir followed by another equal volume 1 h later, the AUC increased by 50%.

This interesting food–drug interaction was discovered completely by accident over a decade ago. Researchers were investigating whether alcohol could interact with felodipine (Plendil) and used a solution of alcohol with grapefruit juice to mask the taste of alcohol for the study. The investigators discovered that blood levels of felodipine were increased several fold more than in previous studies.

In published studies with other drugs (triazolam, midazolam, cyclosporin, coumarin, and nisoldipine), grapefruit juice had comparable effects. Orange juice, however, had no effect. Research about the interaction of grapefruit juice with drugs suggests that compounds in grapefruit juice,

TABLE 4.4

Summary of Adverse Interactions of Drugs with Alcoholic Beverages

Drug	Adverse Effect with Alcohol
Anesthetics, antihistamines, barbiturates, Benzodiazepines, chloral hydrate, meprobamate, narcotics, phenothiazines, tricyclic antidepressants	1. Increased central nervous system depression due to additive effects 2. Decreased sedative or anesthetic effects with chronic use due to tolerance
Pnenothiazines	Increased extrapyramidal effects, drug-induced parkinsonism
Diazepam	Increased diazepam blood levels, varying with beverage
Amphetamines and cocaine	Increased cardiac work; possible increase in probability of cerebrovascular accident
Calcium channel antagonists— felodipine, verapamil, nifedipine	Increased bioavailability; possible toxicity
Acetaminophen	Hepatotoxicity
Anticoagulants	Chronic decreased anticoagulant effect Acute increased anticoagulant effect
Bromocriptine	Nausea, abdominal pain (due to increased dopamine-receptor sensitivity?)
Disuifiram, chloramphenical, oral hypoglycemics, cephalosporins, metronidazole, quinacrine, moxalactam	Disulfiram-alcohol syndrome reactions
Cycloserine	Increased seizures with chronic use
Imipramine (see also above)	Lower blood level with chronic alcohol consumption
Isoniazid	Increased hepatitis incidence, decreased isoniazid effects in chronic alcohol use due to increased metabolism
Propranolol	Decreased tremor of alcohol withdrawal; decreased propranolol blood levels
Sotalol	Increased sotalol blood levels
Phenytoin	Decreased metabolism with acute combination with alcohol; but increased metabolism with chronic alcohol consumption; increased risk of folate deficiency
Nonsteroidal anti-inflammatory agents (aspirin and related)	Increased gastrointestinal bleeding

Source: From *Essentials of Pharmacology*, C. Smith and Reynard (Eds.), W.B. Saunders Company, Philadelphia, 1995 (with permission).

called furanocoumarins (e.g., bergamottin), may be responsible for the effects of grapefruit juice. Researchers believe that furanocoumarins block intestinal P450 that normally breaks down the drugs. One glass of grapefruit juice can elicit the effect, and the effect may persist for longer than 24 h. Since the effect can last for such a prolonged period of time, grapefruit juice does not have to be taken at the same time as the medication in order for the interaction to occur. Therefore, administration of grapefruit juice with a susceptible drug should be separated by 24 or more hours to avoid the interaction. Since this is not practical for individuals who are taking a medication daily, they should not consume grapefruit juice when taking medications that are affected by grapefruit juice. A summary of grapefruit juice–drug interactions is shown in Table 4.5.

SUMMATION AND POTENTIATION

When the effect of two drugs given concurrently is additive, this is referred to as *summation*. However, if the effect of two drugs exceeds the sum of their individual effects, this is referred to as *potentiation* or *synergism*. Potentiation requires that the two drugs act at different receptors or

---

TABLE 4.5
Grapefruit–Drug Interactions*

- Calcium channel blockers (felodipine, nifedipine, amlodipine, diltiazem, verapamil, and pranidipine)
- Tranquilizers/Psychiatric Medications (benzodiazapam, buspirone, triazolam, carbamazepine, diazepam, midazolam, and sertraline)
- Antihistamines (Hismanal®)
- AIDS drugs (protease inhibitors Crixivan® and Sanquinavir®)
- Antifungal (Sporanox®)
- Statins (cholesterol-lowering drugs)
- Immune suppressants (cyclosporine, tacrolimus)
- Impotence drug (sildenafil)
- Antiarrhythmics (amiodarone)

* High blood levels of these drugs can occur following the ingestion of grapefruit juice.

TABLE 4.6
Factors Complicating Assessment of Drug Interactions with Herbal Products

- Failure to inform physician or pharmacist of concomitant use of herbal products
- Incomplete and inaccurate product information (FDA analysis of 125 products containing ephedra alkaloids revealed a range of 0–110 mg/dose)
- Lack of standardization of product purity or potency (the fungal hepatotoxin aflatoxin often found as a natural contaminant)
- Multiple ingredients in product (the presence of a cardiac glycoside has been found in Chinese herbal preparation)
- Product adulteration (up to seven adulterants have been found in a single product)
- Product dosage not standardized
- Product misidentification
- Variations between labeled and actual product content
- Variations in crop conditions and yield (batch-to-batch variability)

---

effector systems. An example of potentiation involves the multiple uses of drugs in the treatment of AIDS. Significant improvement in virtually all criteria relating to the disease has been achieved with the combination of AZT and 3TC (nucleoside analogs that can inhibit the HIV reverse transcriptase) as well as a protease inhibitor (a protease plays a vital role in the virus's replication in T-cells). It has been estimated that in order for HIV to develop resistance to a protease inhibitor alone, one mutation could suffice; for AZT and 3TC, the virus would have to produce progeny with four mutations. However, in order to survive against all three drugs, eight mutations appear to be necessary.

DRUG INTERACTIONS WITH NATURAL (HERBAL) PRODUCTS

Because as many as 70% of patients may not be informing their physician or pharmacist of complementary medicine use, including herbal products, the real potential for interactions is not adequately monitored. Making informed decisions regarding drug interactions with herbal products requires *accurate and complete* information. Because the contents of herbal products are not standardized, the information needed to determine the potential for drug interaction is often not readily available. See Table 4.6 for some of the factors complicating assessment of drug interactions with herbal products.

It should be kept in mind that there exists numerous opportunities for interaction between herbal preparations and prescription drugs. The most potentially serious of these involve drugs with

TABLE 4.7
Examples of Interaction of Popular OTC Drugs with Other OTC Products and Prescription Drugs

- *Ibuprofen*-anticoagulants and aspirin-containing drugs—abnormal bleeding gastric irritation
- *Naproxen*-anticoagulants; any drug containing aspirin—abnormal bleeding and stomach irritation
- *Aspirin*-anticoagulants; any drug containing ibuprofen—abnormal bleeding and stomach irritation
- *Diphenhydramine*-antihistamines, sedating drugs, muscle relaxants—over sedation
- *Famotidine*—OTC antacids and antifungal drugs (ketoconazole, itraconazole)—antacids can reduce the effectiveness of famotidine while famotidine itself can reduce the effectiveness of these antifungals
- *Dextromethorphan*-monoamine oxidase inhibitors—elevated blood pressure and tremors as well as more severe responses possible
- *Calcium carbonate*—tetracycline—reduces absorption

narrow therapeutic indexes (i.e., low margin of safety; see Chapters 6 and 7) and those drugs used in life threatening situations. For example, it has been reported that the concomitant use of St. John's Wort with a protease inhibitor (indinavir) results in a significant reduction of plasma concentration of the anti-AIDS drug. Apparently, some component in the St. John's Wort is capable of inducing the cytochrome P450 that degrades indinavir. Obviously, a consequence of this interaction could be a curtailment of indinavir's efficacy.

OVER-THE-COUNTER (OTC) DRUG INTERACTIONS WITH PRESCRIPTION DRUGS

There are hundreds of drugs available as OTC preparations that are used for self-medication. Obviously, these drugs also lend themselves to interacting with not only prescription medications but herbal preparations as well. Table 4.7 lists the generic name of some of the most popular OTC medications followed by the prescription drug they are most likely to interact with, followed by the effect (s).

SELECTED BIBLIOGRAPHY

Brody, T.M., Larner, J., Minneman, K.P., and Neu, H.C. (Eds.) (1994) *Human Pharmacology: Molecular to Clinical*, 2nd ed., St. Louis: Mosby.
Drug Interactions and Side effects Index. Oradell, NJ: Medical Economics Co, 1994.
Goldstein, A., Aronow, L., and Kalman, S. (1974) *Principles of Drug Action: The Basis of Pharmacology*, 2nd ed., New York: John Wiley & Sons.
Mutschler, E. and Derendorf, H. (Eds.) (1995) *Drug Actions:Basic Principles and Therapeutic Aspects*, Boca Raton: CRC Press.
Smith, C.M. and Reynard, A.M. (Eds.) (1995) *Essentials of Pharmacology*, Philadelphia: W.B. Saunders.

QUESTIONS

1. Which of the following population groups are most likely to experience a drug reaction?
   a. Neonates
   b. Teenagers
   c. Geriatric
   d. The indigent
   e. All are equal

2. Competition for albumin-binding sites by two drugs is really only *clinically* significant if which of the following is/are true?
   a. If they are both of the same pharmacological class
   b. If they are both highly bound
   c. If they have a low margin of safety
   d. If they have a relatively small volume of distribution
   e. All but "a" above

3. Which of the following is/are possible types of drug interactions
   a. Displacement from albumin binding sites
   b. Alteration of drug metabolism
   c. Complex formation in the GI tract
   d. Interaction with food
   e. All of the above

4. When the pharmacological effect of drug A and drug B given concurrently is greater than the sum of each given alone, this process is referred to as
   a. Induction
   b. Additive
   c. Activation
   d. Potentiation
   e. None of the above

5. Which of the following is/are factors contributing to the difficulty in assessing drug interactions with herbal products?
   a. Physician may not be aware of concurrent use
   b. Product labeling may not be consistent with actual contents of main ingredient
   c. Product purity may vary from batch to batch
   d. Product may contain adulterants
   e. All of the above

6. Which of the following effect (s) is/are <u>most commonly</u> produced by aspirin and ibuprofen containing drugs when interacting with prescription drugs?
   a. Tremors
   b. Incontinence
   c. Skin discoloration
   d. Abnormal bleeding and gastric irritation
   e. Constipation

7. An example of <u>potentiation</u> involves which of the following drug/herb pairs?
   a. Diphenhydramine–phenobarbital
   b. St. John's Wort-indinavir
   c. AZT (reverse transcriptase inhibitor)-3TC (protease inhibitor)
   d. Grapefruit juice-aspirin
   e. Phenobarbital–phenobarbital

8. Which of the following foods can interact with tetracycline to reduce its effectiveness?
   a. Licorice
   b. Dairy products containing calcium
   c. Caffeine
   d. Grapefruit juice
   e. None of the above

9. Which of the following has the <u>least</u> percentage bound to plasma protein?
    a. Ethanol
    b. Phenobarbital
    c. Penicillin G
    d. Warfarin
    e. Phenylbutazone

10. Which of the following has the <u>highest</u> percentage bound to plasma protein?
    a. Ethanol
    b. Phenobarbital
    c. Penicillin G
    d. Procainamide
    e. Warfarin

Part II

Fundamentals of Pharmacodynamics and Toxicodynamics

5 Drug Receptors

INTRODUCTION

Part I of this book began by stating that the science of pharmacology involves the measurement of drug effects (i.e., pharmacodynamics). The beginning of pharmacodynamics as a component of pharmacology is attributed to the efforts of *Rudolf Buchheim* (1820–1879). As mentioned previously, Buchheim is believed to have established the world's first pharmacological laboratory at the *University of Dorpat* in Hungary during the mid-nineteenth century.

While Oswald Schmiedeberg is the scientist who brought worldwide recognition to this new science, it was Buchheim who was the father of pharmacology. He wrote one of the first papers devoted to supporting the role of pharmacology in the training of medical students, in 1876. In fact, Buchheim is less known for his pharmacological studies than his efforts to develop a new, independent discipline.

Buchheim believed that the mode of action of drugs should be investigated by scientific means in order to quantify their effects and introduce a more rational basis for therapy. Buchheim introduced two basic principles that now appear self-evident to us: (1) the concept of a "natural system for the classification of drugs" based on their mode of action and (2) the definition of pharmacology as an independent science.

After he had accepted the chair of Materia Medica, Dietetics History, and Encyclopedia of Medicine at Dorpat University, now Tartu State University (Tartu-Estonia), he established the first laboratory of pharmacology at this institute. In 1860, the *Pharmacologisches Institute* was created to reward Buchheim's efforts in research. His pupils worked in many areas of pharmacology and nutrition, such as metabolism, alkaloids, **anesthetics**, laxatives, anthelminthics, arsenical compounds, and other heavy metals that were in vogue at the time. Nearly 100 papers emanated from Buchheim's institute between 1847 and 1867.

The second part of this book will deal with drug-receptor interactions within the body and the quantitation of these resulting effects. In addition, toxicological aspects of drug–receptor interactions, as well as the treatment of toxicological problems, will also be discussed.

HISTORY

The earliest pharmacological receptor models were operational black boxes that preceded accurate knowledge of receptors by many years. In these early schemes, drugs were envisioned as binding to specific *recognition units*. Despite the imprecision of these schemes, they enabled the construction of rudimentary receptor theory, because the receptor was defined as the minimal unit to characterize drug effects.

The development of the concept that *receptors* mediate the effect of drugs was primarily based on a series of observations made during the late-nineteenth and early-twentieth centuries. These observations correlated chemical structure with biological activity, as well as demonstrated the fact that relatively small amounts of drug can elicit an effect. One of the earliest proposals associating chemical structure with function was that of Blake in 1848. Blake suggested that the biological activity of certain metallic salts was due to their metallic component, rather than the complex in its entirety (e.g., the lead moiety in lead acetate or lead nitrate). This important concept received theoretical support in 1884 when Arrhenius introduced his theory of electrolytic dissociation, whereby salts dissolved in water become dissociated into oppositely charged ions.

The effect of *ionization* on the pharmacological action of drugs was also recognized in the latter half of the nineteenth century. In Scotland, Crum Brown and Fraser demonstrated that quarternization (i.e., the addition of a fourth alkyl group) of several alkaloids resulted in their transition from muscle contractors to muscle relaxants. These researchers concluded "… a relation exists between the physiological action of a substance and its chemical composition and constitution; understanding by the latter term the mutual relations of the atoms in the substance."

It was at the turn of the twentieth century that the importance of lipid solubility in drug action was independently described by *Meyer and Overton* (the significance of the oil: water partition coefficient was discussed previously in Chapter 2). The importance of lipid solubility in drug action subsequently became manifested in the "lipoid theory of cellular depression." In essence, this theory correlates a pharmacological effect (e.g., CNS depression) with a *physical* property (i.e., lipid solubility) rather than a structure–activity relationship, and in the process, attempts to explain the diverse chemical structures that exist within the hypnotic and general anesthetic classes of drugs (see Chapter 11). Today, we realize the limitations of the "lipoid theory" and appreciate that the distinction between physical and chemical factors is illusory, since chemical structure is a determinant of physical properties.

Despite the undeniable importance of Meyer and Overton's observations, a number of experimental reports of drug action were emerging in the literature, which clearly indicated that drug molecules must be concentrating on *small, specific areas* of cells in order to produce their effects. These characteristics included (1) the fact that some drugs can express an effect despite *significant dilution* (e.g., 10^{-9} M), (2) drugs can be effective despite interacting with only a *small fraction of tissue* (e.g., acetylcholine decreases frog heart rate when only 1/6000 of the surface is covered), (3) high *chemical specificity* exists (e.g., discrimination between drug stereoisomers), and (4) high *tissue specificity* (e.g., opiates have a significantly greater effect on smooth muscle than on skeletal muscle).

The actual concept of drugs acting on receptors to produce their effect is generally attributed to John Langley, who alluded to their existence in 1878. While studying the *antagonistic effect of atropine* against pilocarpine-induced salivation, Langley wrote, "that there is some substance or substances in the nerve endings or gland cells with which *both* (emphasis mine) atropine and pilocarpine are capable of forming compounds" (i.e., complexes). In 1905, Langley subsequently referred to this factor as "receptive substance." Despite this observation, the specific word "receptor" was not introduced into the medical literature until the turn of the century, by *Paul Ehrlich*.

Ehrlich based his hypothesis on his experiences with *immunochemistry* (i.e., the selective neutralization of toxin by antitoxin) and *chemotherapy* (e.g., the treatment of infectious diseases with drugs derived from the German dye industry; see Chapter 10). Ehrlich believed that a drug could have a therapeutic effect only if it has "the right sort of affinity." He specifically wrote, "that combining group of the protoplasmic molecule to which the introduced group is anchored will hereafter be termed receptor." (It might be appropriate at this point to give credit to the Italian Amedo Avogadro (1776–1856), who coined the term molecules [Latin = "little masses"]). At that time, Ehrlich conceived of receptors as being part of "side-chains" in mammalian cells. As we shall see later in this chapter, Ehrlich was not far-off in his visualization.

Today, we realize that drug binding to sites that produce pharmacological effects may be part of any cellular constituent, for example, nuclear DNA, mitochondrial enzymes, ribosomal RNA, cytosolic components, and cell membranes and wall, to name the most obvious. Nevertheless, in contemporary pharmacology, some authors and researchers apply a more restricted use of the term receptor, reserving it for protein complexes embedded in, and spanning *cellular membranes* (e.g., the adrenergic receptor). However, exceptions to this classification system clearly exist, and students should keep this fact in mind. For example, steroids are known to interact with cytosolic receptors that transport them into the *nucleus* (their site of action), certain anticancer drugs bind to *nucleic acids* to produce their effects, and bile acids interact with *nuclear receptors* to modulate cholesterol synthesis. Regardless of how rigid one's definition of receptor is, receptor theory provides a unifying concept for the explanation of the effect of endogenous or xenobiotic chemicals on biological systems.

Although the great preponderance of drugs interact with membrane receptors or some intracellular sites, there are, however, a few exceptions. Examples of *nonreceptor*-mediated drug action include antacids such as sodium bicarbonate, which act to *buffer* excess hydrogen ions; chelating agents such as ethylenediaminetetraacetic acid, which *form inactive complexes* with inorganic ions; and osmotic cathartics such as magnesium sulfate, which produce their pharmacological response by *attracting water*.

NATURE OF RECEPTORS

Proteins, glycoproteins, proteolipids, and associated proteinaceous species appear to be particularly suited to act as receptors because they can assume three-dimensional configurations. The three-dimensional shape is the net result of primary, secondary, and tertiary structures. Three-dimensionality requires that drugs, or any binding ligand, achieve binding specificity, referred to as "induced fit." If the drug is an active one, the result of this binding is believed to be a conformational change in the receptor, with subsequent modification of membrane permeability or activation of intracellular enzymes "downstream."

The concept of a "lock and key" relationship between drug and receptor is based on the analogous hypothesis of the German chemist and enzymologist Emil Fischer who originally developed the theory in relation to the interaction between enzymes and substrates. In 1895, Fischer wrote that an enzyme's specific effect might be explained, "by assuming that the intimate contact between the molecules necessary for the release of the chemical reaction is possible only with similar geometrical configurations. To use a picture, I would say that the enzyme and the substrate must fit together like lock and key." This lock and key relationship implies extreme precision in the interaction, since extra or improperly placed atoms in the drug, like an additional tooth on a key, can exclude its binding. Failure to achieve "induced fit," therefore, precludes optimal conformational change in the receptor.

The specificity inherent in achieving appropriate geometrical configurations between ligand (i.e., drug) and receptor can extend to *stereoisomerism*. For example, there are many drugs whose chemical structure contains an asymmetric carbon atom and can thus exist as mirror-image isomers: asymmetry is possible only if all four valences of carbon are utilized by different groups. These asymmetric carbon atoms are often referred to as *chiral centers* or, conversely, centers of chirality (as discussed previously). An example of an optical isomer is the antitussive drug dextromethorphan (found in many OTC cough and cold preparations) that is the *d* isomer of the codeine analog levorphanol. However, unlike the *l* isomer levorphanol, dextromethorphan has no analgesic or addictive properties and does not act through opioid receptors.

Although most drug preparations exist as a racemic mixture (i.e., equimolar mixture of optical isomers), often only one of the isomers produces the desired pharmacological effect. Therefore, although racemic mixtures are commonly regarded as single drugs, this may not be technically correct. In fact, the two racemic components may have similar or quite different receptor specificity and exert independent pharmacological effects. Considerable research is presently being carried out in this area and is discussed in more detail in Chapter 15.

Chemists have long appreciated that a protein's primary amino acid sequence determines its three-dimensional structure. It has also been known for some time that proteins are able to carry out their diversified functions only when they have folded up into compact three-dimensional structures; the significance of protein-folding first gained prominence in the 1950s and 1960s, when Christian Anfinsen demonstrated that the enzyme ribonuclease could be *denatured* (unfolded) and *renatured reversibly*.

During the 1960s and 1970s, receptor proteins, primarily membranous in nature, were isolated and the amino acid sequences of various receptor subunits were determined. In the last two decades, complete amino acid sequences of receptors as well as their successful cloning have been determined. Today we recognize that various types of receptors exist, which can be further divided into different subtypes that, if acted upon by the same ligand (e.g., acetylcholine), can produce either ion channel changes or the generation of *secondary messengers* (see below). Some general features of receptors are listed in Table 5.1. A pictorial summary of the development of our conceptual understanding of receptors from Ehrlich's time to the present is shown in Figure 5.1.

TABLE 5.1
General Features of Membrane Receptors

Protein: Generally lipoprotein or glycoprotein in nature

Typical Molecular weight in the range of 45–200 kDa

Can be composed of subunits

Frequently glycosylated

K_d of drug binding to receptor (1–100 nM); binding reversible and stereoselective

Receptors saturable because of finite number

Specific binding of receptor results in change in ion flow signal transduction to intracellular site

Specificity of binding not absolute, leading to drug binding to several receptor types

May require more than one drug molecule to bind to receptor to generate signal

Magnitude of signal depends on number of receptors occupied or on receptor occupancy rate; signal can be amplified by intracellular mechanisms

By acting on receptor, drugs can enhance, diminish, or block generation or transmission of signal

Drugs are receptor modulators and *do not* confer new properties on cells or tissues

Receptors must have properties of recognition *and* transduction

Receptor populations can be upregulated, downregulated, or sequestered

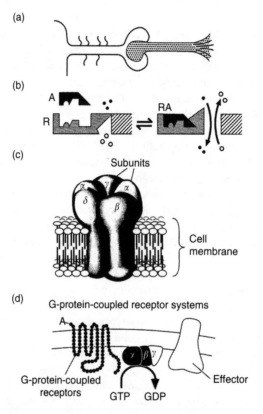

FIGURE 5.1 Comparison of receptor models beginning with (a) Ehrlich's first pictorial representation of his "side-chain" theory in 1898, (b) scheme of drug–receptor interaction in 1971, (c) acetylcholine ion-channel in 1982, and (d) G-protein-coupled receptor system in 1989. (From L.L. Brunton, J.S. Lazo, and K.L. Parker (Eds.) (2006), *The Pharmacological Basis of Therapeutics*, 11th ed., New York: McGraw-Hill. Reproduced in part with permission.

IMPORTANCE OF MEMBRANE-PROTEIN DRUG TARGETS

Membrane proteins are encoded by >25% of the genes present in typical genomes, and many have pharmaceutical and/or medical importance. The pharmaceutical importance of membrane proteins stems from the fact that they include structural proteins, channels, and receptors that are accessible through the exterior of cells and thus present formidable drug targets. For example, the G-protein-coupled receptor (GPCR) family is the largest known family of cell-surface receptors, responding to diverse stimuli such as hormones, neurotransmitters, odorant molecules, and light. The GPCR family thus has a role in virtually all physiological processes and is one of the most important groups of pharmaceutical targets, with 40–60% of drugs used in medicine targeting GPCRs. Membrane proteins also have medical importance, because mutations in genes encoding membrane proteins are the causative agents of various diseases, including cystic fibrosis, retinitis pigmentosa,congenital nephrogenic diabetes insipidus, arrhythmias, and hearing loss. Often, these mutations have been shown to result in misfolded protein or defective signaling. The precursor of the peptide that forms amyloid proteins in Alzheimer's disease is a membrane protein.

CHEMICAL BONDS

If most drugs achieve their effects via interaction with a receptor, then by what chemical binding force(s) is/are this/these achieved? (Ehrlich recognized very early that the combining forces must be very loose. He wrote in 1900 "If alkaloids, aromatic amines, antipyretics or aniline dyes be introduced into the animal body, it is a very easy matter, by means of water, alcohol or acetone, to remove all of these substances quickly and easily from the tissues." This is the reason why isolated organ tissue baths containing smooth muscle preparations, such as the guinea pig ileum, can be used experimentally for the sequential assessment of drug activity, since "wash-out" phases can reversibly restore the tissue essentially to its original condition.)

On the basis of the development of knowledge relating to chemical bonds during the first half of the twentieth century, we can now identify the principle binding forces involved in drug receptor interaction. Of particular importance to this field was some of the research carried out by Linus Pauling in the 1930s. Pauling described (1) a scale of electronegativity that could be used to determine the ionic and covalent character of chemical bonds; (2) the concept of bond-orbital hybridization (the organization of electron clouds of atoms in molecules in configurations that favor bonding); and (3) the theory of resonance (distribution of electrons between two or more possible positions in a bond network).

Simple organic compounds such as hydrocarbons, which by definition only contain carbon and hydrogen atoms, are *electrically neutral* since the valence electrons comprising the bond are shared equally between the carbon and hydrogen atoms. In contrast, more sophisticated molecules comprising pharmacological receptors in cellular membranes, for example, contain atoms such as oxygen, nitrogen, sulfur, or phosphorus, *in addition* to carbon and hydrogen.

The presence of these additional atoms produces an unequal sharing of electrons due to the differing electronegativities of the elements involved (as Pauling described). Such bonds have the overall effect of shifting the distribution of electrons within the molecule such that areas of positive and negative charge are created (thereby introducing polarity and reactivity into the molecule). Drugs also require the presence of similar atoms in their structure in order to possess areas of positivity and negativity.

The binding of a ligand to a membrane-bound receptor in the aqueous environment of the body is an exchange process, whereby ligand and receptor, both solvated by water molecules, bind together releasing some of the water molecules. Therefore, both the ligand and the receptor lose their interactions with water in favor of interaction with one another. This exchange process includes both favorable and unfavorable free energy changes.

The four most favorable forces in chemical bond formation between ligand and receptor in pharmacology are (1) ionic bonds (i.e., electrostatic); (2) hydrogen bonds; (3) van der Waals forces; and (4) covalent bonds. The first three bond types are easily reversible by energy levels normally present in biological tissue at temperatures between 20 and 40°C (i.e., approximately 5 kcal/Mole). Therefore, they are the principle bond forces involved in normal reversible drug action. Covalent bonds are an exception, however, since they require approximately 50–100 kcal/Mole to break. This can have significant implications for both the duration of a drug's effect and its toxicity, as described below.

IONIC BONDS

These are the principle electrostatic bonds that are formed between two ions of opposite charge (e.g., Na^+ and Cl^-) in which the atom lacks or has surplus electrons. The extent to which ionic bonds may be formed depends on the degree of ionization of groups that form cations (e.g., amino groups) and groups that form anions (e.g., carboxyl groups), and this in turn depends, of course, on the pH of the medium and the pK value of the ionizable groups.

Ligands that bind to catecholamine receptors, for example, all contain an amino group that has a dissociation constant >7 so that the ligand will be partly or fully positively charged at neutral pH. It has been assumed, therefore, that the binding of these ligands to their receptors will involve an electrostatic interaction to a negatively charged group on the receptor. A leading candidate to fulfill this role is the *carboxyl* group of an aspartic acid residue within the binding domain.

Because the intermolecular binding force of the ionic bond decreases only with the square of the interatomic distance (r^2), it is the *most* effective bond type in attracting a drug molecule from the medium toward the receptor site. In a biological environment, the duration of an ionic bond at a receptor might last for only 10^{-5} S, owing to the presence of inorganic salts present in the medium that can compete for binding sites. However, when an ionic bond is reinforced by the presence of bonds that act over shorter ranges, the union can become stronger and last for a longer duration.

HYDROGEN BONDS

The hydrogen nucleus is strongly *electropositive*, being essentially a bare proton. This high concentration of electropositivity enables the hydrogen atom to act as a bond between two electronegative atoms (e.g., O, N, and F); assuming the interatomic distance is appropriate. Extensive structure-activity studies using dopamine receptors have shown that one or more *hydroxyl groups* on the benzene ring of an agonist are desirable for activity. It is assumed that these hydroxyl groups are involved in hydrogen bonds with amino acid side chains on the receptor (most likely O or N).

Hydrogen bonds are expressed over a short distance with binding force decreasing by the fourth power of the interatomic distance (r^4). For this reason, hydrogen bonds are considered to be important at the *more intimate levels* of drug receptor interactions and can act in support of ionic bonds. Individually, hydrogen bonds are weak but, collectively, they can significantly stabilize the association of a drug with its receptor.

VAN DER WAALS FORCES

These are the most common of all attractions between atoms. van der Waals forces are the result of the formation of "induced dipoles" when atoms of different electronegativity are bonded together. The *intermolecular attraction* arises from the fluctuations of charge in two atoms or molecules that are close together. Since the electrons are moving, each molecule has an instantaneous dipole moment that is not zero. If the electron density fluctuations in the two atoms or molecules were unrelated, there would be no net attraction. However, an instantaneous dipole in one atom or molecule induces an oppositely oriented dipole in the neighboring atom or molecule, and these instantaneous dipoles attract each other. van der Waals forces are significant only over *very short distances*, since their power

---

TABLE 5.2
Examples of Drugs/Metabolites Forming Covalent Bonds

- Nitrogen mustards—cyclophosphamide
- Anticholinesterase—malathion
- α-Adrenoreceptor antagonist—phenoxybenzamine
- Hepatotoxic drugs—acetaminophen, halothane

---

varies inversely with the seventh power of the interatomic distance (r^7). However, when a number of atoms become closely juxtaposed, significant attraction can occur and confer stability to a drug–receptor association.

COVALENT BOND

As mentioned above, the covalent bond is the most tenacious type of chemical bond, since it involves the *mutual sharing* of orbital electrons. It is the type of bond that holds organic compounds such as proteins, carbohydrates, and lipids together. Fortunately, for these important biochemical entities, it normally does not lend itself to easy reversibility; otherwise we would end up as a pool of protoplasm on the floor. However, it is not the typical drug–receptor bond type. If it were the typical bond formed between drugs and their receptors, all pharmacological effects would have an inordinately long duration of action.

The strongest bond that can be broken nonenzymatically at body temperature requires approximately 10 kcal/Mole. Therefore, covalent bonds (50–100 kcal/Mole) are not examples of reversible drug–receptor interactions. We have seen that conjugation reactions occurring in type II biotransformation reactions can involve the formation of covalent linkage (e.g., glucuronidation). This is an example of a "good" type of covalent bond virtually assuring that the conjugate will be successfully excreted. However, certain bioactivated metabolites can form "bad" covalent bonds with normal macromolecular complexes and produce tissue injury. This will be a focus in Chapter 7 dealing with drug toxicity. Table 5.2 presents examples of drugs forming covalent bonds with biological molecules.

RECEPTOR CLASSES

Table 5.3 presents a representative list of major receptor classes with their respective subtypes and endogenous transmitters. The receptors are further divided into either ion channel or second messenger categories.

LIGAND-GATED ION CHANNEL RECEPTORS

The nicotinic acetylcholine (Ach) receptor is a well-characterized receptor of this type, consisting of five subunits. It is present on the *skeletal muscle cell end plate* in the *neuromuscular junction*, at *all autonomic ganglia*, and in the *CNS*. The function of this receptor is to convert Ach *binding* into an electrical signal via increased Na^+ or K^+ permeability across the cell membrane (i.e., membrane depolarization). When two molecules of Ach bind to the α subunit of the receptor, a conformational change in the receptor induces opening of the channel to at least 0.65 nm for approximately 1–2 ms.

Another important ligand-gated ion channel receptor is the type A γ-aminobutyric acid (GABA) receptor. The GABA receptor is extremely important because it is the primary endogenous *inhibitory* transmitter in the CNS. The inhibitory action of the GABA receptor system is *enhanced* by drugs such as the *benzodiazepine class* (e.g., minor tranquilizers) that are believed to augment *opening* of a chloride-ion channel via interaction at an *allosteric* site.

TABLE 5.3
Examples of Classical Receptors

Type	Subtype[a]	Endogenous Transmitter	Ion Channel	Secondary Messenger
Acetylcholine	Nicotinic	Acetylcholine	X	—
	Muscarinic: M_1, M_2, M_3, M_4, M_5	Acetylcholine		X
Adrenergic	α_1, α_2	Epinephrine and norepinephrine		X
	β_1, β_2, β_3	Epinephrine and norepinephrine	—	X
GABA	A	GABA	X	—
	B	GABA	?	X
Acidic amino acids	NMDA, kainate, quisqualate	Glutamate or aspartate	X	?
Opiate	5-HT_1, 5-HT_2, 5-HT_3	Enkephalins	X^b	X
Serotonin	D_1, D_2, D_3, D_4, D_5	5-HT	—	X
Dopamine	A_1, A_2	Dopamine	—	X
Adenosine	—	Adenosine	—	X
Glycine	H_1, H_2, H_3	Glycine	X	—
Histamine	—	Histamine	—	X
Insulin	—	Insulin	—	X
Glucagon	—	Glucagon	—	X
ACTH	—	ACTH	—	X
Steroids	—	Several	—	Special

Notes: [a] Other subtypes in various stages of documentation have been proposed, especially where no endogenous transmitter is defined yet; [b] Results not clear.
Source: Brody et al. (1994), *Human Pharmacology: Molecular to Clinical.* 2nd ed. St Louis, MO: Mosby. Reprinted with permission.

VOLTAGE-DEPENDENT ION CHANNEL RECEPTORS

These types of receptors are typically present in the membranes of excitable nerve, cardiac, and skeletal muscle cells and are subject to voltage-mediated channel opening. In this situation, *membrane depolarization* induces conformational opening of channels and allows a transient influx of ions such as Na^+ and Ca^{++}. Blockade of these respective ion channels is believed to explain the mechanism of action of local anesthetics and certain antihypertensive agents (e.g., calcium channel blockers), for example. In certain situations, prolonged opening of a channel can result in hyperpolarization of a cell (e.g., Cl^- influx), resulting in resistance of the cell to subsequent depolarization. Human disorders associated with known mutations of genes encoding for K^+ channels now numbers 14 and includes episodic ataxia, certain forms of epilepsy, and hyperinsulinemia hypoglycemia of infancy.

G-PROTEIN-COUPLED SECOND MESSENGER RECEPTORS

Ligand binding to cell surface receptors initiates a series of events known collectively as *signal transduction*. In this process, receptors alter the status of other proteins that in turn leads to a cascade of changes inside the cell. The cell uses this cascade of information to describe what is occurring in the cellular environment and then make the necessary alterations. Without the ability to transduce the initial receptor signal, the cell would be unresponsive to many environmental changes, making homeostasis more difficult to maintain. Understanding signal transduction is critical to gaining insight into how cells communicate with each other as well as how we can influence cell activity pharmacologically.

A very important class of membrane receptors transmits its signal by *coupling* with guanine nucleotide-binding proteins (G-proteins). In fact, GPCRs are the largest family of cell-surface molecules involved in signal transmission. As mentioned above, these receptors are activated by a wide variety of ligands, including peptide and nonpeptide neurotransmitters, hormones, growth factors, odorant molecules, and light. These receptors are the target of approximately 60% of the current therapeutic agents on the market, including more than a quarter of the 100 top-selling drugs, with sales in the range of several billion dollars per year.

Additional examples of GPCR systems include the β-adrenergic receptor (involved in regulating cardiac contractility), the opioid and dopamine receptors (involved in brain function), and the N-formyl peptide receptor (involved in the immune response). Abnormalities in GPCR signaling are involved in numerous diseases and disorders and are, therefore, a major target for future therapeutic intervention.

G-proteins consist of three subunits (α, β, and γ) in one of two states: an inactive form in which guanosine on the α subunit is in the diphosphate form (GDP) or an active state in which GDP is displaced by guanosine triphosphate (GTP). Activation results in dissociation of the α subunit and interaction of its C-terminal region with the appropriate enzyme. Because G-proteins have intrinsic GTPase activity, they are capable of rapid transformation from active to inactive status.

GPCRs are known to generate *second messengers* as the method of transducing their transmembrane signaling mechanism. The principal messengers formed are cyclic adenosine monophosphate (cAMP), inositol triphosphate (IP_3), and 1,2-diacylglycerol (DAG). G-proteins provide the link between ligand interaction with the receptor and formation of the second messenger, generally via enzyme activation of adenylate cyclase and phospholipase C. However, an inhibitory G-protein for adenylate cyclase does exist.

The generation of all three second messengers (cAMP, IP_3, and DAG) leads to the activation of protein kinases and the subsequent phosphorylation of important cellular enzymes. (Note: nine amino acids have the potential for being phosphorylated, but in biological systems phosphorylation has been described primarily on three of these: serine, threonine, and tyrosine.) The phosphorylation of these key enzymes, in turn, produces activation or inactivation of significant cellular biochemical pathways. In summary, the process is a cascade, resulting in amplification of the original receptor signal through a series of four steps: (1) binding of the ligand to the membrane bound receptor; (2) activation of the membrane bound G protein; (3) activation of the membrane bound enzyme; and (4) activation of intracellular kinases.

Receptors with Tyrosine Kinase Activity

A group of receptors that respond to so-called growth factors such as insulin, epidermal growth factor, platelet-derived growth factor, and so forth, exists. These receptors have an *extracellular domain* that binds the growth factor and an *intracellular domain that possesses latent kinase activity*.

Nearly 2% of human genes are devoted to just one class of protein. These powerful enzymes, called kinases, activate other proteins, making them prime movers in basic cellular functions; they are believed to control well over half of all such processes. Kinases are implicated in cancer, immunity, neurobiology, and more. Determining which kinases are affected by drugs and which are not, has been facilitated since the publication of the *kinome*: a collection of more than 500 human protein kinase genes and their fly, worm, and yeast equivalents. With this kinome inventory, companies can now systematically study the effects of kinases and the influence of drugs on them.

The interaction of insulin, for example, results in autophosphorylation of the intracellular domain and subsequent internalization of the insulin receptor complex. The internalized complex now possesses the properties of a tyrosine kinase and can phosphorylate cell substrates that produce the appropriate intracellular effect. However, these kinases differ from the usual protein kinases in that they phosphorylate proteins exclusively on *tyrosine hydroxyl* residues. The ensemble of proteins phosphorylated by the insulin receptor has not yet been identified, but there is supportive evidence that tyrosine kinase activity is required for the major actions of insulin. For example, it is possible that a membrane-linked glucose transport system becomes activated following insulin-stimulated phosphorylation.

RECEPTOR DYNAMISM

An important concept to appreciate regarding receptors is that they are not static, stand-alone components of a cell. Quite the contrary, they are an integral part of the overall homeostatic balance of the body. For example, receptors can become *desensitized* on continuous exposure to an agonist. When desensitization involves a specific class of agonists, it is referred to as *homologous* desensitization. If disparate classes of drugs reduce response, the term *heterologous* desensitization is applied.

GPCR-mediated signal transduction can be attenuated with relatively fast kinetics (within seconds to minutes after agonist-induced activation) by a process called *rapid desensitization*. Rapid desensitization is characterized by *functional uncoupling* of receptors from the heterotrimeric G-proteins that occur without any detectable change in the total number of receptors present in cells or tissues. Rapid desensitization of certain GPCRs is associated with a process called *sequestration* that involves a physical redistribution of receptors from the plasma membrane to intracellular membranes via endocytosis. The process of internalization is thought to promote dephosphorylation by an endosome-associated phosphatase. Dephosphorylation and subsequent recycling of receptors back to the plasma membrane contributes to a reversal of the desensitized state (resensitization) that is required for full recovery of cellular signaling potential following agonist withdrawal.

GPCRs are also regulated by mechanisms that operate over a much longer timescale. A process called *downregulation* refers to an actual decrease in the total number of receptors in cells or a tissue, which is typically induced over a period of hours to days after prolonged or repeated exposure to an agonist ligand. Downregulation of GPCRs can be differentiated in at least three ways from the process of sequestration: (1) downregulation typically occurs much more slowly than rapid internalization, (2) downregulation is characterized by a reduction in the total number of receptors present in cells or tissues, and (3) internalization is characterized by a physical redistribution of receptor status (uncoupling) without a detectable change in total receptor number.

In addition to the possibility of decreases in receptor number, a corresponding condition of *upregulation* can take place. In this case, sensitization can occur by an increase in receptor number. For example, chronic exposure to high levels of thyroid hormone (i.e., thyroxin) can lead to an increase in myocardial β-receptors with corresponding increased sensitivity to β agonists. A corresponding result will be elevated heart rate that is often present in hyperthyroidism.

The question of how receptor numbers can be modified is an intriguing one. Because transmembrane receptor proteins are amphipathic in nature (i.e., they possess both extracellular and intracellular polar groups), they are prevented from moving into or out of the membrane lipid bilayer or changing their orientation. However, they can freely diffuse laterally in the plane of the membrane. One theory proposes that on binding drug–receptor complexes rapidly migrate to specialized membrane areas called "coated pits." Here they hypothetically undergo a sequence of internalization and recycling. Presumably, there is some feedback mechanism that either accelerates or decelerates the process and, hence, the number of regenerated free receptors available.

Disease states can also influence normal receptor function. For example, modified receptor function occurs in certain autoimmune diseases. *Myasthenia gravis* is a neuromuscular disease characterized by weakness and marked fatigability of skeletal muscles. The defect in myasthenia gravis is in synaptic transmission at the neuromuscular junction. Initial responses in the myasthenic patient may be normal, but they diminish rapidly, which explains the difficulty in maintaining voluntary muscle activity for more than brief periods.

Animal studies performed during the 1970s indicated that the disease represented an *autoimmune* response directed toward the acetylcholine receptor. Antireceptor antibody was soon identified in patients with the disorder. In fact, receptor-binding antibodies are detectable in sera of 90% of patients with the disease. The result of the autoimmune reaction is receptor degradation with loss of function at the motor end plate.

Treatment of the disorder usually involves the administration of acetylcholinesterase inhibitors (see Chapter 11). Drugs such as neostigmine increase the response of myasthenic muscle to nerve impulses primarily by preserving endogenously released acetylcholine from enzymatic inactivation.

With release of acetylcholine, receptors over a greater surface of the motor end plate are exposed to the transmitter. *Grave's disease* (hyperthyroidism) is another receptor-mediated autoimmune disease. However, in this case, the antibodies developed against thyrotropin receptors in the thyroid behave like *agonists rather than antagonists*. The result is enhanced thyroid hormone production by the gland, producing elevated levels of circulating thyroid hormone.

OPIATE AND TETRAHYDROCANNABINOL RECEPTORS

One of the more interesting chapters in the history of receptors has been their impact on the discovery of endogenous substances. The fact that substances of plant origin such as curare, nicotine, and muscarine could produce neuropharmacological effects suggested that there might exist corresponding endogenous substances. Eventually, this led to a deliberate search for unknown neurotransmitters as a counterpart of neuroactive plant products. One of these is the classic study of Otto Lowi and the discovery of "vagusstoffe" (see Chapter 11).

It was only a matter of time, several decades later, when neuropharmacologists began to wonder, if endogenous mediators existed, and if they had their own receptors. It seemed reasonable to propose that neuroactive drugs such as morphine, for example, might be interacting with receptors that normally accommodate endogenous ligands. The concept of specific opioid receptors became firmly entrenched more than 40 years ago. The extraordinary potency of some opiates, the availability of selective antagonists, and the stereospecificity of opiates all favored the existence of specific receptors.

A critical breakthrough in the biochemical identification of receptors in nervous tissue was the development of an extremely potent snake toxin (α-bungarotoxin) that acts selectively at nicotinic acetylcholine receptors. During the early 1970s, several groups began to study the electric organ of the eel, where the receptors constituted almost 20% by weight of the organ. In contrast, similar calculations indicated that opioid receptors ought to be only approximately one millionth by weight of the brain. Despite these seemingly overwhelming odds, intensive research on both sides of the Atlantic did establish the existence of opioid receptors in the brain. The question then became "Is it sensible to suppose that such highly specific receptors developed, over the long course of evolution, only to combine with morphine, which is a product of the opium poppy? Was it not more likely that there were natural morphine-like neurotransmitters in the brain, and that these receptors had evolved to accommodate them?"

In 1975, Hans Kosterlitz and John Hughes in Scotland were able to isolate from thousands of pig brains two endogenous active substances that acted just like morphine. Surprisingly, the chemical composition of these substances was peptide in nature, being only five amino acids in length. They were given the name *enkephalins*. A database analysis of all known amino acid sequences revealed the presence of this 5 amino acid sequence in a larger 31 amino acid peptide found in the pituitary and designated *β-endorphin*. Another 17 amino acid opioid peptide was subsequently isolated several years later and named *dynorphin*. These endogenous opioid peptides play important physiological and pharmacological roles in analgesia, behavior, emotion, learning, neurotransmission, and neuromodulation by interacting with a number of opioid receptor subsets (e.g., μ, κ, and δ).

A similar situation has occurred with tetrahydrocannabinol (THC, the active ingredient in marijuana). THC acts on a seven-helix receptor that has been identified in those parts of the brain that could reasonably mediate changes in mood and perception caused by marijuana. The receptor was eventually isolated and its amino acid sequence determined. As was the case with the opiates, the question of an endogenous THC-like material was raised. At the present time, the most likely candidate for an endogenous ligand for the THC receptor is known as *anandamide* (the ethanolamide of arachidonic acid). Interestingly, anandamide has been found to be present in chocolate and cocoa powder. This discovery may be relevant to the well-known phenomenon of "chocolate craving." Can people become dependent on this confection? Do they periodically need an anandamide fix?

SELECTED BIBLIOGRAPHY

Albert, A. (1979) *Selective Toxicity, The Physico-Chemical Basis of Therapy*, 6th ed., London: Chapman & Hall.

Beckett, A.H. and Casey, A.F. (1954) Synthetic analgesics: Stereochemical considerations. *J. Pharm. Pharmacol.*, 6: 986–1001.

Brody, T.M., Larner, J., Minneman, K.P., and Neu, H.C. (Eds.) (1994) *Human Pharmacology: Molecular to Clinical*, 2nd ed., St. Louis: Mosby.

Kenakin. T. (2004) Principles: Receptor theory in pharmacology, *Trends in Pharmacol. Sci.*, 25: 186–192.

Kenakin, T.P., Bond, R.A., and Bonner, T.I. (1992) Definition of pharmacological receptors, *Pharmacol. Rev.*, 44: 351–362.

Woolf, P.J. and Lindeman, J.J. (2001) From the static to the dynamic: Three models of signal transduction, in *G Protein-Couple Receptors in Biomedical Applications of Computer Modeling*, A. Christopoulos (Ed.), Boca Raton: CRC Press.

Wyman, J. and Gill, S.J. (1990) *Binding and Linkage. Functional Chemistry of Biological Macromolecules*, Mill Valley: University Science Books.

QUESTIONS

1. Which of the following individuals first referred to drugs acting on a "receptive substance"?
   a. Crum Brown
   b. John Priestly
   c. John Langley
   d. Paul Ehrlich
   e. c and d

2. The concept of a "lock and key" relationship between drug and receptor is based on work done by which of the following?
   a. Paul Ehrlich
   b. John Langley
   c. William Withering
   d. Paracelsus
   e. Emil Fischer

3. Which of the following bond types can be broken by energy levels normally present in biological tissues?
   a. van der Waals
   b. Ionic (electrostatic)
   c. Hydrogen
   d. Covalent
   e. a, b, and c

4. Which is/are true regarding receptors?
   a. Can be located in the nucleus
   b. Can be located in the mitochondrion
   c. Can be located in the cell membrane
   d. Can be located in the cell cytosol
   e. All of the above

5. Which of the following is/are classified as ligand-gated ion channel ligands?
   a. Cyclic AMP
   b. Inositol triphosphate

    c. Acetylcholine

    d. GABA

    e. c and d above

6. Which of the following is/are second messengers that transduce G-protein membrane receptors?

    a. Cyclic AMP

    b. 1,2 Diacylglycerol

    c. Inositol triphosphate

    d. All of the above

    e. Guanosine triphosphate

7. Successful generation of second messengers results in which of the following?

    a. Phosphorylation of certain enzymes

    b. An amplification cascade

    c. Activation of protein kinases

    d. All of the above

    e. a and c only

8. Rapid desensitization of β-receptors is believed to involve which of the following?

    a. Functional uncoupling of the receptor from its G-protein

    b. No change in receptor number

    c. Increased degradation of receptor

    d. Increase in receptor number

    e. a and b above

9. Sensitization of β-receptors can involve which of the following?

    a. Development of Myasthenia gravis

    b. Chronic exposure to thyroid hormone (e.g., thyroxin)

    c. Reduction of receptor number

    d. Increased sequestration into endosomes

    e. None of the above

10. Which of the following endogenous peptides play an important role in analgesia by interacting with opioid receptors?

    a. Enkephalins

    b. β-endorphin

    c. Dynorphin

    d. All of the above

    e. None of the above

6 Dose–Response Relationship

BACKGROUND

As mentioned in the previous chapter, the concept of biological receptors mediating the effect of drugs provided a useful conceptual framework to understand the action of most drugs. In fact, the foundation of receptor pharmacology is the *dose–response curve*, a graphical representation of the observed effect of a drug as a function of its concentration at the receptor site.

As drug development became of greater importance during the first half of the twentieth century, a more quantitative and analytical foundation was needed in order to assess drug potency per se, as well as *comparative* drug potency. The standardization and quantification of technique and experimental design, as well as the rigorous application of statistical analysis, has provided pharmacodynamics with a necessary solid base.

In order for models to be useful, they must describe data and predict results. To accomplish this, a mathematical formalism is necessary. The individual most associated with the development of early quantitative expressions of drug–receptor interactions is *Alfred Joseph Clark*. Clark was the first to apply the mathematical approaches used in enzyme kinetics systematically to the effects of chemicals on tissues. He said, "The general aim … has been to determine the extent to which the effects produced by drugs on cells can be interpreted as processes following known laws of physical chemistry." (1937).

Clark published most of his proposals between the world wars, based on his studies of atropine and the cholinergic system. It is significant to appreciate the scientific environment in which Clark published his ideas. The prevailing concepts in the years 1895–1930 were rooted in homeopathic theories and others lacking a physicochemical basis; Clark's insight into receptor theory cannot be overestimated.

Clark proposed that drugs combined with receptors in proportion to their concentration and then dissociated from the receptor in proportion to the concentration of the drug–receptor complexes. In essence, Clark envisioned that the interaction between drug and receptor was analogous to the *reversible* adsorption of a gas to a metal surface and, therefore, follows the law of mass action. This relationship can be illustrated in a hyperbolic curve, referred to as a *Langmuir adsorption isotherm*, when depicted using arithmetic scales on both coordinates (Figure 6.1).

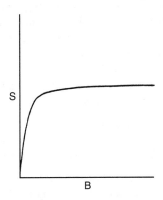

FIGURE 6.1 Typical Langmuir isotherm: S, concentration of substance adsorbed; B, total concentration of substance. (From A. Albert (1979), *Selective Toxicity: the Physico-Chemical Basis of Therapy*. With permission.)

Mathematically, the interaction between drug and receptor can be represented by the following basic relationship:

$$[X] + [R] \leftrightarrow [XR] \rightarrow E$$

Where [X] is the concentration of drug at the receptor, [R] is the concentration of free receptors, and [XR] is the concentration of the drug–receptor complex. Because the law of mass action states that the *velocity* of a chemical reaction is proportional to the concentration of the reacting substances, the *dissociation constant*, K_d, of a drug–receptor complex is expressed by the following relationship:

$$K_d = [X][R]/[XR]$$

The above two equations indicate, therefore, that the fraction of all receptors that is combined with a drug is a function of *both* drug concentration and the dissociation constant of the [XR] complex. K_d is, therefore, basically an indication of strength of binding and can be determined by many methods that are beyond the scope of this book.

From the basic drug–receptor relationship described above, it may be apparent that there are several implicit assumptions: (1) that the magnitude of the pharmacological effect (E) is directly proportional to [XR] and (2) that the maximal effect (E_m) occurs when the drug (X) occupies 100% of the receptors. These assumptions embody the classical receptor theory developed by Clark. Although the validity of these assumptions has been justifiably questioned from time to time (e.g., some experimental data indicates that maximal effect can be achieved with <100% occupancy; leaving "spare receptors"), the Clark "occupancy" model has, nevertheless, found wide validation and provided the framework for subsequent development of concepts such as agonism, antagonism, affinity, and efficacy.

Early formulations of receptor theory presented a simple model consisting of a single receptor that is activated by agonists. Inherent in this paradigm is the assumption that there are only two receptor states, active and inactive. However, the idea that agonists can stabilize different receptor active states has arisen on theoretical grounds based on experimental findings; therefore, receptors are not constrained to only two conformational states.

MEASUREMENT

Experimentation on isolated organs offers several advantages in quantifying drug effects including (1) the drug concentration in the tissue is usually known; (2) reduced complexity and ease of relating dose and effect; (3) it is possible to circumvent compensatory physiological responses that may partially cancel the primary effect in the intact organism (e.g., the heart rate increasing action of norepinephrine cannot easily be demonstrated in the intact animal because a simultaneous compensatory response occurs that slows heart rate); and (4) the ability to examine a drug effect over its full range of intensities. Disadvantages include (1) unavoidable tissue injury during dissection; (2) loss of physiological regulation of function in the isolated tissue; and (3) the artificial milieu imposed on the tissue. Obviously, some drug effects that are being studied require use of the whole animal (e.g., sedation).

Before the widespread availability of radiolabeled ligands, pharmacologists were restricted in terms of the systems at their disposal. Most receptor work was performed on relatively few isolated tissues such as guinea pig ileum, rat atria, and trachea.

> The guinea pig longitudinal muscle is a great gift to the pharmacologist. It has low spontaneous activity; nicely graded responses (not to many tight junctions); is highly sensitive to a very wide range of stimulants; is tough, if properly handled, and capable of hours of reproducible behavior. (W.D.M. Paton, 1986).

Characterization of ligand interaction with tissue receptors can also be carried out by studying concentration–binding relationships. The analysis of drug binding to receptors aims to determine the affinity of ligands, the kinetics of interaction, and the characteristics of the binding site itself. In studying the affinity and number of such binding sites, membrane suspensions of different tissues are used. This approach is based on the expectation that binding sites will retain their characteristic properties during cell homogenization.

In the case of binding studies, the drug under study is radiolabeled (enabling low concentrations to be measured quantitatively), added to the membrane suspension, and allowed to bind to receptors. Membrane fragments and medium are then separated by filtration over filter discs, and the amount of drug bound is determined by measuring the radioactivity remaining on the dried filter disc. Binding of the ligand increases in proportion to concentration as long as a significant number of free binding sites remain. However, as binding sites approach saturation, the number of free sites decreases and the increment in binding is no longer proportional (i.e., linear) to the increase in concentration, and a hyperbolic relationship develops.

The law of mass action describes the hyperbolic relationship between binding and concentration. The relationship is characterized by the drug's affinity and maximum binding. Affinity is expressed as the equilibrium dissociation constant and corresponds to that ligand concentration at which 50% of the binding sites are occupied (K_d). Maximum binding (B_{max}) is the total number of binding sites per unit weight of membrane homogenate (e.g., mg protein) represented by the upper limit of the curve.

The differing affinity of various ligands for a binding site can be demonstrated quite elegantly by binding assays. Although simple to perform, these binding assays pose the difficulty of correlating binding site data with pharmacological effect; this is particularly difficult when more than one population of binding site is present (a not unusual situation). In addition, receptor binding must not be implied unless it can be demonstrated that: (1) binding is saturable (*saturability*), (2) the only substances bound are those possessing the same pharmacological mechanism of action (*specificity*), and (3) binding affinity of various ligands correlates with their pharmacological potency (see below). Although binding assays provide information about the affinity of ligands, they do not provide evidence as to whether a ligand is an agonist or antagonist (see below).

GRAPHICAL REPRESENTATION-GRADED RESPONSE

In pharmacology, it is conventional to plot the dependent variable, response, or effect, against the independent variable, dose (total amount), or dosage (e.g., mg/kg body weight). This can be done by expressing dose on either an arithmetic scale (Figure 6.2a) or a logarithmic scale (Figure 6.2b).

However, there are practical difficulties associated with fitting pharmacological data with appreciable scatter to a curved arithmetic line (Figure 6.2a). For example, a plot of arithmetic dose reaches

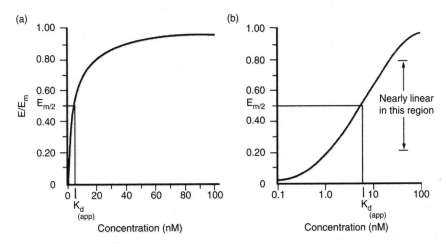

FIGURE 6.2 Concentration–response curve for graded response: (a) arithmetic scale; (b) log concentration scale. K_d (app) is arbitrarily taken to be 4.5 nM. (From T.M. Brody, J. Larner, K.P. Minneman, and H.C. Neu, (Eds.) (1994), *Human Pharmacology: Molecular to Clinical*. With permission.)

a maximal asymptote value when the drug occupies all of the receptor sites. In addition, the range of concentrations needed to fully depict the dose–response relationship usually is too wide to be useful in the format shown.

Most dose–response data are routinely transformed, therefore, to a nearly straight line, by plotting dose on the x-axis on a logarithmic scale (Figure 6.2b). The result is essentially a linear relationship between approximately 20 and 80% of the maximum response. Depicting the data in this manner allows a more accurate determination of a drug's ED_{50} (i.e., the concentration of a drug required to produce 50% of the maximal response possible and is conventionally used as a criterion for drug comparison).

A binding constant for ligand attaching to receptor or inhibitor constant for an enzyme reaction may also be determined. These quantities are usually expressed in terms of the dissociation constant of the ligand–receptor complex (K_d) or enzyme–inhibitor complex (K_i). For the ligand–receptor interaction, this constant is equal to the ligand concentration at which 50% of the receptors are occupied by the ligand and it is assumed, although it is not always correct, that the measured response has fallen to half its maximum value. For typical drug–receptor interactions, the dissociation constants are generally on the order of 10^{-7} to 10^{-10} M (i.e., generally in the nanomolar range).

The measurement of the reversible binding of a radioactive ligand to a receptor preparation (radioligand binding) has greatly increased our understanding of receptors, and, provided it is understood that the binding occasionally may have to be discounted because it is an artifact of the preparation, the knowledge gained has been of great value in identifying, quantifying, and in some cases, isolating a receptor. Two of the greatest challenges in pharmacology are (1) to link binding data with pharmacological effect and (2) to understand in molecular terms how the signal is transduced in a given cell to produce a given response.

QUANTAL RESPONSE

The data plotted in Figure 6.2 represents a *graded* response. That is, the response occurs in gradations in proportion to the number of receptors occupied. However, drug responses can also be classified as *quantal*. That is, the observable response is described on an all-or-none basis. Figure 6.3 depicts a quantal drug response in which the *number of individuals* responding becomes

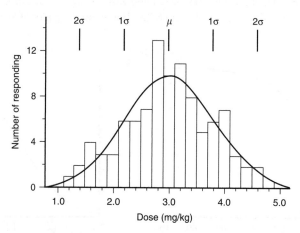

FIGURE 6.3   Quantal effects. Typical set of data after administration of increasing doses of drug to a group of subjects and observation of minimum dose at which each subject responds. Data shown are for 100 subjects: dose increased in 0.2 mg/kg of body weight increments. Mean ($\propto$) (and median) dose is 3.0 mg/kg; standard deviation (V) is 0.8 mg/kg. Results plotted as histogram (bar graph) showing number responding at each dose; smooth curve is normal distribution function calculated for $\propto$ of 3.0 and v of 0.8. (From T.M. Brody, J. Larner, K.P. Minneman, and H.C. Neu, (Eds.) (1994), *Human Pharmacology: Molecular to Clinical*. With permission.)

the dependent variable in response to the minimum dose required. Because the shape of the histogram (i.e., the bell curve), in this example, is in reasonably good agreement with that of a normal or gaussian distribution, statistical parameters for normal distribution can be used to predict variability of drug response in the general population.

AGONISTS

The term *agonist* (derived from the Greek word meaning "to contend" or "to act") was introduced by J. Reuse in 1948 and refers to compounds that *activate* receptor-based processes via reversible interactions based on the laws of mass action described above. An example of typical log concentration–response curves for a series of agonist drugs that bind to the *same* receptor type is shown in Figure 6.4. In this schema, the *x*-axis reflects the relative *affinity* of four agonists for the receptor type in question. Affinity is a chemical property, mandated by chemical forces (see Chapter 5) that cause the drug to associate with the receptor. It should be obvious from the relationship of the four agonists that agonist A has greater affinity for the receptor than the other agonists. In other words, it takes less of agonist A to produce a given effect than agonists B, C, or D. In fact, we can quantify this difference by determining the respective ED_{50} values (in this case agonist A is approximately 20–30 times more *potent* than D). Potency is, therefore, a comparative term and is most appropriately used when comparing agonists that interact with the same receptor type.

As mentioned above, there are several assumptions made in the classic Clark occupancy model. While these assumptions may be true in some cases, there are many exceptions. One of the main problems is that sometimes there is a nonlinear relationship between occupancy and response. In order to explain this seemingly anomalous situation, Ariens (1954) and Stephenson (1956) introduced the terms *intrinsic activity* and *efficacy*, respectively. These terms refer to inherent qualities of the drug that modulate the effect, independent of concentration. Today, the terms are commonly used interchangeably and are operationally synonymous (some authors have, in fact, combined the terms into a new hybrid, namely, *intrinsic efficacy*). These terms have been treated functionally as a proportionality constant that quantifies the extent of change imparted to a receptor on binding an agonist. Thus, the amplitude of the signal for each receptor type is a *product of the efficacy of the agonist and its concentration at the receptor site.*

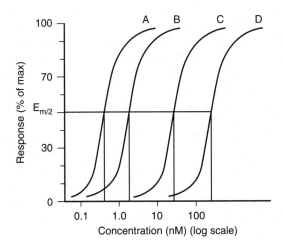

FIGURE 6.4   Schema of log concentration–response curves for a series of agonists (A, B, C, and D). Note that all the drugs are shown having the same maximum response. The most potent drug produces $E_{m/2}$ at the lowest concentration; thus drug A is the most potent. Concentration of each drug needed to produce 50% of maximum response (ED_{50}) also shown. Concentration values are arbitrary. (From T.M. Brody, J. Larner, K.P. Minneman, and H.C. Neu, (Eds.) (1994), *Human Pharmacology: Molecular to Clinical*. With permission.)

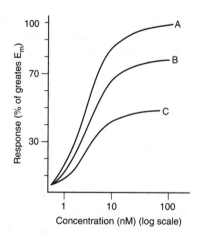

FIGURE 6.5   Series of agonists that vary in efficacy (E_m) at essentially constant potency. Drug A is the most efficacious and drug C the least. Concentrations are arbitrary but in therapeutic plasma concentration range for many drugs. (From T.M. Brody, J. Larner, K.P. Minneman and H.C. Neu (Eds.) (1994), *Human Pharmacology: Molecular to Clinical*. With permission.)

While the *x*-axis reflects an agonist's affinity for the receptor type, the *y*-axis provides us with information regarding the *efficacy* of the agonist. That is, how high will its maximal effect go? In essence, does the drug do anything? For drug development companies this is an important question, since the 1962 Kefauver–Harris amendments to the Federal Food, Drug, and Cosmetics Act require *proof of efficacy* before a new drug can be marketed. Affinity and efficacy characterize an agonist.

In Figure 6.4, all four agonists produce the same level of maximal response. Therefore, although the agonists differ in their affinity for the receptor, they can be equally efficacious if given in adequate amounts. In summary, agonist D can produce the same effect as agonist A, but its lesser affinity for the receptor must be compensated for by increasing its concentration in the vicinity of the receptor. In essence, increasing its probability of a "hit."

There are situations in which agonists can have a relationship the reverse of that described above. Figure 6.5 depicts three agonist that have the same affinity for the receptor type (i.e., the same ED_{50}) but not the same efficacy. In this schema, agonist A is approximately 2.5-fold more efficacious than agonist C. Therefore, agonist C may be thought of as a *partial agonist*. Partial agonists, in fact, have a dual effect, since they can also have *antagonistic* properties. That is, in the presence of agonists with greater efficacy, they can reduce the effectiveness of the latter (i.e., they have mixed agonist–antagonist properties, depending on the situation). Interestingly, because all three agonists have the same ED_{50} they are equally potent, *by definition*. It should be obvious that simply knowing a drug's potency is not the whole story.

By this point, the introductory student may realize that the occupation theory may not be the end of all. During the past 25 years, several new concepts have been developed to bring receptor theory to its present state. These involve the isolation and biochemical study of receptors, application of allosteric theories, and use of recombinant receptor systems and development of the "operational model" of receptor function. The latter model has gained widespread acceptance in the pharmacological community and is the model of choice for describing functional receptor pharmacology.

ANTAGONISTS

Antagonists are compounds that can (partially) diminish or prevent (totally) agonistic effects and are usually classified as *competitive*, *noncompetitive*, or *allosteric*. Competitive antagonists have the

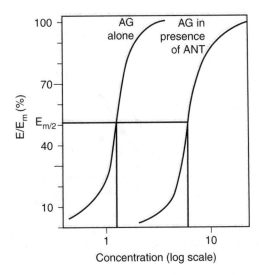

FIGURE 6.6   Competitive antagonism, where both the agonist (AG) and the antagonist (ANT) compete to bind reversibly to the same subtype of receptor sites. (From T.M. Brody, J. Larner, K.P. Minneman, and H.C. Neu, (Eds.) (1994), *Human Pharmacology: Molecular to Clinical*. With permission.)

capacity to bind to the same set of receptors as an agonist (i.e., also have affinity), but do *not* possess efficacy. Because agonist and antagonist compete for the same receptor binding site, it is possible for an agonist to reassert its efficacy if its concentration is sufficiently increased to compensate for the antagonist present.

An example of such competitive displacement is illustrated in Figure 6.6. This figure illustrates a typical parallel shift to the right of the original agonist curve in the presence of a competitive antagonist. The magnitude of the shift to the right on the *x*-axis is an index of the relative affinity of the antagonist, with no change in maximal response. Competitive antagonists with high affinity for the receptor will produce a greater shift to the right than weaker compounds, since higher concentration of the agonist is required to successfully compete. Note that the ultimate potential efficacy of the agonist is not diminished in the presence of a competitive inhibitor. Such is not the case when noncompetitive or allosteric inhibition occurs.

NONCOMPETITIVE AND ALLOSTERIC INHIBITORS

Noncompetitive antagonism can occur if the antagonist binds to the *same site* as the agonist, but does so irreversibly or pseudo irreversibly (i.e., very slow dissociation but no covalent binding). It also causes a shift in the dose–response curve to the right, but does cause depression of the maximal response (not shown).

Some noncompetitive antagonists do *not* interact with the agonist receptor-binding site but, rather, interact with a different site on the receptor molecule such that the receptor is altered. This is sometimes referred to as *allosteric inhibition*. The impact of allosteric inhibition on agonist action is shown in Figure 6.7. In this case, the response to the agonist is plotted in the absence or presence of increasing concentrations of the allosteric noncompetitive antagonist. The result is a decrease in *both* the slope of the agonist dose–response curve as well as the maximum effect produced by the agonist. If high enough concentrations of the noncompetitive antagonist are used, agonist effect can be abolished, even though it may be occupying the receptor. Therefore, in contrast to competitive antagonism, the effect of an allosteric noncompetitive antagonist *cannot* be reversed by simply increasing agonist concentration, since the law of mass action does *not* apply.

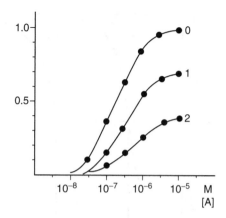

FIGURE 6.7   Concentration–effect curves of: (0) A in the absence of B; (1) A in the presence of B; and (2) A in the presence of three times the amount of B used for curve 1. (From E. Mutscher and A. Derendorf, (Eds.) (1995), *Basic Principles and Therapeutic Aspects*. With permission.)

INVERSE AGONISM

The discovery that some receptor blockers alter the activity of receptors in the absence of agonists has led to the concept of *inverse agonism*. Many drugs such as haloperidol, cimetidine, and prazosin, which were initially characterized as antagonists, are now characterized as inverse agonists. Because so many drugs used in clinical practice are inverse agonists and not neutral antagonists, constitutive receptor activity might be involved in the pathophysiological mechanism that underlies diseases treated with these inverse agonists.

Perhaps the best known natural inverse agonist is retinal. In the dark, retinal minimizes spontaneous rhodopsin receptor activity by keeping this receptor in the inactive conformation. Some natural ligands for chemokine receptors are also inverse agonists.

It may be useful at this point to acknowledge the fact that there are other types of antagonisms involving drug effects. *Physiological antagonism* involves those compensatory biological mechanisms that exist to maintain our homeostasis. For example, if we inject a sufficient amount of norepinephrine to increase blood pressure, baroreceptors located in the carotid arteries will be activated and heart rate slowed via cardiovascular centers in the brain. *Chemical antagonism* occurs when a substance reduces the concentration of an agonist by forming a chemical complex (see Chapter 8). *Pharmacokinetic antagonism* is present when one drug accelerates the metabolism or elimination of another (e.g., enzyme induction by phenobarbital as described in Chapter 3).

SELECTED BIBLIOGRAPHY

Albert, A. (1979) *Selective Toxicity, The Physico-Chemical Basis of Therapy*, 6th ed., London: Chapman & Hall.

Brody, T.M., Larner, J., Minneman, K.P., and Neu, H.C. (Eds.) (1994) *Human Pharmacology: Molecular to Clinical*, 2nd ed., St. Louis: Mosby.

Clapham, D.E. (1993) Mutations in G protein-linked receptors: novel insights on disease, *Cell*, 75: 1237–1239.

Mutschler, E. and Derendorf, H. (Eds.) (1995) *Drug Actions: Basic Principles and Therapeutic Aspects*, Boca Raton: CRC Press.

Pratt, W.B. and Taylor, P. (1990) *Principles of Drug Action. The Basis of Pharmacology*, 3rd ed., [Revised edition of Goldstein, A., Kalman, S.M. and Aronow, L., 2nd ed., 1973, 1974] New York: Churchill Livingstone.

Smith, C.M. and Reynard, A.M. (Eds.) (1995) *Essentials of Pharmacology*, Philadelphia: W.B. Saunders.

Stephenson, R.P. (1956) Modification of receptor theory, *Br. J. Pharmacol.*, 11: 379–393.

QUESTIONS

1. The individual most associated with the early *quantitative* expressions of drug–receptor interactions is which of the following
   a. A.J. Foyt
   b. A.J. Clark
   c. Paul Ehrlich
   d. Claude Bernard
   e. William Withering

2. The "occupancy" model of drug–receptor interaction is based on which of the following?
   a. Fick's law
   b. The principle of LeChatelier
   c. The law of mass action
   d. The law of diminished returns
   e. None of the above

3. Most pharmacological dose–response curves are plotted on which of the following?
   a. Arithmetic scale
   b. Linear scale
   c. Logarithmic scale
   d. Nonlinear scale
   e. Gaussian curve

4. Quantal drug responses refer to which of the following?
   a. % of maximal response
   b. Log of % maximal response
   c. Number of individuals responding
   d. Number of receptors occupied
   e. a and c above

5. When a series of agonist dose–response curves are plotted on a log-scale, the X-axis reflects which of the following?
   a. Intrinsic activity (Efficacy)
   b. Lipophylicity
   c. Potency
   d. The number of receptors occupied
   e. Affinity

6. Which of the following is/are true regarding competitive inhibitors?
   a. Cause a shift to the right of the agonist dose–response curve
   b. Cause a shift to the left of the agonist dose–response curve
   c. Bind to the same receptors as the agonist
   d. Bind to allosteric receptor sites
   e. a and c above

7. Which of the following is/are true regarding allosteric inhibitors?
   a. Bind to the same sites as agonists
   b. Can be displaced by increasing concentration of agonist
   c. Have significant intrinsic activity
   d. Probably produce conformational change in the agonist receptor
   e. a and d above

8. A graded dose–response curve for a series of agonists can provide which of the following data?
   a. ED_{50}
   b. Potency
   c. Affinity
   d. Intrinsic activity
   e. All of the above

9. Which of the following factors contribute to a β-agonist's response?
   a. Concentration at the receptor site
   b. K_d
   c. Intrinsic activity
   d. Signal transduction
   e. All of the above

10. Activation of baroreceptors (blood pressure) is an example of which of the following?
    a. Pharmacokinetic antagonism
    b. Allosteric antagonism
    c. Physiological antagonism
    d. Chemical antagonism
    e. None of the above

7 Drug Toxicity

BACKGROUND

Toxicology is the field of science that focuses on the deleterious effects of chemicals (i.e., xenobiotics) on biological systems. Pharmacology has a rather positive image being concerned with the treatment of disease by natural products, structural modifications of natural products, and by synthetic drugs designed for the treatment of a particular disease. In contrast, toxicology is sometimes regarded in a negative way. Toxicology and pharmacology are, however, complementary and represent both sides of a coin, and the thought processes involved in each discipline are often identical (i.e., toxicokinetics, toxicodynamics, receptors, and dose–response).

Among tens of thousands of chemicals produced each year are those developed for medicinal purposes. Although the actual percentage that drugs represent of the total is quite small, the medical armamentarium that has evolved over the years also numbers in the thousands. Therefore, the possibility of drugs producing toxic effects is a constant concern and represents the other side of the therapeutic coin. It is estimated that each year approximately 2 million hospitalized patients have serious adverse drug reactions, and about a hundred thousand have fatal adverse drug reactions. If this estimate is correct, then more people die annually in the United States from medication errors than from highway accidents, breast cancer, or AIDS.

Every year, 17 million prescription errors such as the wrong drug or the wrong dose occur. One recent survey of pharmacists found that approximately 16% of physician's prescriptions were illegible. Medical abbreviations can also be a problem. For example, the physician may mean to write "QD" (once-a-day) and accidentally write "QID" (four times daily). Similarly, since some drugs such as insulin are prescribed in units (U), if written hastily the U can be misinterpreted as a 0. A prescription for 100 U could, therefore, result in 1000 U being delivered. Drug errors can also happen when a doctor prescribes a medication with a name similar to another drug. The potential for medication mix-ups has increased dramatically over the past two decades as more and more drugs—each with one or more generic and brand names—have flooded the market. There are more than 15,000 drug names in general use in the United States. With only 26 letters in the alphabet, some of these names will inevitably sound alike.

For example, soon after the new arthritis drug *Celebrex* entered the market, the Food and Drug Administration (FDA) received 53 reports of dispensing errors that occurred when it was mistaken for the antiseizure drug *Cerebyx* or the antidepressant drug *Celexa*. Other commonly confused drugs include Flomax (used to treat an enlarged prostate) and Fosamax (osteoporosis), Adderall (attention-deficit-disorder) and Inderall (hypertension or other heart problems), Lamisil (fungal infections) and Lamictal (epilepsy), and Prilosec (acid reflux) and Prozac (depression). The problem of drug misidentification due to name similarity has become such a problem that a nonprofit organization has been founded to address the issue: the *Institute for Safe Medication Practices* independently reviews errors reported through the *U.S. Pharmacopoeia's Medication Errors Reporting System* and publicizes the findings in the media.

Fingl and Woodbury have cogently summarized the significance of drug side effects in 1966: "Drug toxicity is as old as drug therapy and clinicians have long warned of drug-induced diseases. However with the introduction into therapeutic practice of drugs of greater and broader efficacy, the problem of drug toxicity has increased, and it is now considered the most critical aspect of modern therapeutics. Not only is a greater variety of drug toxicity being uncovered, but the average incidence of adverse effects of medication is increasing, and unexpected toxic effects occur relatively frequently."

The incidence of drug toxicity in the general population is unknown. However, there have been reports that 5–10% of hospitalized patients report some drug side effects. Fortunately, life-threatening toxicity from drugs is *relatively* rare. On the other hand, drug toxicity may manifest itself via seemingly innocent forms. For example, in 1996, the FDA warned that dietary supplements such as Herbal Ecstasy also pose "significant health risks." Many of the labels on these products do not list ingredients such as the cardiovascular stimulant *ephedrine* (as mentioned previously).

Most cases of human lethality from drugs are due to either accidental or intentional *overdose*. An example of the former occurred in 1994 in one of the nation's most prestigious cancer institutes. In that case, a dosage error in an experimental chemotherapy regimen resulted in the death of one patient and the crippling of another. The error revolved around ambiguous dosage guidelines of whether 4000 mg of the anticancer drug (times the patients body surface in square meters) was intended as the daily dosage or as the cumulative, 4-day dose. Unfortunately, it was the latter.

The experience with medication errors associated with *methotrexate*, an anticancer drug that is sometimes used for other disorders, in the United Kingdom closely mirrors that recently reported in the United States. In July 2004, the *United Kingdom's National Patient Safety Agency* alerted the *National Health Service* (NHS) in England and Wales about the risks associated with oral methotrexate.

Annually, approximately 50,000 patients receive oral methotrexate treatment from NHS in England and Wales. One hundred thirty-seven patient-safety incidents were reported during a 10-year period (1993–2002), of which 25 resulted in death and 26 in serious harm requiring hospitalization. Overall, 67% of the reported errors involved an overdose of the drug, usually because an intended weekly dose had been prescribed as a daily dose. A further 19% were due to a lack of clinical management and failure to perform the required tests. A third group of errors, accounting for 7% of the total, involved misidentification of the drug and other problems associated with product packaging and labeling. The most frequent indications for methotrexate were rheumatoid arthritis (75%) and psoriasis (17%). Patients for whom safety incidents were reported had a mean age of 59.8 years.

Physicians who make a medical mistake can be charged with a criminal act in the United Kingdom, and the frequency of such charges is increasing, according to an editorial in the November 15, 2003 issue of the *British Medical Journal*. Previous research on the topic found only seven cases reported between 1867 and 1989. But in the decade after that 122-year span, 13 cases involving 17 doctors were reported.

Accidental poisoning with a xenobiotic sometimes has assumed the character of a genuine disaster. An example is poisoning by the fungus *Claviceps purpurea*. This fungus grows as a parasite in grain, particularly rye, and causes the malady known as ergotism. The fungus produces the highly toxic alkaloid known as ergot (from which LSD is derived). In the past, this type of epidemic has killed thousands of people who ingested the fungus with their bread. There are detailed accounts of such calamities. For example, in the year 992 an estimated 40,000 people died of ergotism in France and Spain. As recently as the 1950s, similar outbreaks were still occurring.

One of the most significant historic figures in the development of the science of toxicology was the Swiss physician Paracelsus (1493–1541), mentioned in Chapter 1, who recognized the requirement for appropriate experimentation and gave the discipline a scientific foundation. One of the important distinctions that Paracelsus made was between the therapeutic and toxic properties of chemicals and appreciated the fact that these characteristics are generally manifested by dose. Today, his views remain an integral part of the structure of pharmacology and toxicology.

Paracelsus promoted a focus on the "*toxicon*," the primary toxic agent, as a chemical entity, as opposed to the Grecian concept of the mixture or blend of factors. A concept initiated by Paracelsus that became a lasting contribution embodied in a series of corollaries: (1) experimentation is essential in the examination of responses to chemicals; (2) one should make a distinction between the therapeutic and toxic properties of chemicals; (3) the properties are sometimes but not always indistinguishable except by dose; and (4) one can ascertain a degree of specificity of chemicals and therapeutic or toxic effects.

These principles led Paracelsus to introduce *mercury* as the drug of choice for the treatment of *syphilis*, a very prevalent malady of the day, but led to his famous trial for malpractice. Nevertheless, the practice of using mercury for syphilis survived for 300 years. The use of a *heavy metal* as a therapeutic agent presages the "*magic bullet*" (arsphenamine that contained arsenic) of Paul Ehrlich and the introduction of the *therapeutic index* (TI). In addition, in a very real sense, this was the first sound articulation of the dose–response relationship; a bulwark of pharmacology/toxicology.

Another important contributor to the development of toxicology was the Spanish physician *Orfila* (1787–1853). He was one of the first scientists to make systematic use of test animals and autopsy material. Orfila was the first to treat toxicology as a separate scientific subject and was also responsible for the development of numerous chemical assays for detecting the presence of poisons, thus providing an early foundation for forensic toxicology. Orfila published the first major work dealing with the toxicity of natural agents in 1815.

As mentioned above, Paracelsus recognized the correlation of dose with toxicity. In fact, his statement that "*all substances are poisons; there is none which is not a poison. The right dose differentiates a poison and remedy*" is the most frequently quoted declaration in the field of toxicology. However, as we shall see, there are a number of other factors that can influence the toxic manifestations(s) of a drug. The major factors include dose, the underlying genetic makeup of an individual (both within a given gender and between), the age of the individual, the presence of underlying pathology, and the status of one's immune system.

DOSE

Because most, but not all, toxic reactions to drugs are related to dose, this subject is the most logical to begin with. Fortunately, many of the principles that we have discussed previously can be applied to questions dealing with the dose (dosage)–response relationship. Although there are numerous potential parameters that can be used to measure drug toxicity, a traditional, unmistakable standard in industry deals with *lethality*. In experimental animals, it is obviously all-or-none and is easily quantifiable. While there are serious reservations about this approach, and attempts are underway to limit its application (see Chapter 17), it is, nevertheless, still utilized to a certain extent. The basic relationship between pharmacology and toxicology on the basis of dose–response is shown in Figure 7.1.

In Chapter 6, the concept of a dose–response relationship was introduced (equivalent to the concentration–response curves seen in Figure 6.2). In that context, we were concerned with drug

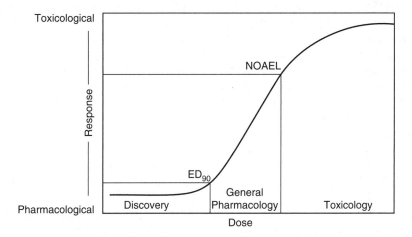

FIGURE 7.1 Representation of departmental responsibility in the evaluation of a drug dose–response curve. ED_{90}, efficacious dose that produces 90% of the intended effect; NOAEL, no observable adverse effect level.

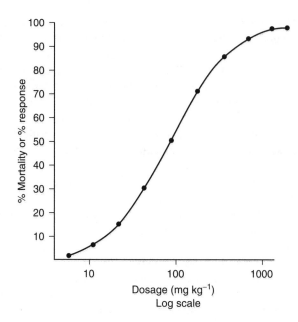

FIGURE 7.2 A typical dose–responsive curve where the percentage response or mortality is plotted against the log of the dosage.

effectiveness (i.e., efficacy) as the response. In the present context, we are concerned with drug toxicity. When comparing Figure 7.2 in this chapter with Figure 6.2b, we can see that the same type of typical sigmoidal curve is produced when plotting drug dosage versus percent mortality.

Once a drug's dose–response relationship for lethality has been established, there are several ways in which this information can be utilized. For example, from the data in Figure 7.2 we can obtain a numerical index of toxicity analogous to the way we obtained a numerical index of effectiveness in Chapter 6. If you remember, we chose to select the ED_{50} as a standard index of effectiveness. In the present example, if we apply the same method our drug can be seen to have an LD_{50} of 100 mg/kg.

The LD_{50} is a routinely utilized index (although not the only one) defined as the dosage of a substance that kills 50% of the animals over a set period of time following an acute exposure. During drug development, multiple routes of administration are usually examined, which generally, but not always, yield different LD_{50} values. For example, the LD_{50} of procaine when administered orally is approximately tenfold higher than when given intravenously. On the other hand, the LD_{50} of isoniazid is virtually identical when given by five different routes.

The examples that have been utilized for determining both ED_{50} (in Chapter 6) as well as LD_{50} values in this chapter have been based on visual inspection of graphical data. In actuality, in the pharmaceutical industry, acute LD_{50} as well as ED_{50} values are obtained by employing one or more of several statistical formulas/methods (e.g., Litchfield and Wilcoxan). These analyses provide a more accurate determination of the value in question.

Standing alone, the LD_{50} provides us with insufficient information to evaluate a drug's potential usefulness. However, if we compare its LD_{50} to its ED_{50} we can obtain some measure of the margin of safety that exists for the drug. By convention, calculation of the LD_{50}/ED_{50} ratio yields what is referred to as the TI of the drug. Obviously, the higher a drug's therapeutic index (TI) the greater the margin of safety.

If a drug's TI is 2.0 or less, however, the compound will probably be difficult to use clinically in patients without encountering significant toxicity. An example of a drug with a TI close to 2.0 is the cardiac drug digoxin (an early toxic effect being vomiting). Other drugs with a relatively low TI are anticancer drugs and the antiasthma drug theophylline. The use of drugs with relatively low TIs can

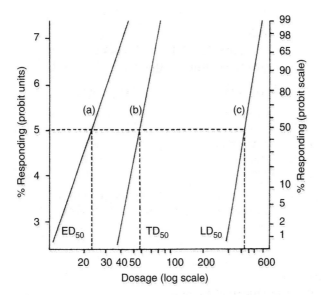

FIGURE 7.3 Comparison of dose–response curves for efficacy (a), toxicity (b), and lethality (c). The effective, toxic, or lethal dosage for 50% of the animals in the group can be estimated as shown. This graph shows the relationship between these parameters. The proximity of the ED_{50} and TD_{50} indicates the margin of safety of the compound. (Probits are units of standard deviation, where the median is probit 5.) (From J.A. Timbrell (1991), *Principles of Biochemical Toxicology*. With permission.)

be justified on the basis of risk versus benefit. It should be pointed out that since no drug has a single toxic effect and many drugs have more than one therapeutic effect, the possibility exists for a given drug to have numerous TLs or toxic effects (i.e., spectra) other than lethality.

Sometimes, in addition to lethality, some other aspect of drug toxicity can be measured. In this situation, one could then determine a TD_{50} (toxic dose producing the effect in 50% of the population) as well as an ED_{50} and LD_{50}. In this situation, the data is often plotted in a comparative fashion using *probit* analysis. It is not necessary that you understand the underlying mathematical transformation of biological data to a probit analysis. Suffice it to say that it is merely a tool to enable the data to be plotted as a straight line. By definition, the 50% value is probit 5.

When expressing efficacy and toxicity data using probit analysis, comparison of the data is facilitated. This is illustrated in Figure 7.3. In this case, we can see that the TI for the drug in question is approximately 18, while the ratio of toxicity for a nonlethal toxic effect (e.g., gastric irritation) to efficacy is approximately 2.4. By obtaining this type of data, we can now express toxicity in a quantitative manner. It should also be reemphasized at this point that there is a continuum of side effects that could conceivably be plotted between lines A and C.

However, one caveat should be mentioned at this point. If you examine Figure 7.3 closely, you will observe that the lines for lethality and efficacy do not exactly follow the same slope. In cases where the mortality/toxicity dose–response curve(s) follows a shallower slope, the TI will necessarily be lower in the lower dosage range. This is particularly significant in hyperresponsive individuals who respond to lower dosage (see below). Therefore, in cases where efficacy and toxicity lines do not parallel each other, a more conservative index of safety can be ascertained by determining the ratio of LD_1/ED_{99} that is sometimes referred to as the margin of safety or the *certain safety factor.*

In addition to providing information relative to a drug's TI, an LD_{50} value can also have utility when comparing the toxicity between drugs. Table 7.1 illustrates this point. In comparing the LD_{50} values of a number of drugs, we can see that they can vary by several orders of magnitude. But what do these data mean? Perhaps one way to put the data in perspective is to apply a classification system based on acute lethality.

TABLE 7.1

Approximate Oral LD$_{50}$ Values for a Variety of Drugs in the Rat

Compound	LD$_{50}$ (mg/kg)
Ethanol	13,600
Acetaldehyde	1,900
Amitriptylline	530
Digitoxin	24
Protoveratrine	5

Source: Hollinger, M.A. (1995), *CRC Handbook of Toxicology* Chapter 22, Boca Raton, FL: CRC Press.

TABLE 7.2

Toxicity Classification System

Toxicity Rating	Commonly Used Term	LD$_{50}$ Single Oral Dosage Rats
1	Extremely toxic	<1 mg/kg
2	Highly toxic	1–50 mg/kg
3	Moderately toxic	50–500 mg/kg
4	Slightly toxic	0.5–5 g/kg
5	Practically nontoxic	5–15 g/kg
6	Relatively harmless	>15 g/kg

Table 7.2 presents a toxicity classification system based on an LD$_{50}$ single oral dose in rats. In applying this system to the drugs listed in Table 7.1, we can see that these drugs would be classified from practically nontoxic to highly toxic. However, it must be emphasized that caution be exercised when using such classification systems to communicate risk information.

Classification based on lethality can communicate a false sense of security because other determinants of toxicity are not addressed in a classification system based solely on lethality. For example, a teratogenic substance such as *thalidomide* could be classified as "slightly toxic" based on its LD$_{50}$, but highly toxic on the basis of producing fetal malformations. Therefore, classification schemes must always be assessed with their inherent limitations in mind.

It should also be borne in mind that it is difficult to extrapolate the LD$_{50}$ of a drug for a particular population of an animal species to other populations of that species, under slightly different conditions. Obviously, extrapolation to a different species, for example, man, gives extremely uncertain results in predicting teratogenic effects. Furthermore, comparisons of LD$_{50}$ values determined in various laboratories often show significant variability. For example, in an interesting study, when the LD$_{50}$ of a test drug was determined in rats by 65 laboratories worldwide, the variation in reported LD$_{50}$ was more than tenfold.

Toxicologists/pharmacologists routinely divide the exposure of experimental animals to drugs into *four* categories: *acute*, *subacute*, *subchronic*, and *chronic*. Acute exposure is defined as exposure to a drug for less than 24 h, and examples of typical exposure routes are intraperitoneal, intravenous, and subcutaneous injection, oral intubation, and dermal application. While acute exposure *usually refers to a single administration*, repeated exposures may be given within a 24-h period for some slightly toxic or practically nontoxic drugs. *Acute* exposure by inhalation refers to continuous exposure for less than 24 h, most frequently for 4 h. *Repeated* exposure is divided into *three* categories: subacute, subchronic, and chronic. Subacute exposure refers to repeated exposure to a drug for 1 month or less, subchronic for 1–3 months, and chronic for more than 3 months.

In some cases, drug exposure may be followed for the lifetime of the animal. In these situations, clinical chemistry measurements as well as pathological examination of postmortem samples can be made. Chronic studies can be carried out in animals at the same time that clinical trials are undertaken.

The importance of chronic testing can be illustrated by an experience that occurred with an antiviral drug, a nucleoside analog in this case, being developed for the treatment of hepatitis. In this particular case, a delayed toxic liver reaction occurred *months* after treatment was begun and, in fact, continued to manifest itself even *after* administration of the drug was discontinued. Initial *short-term* clinical tests had missed the toxicity. Development of the antihepatitis drug was halted when 5 of 15 patients being tested died suddenly from liver failure.

In certain cases, drug toxicity has manifested itself under circumstances that are even more bizarre and could not have been reasonably anticipated. For example, daughters of mothers who took *diethylstilbestrol* (DES) during pregnancy have a greatly increased risk of developing vaginal cancer, in young adulthood, some *20–30 years after their in utero* exposure to DES.

For all the four types of duration-based toxicity testing described above, selection of dosages, species, strain of animal, route of exposure, parameters measured, and numerous other factors are extremely important. Although the type of data generated by acute, subacute, subchronic, and chronic toxicity tests can be useful, there are other types of tests that address more specific toxicity questions. For example, reproductive studies determine the effect of a drug on the reproductive process; mutagenicity tests determine whether a drug has the potential to cause genetic damage; carcinogenicity tests may reveal the appearance of neoplastic changes; and skin sensitization can be useful in determining a drug's irritancy.

The pharmaceutical company developing the drug or a contract research company that specializes in such testing typically carries out toxicity tests. In either case, the conduct of toxicity studies must adhere to strict guidelines codified in national regulatory requirements. Of particular importance is the necessity to carry out the studies in compliance with a system known as *Good Laboratory Practice* (GLP). Violation of these guidelines can jeopardize the successful approval of the drug.

Toxicology studies often involve the quantitative measurement of cell death. Consider, for example, the requirements of cancer therapy. A solid tumor weighing 1 g (which might easily escape clinical detection) already contains as many as 10^9 cells. Any single surving cell may have the potential to regrow into a tumor, so, to be curative, radiotherapy or chemotherapy might require better than 99.999999% killing. Similar considerations apply to the problem of disinfection: to ensure the effective sterilization of contaminated medical instruments, we want to prevent the survival of any bacteria—even a few cells might transfer a disease.

GENETICS

Other than dose, perhaps the most important determinant in influencing our response to drugs (both toxic and therapeutic) is our underlying genetic makeup. This area of pharmacology has been traditionally referred to as *pharmacogenetics* and has helped to explain unexpected drug responses previously referred to as *idiosyncratic* (i.e., occurring for no known reason). The genetic component is pervasive in influencing drug efficacy and toxicity because it affects virtually every phase of pharmacodynamics and pharmacokinetics. From the membranes in our small intestine to the detoxifying enzymes in the liver and systems beyond, there is a succession of genetically regulated factors. You can probably think of many yourself.

Interindividual differences in response to a xenobiotic was probably described first by Pythagorous in 510 BC when he noted that some, but not all, individuals develop hemolytic anemia in response to *fava bean* ingestion. It has been reported that he advised his followers not to eat fava beans.

In a report in 1902, a genetic component was suggested to be involved in biochemical processes, where the cause of interindividual differences in adverse drug reactions (ADRs) was due to enzyme deficiencies. Thirty years later, the first population-based study to identify ethnic differences in a *pharmacogenetic* trait, namely the *phenylthiocarbamate* nontaster phenotype was described. In 1957, it was suggested that interindividual differences in drug efficacy and ADRs were in part due to genetic variation, and in 1959, F. Vogel coined the term *"pharmacogenetics."* Most of the major findings in the P450 field were based on ADRs observed in one individual or a small group of individuals.

The influence of genetic factors is readily apparent when comparing "normal" differences in drug toxicity within a species, between genders of the same species, as well as strain differences within the same species. In addition, there are also examples of drug toxicity related to "abnormal" genetic expression. We will consider significant aspects of both situations in this section.

With regard to species, there are numerous examples of the widely disparate response of different species to a drug. For example, the LD_{50} of ipomeanol ranges from 12 mg/kg in the rat to 140 mg/kg in the hamster. This variability in species response can have significant ramifications when drugs undergo preclinical trials. For example, rats are relatively insensitive to the teratogenic effect of thalidomide while New Zealand White rabbits more closely reflect the human condition. Unfortunately, this fact was not known at the time of the thalidomide disaster when early teratogenic testing in the rat proved negative.

While differences in drug toxicity between species may not be surprising, the more subtle expression of strain differences within a given species can also be significant. For example, the duration of hexobarbital sleeping time to a given dose in mice of the A/NL strain is approximately 48 min while in the SWR/HeN strain it is approximately 18 min. Therefore, strain selection by a pharmacologist/toxicologist can also be a significant factor in preclinical evaluation of a drug's action.

Perhaps the best place to begin analyzing the influence of genetic expression on a population's comparative response to a drug is to apply some basic statistical principles. To begin with, we need to appreciate the concept of *frequency distribution* as it applies to natural phenomena. For example, assume for the moment that we could obtain 100 genetically "normal" college students of a given gender. We could then administer a *fixed* dose of drug X (a sedative) and measure some response, such as sedation. If we plotted the frequency of individuals responding, against the intensity of sedation (i.e., light drowsiness, heavy drowsiness, and sleep) we would, theoretically, obtain a frequency distribution curve similar to that shown in Figure 7.4.

In analyzing Figure 7.4 we can see that it can be arbitrarily divided into three main sections. The ascending limb of the curve represents those individuals who are hyporeactive (i.e., light drowsiness). The crown of the bell represents the most frequent number of responders who comprise the average (i.e., heavy drowsiness). The descending limb of the curve reflects those individuals manifesting greater responsiveness (i.e., sleep). Assuming no other significant variable (e.g., nutritional status, etc.), the most likely explanation for the variability in response is the collective effect of the genetic factors mentioned above.

However, we can take our analysis of the student's response to the drug one step further and attempt to quantify where individuals are within the group's distribution. The statistical expression *standard deviation* is a measure of how wide the frequency distribution is for a given group. For example, if someone says, "My cat is a lot bigger than average." What does this mean? The standard deviation is a way of saying precisely what "a lot" means.

Without going into the mathematics of computing a standard deviation, one can conveniently think of it as the average difference from the mean. This can be graphically depicted as shown in Figure 7.5. In any true normal distribution, 68.27% of all the responders fall in the interval between 1 standard deviation above the mean and 1 standard deviation below it. Applied to Figure 7.4, this would correspond to approximately those individuals showing a biological response between 2X and 3X. In addition, the range within ±3 standard deviations encompasses 99.7% of a

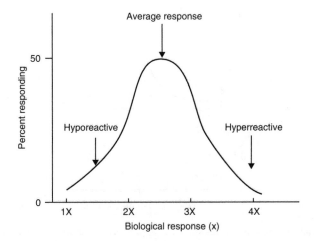

FIGURE 7.4 Typical frequency distribution of a population response to an equivalent dose of a biologically active agent. This type of response represents the variability that occurs within biological systems and is the basis for the concept of dose response in pharmacology and toxicology. This figure demonstrates that within any population, both hyporeactive and hyperreactive individuals can be expected to exist and must be addressed in a risk assessment.

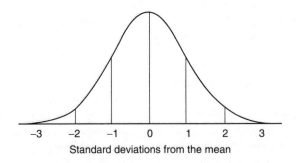

FIGURE 7.5 Typical frequency distribution with the demarcations of standard deviations from the mean.

normally distributed population. Obviously, the standard deviation within a population can be narrow or wide, depending on whether the corresponding frequency distribution is narrow or wide.

In some cases, the variability in response to a drug within the normal population can be quite significant and present a therapeutic challenge. For example, the anticoagulant drug warfarin (also known as coumarin) shows a 20-fold range in the dose required to achieve controlled anticoagulant therapy in humans. Obviously, care must be exercised in administering this drug, since a number of people can be predicted to experience excessive bleeding episodes while others will be refractory to a given dose. The relative sensitivity or resistance to the anticoagulant action of warfarin is due to *altered expression of vitamin K epoxide reductase*. This enzyme is the site of warfarin drug action (inhibition) and is critically involved in the regeneration of reduced vitamin K used in the synthesis of important coagulation proteins.

As mentioned above, in addition to the variability imposed by genetic factors within the "normal" population, there are also examples of genetically mediated drug toxicity outside this constraint. In these situations, the population distribution curve becomes bimodal (or sometimes multimodal), indicating statistically separate populations that can be more or less sensitive for a given parameter and have their own frequency distribution. An example of a bimodal distribution in drug metabolism is shown in Figure 7.6b. In this situation, the left and right hand curves represent fast and slow metabolizers, respectively, of a hypothetical drug.

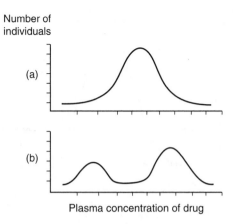

FIGURE 7.6   Frequency distribution curves showing (a) the normal variability in plasma concentration when a fixed dose of drug X is administered to a large population of patients and (b) a bimodal distribution typical of a pharmacogenetic alteration when drug Y is administered under the same conditions.

Genetic modification of enzyme activity associated with the detoxification of certain drugs is a significant factor in pharmacogenetics. A classical example is *N-acetylation polymorphism* (i.e., variation in a particular type of conjugation reaction that would fit Figure 7.6b), originally discovered in tuberculosis patients treated with *isoniazid*. Because of patient variability in response to isoniazid, plasma concentrations were determined at a specific time following a fixed dose of the drug. It was found that patients could be separated into two distinct populations based on remaining isoniazid plasma levels. These two groups are referred to as "slow" and "rapid" acetylators and correspond to the frequency distribution curves shown in Figure 7.6b.

Since the discovery of this phenomenon with isoniazid in 1960, nearly a dozen related drugs and chemicals have been found to be similarly influenced by genetic variation in this acetylase enzyme alone. Therefore, the likelihood of a "slow" acetylator encountering such a chemical/drug has increased. Presently, DNA amplification assay techniques (polymerase chain reaction) of samples obtained from leukocytes, single hair roots, buccal epithelia, or other tissues have been developed, which can be used to predict the *acetylation phenotype* of an individual. The availability of such information could, theoretically, be used to assess workers at high risk for toxicity (e.g., chemical workers exposed to arylamines normally inactivated by acetylation).

N-acetylation polymorphism varies considerably depending on racial genetic predisposition; 45% of the U.S. population (Caucasian and African-American) are slow acetylators and 55% are rapid, whereas 90% of Orientals are fast acetylators. Separation of individuals into either "rapid" or "slow" acetylators is determined by variation at a single autosomal locus and constitutes one of the first discovered genetic polymorphisms of drug metabolism. In general, Eskimos are fast acetylators, while Jews and white North Africans are slow. The half-life of the acetylation reaction for isoniazid in fast acetylators is approximately 70 min, whereas in the slow acetylators, this value is in excess of 3 h.

MALARIA

Another example of a genetically predisposed toxic reaction to drugs is a condition known as *primaquine sensitivity* (primaquine is an *antimalarial* drug). Malaria was a major impediment to the expansion of European colonial empires into tropical countries in Africa, South America, and Asia. Native people in South America knew that the bark of the indigenous *cinchona tree* could be brewed to make a tea that alleviated the symptoms of the disease. The Spanish colonialists quickly appreciated the value of this remedy, which became known in Europe as "Jesuit tea" (in honor of

Catholic missionaries), and they were desperate to prevent acquisition of the plant by competing European powers. The active ingredient of cinchona bark is the alkaloid *quinine*.

Malaria again became a crucial factor in warfare in the twentieth century, when allied troops fought in the Pacific theater of World War II and again in the Korean conflict. The United States began an enormous screening and testing program, aimed at finding substances that could combat mosquitoes and thus malaria. These efforts led to the development of the *quinoline* antimalarial drugs, of which primaquine and chloroquine are prototypical—agents that remain in wide use today. Many antimalarial drugs induce red cell oxidative stress, methemoglobinemia, glutathione depletion, and hemolysis.

Primaquine sensitivity relates to a genetic alteration of the X chromosome that affects approximately 10% of African-American *males* as well as darker-hued Caucasian ethnic groups including Sardinians, Sephardic Jews, Greeks, and Iranians. When U.S. soldiers were administered primaquine as a routine antimalarial prophylactic during the war in Korea, primaquine sensitivity manifested itself as hemolytic anemia. Excessive hemolytic anemia in the presence of oxidizing drugs such as primaquine, or some 50 other known drugs, was found. The hemolytic anemia occurred at approximately one-third the normal dose.

When primaquine is incubated *in vitro* with erythrocytes, neither methemoglobin formation nor hemolysis occurs, suggesting that the toxicity is due to metabolites—presumably formed in the liver—rather than the parent compound. Eventually, two human metabolites that qualified were identified as 6-methoxy-8-hydroxyaminoquinoline and 5-hydroxyprimaquine. Another potential human metabolite is 5-hydroxy-6-desmethylprimaquine.

The mechanism of hemolysis relates to the paucity of *glucose-6-phosphate dehydrogenase* (G6PDH) in the erythrocytes of sensitive individuals. G6PDH is the first of the two pentose phosphate enzymes that generate NADPH for the reduction of hydrogen peroxide in red blood cells. G6PDH deficiency is probably the most common genetic disease or genetic polymorphism in the world, affecting at least 400 million people. More than 80 polymorphic gene variants are present at frequencies greater than 1% in the population.

Under *normal circumstances*, this deficiency may not express itself. Hemoglobin, the oxygen carrying component of the erythrocyte, constitutes more than 90% of the cell's total protein; not surprisingly, then, hemoglobin is a critical target of oxidative damage. Hemoglobin is a tetramer with subunit composition $\alpha_2\beta_2$. The binding of oxygen by hemoglobin is highly cooperative; the entire tetramer undergoes a conformational shift from the "tight," low-oxygen-affinity form into the "relaxed," high-oxygen-affinity form. Therefore, the presence of even a single *ferric* monomer subunit in a hemoglobin molecule greatly *reduces* the oxygen affinity and oxygen-carrying capacity of the entire tetramer. Besides hemoglobin, other erythrocyte proteins, including enzymes and the cell membrane, are also potential targets for oxidative damage.

In the presence of oxidative stress within the erythrocytes, their capacity to generate the very important antioxidant reduced glutathione (GSH) is compromised due to inadequate G6PDH formation (see simplified reaction sequence below). The result is oxidative damage (membranes, hemoglobin, etc.) due to its failure to scavenge superoxide and hydrogen peroxide, culminating in cell death due to failure to replenish NADPH and, hence, GSH; protection against the malaria parasite is also diminished.

$$G6P + G6PDH \rightarrow 6\text{-phosphogluconolactone} + NADPH$$

$$2NADPH + GSSG \rightarrow 2GSH + 2NADP$$

If one were to plot the frequency distribution of erythrocyte G6PDH in the general population, a trimodal distribution would be revealed. This would reflect (1) males and females not carrying the affected gene; (2) males carrying the affected gene; and (3) heterozygous females. Hemolysis is often of intermediate severity in the latter group, since they have two populations of red blood cells, one normal and the other deficient in G6PDH.

Another important example of "abnormal" gene expression occurs in the syndrome known as *succinylcholine apnea*. This malady expresses itself with a frequency of approximately 1 in 6000 and involves serum cholinesterase variants called "*atypical cholinesterase*." Plasma cholinesterase is capable of hydrolyzing a number of drugs including cocaine and heroin, but its most important clinical importance is inactivating the muscle relaxant *succinylcholine*. Normally, this drug is given to reduce skeletal muscle rigidity and facilitate operative procedures; its duration of action is normally a matter of minutes. However, in the presence of an atypical enzyme, the action of an ordinary dose of succinylcholine can last for approximately an hour.

Expression of the atypical enzyme can be monitored in humans by exposing serum samples from them to a substrate (benzoylcholine) and a competitive inhibitor (dibucaine) and measuring the percent inhibition of benzoylcholine hydrolysis. In the presence of the atypical enzyme, dibucaine produces less inhibition of substrate hydrolysis due to lower affinity of the atypical serum cholinesterase for benzoylcholine. The result is a trimodal distribution reflecting 20, 60, and 80% inhibition (i.e., the so-called *dibucaine number*).

The most obvious manifestation of genetic expression is gender identity. In addition to the obvious differences between males and females, there are also differences in genetic expression that affect drug toxicity. We have mentioned previously that after consuming comparable amounts of ethyl alcohol, women have higher blood ethanol concentrations than men, even after correcting for body weight and body water content. Much of the first-pass metabolism of ethanol occurs in gastric tissue even before it reaches the liver. The first-pass metabolism of ethanol in women in this organ is approximately 50% less than in men because of the presence of lower alcohol dehydrogenase activity in the female gastric mucosa. This largely explains the increased hyperresponsiveness of women to the acute effects of alcohol.

In addition to differences in metabolic transformation between genders, there are also examples of gender differences in routes of excretion that can influence xenobiotic toxicity. For example, 2,6-dinitrotoluene-induced hepatic tumors occur with a greater frequency in males of some rodent species. This is due to the fact that the biliary excretion of the glucuronide conjugate of the carcinogen is favored in males, where it is hydrolyzed by intestinal microflora, reabsorbed, transported to the liver, forms a reactive metabolite (see below), binds to DNA, and causes a mutation. In the female, urinary excretion predominates and results in greater clearance. Male mice are also more susceptible to chloroform-induced kidney damage. Endocrine status obviously plays an important role since castration diminishes the effect while androgens restore it. Testosterone may be mediating this effect by enhancing the formation of a toxic metabolite.

AGE

Pharmacokinetic as well as pharmacodynamic differences can exist between infant, adult, and geriatric populations. This is due to the fact that many physiological changes take place during one's life span. The changes that principally affect drug toxicity include (1) liver metabolic function; (2) renal elimination; and (3) body composition. Although we know that differences can exist in drug effects due to age, drug screening is still generally *not* carried out in neonates, infants, or extremely old animals.

Liver metabolism of drugs is typically reduced at the extremes of age. Hepatic drug metabolizing as well as glucuronidation conjugation enzymes are generally present in significantly decreased amounts in the newborn infant due to incomplete genetic expression. In fact, the unique physiology of the newborn, particularly premature infants, can lead to clinical disorders such as *gray baby syndrome*. This pediatric entity is due to inadequate glucuronidation of excessive doses of the antimicrobial agent chloramphenicol. The syndrome usually begins 2–9 days after treatment is started. It is characterized by cyanosis producing an ashen-gray color. At times of physiologic change, corresponding alterations can occur in pharmacokinetics. This can be reflected in variability in response and the need for dosage adjustment. Unusual, paradoxical pharmacodynamic differences can occur in children, for example. While antihistamines and barbiturates generally sedate adults, these drugs may cause some children to develop hyperexcitable behavior. *Conversely,* the use of stimulants such as methylphenidate (Ritalin) in adolescents may stabilize attention deficit disorder in some children. These unusual responses may be due to differences between receptors and transduction pathways in the two age groups and may reflect the imbalance toward excitation in the young brain.

As noted above, variation in kidney function can affect drug toxicity. Regardless of whether renal function is normalized to body weight or body surface area, it is lower in the neonate compared to adult. As the infant matures, renal blood flow increases as a consequence of increased percent of the cardiac output going to the kidneys as well as decreased peripheral vascular resistance. Renal plasma flow increases approximately 8-fold within 1–2 years of birth.

In addition to renal blood flow, development of the glomerulus results in an increase in glomerular filtration rate (GFR). Adult values for GFR are generally reached within 2.5–5 months of age. For drugs eliminated virtually entirely by glomerular filtration, such as the antibiotic gentamicin, significant reductions in half-life occur within the first several weeks of life. In summary, developmental changes affecting presentation of the drug via renal blood flow as well as processing by glomerular filtration contribute to relatively rapid changes in the elimination kinetics of drugs cleared by the kidneys.

Decline in physiological function as part of the normal aging process can also lead to altered drug disposition and pharmacokinetics, as well as altered pharmacodynamic response to drugs. This field of study is often referred to as *geriatric pharmacology.* It should be appreciated in discussing this area, however, that physiological changes in the elderly are highly individualized.

Among the factors that can influence pharmacokinetic changes in older people are decreased percentage of total body water, increased percentage of body fat, decreased liver mass and blood flow, decreased cardiac output, and reduced renal function. For example, total body water decreases by 10–15% between 20 and 80 years of age. Coincidentally, the fat portion of body weight increases from mid-life averages of approximately 18% for men and 33% for women, to 36% and 48%, respectively, for individuals aged 65 and over. As a result, the volume of distribution for water-soluble drugs decreases with age, whereas that for fat-soluble drugs increases.

After 40 years of age, liver mass decreases at a rate of approximately 1% per year, in addition to a reduction in blood flow (40–50%), resulting in a diminished ability to metabolize drugs. However, since hepatic drug metabolism varies widely among individuals, there are no absolute age-related alterations in this regard. Cardiac output also decreases by approximately 1% per year, beginning at 30 years of age, and contributes to the decrease in hepatic blood flow. Glomerular filtration rate, renal plasma flow, and tubular secretory capacity also become reduced.

Reduced total body water in conjunction with elevated body fat in the geriatric population can lead to alterations in drug distribution and, hence, pharmacokinetic and possible toxic effects. As mentioned above, lipid-soluble drugs such as the tranquilizer valium will have a potentially larger volume of distribution in a typical elderly person, while water-soluble drugs such as acetaminophen, alcohol, and digoxin (a drug used to treat congestive heart failure) will have a smaller volume of distribution. Therefore, the geriatric population will generally be more sensitive to the effects of alcohol consumption because a given dose will be concentrated in a smaller compartment. Similarly, the dose of digoxin will probably have to be monitored particularly carefully in order to avoid toxicity, since it has a relatively low TI.

In view of the fact that several aspects of kidney function decline with age (e.g., 35% in GFR by the 7th–8th decade), it should not be surprising that the rate of elimination of those drugs primarily dependent on the kidney is reduced. Unlike hepatic clearance, the GFR reduction leads to predictable, directly proportional decreases in the clearance of drugs dependent on the kidney for excretion. In order to minimize toxicity for drugs frequently prescribed in the geriatric population, such as lithium carbonate (used in manic depression), chlorpropamide (used in maturity-onset diabetes), and digoxin, it may actually be necessary to assess renal drug clearance including glomerular filtration rate (i.e., creatinine clearance; see Chapter 3). Determinations are usually achieved using either normograms or mathematical equations adjusting for age, body weight, and gender.

Changes in pharmacodynamic responses in the elderly have been less well studied than pharmacokinetic changes. However, drug responses can be altered due to factors such as age-related changes in receptors and transduction pathways. For example, reduced sensitivity of β-receptors to β-agonists in the hearts of the elderly may be the result of reduced formation of the second messenger cyclic adenosine monophosphate. The fact that the elderly are more prone to experience depression after taking valium, despite a larger volume of distribution for this drug, also suggests that altered tissue sensitivity at the receptor/transduction level may play a role.

ALLERGY

Perhaps the most common type of allergy is *hay fever*, affecting 20% of the population. The term is actually a misnomer and probably denotes our agrarian past when hay was a principal product of farm agriculture and a common source of allergens. Early descriptions of the symptoms caused by working with dry, cultivated field hay (sneezing, nasal congestion, and eye irritation) promoted this popular expression. The correct term is *"allergic rhinitis"* (i.e., irritation of the nose). When the symptoms occur during a specific season, the malady is called "seasonal allergic rhinitis." When the symptoms occur throughout the year, it is called "perennial allergic rhinitis."

The eye symptoms are referred to as "allergic conjunctivitis." These allergic symptoms routinely interfere with the quality of life and can lead to other problems such as sinusitis and asthma.

A hay fever allergic reaction occurs when the immune system of a *sensitive* individual attacks a usually harmless substance (the antigen) by generating an antibody that complexes with the antigen on the cell surface of *mast cells* in the nose, for example. This is an example of a type I reaction as illustrated in Figure 7.8. When a mast cell is injured, it releases a variety of potent chemicals into the tissues and blood. These chemicals are very irritating and cause itching, swelling, and fluid to leak from cells.

After a period of sensitization (discussed below), when a person with allergic rhinitis comes in contact with the protein (usually in the form of pollen) from many trees, grasses, and weeds, the pollen lodges in the respiratory tract. Since allergic rhinitis is usually associated with pollen, symptoms are at their worst when pollen is in the air. Trees primarily pollinate in the spring, while grasses pollinate in the spring and summer. Of all allergy sufferers in the United States, 75% are allergic to ragweed, 50% are allergic to grasses, and 10% to trees. If you wish to know the pollen count in your area, this information can be found by calling the *National Allergy Bureau's Hotline at 1-800-9-POLLEN*.

IDENTIFICATION OF ANTIGENS

Most people identify their allergies by exposure to the offending agent, be it ragweed or their cat. Because the identification of allergens is important and often difficult to pinpoint, *skin testing* is often needed to identify exactly the specific substance causing the response. Skin testing is now routinely carried out as follows:

- A small amount of the suspected allergy substance is placed on the skin.
- The skin is then gently scratched through the small drop with a special sterile needle.
- If the skin reddens and, more importantly, swells (wheal formation) then allergy to that substance is probable.
- This type of testing is well tolerated by young patients and is considered the standard of testing.

Drugs play an important role in allergic reactions because some are used to treat allergic responses while others can actually cause them. Drug-induced allergic reactions are responsible for approximately 6–10% of all adverse drug reactions. Although an estimated 5% of the population is allergic to one or more medications, approximately 15% of the population believe themselves to have medication allergies or have been incorrectly labeled as having a medication allergy.

It might be appropriate, at this time, to expand on a caveat alluded to previously in this chapter. In the section dealing with dose, it was indicated that most toxic reactions to drugs generally follow a conventional dose–response relationship (the *Paracelsus dictum*). The word *most* was intentionally used because allergic *reactions* to drugs do not really follow a clear-cut dose–response relationship. This is basically due to the fact that many allergic reactions can involve the explosive release of mediators in response to minute levels of the drug, bee venom or environmental toxin—akin to an all-or-nothing effect. The classic example of a drug that can cause a whole body allergic response is penicillin (see below). The same principle holds true for environmental toxins. An example in humans is chronic beryllium disease (CBD). CBD is an allergic lung disorder caused by exposure to beryllium, primarily in mining, which has been demonstrated to be not strictly dependent on beryllium concentration. It should be pointed out, however, that putative exceptions such as these to the dose–response rule are not universally accepted. A further list of distinguishing characteristics between various types of drug side effects is shown in Table 7.3.

As mentioned above, the reason for the lack of clear correlation between dose and response in allergic reactions has to do with the underlying mechanism(s). This will be described in more detail below. Suffice it to say at this point that allergic responses can involve *explosive mediator release in response to minute quantities of drug*; there is a magnifying effect rather than a simple one-to-one relationship, much in the same way that one well-placed canon shot at a snow-covered mountain can start an avalanche.

Normally, we consider the immune system as playing a vitally important role in protecting us against the invasion of pathogenic organisms. This protective function is accomplished via the formation of antibodies in response to antigenic determinants residing on the bacteria or viruses. Similarly, antibody formation is also the underlying factor in immune disorders such as hay fever—as described above—which serves no apparent useful function. In both cases, the immune system is responding to relatively large protein molecules of many thousands of Daltons, if not millions. How then do drugs, whose molecular weight usually ranges between 250 and 500 Da, achieve antigenicity?

TABLE 7.3
Distinguishing Characteristics of Toxic, Idiosyncratic, and Allergic Responses to Drugs

	Toxic Response	Idiosyncratic Response	Allergic Response
Occurrence			
Incidence in population	In all subjects, if dose high enough	Only in genetically abnormal subjects	Varies widely
Incidence among drugs	All drugs	Few drugs	Many drugs
Circumstance	Prior exposure unnecessary	Prior exposure unnecessary	Prior exposure essential
Dose–response relationship	Dose related	Dose related	Independent of dose; erratic relationship
Mechanism	Drug–receptor interaction	Drug–receptor interaction	Through antigen–antibody reaction; specific antibody formed in response to first dose of antigen
Effect produced	Determined by drug–receptor interaction; depends on eliciting drug	Determined by drug–receptor interaction; depends on eliciting drug	Independent of eliciting drug; determined by mediators released by antigen–antibody complex
Effect antagonized	By specific antagonists	By specific antagonists	By antihistamines, epinephrine, or anti-inflammatory steroids, like cortisone

We now know, based on the pioneering work of Landsteiner, that certain drugs or drug metabolites can bind to *endogenous proteins* (carriers). In this context, the binding ligand is referred to as a *hapten*. The resulting hapten–protein complex can be sufficiently different in nature that it is perceived by the body to be foreign and becomes an antigenic determinant, or *epitope.*

A classic example of a drug that forms haptenic derivatives is penicillin. Penicillin and its structural analogs are widely used antibiotics that are, unfortunately, responsible for more allergic reactions than any other class of drug (1–10% of the population). Although all four types (see below) of allergic reactions have been observed with penicillin, type I *anaphylactic* reactions, which can occur with a frequency of 1/15,000 patients, may be life threatening.

Among the metabolites that can be formed during penicillin metabolism are those containing *penicilloyl groups* (Figure 7.7). These particular metabolites have been shown to bind to endogenous protein. Studies in humans have shown that the antibodies most often associated with sensitivity in penicillin-treated patients are specific for the penicilloyl groups.

Like most immune responses, a characteristic feature of drug allergy is that a response occurs only after a sufficient interval follows initial exposure. This period of *sensitization* is normally on the order of 7–10 days and represents the requisite time for antibody synthesis. The manifestations of drug allergy are numerous. They may involve various organ systems and range in severity from minor skin irritation to death. The pattern of allergic response differs in various species. In humans, involvement of the skin (e.g., dermatitis, urticaria, and itching) and involvement of the eyes (e.g., conjunctivitis) are most common, whereas in guinea pigs, bronchoconstriction leading to asphyxia is the most common.

While *sensitization* is required for the priming of the immune response in allergic rhinitis, the opposite process, *desensitization*, can provide a palliative effect in sensitive individuals showing symptoms. The therapeutic procedure known as desensitization or *immunotherapy* is widely established by over 3000 allergy specialists in the United States. Immunotherapy is designed to help the immune system develop a tolerance for the culprit substance, by exposing the body to tiny amounts of it over time.

Historically, the regimen of desensitization developed largely as a result of empirical observations; the injections of allergic extracts could, in certain cases, reduce the severity of a patient's symptoms to seasonal allergies. However, the concept of an *allergic* process was not involved in these original attempts but, rather, the notion that pollen contained *toxins* that could provide immunity to such patients with a vaccine composed of pollen extract. As our knowledge of allergy developed, the process of inoculation became known as desensitization.

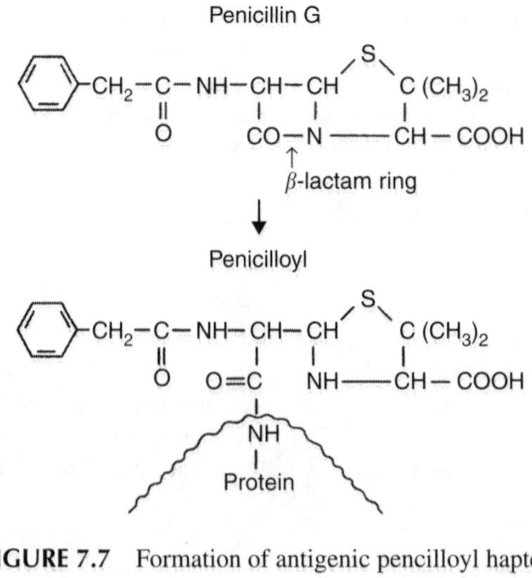

FIGURE 7.7 Formation of antigenic pencilloyl hapten.

Desensitization implies the administration of graduated doses of an allergen over a several-month period of time, with diminishing responses. In practice, the success achieved is variable, and the success depends on the patient and on the allergen in question. When effective, the therapeutic mechanism appears to involve an interaction between IgG and IgE immunoglobins. It has been suggested that the process of desensitization may result in the formation of IgG antibodies that either compete with mast cell-bound IgG for the allergen or possibly interfere with the synthesis of IgE.

This form of treatment is very effective for allergies to pollen, mites, cats, and stinging insects such as bees. Unfortunately, allergy immunotherapy usually requires inconvenient office visits for weekly injections of the offending allergen for several months, followed by monthly injections for several years. However, the success rate of an allergy desensitization program in significantly reducing symptoms can approach 80%. Rarely, serious allergic reactions can occur while receiving allergy injections (1 in 2–5 million injections).

A potentially important breakthrough in the treatment of allergic rhinitis has been reported in 2006 by a European study. The research supports the effectiveness of an *oral* form of immunotherapy using a rapidly dissolving grass allergen tablet (under the tongue) called *Grazax*. Overall, the research team found patients on Grazax had symptom scores that were 30% lower than placebo patients, and they needed their standard hay fever medication about one-third less often. The Grazax group also had more symptom-free, medication-free days during allergy season. This product has already been approved in Sweden.

It may be useful, at this time, to consider the various types of allergic responses that have been ascribed to drugs. They are summarized in Figure 7.8.

Type I, or immediate immune response, involves the production of *IgE antibodies* in lymphatic tissue, which bind to the surface of *mast cells and basophils* and prime them for action. The antibodies are produced in B-lymphocytes during the period of sensitization. Sensitization occurs as

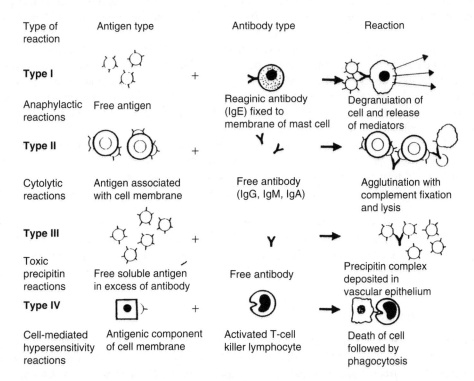

FIGURE 7.8 Mechanisms of stimulation of immune responses. (From Timbrell, J.A. (1989), *Introduction to Toxicology*, London: Taylor & Francis. Adapted from W.C., Bowman and M.J. Rand (1980), *Textbook of Pharmacology*, 2nd ed., Oxford: Blackwell Scientific.)

the result of exposure to appropriate antigens through the respiratory tract, dermally, or by exposure via the gastrointestinal tract. Subsequent cross-linking of the antibodies with the *hapten–protein complex* results in the release of *preformed*, granule-stored mediators (e.g., histamine, heparin, and tryptase) as well as *newly generated* mediators (e.g., leukotrienes, prostaglandins, and cytokines).

These mediators can produce a number of effects including bronchiolar constriction, capillary dilatation, or urticaria (i.e., hives). In severe episodes of type I reactions, a life-threatening *anaphylaxis* can develop in humans due to the development of (1) extreme bronchoconstriction and (2) severe hypotension. Epinephrine is a principal drug used in the acute management of these critical effects, since epinephrine achieves (1) an elevated blood pressure via activation of alpha receptors in peripheral resistance blood vessels and (2) relaxation of bronchiolar smooth muscle via activation of $beta_2$ receptors in the lung. Relief from the dermatological problem (i.e., hives) is also achieved via vasoconstriction of capillaries in the skin, which reduces permeability and, hence, fluid accumulation. Penicillin is a classic example of a drug that can cause a type I reaction.

Type II, or cytotoxic immune responses, can be compliment-independent or compliment-dependent in nature. In the former case, IgG antibodies bind to antigens attached to the surface of normal cells (e.g., erythrocytes, platelets, etc.). Cytotoxic cells (macrophages, neutrophils, and eosinophils) then attach to the Fc portion of the antigen, release cytotoxic granules, and lyse the cell.

The compliment system is a series of approximately 30 serum proteins that promote the inflammatory response. In compliment-dependent responses, after IgG antibodies bind to the cell surface antigens, compliment fixes to compliment receptors on the target cell membrane, inducing lysis. Drugs such as methydopa and quinidine may cause hemolytic anemia and thrombocytopenia, respectively, via type II responses.

Type III hypersensitivity reactions also involve IgG immunoglobins. The distinguishing feature of type III reactions is that, unlike type II reactions, in which immunoglobin production is against specific tissue-associated antigen, immunoglobin production is against *soluble* antigen in the serum. Hence the term serum sickness is often used. The formation of circulating immune complexes composed of a lattice of antigen and immunoglobin may result in widely distributed tissue damage in areas where immune complexes are deposited. The most common location is the vascular endothelium in the lung, joints, and kidneys. The skin and circulatory system may also be involved. Pathology occurs from the inflammatory response initiated by the activation of compliment. Macrophages, neutrophils, and platelets attracted to the deposition site contribute to the tissue damage. Examples of drugs that can cause serum sickness include sulfonamides, penicillins, and certain anticonvulsants.

Type IV, or cell-mediated, response involves a delayed reaction to the antigenic material. Contact dermatitis is an example of a type IV response. Sensitization occurs when the antigen penetrates the epidermis and forms a complex with a protein carrier that subsequently migrates to local lymph nodes where activated; memory *T lymphocytes* are expressed. *No* serum antibodies are formed. When these *activated T lymphocytes* subsequently encounter the original antigenic material, they release lymphokines that activate inflammatory cells such as macrophages and neutrophils, resulting in erythema and the formation of papules and vesicles. The infiltration of these cells into an internal organ can produce an analogous response. An example is believed to be halothane-induced hepatitis, the mechanism of which will be described in more detail in a subsequent section on covalent binding.

ANTIHISTAMINES

As mentioned above, one of the principal mediators involved in certain allergic reactions (e.g., type I-anaphylactic) is histamine. *Histamine* is an endogenous substance that is synthesized, stored, and released primarily from *tissue mast cells* and *circulating basophils*. The actions of histamine are mediated by at least three distinct receptor subgroups H_1, H_2, and H_3. Of these, H_1 receptors mediate the major actions in humans related to allergic responses. A list of some of the principal actions of histamine in humans is shown in Table 7.4.

TABLE 7.4

Principal Effects of Histamine Related to Allergic Reactions in Humans

Organ/Tissue	Effect	Receptor Subtype
Cardiovascular	Decreased peripheral resistance	H_1, H_2
Respiratory	Increased permeability postcapillary venules	H_1
Skin	Increased contraction bronchiolar smooth muscle	H_1
	Increased pain and itching	H_1

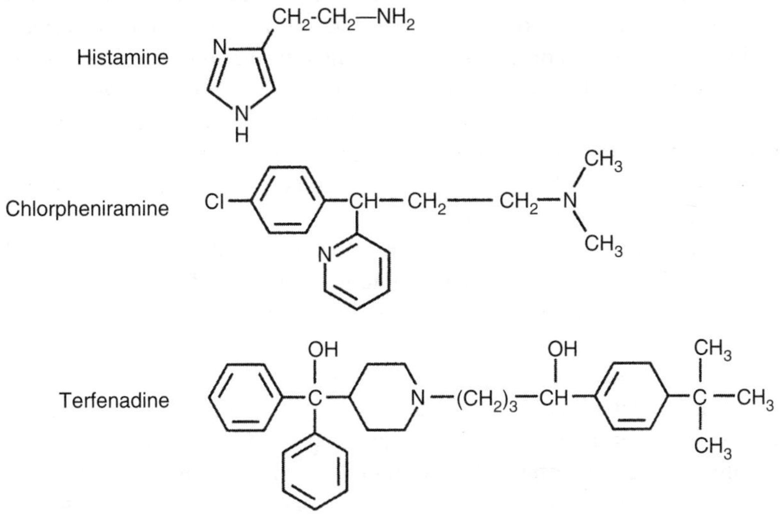

FIGURE 7.9 Comparison of "old" and "new" antihistamine structures with histamine.

Histamine is formed *in vivo* via the decarboxylation of the amino acid L-histidine. As indicated previously, it is stored in an inert, ionically bound complex with proteoglycans, such as heparin and chondroitin sulfate, within granules at its site of synthesis. Histamine is distributed throughout the body. However, the greatest concentration in humans occurs in the skin, lungs, and gastrointestinal mucosa. It is the latter site that is the locus of action of *H₂ blockers*, such as *cimetidine* (introduced during the 1970s), to inhibit gastric acid secretion in cases of acid indigestion or ulcers (see Chapter 14 for more information). The H_1 and H_2 receptors have been cloned and shown to belong to the superfamily of G protein-coupled receptors. H_3 receptors are believed to play a role in histaminergic neurons *in vivo*. To date, no H_3 agonist or antagonist has found clinical use.

Agents generally referred to as antihistamines are those that antagonize the action of histamine at H_1 receptors. They act in a competitive manner and are primarily used in situations such as urticaria, hay fever, and insect bites. They are available for both local and oral administration. At the time of the development of the first antihistamines in the 1940s, they were hailed as the cure for the common cold. Antihistamines do not stop the formation of histamine nor do they block the interaction between IgE and antigen.

The original antihistamines bore a relatively close structural similarity to histamine (Figure 7.9). One of the most significant structure–activity relationships is the *ethylamine side chain* present as a *substituted derivative* in chlorpheniramine, a common component in OTC preparations. Newer, second-generation antihistamines, such as terfenadine (subsequently withdrawn from the market for drug interaction problems), *loratadine* (Claritin), fexofenadine (Allegra), and cetirizine (Zyrtec) show more significant structural divergence.

Antihistamines differ primarily in terms of their potency, selectivity of action, and side effects. The newer second-generation H_1 blockers, *loratadine and fexofenadine*, for example, are more specific for H_1 receptor antagonism than the older generation that can also block cholinergic and muscarinic receptors. In addition, the second-generation drugs do not cross the blood-brain barrier as readily and are, therefore, generally devoid of sedative properties (hence the term *nonsedating antihistamines*).

Several of the older generation antihistamines are used exclusively for situations that do not involve an allergic reaction. For example, some demonstrate significant antiemetic, antimotion sickness, antiparkinsonan, antitussive, and local anesthetic actions (some H_1 antagonists are more potent than procaine). They can be found in many OTC products, particularly for the relief of symptoms from the common cold and allergies, as well by prescription. The effectiveness of the agents in the treatment of motion sickness and Parkinson's disease may be attributed to their *anticholinergic* actions.

One of the interesting aspects of the marketing of first generation antihistamines has to do with their propensity to induce sedation. The ethanolamines (e.g., *diphenhydramine*) are particularly prone to cause sedation. While this is generally an undesirable side effect that has been basically eliminated in newer generation antihistamine drugs, this property does have commercial value. For example, most OTC sleeping aides contain older generation antihistamines that are quite useful because of their tendency to produce sedation.

OTC antihistamines include diphenhydramine (Benadryl), chlorpheniramine (Chlortrimaton), clemastine fumarate (Tavist), and dexbrompheniramine (Drixoral). The newer "nonsedating" antihistamines include loratadine (Claritin), fexofenadine (Allegra), cetirizine (Zyrtec), and azelastine (Astelin Nasal Spray).

Some people with allergic rhinitis need specialized prescription medication such as one containing a cortisol-like anti-inflammatory nasal spray; cromolyn or ipratropium (atropine-like) are also available (see Chapter 13 for more details). These nasal sprays do not cause the rebound effect common to many adrenergic decongestants. Corticosteroid nasal sprays are very effective in reducing the inflammation that causes swelling, sneezing, and running nose. Many corticosteroid nasal sprays are on the market through prescription only.

Although cromolyn can also act as an anti-inflammatory medication, it is not as potent as corticosteroids. In allergic rhinitis, it can act prophylactically. Because its mechanism of action involves stabilization of mast cell membranes and prevention of mediator release, it needs to be taken before the allergy season gets in full "bloom." Ipratropium is an atropine derivative and, as such, can block certain cholinergic receptors, like the ones on nasal blood vessels that control fluid leakage (i.e., a running nose). Ipratropium nasal spray is available for drying a wet running nose.

DECONGESTANTS

Decongestants help control allergy symptoms, rather than the cause. The mucous membrane of the nose is a common site for irritation and infection, because it is the first tissue contacted by all respirable materials. Lysis of antibody-bearing host cells (i.e., mast) during common allergy attacks destroys upper respiratory membranes, resulting in local inflammation caused by mediator release, with attendant capillary dilation leading to interstitial edema, and with a reflex increase in mucous secretion and mucosal permeability. Edema of the nasal mucosa can be particularly bothersome, because this area has a rich vascular supply that forms subepithelial plexuses of arterioles. The large volume of blood that can be diverted into these plexuses during inflammation can produce significant engorgement of the nasal mucosa. Therefore, both capillary dilation and the mucus contribute to nasal congestion. When the nasal mucosa is significantly congested, the passageway through the turbinated airway becomes a major factor in air flow resistance.

Sympathomimetic decongestant compounds are used topically and orally because of their *vasoconstrictor* property (*α-receptor activation*), which produces a physiological antagonism to vasodilation. By causing capillary vasoconstriction, pore size is reduced and fluid loss is decreased.

Chronic use of topical preparations is not recommended for more than 5 days because of the possibility of a "rebound" effect, the result of tachyphylaxis (acute tolerance due to a compensatory decrease in α-receptors).

Although the oral route of administration affords a potentially longer duration of action, with no nasal irritation or associated "rebound" congestion, oral sympathomimetics are, nevertheless, not considered to be as effective or safe as topical preparations (e.g., phenylpropanolamine [PPA]). In fact, oral vasoconstrictor drugs rarely do much to relieve the nasal stuffiness associated with allergic rhinitis, mainly due to inadequate dosage, nonlocalized deposition, and disseminated distribution.

The FDA is in the process of removing PPA from all drug products including OTC decongestants; it will be reclassified as a Category II drug—not generally recognized as safe and effective. Concerns exist regarding PPA increasing the risk of hemorrhagic stroke in the brain.

IMMUNE-RELATED DRUG INJURY

The past decade has seen an increasing number of indications that human exposure to substances suppressing the immune system results in an increased incidence of infections and neoplastic disorders. In this regard, the most provocative theory regarding the etiology of AIDS relates to a proposed immunotoxicity of drugs of abuse rather than the human immunodeficiency virus (i.e., the so-called Duesenberg Hypothesis). While this is a "radical" theory and not generally accepted, we do know of studies of transplant patients who have received long-term treatment with immunosuppressants, such as glucocorticoids or azathioprine (to prevent organ rejection), showing a marked increase in the incidence of tumors.

Apart from the process of haptenization discussed above, certain drugs are also capable of modifying the antigenic potential of endogenous molecules, *without binding*. In unknown ways, the tissue becomes modified and is recognized as foreign and induces an autoimmune disorder. Table 7.5 lists drugs that can give rise to a syndrome known as *systemic lupus erythematosus* (SLE). SLE is characterized by skin eruptions, arthralgia, leukopenia, and fever.

A particularly good example of a drug inducing SLE is the vasodilator hydralazine, sometimes used for the treatment of hypertension. The drug-induced lupus syndrome usually occurs after at least 6 months of continuous treatment, and its incidence is related to dose, gender, and race. In one study, after 3 years of treatment with hydralazine, drug-induced lupus occurred in 10.4% of patients who received 200 mg daily, 5.4% who received 100 mg daily, and none who received 50 mg daily. The incidence is approximately four times higher in women then in men, and the syndrome is seen more commonly in Caucasians than in African–Americans.

PRIMARY MECHANISMS OF DIRECT DRUG-INDUCED CELL INJURY

Advances in techniques used in the biological sciences (e.g., histopathology, electron microscopy, subcellular fractionation, and analytical methods) have provided the framework for identifying

TABLE 7.5
Drugs Known to Produce Systemic Lupus Erythematosus

Drug	Class
Practolol	β-Adrenergic receptor blocker
Chlorpromazine	Antipsychotic
Hydralazine	Antihypertensive
Isoniazide	Antibacterial agent
Diphenylhydantoin	Anticonvulsant
Ethosuximide	Anticonvulsant

LIVERPOOL JOHN MOORES UNIVERSITY
LEARNING SERVICES

mechanisms of toxicity at the cellular level. One of the underlying principles driving this type of inquiry is the concept of a "biochemical lesion," first proposed by Rudolf Peters in 1931. In essence, the term biochemical lesion refers to the initial metabolic alteration produced by a xenobiotic that is ultimately expressed in morphological change.

While antihistamine-induced sedation may be a side effect that can have a commercial "spin" put on it, there are several more fundamental toxic effects at the cellular level that can jeopardize cellular function as well as produce cell death. Although any organ or tissue may be a target for a toxic drug effect as a result of differences in anatomical structure (e.g., blood-brain barrier), blood flow (e.g., liver and kidney), oxygen tension (e.g., lung), and highly specialized binding affinity (e.g., adriamycin in the heart), there are several primary mechanisms that can produce cellular damage.

The principle mechanisms underlying the primary events of drug toxicity include (1) covalent binding; (2) lipid peroxidation; and (3) oxidative stress. The dividing line between these types of mechanisms is not always clear. For example, a reactive intermediate may cause death via covalent binding, while the necrotic cells may release toxic oxidative products. The reverse scenario is also conceivable.

COVALENT BINDING

In Chapter 5, the four major types of chemical bonds involved in drug receptor interaction were described. One of these is the covalent bond. Being practically irreversible, covalent binding is of great toxicological significance because it results in the permanent alteration of endogenous molecules. Some chemicals can form covalent adducts directly, whereas most appear to require metabolic activation. In Chapter 3, it was indicated that certain drugs can undergo bioactivation (often catalyzed by the P450 system) yielding metabolites with the capacity to form covalent bonds with endogenous macromolecules. Covalent adduct formation is common with electrophilic metabolites (molecules containing an electron-deficient atom) interacting with endogenous electron-rich atoms (nucleophiles). Nucleophilic atoms are abundant in biological macromolecules such as proteins and nucleic acids.

Covalent adducts to DNA and proteins mediate the toxic effects of many carcinogens and cytotoxic agents. Protein modification by xenobiotics can lead to cytotoxicity, toxic immune-mediated reactions, and idiosyncratic reaction to drugs. DNA modifications (e.g., covalent adducts, strand breaks, and loss of bases) may constitute premutagenic lesions, alterations that can cause mutations. Unpaired DNA damage may kill the cell. Protein adducts have been less studied than DNA adducts, even though they are usually *more* abundant.

Proteins have many nucleophilic sites that are potential targets for electrophiles. One target is the terminal amino group. Aside from the aliphatic side chains, most amino acid side chains have nucleophilic functional groups. Among the most important targets are (1) cysteine thiol SH; (2) histidine imidazole NH; (3) lysine ε-NH$_2$; and (4) tyrosine phenolic OH. As with DNA adduction, steric factors are important determinants of sites of damage.

Protein function is impaired when conformation or structure is altered by interaction with such toxic metabolites. Many proteins contain critical moieties, particularly thiol (SH) groups, that are essential for catalytic activity or assembly of macromolecular complexes. Proteins that are sensitive to covalent modification of their thiol groups include enzymes involved in metabolism, Ca^{++} pumps, and transcription factors.

As mentioned previously, one of the key protectants in cells against toxic covalent binding is *glutathione*. This sulfhydryl-containing substance can serve as an alternate binding site in the cytosol to reactive intermediates and protect more significant cellular sulfhydryl moieties. An example of the inverse relationship between sulfhydryl availability and covalent binding can be demonstrated using radioactive thiourea.

Thiourea is a potent edematogenic agent in rats causing pulmonary edema and death. When rats are exposed to diethylmaleate *in vivo*, this chemical causes the lung content of glutathione to

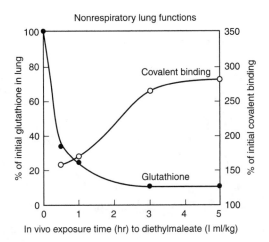

FIGURE 7.10 Effect of glutathione depletion *in vivo* on covalent binding of radioactivity from ^{14}C-thiourea to lung protein *in vitro*. (From M.A. Hollinger, S.N. Giri, and F. Hwang (1976), *Drug Metab. Dispos.*, 4: 121. With permission.)

become depleted. Conversely, during the same time interval, the covalent binding of ^{14}C-thiourea to lung protein is allowed to increase (see Figure 7.10).

The covalent binding of highly reactive drug metabolites to DNA could, conceivably, cause nucleotide mispairing during replication. For example, covalent binding to the reactive N at the 7 position of guanine could result in pairing of the adduct-bearing guanine with adenine rather than cytosine, leading to the formation of an incorrect codon and the insertion of an incorrect amino acid into protein. Such a sequence of events is known to occur with *aflatoxin* 8,9-oxide in the liver.

Historically, drug-induced liver injury has been a relatively rare, often an idiosyncratic event. But according to the FDA, such injuries have become the leading cause of liver failure in the United States and the most common single cause for withdrawal of drugs from the market. Furthermore, more than 75% of cases of idiosyncratic drug reactions result in liver transplantation or death.

The statistical infrequency of drug-related hepatotoxicity is an important part of the problem. The reactions to many drugs may occur in less than 1 in 10,000 patients. But a typical phase III clinical trial can involve only about 3000 patients—or less. Significantly, detecting a single case of an adverse drug reaction to a drug (with 95% confidence) requires that the number of patients studied be three times the incidence of reaction, or about 30,000. Therefore, many drugs are approved before liver effects can be identified. This puts the responsibility on observant postmarketing monitoring. In addition to individual patient safety, it is vital for health care professionals to detect occurrences of drug-induced liver damage to provide an accurate record to the FDA.

Recently, a new use for caffeine has been introduced clinically. It is called the *caffeine breath test (CBT)*; it may prove to be a complementary, noninvasive test for *liver function*. Using orally administered ^{13}C-caffeine, CBT values were found to be decreased in cirrhotic patients and patients with hepatitis. The investigators carrying out the study suggest that CBT in conjunction with other data may obviate the need for liver biopsy.

Hepatotoxic drug reactions, when they occur, are characterized by rapid onset of malaise and jaundice in association with elevated serum *aminotransferase* levels.

An example of a drug that can undergo metabolic activation with subsequent liver injury is the widely used anesthetic agent halothane. Actually, there are believed to be two types of hepatic damage that halothane can produce, depending on whether an oxidation or reduction pathway is involved. Oxidative dehalogenation is the primary mechanism in humans while reductive dehalogenation predominates in the rat. In the final analysis, covalent binding is a common feature. *Halothane hepatitis*

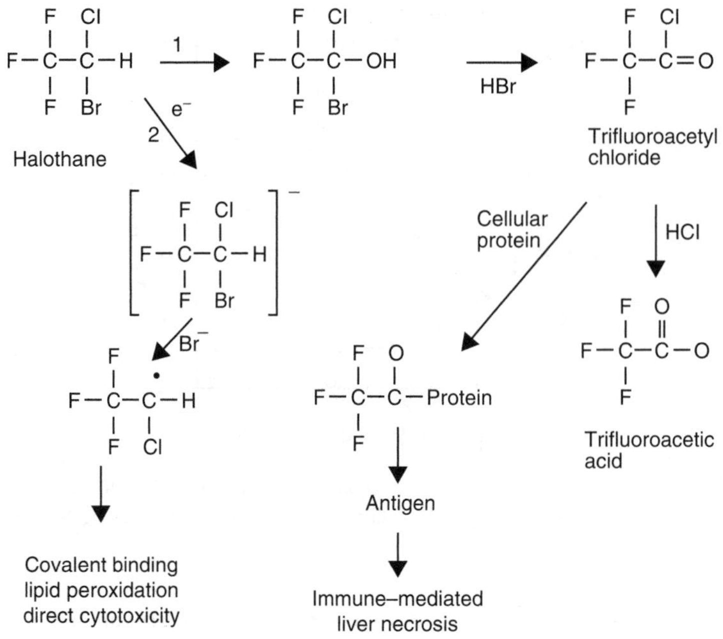

FIGURE 7.11 The metabolism of halothane and its proposed involvement in liver toxicity. Pathway 1 (oxidative) and pathway 2 (reductive) are both catalyzed by cytochrome P450. (From J.A. Timbrell (1991), *Principles of Biochemical Toxicology*, 2nd ed., London: Taylor & Francis. With permission).

in humans is a rare (1 in 20,000) but severe form of liver necrosis associated with repeated exposure to this volatile anesthetic.

Halothane, as the name implies, contains halogen atoms within its molecular structure (e.g., 3 F, 1 Br, and 1 Cl). Within the human liver, halothane undergoes a dechlorination reaction that leads to the production of an *unstable free radical* intermediate (Figure 7.11). A free radical is a molecule or molecular fragment that contains one or more unpaired electrons in its outer orbital shell and is highly electrophilic. Most of the free radical formed in the human liver is *trifluoroacetylchloride*.

Some of this free radical covalently binds to specific liver protein and elicits an immune response. This scenario is supported by data obtained in human subjects. Serum samples from patients suffering from halothane hepatitis contain antibodies directed against neoantigens formed by the trifluroacetylation of liver proteins. In addition, the administration of radiolabeled halothane to a patient undergoing a transplant operation resulted in the detection of covalent binding in liver protein.

The principle antigenic proteins seem to be associated with the smooth endoplasmic reticulum. This is not particularly surprising since it is the probable site of metabolite formation via P450. Trifluoroacyl adducts have also been detected on the outer surface of hepatocytes, although it is not clear how they arrive there. In halothane-induced hepatitis, the number of exposures does seem to be important, with about four being optimum.

Perhaps the best-studied example of drug toxicity resulting from covalent binding involves the widely used analgesic drug acetaminophen (known as paracetamol in the United Kingdom), introduced in the consumer market in the 1950s.

Acetaminophen overdose is the most common cause of acute drug-related liver failure (ALF) in the United States and the United Kingdom. Under normal circumstances, the drug poses little risk. However, if extremely large amounts are taken, the liver's capacity to detoxify it via sulfation and glucuronidation is exceeded, while, coincidentally, there is increased formation of a toxic metabolite. The result is death and necrosis of liver and kidney cells.

Since acetaminophen pills were often found in household medicine cabinets, children occasionally opened the bottles and swallowed the contents, particularly before the introduction of "childproof" packaging for hazardous products in the 1970s. In 1977, the *Analgesic Review Panel* of the U.S. FDA recommended that all acetaminophen products carry a warning label stating that overdose can cause liver damage. Unfortunately, acetaminophen continues to be chosen as a poison by suicidal individuals. In the United Kingdom, about 500 deaths occur annually due to acetaminophen overdose, accounting for approximately 15% of fatal poisonings.

Because of the high incidence of acetaminophen poisoning cases, there have been ongoing research efforts to understand the mechanisms of acetaminophen hepatotoxicity and to develop therapeutic interventions that can be applied to victims of acetaminophen overdoses.

The mechanism of acetaminophen toxicity has been extensively studied in experimental animals. We know that oxidation of acetaminophen in the liver via cytochrome P450 results in the formation of a cytotoxic electrophile *N-acetyl-p-benzoquinoneimine* (NAPQI), catalyzed by prostaglandin H synthase, that binds to hepatic proteins; this adduct damages liver cells.

Evidence from rodent studies further indicates that NAPQI covalently binds with cysteinyl sulfhydryl groups yielding 3-(cystein-S-yl) acetaminophen protein adducts (3-Cys-A) on more than 15 proteins. Studies in humans indicate a similar pathogenesis. This forms the rationale for using *N-acetylcysteine* as a glutathione donor in early acetaminophen poisoning. The primary target for NAPQI covalent binding appears to be a 58 kDa binding protein. This protein may function as an electrophile sensor that signals the nucleus that an electrophile is present and that alterations in cellular homeostasis are necessary. The NAPQI adduct may also function as a hapten and elicit an immunological response.

A recent study has demonstrated that cocaine, a common drug of abuse, can bind to proteins. In this case, the parent drug is active. *In vitro* experiments with amino acids suggest that the ε-amino group of lysine is the main target. Cocaine-adducted proteins have been detected in blood plasma samples from cocaine users.

The final example of covalent binding does not really involve a drug but, rather, chemical warfare agents known as organophosphates. Diflurophosphate (DFP) is probably the most extensively studied compound of this class. DFP functions by irreversibly inhibiting esterases such as *acetylcholinesterase* via alkylphosphorylation to become covalently bound. The result is an accumulation of acetylcholine at cholinergic synapses, both in the periphery and CNS, with the attendant exaggeration of cholinergic effects (see Chapter 11).

LIPID PEROXIDATION

As indicated above, some drugs are bioactivated to reactive intermediates that interact with cellular constituents. One specific type of reactive substance mentioned previously is the *free radical*. Free radicals are highly reactive chemical species containing, in the outermost or bonding orbital, a single *unpaired electron*. As a result, this is an extremely reactive *electrophilic species* with a very short half-life. Free radicals seek other electrons to make a new pair. A free radical may collide with another free radical to create a stable electron pair (a process termed annihilation) or it may obtain the transfer of another electron from a compound more susceptible to electron donation, thus eliminating the original free radical but replacing it with another (perpetuation). Free radicals cause cellular damage when they pull electrons from components of normal cells of the body (e.g., cell membrane lipids).

An example of free radical formation is molecular oxygen that can accept electrons from a variety of sources to produce reactive oxygen species (ROS) such as *superoxide radical, hydroxyl radical, and nitric oxide radical*. The superoxide anion radical is formed when one electron is taken up by one of the 2p-orbitals of molecular oxygen. Certain drugs, as well as other xenobiotics, have the capacity to undergo so-called redox cycles, whereby they provide electrons to molecular oxygen and form superoxide.

The generation of free radicals in mammalian cells is continuous and occurs as a result of *both* normal and abnormal cellular activity, and also environmental perturbations. It has been estimated that every single one of our body's cells suffers approximately 10,000 free radical "hits" per day. Over a typical 70-year life span, the body generates an estimated 17 tons of free radicals. DNA is a probable target that may partially explain the higher frequency of mutations in the elderly. In addition to DNA, cell membranes, proteins, and fats are also being targeted by free radicals.

Polyunsaturated fatty acids (PUFA) such as those present in *lipid biomembranes* are particularly susceptible to free radical action because of their state of *unsaturation*. When exposed to superoxide or other reactive radicals such as trichloromethylperoxy or hydroxyl, for example, a chain reaction known as *lipid peroxidation* occurs, resulting in a breakdown in membrane structure and function. The term peroxidation is most commonly applied to the incorporation of molecular oxygen into the PUFA of biological membranes. Lipid peroxidation distorts the structure of the lipid bilayer and compromises its integrity and *impermeability*.

All living cells maintain large transmembrane electrolyte concentration gradients. These gradients provide a source of free energy for transport processes that control cell turgor and mediate the import and export of metabolites. One of the primary biological effects of lipid peroxidation is membrane leakage: efflux of potassium, influx of sodium, and concomitant influx of water into the cell. These functional impairments are probably caused by damages both to the membrane lipids themselves and to the transport activities of integral proteins.

After the breakdown has been initiated by the free radical attack, lipid fragmentation is self-propagating due to the successive formation of a series of *highly reactive lipid breakdown products*. Therefore, lipid peroxidation not only destroys lipids in cellular membranes but also generates endogenous free radicals and electrophiles. These substances can readily react with neighboring molecules, such as membrane proteins, or diffuse to more distant molecules such as DNA. Although lipid peroxidation may be a critical mechanism for the cellular injury induced by some drugs, it is not a comprehensive mechanism underlying all toxic drug effects.

OXIDATIVE STRESS

Approximately 50 years ago, it was shown that the discharge of electrical energy into a primordial atmosphere of reduced gases, such as ammonia, methane, hydrogen, and water, yields complex mixtures of organic compounds, including amino acids and sugars. The prebiotic chemical synthesis that made possible the origin of life therefore probably took place under conditions dominated by such reduced gases and driven by sunlight, lightening, or other geological sources of energy. Molecular oxygen did not appear on the scene until a much later time, following the evolution of photosynthetic cells. The atmosphere of the earth today (as far as is known) is unique in containing molecular oxygen as one of its chief components. This store of molecular oxygen is a reservoir of free energy that is continuously consumed by the *oxidation* of organic molecules and replenished from solar energy and water via photosynthesis.

The transformation of the earth's atmosphere from reductive to oxidative conditions presented a new high-octane opportunity for the evolution of more complex life forms. By the same token, however, it presented a threat to all forms of life. Oxidation of organic compounds could be utilized for the release of far more free energy than that yielded by anaerobic processes (e.g., fermentation), *but only if this energy could be controlled and stored in a biologically useable form*. Uncontrolled oxidation threatened the integrity of biomolecules. The relatively unique chemical properties of the oxygen molecule permitted the evolution of biochemical processes that could take advantage of this thermodynamic opportunity without being victimized by the converse threat of excess oxidative activity—under normal circumstances.

As the reader may remember from any introductory chemistry course, the relative strengths of oxidants and reductants are illustrated by *redox potentials* that correspond to free energy changes of the reactions (this can be achieved using electrochemical and spectrophotometric methods).

Pyridine (NADH and NADPH) and flavin (FAD and FMN) coenzymes mediate most biochemical redox processes. As such, these cofactors are the most important oxidizing agents in the reactions of intermediary metabolism.

Under typical cellular conditions, [NAD$^+$/NADH] is more abundant (approximately 1 mM) and mainly oxidized; [NADP$^+$/NADPH] is less abundant (approximately 0.1 mM) and primarily reduced. In view of the fact that reduced nicotinamides are stronger reducing agents than reduced flavins, the path of electron flow in biological electron-transfer chains often goes from a nicotinamide-linked dehydrogenase to a flavoenzyme.

Since mitochondria are the principal site of high oxidative metabolism, they are under continual oxidative stress. In fact, it has been estimated that approximately 2% of mitochondrial O_2 consumption generates ROS. The mitochondrial electron transfer chain is one of the main sources of ROS in aerobic cells, due to electron leakage from energy-transducing sequences leading to the formation of superoxide radicals. The complete reduction of molecular oxygen to water requires four electrons ($O_2 + 4H^+ + 4e^- \rightarrow 2H_2O$); it is sequential and proceeds via four partially reduced intermediates: superoxide anion, hydrogen peroxide, hydroxyl radical, and finally water.

The thermodynamic potential inherent in the reduction of molecular oxygen is released mainly in the final step: reduction of the *hydroxyl radical*. The hydroxyl radical is an extremely potent oxidant and a highly reactive species. It reacts immediately with any available biological substance. For example, it is believed to play a role in the toxicopathology produced by the anticancer drugs bleomycin (lung) and adriamycin (heart) as well as the antibiotic nitrofurantoin.

Redox cycling agents are chemicals that undergo enzymatic one-electron reduction ultimately leading to the formation of superoxide (an oxidative stress mechanism). Numerous xenobiotics cause human toxicity via this process. *Paraquat*, a common herbicide used to control certain weeds, is a pulmonary toxicant in humans. Fatal paraquat poisonings due to accidental, suicidal, or even homicidal exposures have been reported. Paraquat redox cycling generates ROS and depletes cellular NADPH. The particular sensitivity of the lung may result from its exposure to the highest levels of oxygen. Other agents that cause toxicity by redox cycling include quinones, adriamycin, and nitrofurantoin.

The organization of the electron transport chain in the mitochondrial inner membrane allows the thermodynamically favorable flow of electrons (reducing equivalents) from reduced cofactors, through intermediary carriers, to oxygen, to be coupled to the vectorial transport of protons across the membrane. This transport establishes an electrochemical gradient and stores the free energy (ATP) generated by the electron transport chain. Oxidative phosphorylation is driven by the return flow of protons across the membrane, down the electrochemical gradient. Any xenobiotic that deleteriously interferes with this natural generation of energy will have a profound effect on cellular function.

Peroxisomes are organelles present in all nucleated eukaryotic cells. Like mitochondria, peroxisomes specialize in oxidative metabolic processes. For example, fatty acid β-oxidation occurs in both peroxisomes and mitochondria of mammalian cells. However, in distinction to mitochondria, peroxisomes are bounded by a single lipid bilayer membrane and do not produce ATP.

As mentioned previously (Chapter 3), reduced glutathione (GSH) plays an important role as an antioxidant. Oxidative stress is believed to play a key role in a number of neurological disorders including the selective death of motor neurons in *amyotropic lateral sclerosis* (Lou Gehrig's disease). As discussed in Chapter 11, the central nervous system possesses a very high rate of aerobic metabolism and, thus, would be expected to generate considerable ROS. Recent research suggests that GSH may play a vital role in protecting the CNS by functioning as a *free-radical scavenger*. Figure 7.12 shows possible roles for GSH in neurological disease. However, it should be kept in mind that a similar role for GSH as a free-radical scavenger in other tissues is well documented.

There are three classes of enzymes known to provide protection against reactive oxygen species: the *catalases* and *peroxides*, which react specifically with hydrogen peroxide, and the *superoxide dismutases* (a family of enzymes) which react with superoxide anions. If the protective capacity of

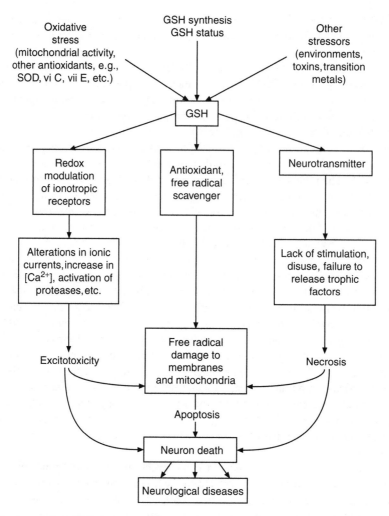

FIGURE 7.12 A model of GSH depletion and neurological disease. GSH is known to play an analogous role in other tissues. (From C.A. Shaw, (Ed.) (1998), *Glutathione in the Nervous System*, Washington, DC. With permission.)

superoxide dismutase and catalase is inadequate, then superoxide anions and hydrogen peroxide can react to form hydroxyl radicals. Oxidant stress, followed by depletion of cellular reducing agents (e.g., thiols, pyridine nucleotides—NADP and NADPH) as well as ATP depletion and elevated intracellular Ca^{++} can lead to cell necrosis. Cells can sometimes avoid this disordered decay by activating a controlled catabolic process that brings about an ordered disassembly and removal of the cell, called apoptosis.

APOPTOSIS

Apoptosis is an orchestrated cell death mechanism that brings about the removal of cells without the inflammation and stress that are associated with other forms of cellular death. It is characterized by the active degradation of chromosomal DNA. The term is derived from the Greek for "a falling away, as leaves in the autumn." It should be distinguished from cellular *necrosis*. Necrosis is a tissue-based form of pathological cell death, mediated mainly by external factors such as traumatic injury, oxygen deficiency, and other gross cellular damage.

Necrosis involves multiple cells and induces an inflammatory response when the plasma membrane ruptures. In contrast, apoptosis is individualized in nature; it is an energy-dependent internally programmed process and the plasma membrane retains its integrity. Single cells undergo apoptosis independent of the fates of their neighbors. Undesirable cells are eliminated by phagocytes without leakage of the intracellular contents to the surrounding medium, and no immune response is therefore triggered.

Apoptosis is far reaching and is responsible for developmental processes such as the brain. In addition to tissue homeostasis in the adult organism, misregulation of apoptosis is a component of several diseases such as autoimmunity, focal ischemia, Huntington's disease, and cancer. Because apoptosis is the mechanism by which the body eradicates mutated cells, the inactivation of apoptotic pathways is central to the success of a cancerous tumor. Moreover, many cancer therapies use apoptotic pathways to kill tumor cells.

Understanding the cell death signaling process and its internal manifestations is the first step to designing better drugs to activate it, in the case of cancer, or stop it, in the case of osteoarthritis, neurodegenerative diseases, type 1 diabetes, and hyperreactions to infection or trauma.

The regulation of apoptosis has been investigated extensively and is incredibly intricate. The release of the electron-transport chain hemeprotein cytochrome C from its normal mitochondrial compartment into the cytosol is a signal that the cell has undergone irreparable damage, and triggers apoptosis. Reactive products of lipid peroxidation, such as 4-hydroxynonenal, induce apoptosis by causing damage to the mitochondrial membrane, and therefore, any drug that induces lipid peroxidation is potentially capable of producing apoptosis. Thus, apoptosis may be, at least in part, a biological response that eliminates cells that have suffered excessive membrane damage due to the effects of oxidative stress.

Drugs such as alkylating agents and doxorubicin can produce DNA damage. DNA damage is potentially mutagenic and carcinogenic, therefore, apoptosis of cells with damaged DNA is an important self-defense of the body against drug-induced oncogenesis. In addition, catecholamines such as epinephrine and norepinephrine, as well as cocaine, are also believed to induce cardiomyopathy, at least partially, via apoptosis.

The apoptotic process is mediated by the *caspace* family of cysteine proteases. Caspaces are implicated both in the induction and execution of the death sentence. Caspaces mediate the protein fragmentation and the activation of DNAases in apoptotic cells by cleaving adjacent to aspartic acid residues in substrate proteins that affect cellular chromatin, cytoskeleton, and nuclear envelope. In the healthy cell, caspaces exist as inactive procaspace molecules.

Apoptosis can be induced by (1) activation of "death" receptors, like Fas, that recruit procaspase-8, via adaptor proteins, and promote its autocatalytic activation and (2) the release of cytochrome C from mitochondria by DNA-damaging drugs and other chemotherapeutic agents (Figure 7.13).

Ajoene, a garlic-derived natural compound, has been shown to induce apoptosis in leukemia cells in addition to other blood cells of leukemic patients. Ajoene induces apoptosis in human leukemic cells via stimulation of peroxide production and activation of nuclear factor κB. Ajoene also affects apoptosis by activation of caspase-3-like activity and caspase-8 activity in leukemic cell lines.

In summary, damage to the mitochondria (in this illustration) causes release of the protein Apaf-1 from their membrane as well as leakage of cytochrome C from the organelle. The released cytochrome C and Apaf-1 bind to molecules of caspase 9. The resulting complex of cytochrome C, Apaf-1, caspase 9, and ATP is called the apoptosome. Caspase is one of a family of over a dozen caspases. They are all proteases; they get their name because they cleave proteins, mostly each other, at aspartic acid (Asp) residues. Caspase 9 cleaves, and in so doing, activates other caspases. The sequential activation of one caspase by another creates an expanding cascade of proteolytic activity (similar to blood clotting) that leads to digestion of structural proteins in the cytoplasm, degradation of chromosomal DNA, and phagocytosis of the cell.

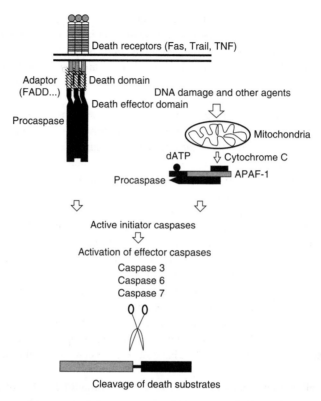

FIGURE 7.13 Activation of the caspase proteases during apoptosis. Caspases are implicated in both the induction and execution of the apoptotic process. Following the apoptotic stimuli, initiator caspases (caspase 8 or 9) are activated by autocatalysis. The initiator caspases then activate the effector caspases (caspase 3, 6, and 7), which are responsible for most of the protein cleavage during apoptosis. (From Szabo, C. (Ed.) (2000), *Cell Death: The Role of PARP*. With permission.)

TERATOGENESIS

From the time that man has been capable of leaving records, "monsters" resulting from biological malformations appear to have been of considerable interest. In early cave paintings, for example, monsters are frequently portrayed. Recent painters have also utilized this theme by using congenitally malformed models in their work (e.g., the painting of a phocomelic infant by the nineteenth-century Spanish painter Francisco de Goya, presently in the Louvre).

The condition of *phocomelia* was so rare prior to 1961 that no photographs were available and Goya's painting was used in medical texts for illustration. The term phocomelia is derived from the Greek words for "seal" and "limb." It is characterized by the hands or feet growing directly from the main joint—like the flippers of a seal.

Early attempts to explain congenital malformations followed two basic premises. Either they were of prophetic significance (a belief held by the Babylonians) or they were manifestations of the "wrath of God." A "modern" twist on this kind of thinking occurred in Iraq in 1965. In this situation, a mother and newborn child were put to death following a family "trial" since the infant was born with a well-developed "tail." The assertion was that the mother must have indulged in obscene sexual practices with a monkey.

In mammals, the first report of induction of congenital malformations *attributed* to extrinsic factors is a single observation in 1921. This report linked a dietary deficiency of a "fat-soluble factor" with rudimentary limb development in pigs (subsequently determined to be vitamin A; see below). It was not until 1929 that x-rays were proved to affect embryonic development.

Chemically related teratogenesis was not finally accepted until 1935, when anophthalmia (failure in eye development) was reported in piglets born to sows fed on a vitamin A–*deficient* diet throughout pregnancy. Further studies of teratogenesis followed in the 1940s, but it was not until 1948 that nitrogen mustard and trypan blue were implicated as positive chemical teratogens. Rubella had been identified as a teratogen in 1941.

In Chapter 2, the significance of the placental transfer of drugs from the maternal circulation into the fetus was discussed. At that time, the prototypic teratogen thalidomide was discussed along with several contemporary drugs such as alcohol and cocaine. By the time that thalidomide was finally removed from the market and the medicine cabinets, it had caused severe deformities in approximately 10,000 children in 46 countries.

Interestingly, almost 40 years after its removal from the market, thalidomide is experiencing a renewed interest in its clinical utility. On the basis of observations made in 1964 by an Israeli physician treating a leprosy patient with a painful condition known as erythema nodosum leprosum (ENL), thalidomide was used as a *sedative*; the drug alleviated the pain symptoms of this painful condition. Thalidomide has become the drug of choice for the treatment of ENL according to the World Health Organization. The company that holds the rights to thalidomide (Celgene) received approval to market the drug in 1998.

Thalidomide has also been reported to display efficacy in the treatment of advanced cases of multiple myeloma that are notorious for being resistant to chemotherapy. The prevailing hypothesis is that thalidomide possesses an antiangiogenesis capacity that can starve rapidly dividing cells from developing the additional blood supply that is necessary for their growth. Celgene has also provided the drug, under FDA approval, to treat more than 70 forms of cancer and various skin, digestive, and immunological disorders. It may also be useful in treating AIDS-associated cachexia (wasting).

In this section, we shall consider some of the underlying principles related to embryotoxicity. A teratogen is an agent that induces structural malformations, metabolic or physiological dysfunction, psychological or behavioral alterations, or deficits in the offspring, either at birth or manifested during the postnatal period. While it is known that approximately 25% of malformations are due to genetic transmission and chromosomal aberrations, the incidence of drug-induced teratogenic effects is not known with precision and estimates vary widely. However, because this toxic potentiality exists, teratogenic assessment of new drugs is required by all regulatory agencies around the world.

In order for a teratogen to express its toxicity, it must be administered at a sufficient dose to a genetically susceptible animal when the embryo is in a susceptible stage of development. Based on material presented in this chapter, the reader should already recognize the obvious implications of (1) the dose–response relationship as well as (2) the influence of an organism's genotype on drug toxicity. With regard to the latter, humans, monkeys, and rabbits appear to produce a toxic metabolite from thalidomide while other species, such as rat and mice, do not. This explains why screening for teratogenicity in the rat proved negative for thalidomide.

In humans, the period during which drugs can affect the morphological development of embryonic organs is relatively short. It is largely completed by the end of organogenesis (approximately 56 days following fertilization; Figure 7.14). The sequence of embryonic events during the period of organogenesis is such that each organ/system undergoes a critical state of differentiation during which it is sensitive to chemical toxicity (Table 7.6).

These periods of sensitivity are referred to as "toxic" or "target" windows. For example, the window for thalidomide in the human is as little as one dose between the 20th and 35th day of gestation. If a drug produces a toxic effect in the fertilized egg prior to differentiation beginning, the effect is usually all-or-none and the embryo fails to reach the differentiation stages.

Although new drugs are screened for teratogenicity, usually in two species, animal experiments give only an approximation of possible effects in humans. One of the reasons for this is that the period of gestation is contracted (e.g., 21 days in rat and mouse and 32 days in rabbit). Therefore, the "target Windows" for some organ systems in some species are sometimes no longer than a 24-h period.

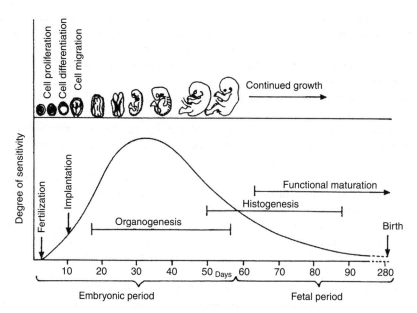

FIGURE 7.14 The stages of mammalian embryogenesis indicating the periods of greatest susceptibility to teratogens. From J.A. Timbrell (1991), *Principles of Biochemical Toxicology*, 2nd ed., London: Taylor & Francis. With permission).

TABLE 7.6

Comparison of Maximum Periods of Teratogenic Sensitivity for Various Organs/Systems in Humans

Organ/system	Days Following Fertilization
Brain	15–60
Eye	15–40
Genetalia	35–60
Heart	15–40
Limbs	25–35

Note: the period of susceptibility in humans occurs primarily in the first 60 days of pregnancy; a time when a woman would not necessarily be aware of her pregnancy.

The number of drugs reported to be teratogenic in *laboratory animals* approximates 1000. Therefore, a working hypothesis within the field is that all chemicals are capable of providing some embryotoxic effect under the appropriate conditions of dose, developmental stage, and species selection. The number of drugs generally considered to have teratogenic potential in *humans* is on the order of several dozen.

The teratogenic effects reported include a wide spectrum including bleeding problems, deafness, discoloration of teeth, masculinization of female offspring, and cleft palate. The major classes of drugs implicated include hormones (e.g., glucocorticoids and progestins with androgenic activity), folic acid antagonists, oral anticoagulants, antibiotics, alkylating anticancer agents, and anesthetic gases. Unfortunately, there are undoubtedly other more subtle toxic effects on brain development affecting intelligence, motor skills, and behavior that are more difficult to ascertain. However, recent data relating to subtle changes in intelligent quotients (IQs) in children exposed to cocaine *in utero* is alarming.

Using a meta analysis, a statistical procedure in which effects from differing studies are pooled to provide a better estimate of the effect size, a study of the effect of prenatal cocaine exposure on IQ was carried out. The investigators reported a decrease of 3.26 IQ points in the cocaine-exposed group. (For more details of study design, consult B.M. Lester, L.L. LaGasse, and R. Seifer, Cocaine exposure and children: the meaning of subtle effects, *Science*, 282, 633–622, 1998.) The societal cost of such children is difficult to assess since estimates of the number of cocaine-exposed children ranges from 45,000 to more than 375,000 per year in the United States. These figures predict that the number of children affected by this 3.26-point deficit in IQ is estimated to be between 1,688 and 14,062. The added costs of the special educational services required of this population has been estimated to be between $4 million and $35 million per year or more.

In response to concerns about the adverse effects of alcohol, the Congress of the United States passed the *Federal Beverage Labeling Act* of 1988. The law requires that all containers of alcoholic beverages display the following warning: **Government Warning**: *(1) According to the Surgeon General, women should not drink alcoholic beverages during pregnancy because of the risk of birth defects; and (2) Consumption of alcoholic beverages impairs your ability to drive a car or operate machinery and may cause health problems.* This legislation was in response to several reports during the 1970s that described a syndrome suitably titled as *fetal alcohol syndrome (FAS)*.

FAS is characterized by a triad of features: (1) pre-and/or postnatal growth deficiency; (2) specific pattern of craniofacial malformations; and (3) evidence of central nervous system dysfunction. Reports of at least two dozen autopsies have appeared in the literature, and they report a wide range of neuropathology. The CNS deficits of FAS appear to be long lasting, since recent studies have shown that they persist in young adults born with FAS, even if other symptoms such as growth retardation and facial characteristics have become diminished. Studies carried out during the 1990s indicate that implementation of the beverage warning label achieves only a *modest reduction* for underage drinkers (pregnant women under the age of 21; older pregnant women were even less aware of the label and gave it less heed).

FAS is now considered a leading cause of mental retardation in the general population. Figure 7.15 shows the comparison between brain growth spurt in humans and rats. It should be

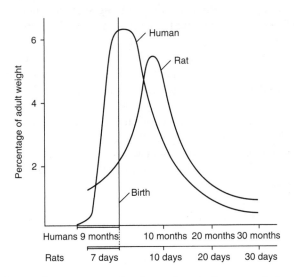

FIGURE 7.15   The brain growth spurt expressed as first-order velocity curves during development in humans and rats. Growth is measured as the percentage of adult weight. In humans, the brain growth spurt commences during early gestation, peaks around birth, and continues in early postnatal life. In rats, the growth curve ascends gradually during the latter part of gestation and peaks around the middle of the postweaning period. Unit scale: months in humans and days in rats. (From E.L. Abel, (Ed.) (1996), *Fetal Alcohol Syndrome: From Mechanism to Prevention*. Boca Raton. With permission.)

TABLE 7.7
CNS Depressants Associated with
Neonatal Withdrawal Syndrome

Opiates/narcotics Methadone
- Heroin
- Codeine
- Pentazocine (Talwin)
- Propoxyphene (Darvon)
- Other narcotics

Other drugs
- Alcohol
- Barbiturates
- Bromine
- Chlordiazepine (Librium)
- Diazepam (Valium)
- Diphenhydramine (Benadryl)
- Ethchlorvynol (Placidyl)

Source: E.L. Abel (Ed.) (1996) *Fetal Alcohol Syndrome: From Mechanism to Prevention.* Boca Raton, FL: CRC Press. Reprinted with permission.

noted that brain development characterized by accelerated synaptogenesis, neuronal proliferation, and myelination commences prenatally during the third trimester in humans and continues into early postnatal life.

It appears likely that the distinctive FAS facial dysmorphology is related to first trimester alcohol exposure. The clinical data is derived from cases of FAS in populations of women reporting heavy alcohol consumption during this period. This is alarming since a majority of women who abuse alcohol may not know they are pregnant for the first 4–6 weeks of gestation.

One of the particularly perplexing aspects of drug-induced teratogenesis is that it may not express itself for considerable time. Concern over subtle effects on brain development was indicated above since decrements in cognitive development can be difficult to discern and may not manifest themselves for decades. Other drug-induced teratogenic effects can also have a substantial latent period. During the 1950s, hormones were often given to pregnant women in an attempt to prevent premature labor. As mentioned previously, one of the agents used in this regard was the synthetic estrogenic compound *diethylstilbestrol* (DES). Following its use during this period, some daughters of treated mothers developed an increased incidence of cervical and vaginal carcinomas approximately 20 years later. An additional unfortunate aspect of the DES tragedy is that the drug did not prove efficacious in preventing miscarriages.

Drugs can also express nonteratogenic effects on delivery. This is particularly true if the mother has been exposed to CNS depressants of licit or illicit drugs. These types of drugs are particularly prone to produce withdrawal symptoms (Table 7.7).

RECENT TERATOGENS

During the 1980s, two drugs used to treat different types of skin diseases were found to be teratogenic. The drugs' generic names are *isotretoin* and *etretinate*, respectively, and are synthetic retinoids (i.e., derivatives of vitamin A). Isotretoin (Accutane) was prescribed for the treatment of acne while etretinate was prescribed for psoriasis.

Isotretoin was recognized as an animal teratogen before it was first marketed in September of 1982. It was, therefore classified as Category X, contraindicated for use during pregnancy. A statement to that effect was included in the package insert. All physicians did not heed this warning, however, and 9 months later, human teratogenicity was reported to the FDA in June 1983. By the late 1980s, approximately 78 babies were reported with birth defects.

Exposure to isotretoin during the first few weeks of exposure results in a characteristic group of birth defects; these include facial abnormalities such as missing ears, or ears developing below the chin, as well as cardiac and brain malformations. A prospective follow-up study revealed a relative risk of 25.6% for the defects associated with isotretoin embryopathy.

Human birth defects have also been observed after prenatal exposure to etretinate. Of particular significance in the case of this drug is that measurable serum concentrations have been documented more than 2 years after cessation of therapy. Suggesting a remarkable example of tissue sequestration. Therefore, the risk of teratogenicity may exist for an extended period of time.

THE BENDECTIN STORY

Although numerous drugs have been shown to have the capacity to induce teratogenic toxicity, there is an example of a drug falsely accused. In 1979, a report appeared in the literature estimating an 80% increase in the prevalence of congenital heart disease among children of women who *recalled* use in early pregnancy of Bendectin, an antinausea medication. Prior to this date, 10–25% of pregnant women were exposed to Bendectin, and over the years the drug was used in as many as 33 million pregnancies. The scientific evidence available pointed to the safety of Bendectin (the relative risk was calculated as being 0.89 with 95% confidence limits of 0.7 and 1.04).

In 1983, Merrell Dow Pharmaceuticals, Inc. voluntarily removed Bendectin from the market because of the many product liability suits pending. However, subsequent in-depth analysis of epidemiological and scientific data indicated that the therapeutic use of Bendectin had no measurable teratogenic effects. Nevertheless, despite the overwhelming scientific evidence, a number of jury decisions were rendered against the company (providing an argument for tort reform).

A generation of pregnant women has been *without* access to this highly effective drug. As a result, hospital admissions for excessive vomiting in pregnancy per thousand live births rose by 50% in 1984. An estimate of excess hospital costs attendant to these admissions over the years 1983–1987 was $73 million in the United States alone.

PREGNANCY CATEGORY

An attempt to develop a system of classifying drugs, according to their established risks, for use during pregnancy has been made. Category A: Controlled human studies have demonstrated no fetal risk. Category B: Animal studies indicate no fetal risk, but no human studies have been carried out. Category C: No adequate human or animal studies have been carried out. Category D: Evidence of fetal risk, but benefits outweigh risks. Category X: Evidence of fetal risk. Risks outweigh any benefits.

SELECTED BIBLIOGRAPHY

Abel, E.L. (Ed.) (1996) *Fetal Alcohol Syndrome*, Boca Raton, FL: CRC Press.

Aldridge, W.N. (1996) *Mechanisms and Concepts in Toxicology*, London: Taylor & Francis.

Brody, T.M., Larner, J., Minneman, K.P., and Neu, H.C. (Eds.) (1994) *Human Pharmacology: Molecular to Clinical*, 2nd ed., St. Louis: Mosby.

Ecobichon, D.J. (1997) *The Basis of Toxicity Testing*, 2nd ed., Boca Raton, FL: CRC Press.

Hardman, J.G., Limbird, L.L., and Gilman, A.G. (Eds.) (2001) *Goodman and Gillman's: The Pharmacological Basis of Therapeutics*, 10th ed., New York: McGraw-Hill.

Hollinger, M.A. and Giri, S.N. (1979) ^{14}C-thiourea binding in the rat lung, *Res. Commun. Chem. Pathol. Pharmacol.*, 26: 611.

Hollinger, M.A., Giri, S.N., and Hwang, F. (1976) Binding of radioactivity from ^{14}C-thiourea to rat lung protein, *Drug Metab. Dispos.*, 4: 121.

Johnstone, R.W., Ruefli, A.A., and Lowe, S.W. (2002) Apoptosis: a link between cancer genetics and chemotherapy, *Cell*, 108: 153–164.

Klassen, C.D. (Ed.) (2001) *Casarett and Doull's Toxicology: The Basic Science of Poisons*, 6th ed., New York: McGraw-Hill.

Niesink, R.J.M., De Vries, J., and Hollinger, M.A. (Eds.) (1996) *Toxicology: Principles and Applications*, Boca Raton, FL: CRC Press.

Raje, N. and Anderson, K. (1999) Thalidomide-A revival story, *New Eng. J. Med.*, 341: 1606–1609.

Rama Sastry, B.V. (Ed.) (1995) *Placental Toxicology*, Boca Raton, FL: CRC Press.

Rama Sastry, B.V. (Ed.) (1996) *Placental Pharmacology*, Boca Raton, FL: CRC Press.

Szabo, C. (Ed.) (2000) *Cell Death: The Role of PARP*, Boca Raton, FL: CRC Press.

Timbrell, J.A. (1991) *Principles of Biochemical Toxicology*, 2nd ed., London: Taylor & Francis.

QUESTIONS

1. Which of the following is generally credited with developing the early concept of the dose–response relationship?
   a. August Busch
   b. Paul Ehrlich
   c. Orafilla
   d. Paracelsus
   e. Oneacelsus

2 The type of allergic reaction most likely to cause death in humans is which of the following?
   a. Type I
   b. Type II
   c. Type III
   d. Type IV
   e. Type A

3. A chemical feature common to first generation antihistamine drugs is which of the following?
   a. Three benzene rings
   b. Halogenation
   c. Ethylamine side chain
   d. Sulfuration
   e. a and c

4. A "hapten" is which of the following?
   a. A serum protein that binds to a drug
   b. A plasma protein that binds to a drug
   c. A drug–lipid complex
   d. Twice a "hapfive"
   e. A drug or metabolite that binds to endogenous protein

5. Antihistamine drugs that block H_2 receptors are most effective against which of the following?
   a. Combining antigen with antibody
   b. Reducing acid indigestion

   c. Blocking release of leukotrienes from mast cells
   d. Relieving bronchiolar smooth muscle contraction
   e. Blocking release of histamine from mast cells

6. The type of antibodies (immunoglobulins) principally involved in type I drug-induced allergy is which of the following?
   a. IgA
   b. IgI
   c. IgG
   d. IgE
   e. IgK

7. Which of the following produces the most prompt alleviation of bronchoconstriction in the airway and hypotension that occurs in anaphylaxis?
   a. H_1 blockers
   b. H_2 blockers
   c. Epinephrine
   d. Leukotrienes
   e. Histamine

8. In humans, which of the following is the period of gestation when a fetus is most susceptible to a <u>teratogenic</u> effect?
   a. First trimester
   b. Second trimester
   c. Third trimester
   d. At implantation
   e. There is equal sensitivity throughout gestation

9. Subchronic administration of a test drug to animals generally involves which of the following?
   a. Repeated daily injections for less than a month
   b. Repeated daily injections for more than 3 months
   c. Repeated daily injections for 1–3 months
   d. Weekly injections for less than 3 months
   e. Weekly injections for 1–3 months

10. Drug X has an ED_{50} of 10 mg/kg and an LD_{50} of 10 g/kg. Which of the following is its TI (therapeutic index)?
   a. 0.1
   b. 1.0
   c. 10.0
   d. 100.0
   e. 1000.0

8 Treating Drug Toxicity

BACKGROUND

As indicated in the preceding chapter, the exact incidence of drug side effects is not known with certainty. However, we do know that among the millions of cases of human poisonings, pharmaceuticals are most frequently involved in fatalities. According to the 1998 Annual Report of the *American Association of Poison Control Centers Toxic Exposure Surveillance System*, analgesics, antidepressants, stimulants, street drugs, cardiovascular drugs, and sedative/hypnotics/antipsychotics were responsible for 264, 152, 118, 118, and 89 deaths, respectively. Most of the people who die are adults, and the deaths often result from intentional rather than accidental exposure.

Ingestion is the most likely route of exposure for human poisoning occurring in 75% of the cases. *Accidental* ingestion is most likely in children under the age of 5 (60%) while *intentional* ingestion is most likely between 18–64 years (6.2%) and 13–17 years (2.2%). Fifty to sixty percent of intentional poisonings in adults are poly-drug exposures.

ASPIRIN

The pattern of drug ingestion hazards parallel the substances required to have child-resistant closures by the *Poison Prevention Packaging Act* (PPPA) of 1970. Before 1972, aspirin was the drug most frequently associated with childhood poisoning, a fact that contributed to the passage of the PPPA. Under the provisions of the act, regulations were issued that require special child-resistant packaging for any aspirin-containing preparations for human use in a dosage intended for oral administration. The regulation also covered liquid preparations containing more than 5% by weight of methyl salicylate, other than those packaged in pressurized spray containers.

The special packaging regulations were devised to protect children less than 5 years of age from serious personal injury or illness resulting from handling, using, or ingesting dangerous drugs. The law required vendors to follow a specific protocol to test the special packaging for its effectiveness with children as well as adults. The child-resistant effectiveness is required to be not less than 85% without a demonstration and not less than 80% after a demonstration of the proper means of opening the package. Adult-use effectiveness is also required, being not less than 90%.

Analyzing the number of aspirin associated deaths after implementation of the program can assess the effectiveness of the program. Between 1972 and 1989, the total number of deaths in the children under 5 years of age category, as a result of aspirin intoxication, decreased from 46 to 2. It has been estimated that a total of 500–620 child deaths have been saved since the PPPA went into effect, from the early 1970s through 1989. Remarkably, there were *no* reported childhood deaths due to aspirin in 1998.

IRON SUPPLEMENTS

The most likely cause of unintentional pediatric fatalities reported between 1983 and 1990 was iron supplements, representing approximately 30% of all deaths (16 of 53). From 1986 to 1995, over 110,000 such pediatric incidents were reported, including 33 deaths. The children who died had swallowed as few as 5 to as many as 98 tablets. Antidepressants represented an additional 18.9% (10 of 53) of fatalities in the pediatric population between 1983 and 1990.

Iron is an essential nutrient that is sometimes lacking in people's diets. For that reason, physicians often recommend iron for people with certain health conditions, such as *iron deficiency anemia*. Some iron products are available without a prescription, either as single-ingredient iron pills or in combination with vitamins or other minerals, including pediatric vitamins with iron. Drugs that contain iron and folic acid are available by prescription and are principally used by women during pregnancy.

Two-year olds account for the majority (53.7%) of ingestions of prescription drugs. Once again, the most frequently ingested is ferrous sulfate. In more than 75% of cases surveyed, nonchild resistant packages or no containers at all were involved in the ingestion. Although parent's prescriptions account for approximately 54% of the ingestions, nearly 30% involve grandparent's medications. Factors responsible for the ineffectiveness of child resistant closures include consumer noncompliance and violations of the Act by the dispensing pharmacist.

The Food and Drug Administration (FDA) has proposed that manufacturers be required to wrap high-potency iron tablets and capsules individually, such as in blister packaging—the type that makes it necessary to punch out each tablet or dosage unit. The FDA believes that the time and dexterity needed to remove tablets from unit-dose packaging would discourage a youngster, or at least limit the number of tablets a child would swallow. The unit-dose packaging requirement would apply to products that contain 30 mg or more iron per dosage unit.

AGE-RELATED DRUG POISONING

Statistics on poisoning deaths vary greatly: *The Poison Prevention Week Council* (PPWC) estimates that adults place one million phone calls yearly for help with childhood poisonings; *Poison Control Centers* (PCC) reported 2.2 million poison exposures in 2000 (of these, 52.7% occurred in children younger than 6; in 1999, national vital statistics databases recorded 19,741 poisoning deaths in adults and children; PCC reported 920 deaths in 2000.

One of the problems in reporting poisoning is that each PCC has its own telephone number. This issue was simplified on January 30, 2002, with the launch of a national toll-free poison control phone number: (800) 222-1222. The number automatically connects the caller to his or her local PCC, 24 h a day, 7 days a week.

Intentional poisoning in *adolescents* (11–17 years of age) is one of the ten leading causes of death and loss of productive years of life in the United States. Alcohol use and abuse obviously play a large role in fatal injuries in this age group. However, drug-related fatalities following the use of *antidepressants* represented nearly one-half of those reported between 1989 and 1991.

It has been estimated that adult aspirin poisonings are approximately 10% accidental, about 10% *planned* suicides, and approximately 80% *impulsive* suicidal gestures. The fatal toxic dose is generally in the range of 20–30 g (60–90 adult tablets) in reported cases. Much larger amounts have been ingested without fatality, however, and the potency varies with the specific preparation. The pharmacodynamics also changes somewhat with the use of enteric-coated tablets, which delays absorption. The degree of intoxication varies with the serum salicylate level. The lethal blood concentration of salicylate is approximately 500 mg/kg/24 h for 2 or more days.

Poisoning in the *geriatric population* is an ongoing public health concern. In the majority of patients older than 64 years of age, accidental poisoning due to dementia and confusion, improper use or storage of a product, and therapeutic errors is the rule. However, approximately one in ten is intentional with suicidal intent. Interestingly, elderly females are approximately three times more likely to commit suicide with drugs than males (who prefer carbon monoxide—running their car in the garage).

As mentioned previously, there are a number of theoretical changes that can occur in the elderly that influence a drug's pharmacokinetics. For aspirin, the two most important alterations in pharmacokinetics that accompany aging are decreases in serum albumin and a decreased glomerular filtration rate. Following absorption, aspirin rapidly deacetylates to salicylate, its circulating form, and is predominantly (80–90%) bound to albumin. Circulating albumin concentrations decrease with age. Therefore, in the presence of other drugs that can displace salicylate or a high initial dose, the binding

TABLE 8.1

Various Therapies Provided in Human Drug Exposure Cases

Initial decontamination	Specific antidote administration
Dilution	Naloxone
Irrigation/washing	*N*-acetylcysteine (oral)
Activated charcoal	Atropine
Cathartic	Deferoxamine
Ipecac syrup	Ethanol
Gastric lavage	Hydroxocobalamin
Other emetic	*N*-acetylcysteine (IV)
Measures to enhance elimination	Pralidoxime (2-PAM)
Alkalinization (with or without diuresis)	Fab fragment
Hemodialysis	Pyridoxine
Forced diuresis	Dimercaprol (BAL)
Hemoperfusion (charcoal)	Methylene blue
Exchange transfusion	Cyanide antidote kit
Acidification (with or without diuresis)	EDTA
Hemoperfusion (resin)	Penicillamine
Peritoneal dialysis	

Each category in decreasing frequency of use.

capacity of albumin can be exceeded, thus contributing to elevated free blood levels (see Chapter 4). Probably of more significance is the association of decreased creatinine clearance (kidney function) with aging. On the average, the elimination time of salicylate in healthy elderly people, mean age 77 years, is 1.5 times the rate of younger people with a mean age of 21 years.

MANAGEMENT TRENDS

The principle therapies employed for the treatment of drug overdose/toxicity are shown in Table 8.1. They can be divided into three major categories: (1) initial decontamination; (2) measures to enhance elimination; and (3) specific antidotes. During the past several years, there has been a change in emphasis within some of these categories. In any event, they are all used within the broader context of appropriate supportive care.

INITIAL DECONTAMINATION

Concerned parents who attempt to purchase nonprescription poison control products soon discover that the range of possibilities is quite restricted. *Syrup of ipecac* was once recommended for every household with young children but recently has fallen into disfavor. Activated charcoal is an effective nonprescription poison adsorbent, but is typically not displayed prominently in retail pharmacies.

During the period from 1983 to 1991, there occurred a continual decline in the use of syrup of *ipecac* to induce *emesis*; this decline was accelerated in 2004 by the burgeoning evidence of widespread abuse of ipecac by people with *anorexia and bulimia*. The ability of ipecac to induce vomiting in the poisoned patient has been thought to limit the extent of toxin absorption. An FDA advisory panel recommended its approval for this use in 1982 and confirmed this recommendation in a 1985 publication. However, a serious challenge to ipecac appeared in the journal *Pediatrics* in 2003 in a paper entitled, "*Home syrup of ipecac use does not reduce emergency department use or improve outcome*." The author researched poisonings in children younger than 6 in 2000 and 2001, as reported to the *American Association of Poison Control Centers, Toxic Exposures Surveillance System Database*. In comparing those who ingested ipecac to those who did not, he found that administration of ipecac did not affect referral to an emergency department, nor did it affect the rate of adverse outcomes.

In the same issue of *Pediatrics* (November, 2003), the *American Academy of Pediatrics* (AAP) Committee on injury, violence, and poison prevention issued a policy statement on poison treatment in the home. It discussed AAP's past recommendation that households with young children keep a 1-oz bottle of syrup of ipecac in the home to be used only on the advice of a physician or poison control center. In light of the 2003 paper, the AAP updated its policy, *recommending against keeping ipecac in the home, further recommending that ipecac presently in the home be disposed of safely.* It cited several reasons for this change in policy:

- Ipecac does not completely remove a toxin from the stomach; in addition, tablets often remain in the stomach after a bout of ipecac-induced vomiting.
- Adverse effects of ipecac include persistent vomiting, lethargy, and diarrhea. Lethargy can complicate assessment of patients who ingest sedative medications.
- Ipecac is mistakenly given to 61% of children who ingest nontoxic substances because their parents or caregivers fail to call a health care professional prior to administration.
- Persistent ipecac-induced vomiting may cause patients to expel needed interventions, such as activated charcoal, *N*-acetylcysteine, or whole-bowel irrigations.
- Ipecac is abused by people with eating disorders and by child caregivers with *Munchausen syndrome* by proxy (a situation where children are intentionally injured or poisoned). The cause of death of musician *Karen Carpenter*, thought for years to be anorexia nervosa, is listed as *emetine* cardiotoxicity on her death certificate due to chronic ingestion of ipecac.

Ipecac contains a number of plant alkaloids, including emetine. It induces emesis through stimulation of the *chemoreceptor trigger zone* in the brain and local irritation of the gastrointestinal tract. The latency period for the induction of emesis by ipecac ranges from approximately 5–20 min, with a single dose successfully inducing vomiting in approximately 85% of patients. Contraindications for the use of ipecac include the presence of coma or convulsions, the ingestion of corrosive substances, and an impaired gag reflex.

While ipecac has been decreasing in popularity in emergency rooms, there has occurred a corresponding increase in the use of *activated charcoal* (AC) to *adsorb* the drug onto the surface of the charcoal. AC is an inert, nonabsorbable, odorless, tasteless, fine black powder that has a high adsorptive capacity (i.e., high surface area). When AC is administered after emesis or lavage, it binds residual drug within the lumen of the gastrointestinal tract and reduces its absorption. A cathartic can be coadministered with AC to prevent constipation.

Normally, AC is mixed with water and administered orally or by nasogastric tube. For optimal binding, a charcoal:drug ratio of 10:1 is recommended. The success with which AC prevents absorption depends on the nature of the drug as well as the time between ingestion and administration of AC. With regard to the latter factor, simultaneous administration of AC with aspirin results in nearly 60% being adsorbed, while a 3-h delay achieves only 9% of the drug being adsorbed.

While the FDA has approved activated charcoal for the treatment of poisoning as an adsorbent agent, the AAP has stopped short of recommending its routine use in the home for the following reasons:

- It is poorly accepted by pediatric patients because of its black color and unpleasant, gritty taste (in emergency rooms, it is usually given via nasogastric tube).
- As a result of long-term storage, particles settle into dense cakes that fail to resuspend with normal efforts when shaking the bottle. Parents may unknowingly give a dose that is mostly vehicle, assuming that it will be effective.
- It is often vomited and stains linens and surface.
- Routine stocking activated at home may lead to inappropriate use.

ENHANCED ELIMINATION

Most techniques used for enhancing the elimination of drugs from the body utilize facilitated *renal* excretion or *extracorporeal* (outside of the body) techniques. Attempts to increase renal excretion of a drug will be successful only if that drug is substantially excreted via the kidneys to a significant extent. Unfortunately, there are relatively few drugs that have significant renal excretion following an acute overdose. Among the drugs that can be managed in this way are the weak acids phenobarbital and acetylsalicylic acid, the weak bases phencyclidine and amphetamine, as well as the ion lithium.

Enhanced renal excretion is usually achieved by *fluid diuresis* in which excess fluid is administered to increase urine flow. Forced diuresis is generally reserved for cases of mild to moderate severity. In some cases, fluid diuresis is supplemented by *ionized diuresis* (discussed previously in Chapter 3). By the appropriate raising or lowering of urine pH, the degree of ionization of acidic and basic drugs, respectively, is increased, and they can be "trapped" in the urine.

Extracorporeal strategies for treating drug overdose include *dialysis* and *hemoperfusion*. Dialysis is usually carried out on blood (*hemodialysis*) while *peritoneal dialysis* is used infrequently. For hemodialysis to be effective, the dialyzing membrane must be permeable to the drug and the drug should equilibrate rapidly between the circulating plasma and the dialysis fluid. Hemodialysis and hemoperfusion are usually reserved for cases of *severe* drug intoxication (e.g., deep and prolonged coma), ingestion of known lethal doses, or the presence of lethal blood concentrations of the drug. Table 8.2 lists some of the drugs that have been treated with hemodialysis and hemoperfusion in drug overdose.

It should be kept in mind that these procedures are invasive, requiring cannulation of a large vessel (usually the femoral vein), systemic anticoagulation, and pumping the blood through a dialysis machine. Complications can include laceration of the cannulated vessel, air embolism, hypovolemia, and thrombocytopenia (depletion of platelets). It should also be pointed out that neither of these procedures is effective for drugs with a high degree of tissue binding (i.e., a large volume of distribution).

Generally, hemodialysis is easier to perform and is associated with fewer complications. It is ideal for low molecular weight, polar, water-soluble molecules such as alcohol, salicylate, or lithium. Hemoperfusion is used for drugs that are poorly soluble in water or relatively higher in protein binding.

Hemoperfusion differs from hemodialysis in that the blood is passed over a resin or charcoal column. The drug becomes bound to the column and the "clean" blood returned to the body. Hemoperfusion units have adsorptive surface areas of *several thousand square meters* while hemodialysis devices have an effective dialysis surface limited to *several square meters*. Obviously, relatively sophisticated technology is required for these procedures and there is the need to prevent clotting in the perfusion circuit, which can produce complications.

TABLE 8.2

Hemodialysis (HD) and Hemoperfusion (HP) in Drug Overdose

Carbamazepine—HP preferred

Ethylene glycol, Methanol—HD preferred

Lithium—HP not effective

Theophylline—both HP and HD are effective

Salicylates—HD indicated for acute overdose

Valproic acid—HD preferred

Source: Adapted from K. R. Olson and B. Roth, *Update on Management of Patient with Poisoning or Drug Overdose*, American College of Chest Physicians, with permission.

ANTIDOTAL THERAPY

Attempts to counteract the effects of poison were undoubtedly being made long before the start of recorded history. It is likely that the earliest method used was to try and empty the stomach of the afflicted individual before too much poison had been absorbed, usually by making the patient vomit, often from exposure to unpleasant smells or the administration of a nauseous substance.

As times progressed, many people of nobility were dying as a result of the deliberate administration of poison, which resulted in the rich and powerful living in constant fear of being murdered by this method. This fear led to the utilization of food tasters and also created a demand for something that would not only cure someone who had been poisoned, but that could be taken as a prophylactic to stop poisons being effective.

In the past, accidental poisoning was much commoner than it is today. The risk of being bitten or stung by a venomous or rabid animal could not easily be dismissed, and there was also the possibility of inadvertently eating poisonous berries, roots, or herbs. Early vegetable poisons, sometimes used medicinally, such as henbane, mandrake, aconite, opium, and cannabis, and available mineral poisons including arsenic trisulfide, mercuric sulfide, and lead monoxide, could also be used with intent to kill. Animal poisons included toads and salamanders. The need to combat such poisons led to the demand for antidotes.

By far, the greatest number of antidotes in use before 1800 was herbal, either singly or in combination, sometimes including a very small proportion of animal and/or mineral ingredients. Few antidotes were for particular poisons because orthodox doctors practiced *humoral* medicine—which treated symptoms rather than specific conditions. This meant that most herbs were used for several different complaints. One of the most popular herbs of the day was *garden rue*. When its seeds were taken with wine it was believed to be an antidote against "all dangerous medicines or deadly poisons."

Humoral medicine was based on early Greek manuscripts formerly believed to have been written by Hippocrates in the fifth century BC, but now accepted as the work of several authors, and known as the *Hippocratic corpus*. The doctrine of the four humours stated that the human body consisted of *blood, phlegm, yellow bile, and black bile*. If these were in correct proportions in strength and quantity, the body was healthy, much like the "vital bodily fluids" in *Dr. Strangelove*.

The four humours were associated with the heart, brain, liver, and spleen. In each individual, every part of the body had a unique natural combination of these humours. Because this balance was different for every person, it was necessary for the physician to determine the patient's normal humoural condition before he could assess the changes that caused the illness.

Medicines had qualities that corresponded to the humors of the body, and to correct a bodily imbalance, a medicine that had the opposite characteristics was employed. For example, a hot, dry drug would be used to counteract a phlegmatic (cold, moist) condition.

By the eighteenth century, dispensaries (pharmacies) still described therapeutic effects in humoural terms; but the goal was always the same. Superfluous humours were often eliminated by *bloodletting*. Probably the most common method was to open a vein with a lancet (a small sharp knife). The blood that flowed from the small cut was collected and measured; the vein being closed when the necessary amount had been taken. The blood was usually taken from one of three veins in the arm, *the cephalic, the median, or the basilica*, but sometimes a vein in the forehead or under the tongue (ouch!) was used.

As an alternative to opening a vein, *cupping* could be employed. In wet cupping, the skin was scarified by using a spring operated "scarificator," which usually had 1, 4, 10, or 12 blades that could be adjusted by a screw to vary the depth of the cuts. A previously heated cupping glass was then applied over the area, and as it cooled, the vacuum created drew blood from the cuts. By the late-eighteenth century, glasses fitted with a valve were made so that the vacuum could be created by using a piston syringe. Blood could also be extracted by leeching, as described in section one.

Another common method of expelling corrupt or excessive humours was by purging. Some laxatives were used for specific humours. *Clysters* (enemas) could be administered instead of laxatives to empty the bowel. Originally made from a pig's bladder attached to a wooden pipe, subsequent variations consisted of a pewter syringe of one-pint capacity terminating in a straight or curved rectal pipe. The nature of the enema could be very simple, such as a solution of milk and sugar, or a complex of more than a dozen ingredients. Tobacco smoke was also used—said to be particularly efficacious for "obstinate" constipation.

As mentioned above, herbs were often mixed together (a precursor to polypharmacy). Like today, that practice is based on the belief that mixing several remedies that are each effective against one poison would produce an antidote that would offer protection against all of them; some preparations contained >70 ingredients.

Although the number of medicines prepared from animals today is relatively small, this has not always been the case. Many of these antidotes appear strange to us now as the following examples illustrate:

- *Blood of animals*. Several ancient antidotes contained the blood of one or more types of animal, including geese, ducks, goats, hares, sea-turtles, and dogs.
- *Vipers*. Vipers were highly valued as an antidote for both venoms and poisons. To treat the bite of a viper, Galen recommended cutting off its head and applying the bloody part to the wound to induce healing. It was also suggested that dried, powdered serpent flesh taken in wine or broth could serve as a counter-poison, particularly for the bites of serpents or other venomous beasts. Viper wine was also used. It was recommended that live female vipers gathered in springtime should be used in its preparation. Viper fat was carried by English viper catchers to anoint any bites as soon as possible, repeating this every hour or less. Vipers were used to treat many other conditions, including leprosy, elephantiasis, barrenness, and plague.
- *Bone of a stag's heart (actually an ossified artery)*. Stag's were believed to hunt snakes by pushing their nostrils into snake holes and sniffing to draw them out. Stags that had been bitten by vipers would then eat the snakes. This was thought to counteract the effect of the venom and prove restorative to the animal. "Bones" beaten into powder could be taken internally and were an ingredient in the seventeenth century. Dr. John Hall, Shakespeare's son-in-law, used this preparation as part of his treatment for a patient who was suffering from "Wind in the Womb."
- *Unicorn's horn*. The unicorn was a mythical beast with a single horn in the middle of its forehead. Belief of the unicorn's existence lasted into the eighteenth century. Eventually, it was discovered that it was the tusk of a narwhal that was used in medicinal preparations. It was usually used in the form of a jelly, but the horn could also be made into a drinking vessel. It was believed that to drink water or wine from one of these tusks, just before or after taking poison, could nullify the effects of the poison; of course, only the very rich could afford to possess such a tusk.

DECLINE IN THE USE OF ANCIENT ANTIDOTES

By the middle of the eighteenth century, the belief in the efficacy of many of these antidotes was declining. The second half of the century saw the introduction of scientific experimentation to determine the effectiveness of the old antidotes, leading to toxicology becoming a science. The publication of the Spaniard Orfila's *Traité des Poisons Tirés des Régnes, Minéral, Végétal et Animal ou Toxicologie Général* in 1815 effectively ended the use of most traditional antidotes. Nowadays, most antidotes are used for specific poisons or groups of poisons.

MODERN ANTIDOTES

Naloxone is a modern drug structurally related to the opioid class of analgesics such as morphine. Naloxone is a drug used to counter the effects of opioid overdose, for example, heroin and morphine.

Specifically, naloxone is used in opioid overdoses for countering life-threatening depression of the central nervous system and the respiratory system. Naloxone has virtually no intrinsic activity but can compete for opioid receptors. By reversibly competing for the μ (primarily) and κ opioid receptors in the brain and spinal cord, it can reverse the sedation and respiratory depression associated with an overdose of morphine-like drugs.

In an emergency setting, naloxone is usually injected intravenously for fastest action. Naloxone has also been distributed as a component of emergency kits to heroin users; this has been shown to reduce rates of fatal overdose. Projects of this type are underway in San Francisco, Chicago, and Scotland.

While Naloxone is still often used in emergency treatments for opioid overdose, its clinical use in the long-term treatment of opioid addiction is increasingly superseded by naltrexone. Naltrexone is structurally similar to naloxone but has a slightly increased affinity for μ receptors over Naloxone; it can be administered orally and has a longer duration of action.

One of the most important relatively new developments in the field of antidotes has been the application of *N*-acetylcysteine. This sulfhydryl-containing compound is specifically used in drug toxicity cases (e.g., acetaminophen) in which an electrophilic drug metabolite (one that seeks electrons to interact with) binds to critical cellular macromolecules after saturating intracellular GSH pools (discussed in Chapter 7). By providing exogenous SH groups for electrophilic attack, endogenous sites are protected.

In adults, *Hepatotoxicity* may occur after ingestion of a single large dose of acetaminophen (10–15 g); doses of 20–25 g or more are potentially fatal. Acetaminophen bottles currently recommend that adults take no more than 4 g a day, or eight extra-strength pills. Severe liver damage occurs in 90% of patients with plasma concentrations of acetaminophen in excess of 300 μg/mL at 4 h or 45 μg/mL at 15 h after ingestion of the drug. The FDA warned in 2003 that more than 56,000 emergency-room visits a year are due to acetaminophen overdoses and that 100 people die annually from unintentionally taking too much, making acetaminophen the leading cause of acute liver failure. Administration of *N*-acetylcysteine is recommended if less than 36 h has elapsed since ingestion of acetaminophen, although the antidote is most effective if administered within 10 h.

As mentioned previously, one of the major sources of pediatric drug poisoning relates to the ingestion of maternal iron preparations taken for the treatment of iron deficiency anemias. An agent useful in the treatment of iron poisoning is the drug *deferoxamine*. This particular drug is a member of an antidotal class of drugs known as *chelating agents* (from the Greek Chele, meaning crab's claw).

Chelating agents act by forming *stable complexes* with inorganic ions. There are naturally occurring chelators in the body, such as hemoglobin, which complex with iron. The therapeutic use of exogenous chelating agents is based on their differential tendency to form various chelate complexes. In essence, each chelating compound has a stability constant for each inorganic ion. Fortunately, the chelating constant of hemoglobin for iron, for example, is greater than that of deferoxamine. Therefore, when deferoxamine is used clinically, it preferentially removes excess iron without disrupting biologically indispensable iron complexes.

Another novel antidotal strategy is the development of *antibody fragments* to certain drugs. For example, treatment of life-threatening digoxin (a drug used to treat certain cardiovascular problems; see Chapter 12) intoxication with digoxin-specific Fab antibody fragments has been found to be useful. Patients with life-threatening digoxin poisoning who receive intravenous digoxin antibody fragments demonstrate an immediate decrease in free digoxin serum concentrations due to binding to the antibody fragment, and favorable changes in cardiac arrhymias within 30 min of administration. This area of research will hopefully prove fruitful for the future development of similar strategies for other drugs.

In 1995, scientists at Scripps Research Institute reported the development of a "vaccine" that elicits antibodies to cocaine. The nature of the antigen is a cocaine analog bound covalently to a

TABLE 8.3
Comparative Serum Concentrations of Drugs at
Therapeutic and Toxic Levels*

Drug	Therapeutic	Toxic
Digoxin	0.0010–0.0022	>0.0025
Diphenylhydantoin	10–20	>25
Phenobarbital	15–30	>40
Procainamide	4–8	>10
Theophylline	10–20	>20

* mg/mL.

protein with a Monty Python-like name, keyhole limpet hemocyanin. Administration of the complex resulted in a reduction of the psychoactive response to subsequently administered cocaine. In experiments in rats, the antibodies bound cocaine in the bloodstream and prevented the drug from crossing the blood-brain barrier. A potential clinical application would be to immunize cocaine abusers trying to abstain from the drug. However, because of the short duration of these foreign antibodies in the body and the fundamental behavioral pathology of drug addiction, immunization may have greater benefit in treating cocaine overdose rather than treating drug addiction itself.

TOXICOLOGICAL TESTING

Toxicological testing of blood, urine, and gastric contents is frequently ordered for patients with suspected drug overdoses. In view of the fact that 10–15 drugs account for more than 90% of all drug overdoses, most clinical laboratories limit the number of drugs tested to the common drugs of abuse and therapeutic agents. These include alcohols, barbiturates/sedatives, antiepileptics, benzodiazepines, antihistamines, antidepressants, antipsychotics, stimulants, narcotics, cardiovascular drugs, and OTC analgesics. A comparison of therapeutic and toxic serum levels of selected drugs is shown in Table 8.3. As can be seen, in certain cases the differences can be relatively small.

A toxicology screen utilizes various methodologies to identify and quantify the drugs most frequently used or abused by the poisoned patient. Drug quantitation in serum is used to monitor the course of the patient, to diagnose whether toxicity is occurring, but not yet clinically apparent, to establish a prognosis, and to determine if extreme methods of drug elimination will be necessary.

ROLE OF THE POISON CONTROL CENTER

There are over 100 regional poison centers in the United States that are members of, or are certified by, the *American Association of Poison Control Centers*. Poison control centers serve several functions including (1) providing expert information and consultation to the public and health professionals; (2) providing public education programs; (3) providing regional professional education programs; (4) interacting with care providers and analytical toxicology laboratories to improve the management of the poisoned patient; and (5) collecting data on poisonings.

Most of the calls received by poison control centers are managed by poison information specialists who are registered nurses, pharmacists, or other health-related professionals. In general, when a poison control center is called regarding drug ingestion, it will want to know the following: (1) the type of ingested drug; (2) the age of the victim; (3) the estimated dose and time taken; and (4) the victim's condition.

SELECTED BIBLIOGRAPHY

Dolgin, J.G. (2001) Human clinical toxicology, in *CRC Handbook of Toxicology*, 2nd ed., Derelanko, M. and Hollinger, M.A. (Eds), pp. 957–999, Boca Raton: CRC Press.

Kalant, H. and Roschlau, W.H.E. (1989) (Eds), *Principles of Medical Pharmacology*, 5th ed., Toronto: B.C. Decker.

Litovitz, T.L., Klein-Schwartz, W., Caravatti, E.M., Youniss, J., Crouch, B., and Lee, S. (1999) 1998 Annual report of the American association of poison control centers toxic exposure surveillance system, *Am. J. Emerg. Med.*, 17: 435–487.

Melmon, K.L., Morrelli, H.F., Hoffman, B.B., and Nierenberg, D.W. (1992) (Eds) *Clinical Pharmacology Basic Principles in Therapeutics*, 3rd ed., New York: McGraw-Hill.

Rawcliffe, C. (1995) Ideas about the body, *in Medicine and Society in Later Medieval England*, Sutton Publishing, pp. 29–57.

QUESTIONS

1. Which of the following is/are most frequently associated with pediatric drug poisoning?
   a. Iron supplements
   b. Birth Control pills and c above
   c. Vitamin C
   d. a and b above
   e. All of the above

2. With regard to aspirin poisoning, which of the following is/are true?
   a. Some are accidental
   b. Some are planned suicides
   c. Some are impulsive suicide gestures
   d. The fatal dose is in the range of 2–3 g
   e. a, b, and c above

3. Which of the following is/are employed for the treatment of drug overdose?
   a. Specific antidotes
   b. Measures to enhance elimination
   c. Measures to enhance metabolism
   d. a and b above
   e. All of the above

4. Which of the following is/are true regarding initial decontamination treatment in drug poisoning over the past 10–15 years?
   a. There has been an increase in the use of ipecac
   b. There has been a decrease in the use of ipecac
   c. There has been an increase in the use of activated charcoal
   d. There has been a decrease in the use of activated charcoal
   e. b and c above

5. Which of the following is/are extracorporeal treatments for drug overdose?
   a. Ionized diuresis
   b. Hemodialysis
   c. Retrograde iontophoresis
   d. Hemoperfusion
   e. b and d above

6. Which of the following is/are considered antidotal treatments?
   a. Deferoxamine
   b. Naloxone
   c. *N*-acetylcysteine
   d. Antibody fragments
   e. All of the above

7. Chelating agents act by which of the following antidotal mechanisms?
   a. Enhancing glomerular filtration rate
   b. Providing increased levels of SH groups
   c. Decreasing renal reabsorption
   d. Increasing hepatic P450
   e. Forming stable complexes with inorganic ions

8. Which of the following is/are true with regard to most laboratory testing for drugs?
   a. They are required to test for at least 100
   b. They are required to test for at least 200
   c. They usually test for about 10–15
   d. They usually test for about 3
   e. None of the above

9. *N*-acetylcysteine is useful in which of the following drug overdoses?
   a. Aspirin
   b. Deferoxamine
   c. Acetaminophen
   d. Digoxin
   e. a and c above

10. Antibody fragments are a provocative relatively new method to deal with which of the following drug poisoning?
    a. Acetaminophen
    b. Morphine
    c. Aspirin
    d. Antidepressants
    e. Digoxin

Part III

Drugs That Replace, Cure, or Treat Symptoms

9 Hormones

BACKGROUND

Regulation of the body's homeostasis is partially under the control of the *endocrine system*. This is a system whereby specialized tissues or glands elaborate hormones (from the Greek *"to urge on"*) into the blood stream for distribution within the body where they regulate organ and cellular function in a *"feedback"* relationship. Without this constant feedback, the human body would be a disorganized mob of 50 trillion cells. Endocrine transmission is relatively slow and diffuse. In comparison, neuronal transmission is rapid and discrete; sometimes delivering a specific signal to an individual cell.

The modern history of endocrine research can be traced back to *Claude Bernard's* introduction of the term *"milieu interieur."* A notable advance in endocrine research was initiated by the invention of radioimmunoassay by Berson and Yalow in 1967. However, to understand how low concentrations of circulating hormones affect the function of their target cells, the equally important concept of cell surface receptors was introduced, together with the idea of signal transducers that transmit the information from the receptors to the cell interior. Much of our current understanding of cellular biochemistry and cell physiology result from the significant expansion of research stemming from these early endocrine and metabolic studies.

Hormones are exceptionally potent chemicals that operate at concentrations so low that they can be measured only by the most sensitive analytical methods. Their concentrations are typically expressed as parts per trillion, one thousand times lower than parts per billion. This magnitude of dilution can be dramatized by thinking of a drop of gin dissolved in a train of tank cars containing tonic. It has been calculated that one drop in 660 tank cars would approximate one part in a trillion; such a train would be six miles long.

The hypothalamus-pituitary, thyroid, parathyroid, pancreas, adrenals, ovary, and testes are considered to be the principle endocrine glands producing hormones. A more complete list of the major endocrine hormones and their primary gland of origin is shown in Table 9.1.

As indicated in Table 9.1, the endocrine hormones can be divided into two major chemical classes: (1) the peptides and amino acid derivatives and (2) the cholesterol-based steroid compounds. In general, the former are believed to interact primarily with membrane-associated receptors while the latter are more lipophilic and are able to gain entrance into target cells. In any event, overactive or underactive endocrine glands may produce syndromes that require treatment with drugs, and/or surgery, or hormone replacement, respectively.

Hormones can be exploited for a variety of therapeutic and diagnostic purposes. However, when considering the clinical applications of hormones, one usually thinks first of their use in replacement therapy. It is the latter aspect of endocrine pharmacology that this chapter will be primarily concerned with. However, when significant pharmacological aspects of glandular products exist, they will be presented over and above replacement roles. In a number of instances, the development of synthetic hormone analogs has actually achieved significant improvements over natural hormones in terms of potency, selectivity, and usefulness.

As mentioned in Chapter 1, perhaps the purest form of drug therapy is the replacement of inadequate amounts of an endogenous substance such as a hormone. Any gland that normally secretes a hormone is a potential target for hypofunctioning. Classical examples include Addison's disease (adrenal cortex), dwarfism (anterior pituitary), juvenile onset, insulin-dependent diabetes (pancreas), and hypothyroidism (thyroid).

When the appropriate hormone is given to replace a physiological inadequacy, it is given as a pharmaceutical preparation at a "physiological" dose. If the appropriate dose is given, no undesired side effects should be expected. However, when hormones are given at supraphysiological levels,

TABLE 9.1
Principle Endocrine Hormones

Hormone	Secreted by	Hormone	Secreted by
Peptide or amino acid derivative		Steroid	
Insulin	Pancreas	Estrogens	Ovary, adrenals
Glucagon	Pancreas	Progesterone	Ovary, testes, adrenals
Somatostatin	Pancreas	Testosterone	Testes, ovary, adrenals
Thyroid hormones(T_3 and T_4)	Thyroid	Cortisol	Adrenals
Antidiuretic hormone (ADH)	Pituitary	Corticosterone	Adrenals
Oxytocin	Pituitary	Aldosterone	Adrenals
adrenocorticotropic hormone (ACTH)	Pituitary		
Thyroid-stimulating hormone (TSH)	Pituitary		
Luteinizing hormone (LH)	Pituitary		
Follicle-stimulating hormone (FSH)	Pituitary		
Growth hormone (GH)	Pituitary		
Prolactin	Pituitary		
Gonadotropin-releasing hormone (GnRH)	Pituitary		
Luteinizing-hormone releasing hormone (LHRH)	Pituitary		
Thyrotropin-releasing hormone (TRH)	Pituitary		
Parathyroid hormone	Parathyroid		
Melatonin	Pineal		
Calcitonin	Thyroid		
Catecholamines	Adrenals		

referred to as "pharmacological" doses, side effects are relatively common and are usually extensions of their physiological properties. This is a particular concern with adrenal glucocorticoids, which are often used in high doses to suppress serious cases of chronic inflammation or the rejection of transplanted organs.

As mentioned above, there are a number of physiological disorders related to glandular hypofunction that require pharmacological intervention. However, the underlying principles of therapeutics are essentially the same. That is, determine the correct replacement dose and deliver the hormone in a manner that most accurately reproduces its normal physiological pattern of release. Among the endocrine replacement disorders, the most prevalent in the world is diabetes mellitus, which will serve as our prototype.

DIABETES MELLITUS

The word *diabetes* is derived from the Greek word of the same spelling, which signifies the copious urine production associated with the affliction (i.e., a siphoning). However, *diabetes mellitus* should be distinguished from *diabetes insipidus*, which also produces excess urine production because of a deficiency of antidiuretic hormone (vasopressin). *Mellitus* is the Latinized Greek word for "honeyed" and reflects the increased concentration of glucose in the urine. Although diabetes has a name that suggests both its symptoms and its nature, physicians were nonetheless unable to stem its debilitating effects until the twentieth century.

In the United States, the number of persons with diabetes has grown twofold since 1997 and is estimated to be over 13 million. An additional 5 million persons have undiagnosed disease. Worldwide, the number of people with diabetes is projected to more than double to 366 million by 2030.

Of the diabetics diagnosed, 5–10% are classified as having *insulin-dependent* juvenile onset (type 1) while the remainder (90–95%) have *non–insulin-dependent* maturity onset (type 2).

One common denominator that both types share is insulin deficiency (absolute or relative). Autoimmune type 1 is an autoimmune disorder. In type 1, a selective destruction of the β-cells of the pancreas by the immune system is the main reason for the decline in insulin secretion.

Triggering of the immune response targeting destruction of the β-cells is the result of genetic and environmental factors. Patients diagnosed with type 1 have been found to have an accumulation of immune cells in the pancreas, on autopsy and biopsy. In addition, autoantibodies against the β-cell or insulin are found in the blood of most patients with type 1. However, the situation can be somewhat more complex than this straightforward definition in that type 1 can occur at any age and type 2 can require the use of insulin.

Type 2 diabetes is characterized by *both* insulin resistance and deficient insulin secretion. The inability of the pancreas to secrete is unmasked when there is increased demand for insulin as a result of resistance to insulin action. These individuals usually have a metabolic syndrome of obesity, hypertension, hyperlipidemia, and hyperglycemia. Some of the known insulin resistance states are pregnancy, Cushing's syndrome (excess cortisol production by the adrenal glands), acromegaly (excess production of growth hormone by the pituitary), and polycystic ovary syndrome. Type 2 is the most complex and prevalent form of diabetes in terms of etiology and genetic predisposition.

The capacity of β-cells to secrete insulin decreases with age; therefore, it is not surprising that there is a higher incidence of type 2 in older adults. Results of a study in the U.K., one of the largest prospective studies of type 2, suggest that nearly 50% of the insulin secretory capacity of the pancreas has already diminished at the time of diagnosis with the gradual loss of the rest within the next 5–10 years. This loss in insulin secretory capacity is the result of progressive loss of β-cell mass, which started months to years before the diagnosis of type 2.

Type 2 is associated with significant microvascular (e.g., retinopathy) and macrovascular (e.g., cardiovascular disease) complications. Unfortunately, many patients can develop these underlying pathologies by the time type 2 diabetes is diagnosed. Annual costs in the United States for treatment of diabetes and its complications are over $130 billion. That equates to nearly 1 out of 5 dollars spent on health care. Strategies to identify individuals at increased risk for development of type 2 diabetes and to intervene before they progress from euglcemia to hyperglycemia (an index of impending pathology) have the potential to limit the complications and lower the costs.

Generally, in the case of type 1, there is inadequate production of insulin that eventually becomes absolute. If left untreated, the body will starve because glucose cannot gain access into key body organs. Type 1 diabetics are typically underweight due to lipid breakdown. Death will occur from *ketoacidosis* due to the unregulated production of acidic lipid breakdown products. In the case of type 2 diabetes, there is often a "relative" lack of adequate insulin production, since these individuals are typified by target cell "resistance" to the hormone. In fact, their circulating insulin levels may be normal or even elevated. Normally, the sugars and starches you eat are converted to glucose (blood sugar), which enters your bloodstream to be transported to the cells where it is burned for energy. This is where insulin comes into play. The pancreas releases insulin in response to the sugar, which then "unlocks" your cell walls so that glucose can enter, but in order for this to work, your cells need to be sensitive to insulin.

Treatment of type 1 diabetes is limited to insulin replacement, while type 2 diabetes is treatable by a number of therapeutic approaches. Many cases of insulin resistance are asymptomatic due to normal, compensatory increases in insulin secretion, and others may be controlled by diet and exercise. Both types of diabetes mellitus can be influenced by diet and exercise, to achieve caloric control as well as exogenous insulin. Drug therapy in type 2 diabetes may also be directed toward (1) increasing insulin secretion, (2) increasing insulin sensitivity, or (3) increasing insulin penetration of the cells.

Antidiabetic drugs may be subdivided into six groups: insulin, sulfonylureas, α-glucosidase inhibitors, biguanides, meglitinides, and thiazolidinediones.

Insulin is an 86-amino acid 6000 Da protein; it is the only medication for glucose control in people with type 1. Most of the people with diabetes, and the fastest growing segment of the population with diabetes, are those with type 2. Because glycemic control is often not met with oral medications (see below), dietary interventions and physical exercise in this population, insulin serves as a last resort. Currently, insulin is viewed not only as a hypoglycemic agent for all patients with diabetes, but also as a medication that slows the progression of diabetic complications and decreases the risk of adverse cardiovascular events.

Years ago, the only insulins available were purified pork and bovine insulins. Human insulins became available in the late 1980s (Humulin line) with the advent of recombinant DNA techniques; the α- and β-chains of insulin were synthesized within *Escherichia coli*. Many diabetics were successfully switched to them because the human insulins cause fewer allergies than the pork insulin do. In 1998, Eli Lilly and Company stopped manufacturing beef and beef-pork insulins, thus completing the shift to human insulins.

The newest insulins are insulin analogs, which appeared on the market after 1995. The first insulin analog of this type, Humalog (insulin lispro), was introduced in 1996, followed several years later by Novolog (insulin aspart). Lispro differs from regular insulin in that the 28th and 29th amino acids of the β-chain of insulin are reversed to form lys-pro instead of pro-lys. Aspart is a recombinant human insulin in which aspartic acid is substituted for proline at B28. In 2001, Lantus (insulin glargine) was launched as a product to avoid nocturnal hypoglycemia. All the changes made influence the pharmacodynamics of the preparations.

Preparations that are rapid-acting, intermediate-acting, long-acting, and various combinations thereof are available. Selection of which one(s) is a clinical decision, dependent on the particular needs of the patient.

ORAL HYPOGLYCEMIC AGENTS

Since the availability of insulin became a reality, the desirability of an alternative method of delivery became obvious. While "improvements" in insulin preparations have become a reality, there have been sluggish improvements in the area of oral alternatives. Some of these are listed below:

Sulfonylureas (chlorpropamide, tolazimide, glipizide, and others) act by increasing insulin release from the beta cells of the pancreas. Glimepiride appears to have a useful secondary action in increasing insulin sensitivity in peripheral cells.

Alpha-glucosidase inhibitors (acarbose, miglitol) do not enhance insulin secretion. Rather, they inhibit the conversion of disaccharides and complex carbohydrates to glucose, thus reducing peak blood glucose levels.

Metformin is the only available member of the biguanide class. This drug decreases liver glucose production, decreases intestinal absorption of glucose, and increases peripheral glucose uptake and use. Metformin may be used alone or in combination with a sulfonylurea.

There are two members of the meglitinide class: repaglinide and nateteglitinide. The mechanism of action of the meglitinides is to stimulate insulin production.

Rosiglitazone and pioglitazone are members of the tiazolidine class. They act by reducing glucose production in the liver and increasing insulin-dependent glucose uptake in muscle cells. They do not increase insulin production.

BLOOD GLUCOSE METERS, INHALED INSULIN, AND INSULIN PUMPS

Blood glucose meters have undergone constant updating and refinement since the introduction of the first meters. Manufacturers continually strive to improve their models, ensuring that they will retain a share of the lucrative market for blood glucose test strips. Manufacturers have also developed new insulin dosing devices. These "pens" come prefilled with insulin, are disposable, and can be dialed with the user's dose.

Research continues to find alternative methods of delivery of insulin to free patients from frequent injections. In 2003, two encouraging findings from two new studies suggest that in the near future *inhaled insulin formulations* will supplant or at least supplement injectable insulin therapy. The therapy involves the *inhalation* of tiny particles that are loaded with regular insulin after the start of meals. Intrapulmonary insulin delivery has been preferred to intranasal delivery, because the latter would require the use of surfactants to allow insulin to cross the nasal mucosa, and the bio-availability of the dose is low at no more than 10%. If long-term studies prove successful, a new era in drug delivery may emerge, freeing some diabetic patients from using a needle.

Several companies have tried to develop successful *insulin infusion kits*. For years, millions of people worldwide had no choice but to take daily insulin injections—sometimes up to ten a day. Today, those same people are offered a new technology that allows them to replace the daily regimen of shots with a continuous flow of insulin in their bodies, through a "pump." These pumps are devices that contain a small syringe that can be filled with insulin and can be programmed using a touchscreen to deliver small hourly doses of insulin (basal needs) as well as insulin boluses before meals through a catheter placed in a subcutaneous site. In addition to not having to endure the pain and inconvenience that multiple daily injections can sometimes cause, pump users have more control of their insulin flow than do people taking injections. With just the press of a button, a pump user can stop or cut down the flow of insulin, as needed.

First introduced in the 1970s, today's pumps are small, sleek, and safe machines, about the size of a beeper. Just like a pancreas, an insulin pump releases small, continuous amounts of insulin into the bloodstream. This is known as "basal" insulin. In addition, just as a pancreas produces insulin quickly in response to sugar intake, an insulin pump allows its wearer to dial in additional insulin to cover an increased amount of carbohydrate ingested.

Today's insulin pumps contain tiny computers and run on batteries. Insulin is delivered through a thin tube that is connected both to the pump and to the person wearing the pump, through a needle or catheter placed under the skin. The tubing needs to be changed every 2–3 days. Most pump users connect at the abdomen, although others use thighs, hips, upper buttocks, or even arms. The tube can be easily detached for some activities such as showering. Many pumps are water resistant, allowing the pump user to remain attached while swimming.

Significantly, at the June 2002 meeting of the American Diabetes Association, three studies demonstrated that pump therapy is the most effective way to maintain tight blood sugar control.

HISTORY OF INSULIN

Of all the hormones, perhaps insulin possesses the most interesting history in endocrine pharmacology. Diabetes mellitus itself has been recognized as a clinical entity for at least 2000 years. However, the discovery of insulin, and its utilization in treating diabetes mellitus, required a combination of circumstances that illustrate the scientific method. For example, the symptoms of the disorder had to be recognized, a hypothesis based on relevant physiological knowledge had to be constructed, appropriate experiments needed to be carried out dealing with both glandular extirpation and extract replacement, and the application of these observations to the human clinical condition had to be assessed. Finally, the utilization of modern genetic engineering has resulted in the synthetic production of the hormone for treatment, thus rendering patients not susceptible to shortages of animal preparations.

In 1889, Austrian scientists Joseph von Mering and Oskar Minkowski observed that if experimental animals were pancreatectomized they developed symptoms identical to diabetes mellitus (e.g., loss of weight, and copious urine production containing glucose) and speculated that an unknown substance in the pancreas could be the missing factor. Support for this hypothesis was based on the general concept of the physiological function of endocrine secretions as well as the specific observation of a correlation between pancreatic β-cell damage and diabetes symptoms. Therefore, by the beginning of the twentieth century, it was widely believed that some type of "internal secretion" of the pancreas played a significant role in the control of carbohydrate metabolism. In 1909, the German scientist Georg Zuelzer developed the first pancreatic extract in an attempt to treat diabetes, but the side effects were too severe to allow further studies.

Despite the widely held belief of pancreatic secretion, early attempts to prove the existence of the missing factor were widely disparate and inconclusive. For example, the early administration of pancreatic extracts to human diabetics would sometimes reduce glycosuria while in other cases the results would be life threatening, the latter probably being the result of the presence of toxic contaminants and subsequent immunological responses to them. However, by 1919, a somewhat more regular hypoglycemic effect was achieved in experimental animals by the intravenous injections of aqueous solutions of freshly ground pancreas. It only remained for Frederick Grant Banting to appear on the scene and complete the discovery process.

In 1920, the 22-year-old Banting accepted a demonstratorship in surgery and anatomy at London, Ontario's Western University. One of Banting's responsibilities involved lecturing on carbohydrate metabolism to medical students. It was in the process of preparing for these presentations that his curiosity was stimulated regarding the relationship of pancreatic islets of Langerhans cells to diabetes.

On returning to his alma mater (University of Toronto) the following year, Banting enlisted the support of J.J.R. Macleod, a professor of physiology, to carry out research on his theories relating to the functional relationship between the pancreas and diabetes. It was Banting's hypothesis that previous attempts to use pancreatic extracts were doomed to failure or mediocre success at best, because they were heterogeneous in nature. That is, they contained material from both *acinar cells* (e.g., digestive enzymes) as well as *β-cells* (presumably containing insulin). In order to circumvent this problem, Banting's strategy was to ligate the pancreatic duct in dogs, keep them alive while their acinar cells degenerated, and then remove the remaining pancreatic tissue for the preparation of an extract. Banting began his work, assisted by Charles Best, in May 1921.

Within 2 months, Banting and Best had succeeded in preparing saline extracts of atrophied pancreas that they administered by intravenous injection to depancreatectomized dogs. Over the course of the next 6 months, Banting and Best accumulated data substantiating that their extract could reduce hyperglycemia in diabetic dogs, most notably with a dog named "Marjorie." Although their saline extracts continued to produce side effects, it was decided that a clinical test in humans was merited. Before the availability of insulin, type 1 diabetes was treated by diet alone—leading to inevitable death.

On January 11, 1922, a 14-year-old severely diabetic boy named Leonard Thompson received a 15 mL saline extract at the Toronto General Hospital. He had appeared at the hospital with a blood glucose of 550 mg% (normal being approximately 90) and he was excreting 3–5 L of urine per day (he obviously was suffering from type 1). After initial failures during the first week and a half, a series of injections begun on January 23 produced immediate results, including significantly decreased glycosuria and ketoacidosis, as well as a general feeling of improvement on the part of the patient. The research team initially feared that some unknown factor may have caused the youngster's amazing recovery, so they withheld insulin for 10 days to determine whether this was indeed so. Once off the insulin, Thompson's condition deteriorated and he displayed all the classic symptoms of diabetes. Insulin injections were resumed and the boy's health improved.

For the first time in history, there was clear, unambiguous clinical evidence in humans that symptoms of diabetes mellitus could be controlled with the exogenous administration of the active factor of the pancreas—insulin. Thus, *replacement therapy* with the newly discovered hormone, insulin, had arrested what was clearly an otherwise fatal metabolic disorder. From that point forward, diabetes mellitus (type 1) became a manageable disease by pharmacological intervention.

Following the treatment of Leonard Thompson, events proceeded rapidly toward the commercial production of insulin. A formal agreement was signed with Eli Lilly and Company on May 29, 1922 for the isolation and processing of insulin from animal sources (pig and beef). By the end of June, Lilly was producing potent batches of pig insulin that were sent to Toronto for testing, and, by the autumn, an improved method for producing large quantities of even purer insulin was developed. By the end of 1923, insulin was being widely used clinically, and Banting and Macleod's work was rewarded with a Nobel Prize in Physiology and Medicine.

On the human side, Banting was outraged that the Nobel Committee decided to split the award with Macleod, whom he had grown to dislike, and had slighted Charles Best, who had assisted Banting throughout the entire research process. In an honorable display, Banting gave half of his $40,000 share of the award to Best (compare to $950,000 awarded for the equivalent prize in 2001). Not to be outdone, Macleod gave half of his award to James Collip, a biochemist, who had also worked closely on the project.

The first commercial insulins, obtained from animals such as cows and pigs, were very impure acidic solutions. Before 1970, injected insulins contained contaminants, particularly proinsulin and other proteins from the islet cells such as glucagon, somatostatin, and pancreatic polypeptide. After the pancreas was collected following slaughter and cooled to –20°C, the frozen glands were chopped up and the insulin extracted with acidified ethanol and water. Then came purification by salting-out, pH adjustment, and recrystallization (impurities were up to 20,000 ppm). Later, insulins were further purified using ion-exchange chromatography and molecular sieving techniques. By this means, contaminants were reduced to 20 ppm or less.

Animal insulins, although they work in humans, are not structurally identical to human insulin. Porcine insulin differs in one amino acid while bovine insulin differs in three amino acids. While these differences may seem small, they may be, nevertheless, sufficient to induce antibody formation and subsequent allergic reactions. Human insulins that are produced are structurally identical to endogenous insulin and are basically devoid of antigenicity. Today, several types of insulin preparations are available, differing primarily in their onset and duration of action. Since diabetics differ in their "brittleness," that is, difficulty in maintaining appropriate glycemic control, some products may not be appropriate for all patients all the time.

For almost a decade, there was a continuing dispute over the exact nature of insulin's chemical composition until it was finally accepted that the hormone was, in fact, a protein. Sanger established the amino acid sequence of insulin in 1960, and this led to the complete synthesis of the protein in 1963, and to the elucidation of its three-dimensional structure in 1972. Insulin was the first hormone for which a radioimmunoassay was developed (1978) and the first to be produced by genetic engineering (given to human volunteers in the summer of 1980).

THE THYROID GLAND

Hypothyroidism

The thyroid gland, which is anatomically located in the neck, is an organ that sequesters iodine (obtained from the diet) from the bloodstream. Uptake, organification, and release of thyroid hormones are largely regulated by thyroid stimulating hormone (TSH) released from the anterior pituitary. Within the thyroid follicular cells, there occurs a sequence of events that results in the formation of iodinated tyrosine that couple to form the principal hormones of the thyroid gland, namely *triiodothyronine*, 20% (T_3), and *thyroxine*, 80% (T_4) (Figure 9.1). T_4 is converted into T_3 in the body. The former is the magical hormone responsible for the metamorphosis of the tadpole into a mature frog. T_3 and T_4 act to regulate TSH release by feedback inhibition. These hormones play decisive roles in regulating cellular metabolism in every cell throughout the body.

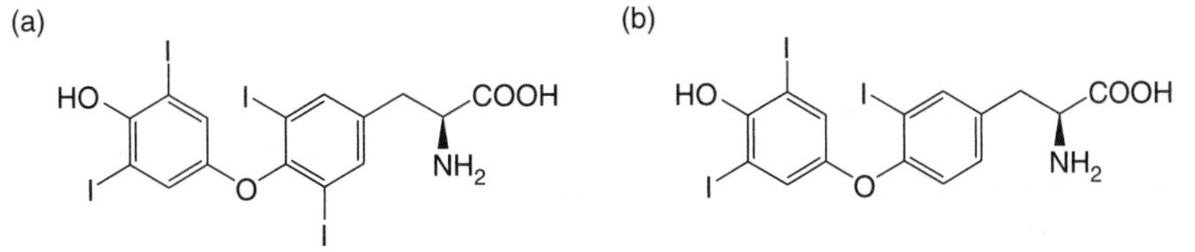

FIGURE 9.1   Structural features of (a) thyroxine (T_4), (b) triiodothyronine (T_3). (Figure selected by Taylor & Francis editorial staff.)

Hypothyroidism, known as *myxedema* in adults, when severe, is the most common disorder of the thyroid gland. More than 5 million Americans have this ailment, and as many as 10% of women may have some degree of thyroid deficiency. Worldwide, hypothyroidism is most often the result of endemic iodine deficiency. In nonendemic areas, where iodine is sufficient in the diet, chronic *autoimmune thyroiditis* (Hashimoto's thyroiditis) accounts for the majority of cases. This disorder is primarily characterized by high levels of circulating antibodies against a key enzyme (thyroid peroxidase) in the processing of iodine in the thyroid gland. Blocking antibodies directed at the TSH receptor may also be present. Thyroid destruction may also occur via apoptotic cell death.

As food enters the body, the thyroid gland extracts iodine, found in many foods, and converts it into the hormones thyroxine, T_4 and triiodothyronine, T_3. Thyroid cells are the only cells in the body that can absorb and sequester iodine. These cells subsequently combine iodine with tyrosine to make T_3 (20%) and T_4 (80%), which are ultimately released into the bloodstream where they influence metabolism. Every cell in the body depends on thyroid hormones for regulating its metabolism—this is why hypothyroidism is so widely expressed in the body (Table 9.2).

Hypothyroidism at birth is known as *cretinism* and is the most common preventable cause of mental retardation in the world. The incidence of cretinism is approximately 1 per 4,000 births. Diagnosis and early intervention with thyroid hormone replacement prevents the development of cretinism. Failure to achieve timely intervention results in irreversible damage to the developing central nervous system as well as other changes. The child is dwarfed, with short extremities, inactive, uncomplaining, and listless. The face is puffy and expressionless, and the enlarged tongue may protrude through the thickened lips of the half-opened mouth. Screening of newborn infants for deficient function of the thyroid is carried out in most industrialized nations. Principle symptoms of hypothyroidism are shown in Table 9.2.

Failure of the thyroid to produce sufficient thyroid hormone is the most common cause of hypothyroidism and is known as *primary hypothyroidism*. *Secondary hypothyroidism* occurs much less often and results from diminished release of TSH from the pituitary. Treatment of hypothyroidism is achieved by the replacement of thyroid hormone, primarily T_4. A *synthetic* preparation of T_4 is available, *levothyroxine (Synthroid®),* which has been a popular choice for hypothyroidism because of its

---

TABLE 9.2
Principle Symptoms of Hypothyroidism

- Fatigue
- Cold intolerance, cold skin; weight gain or increased difficulty losing weight
- Constipation
- Depression
- Coarse, dry hair
- Memory loss
- Bradycardia, excessive menstrual bleeding
- Impaired growth of skeletal tissues
- Impaired growth, development and function of the CNS
- Impaired synthesis of protein
- Impaired absorption of carbohydrates and amino acids
- Impaired lipid metabolism (hypercholesteremia)
- Impaired gonadal function (decreased libido)
- Impaired cardio renal function (diminished peripheral resistance and glomerular filtration rate)
- Impaired overall tissue metabolism (basal metabolic rate)
- Irritability
- Abnormal menstrual cycles
- Decreased libido

consistent potency and prolonged duration of action. No toxicity occurs when given in physiological replacement doses at the proper level (the average *maintenance dosage* being in the 75–125 μg range daily).

Although treatment of hypothyroidism is easy in some individuals, others may have a difficult time finding the right type and dosage. Desiccated animal thyroid is also available at a lesser cost and has been used by low-income patients. *Overdoses* cause symptoms of *hyperthyroidism* and can be used as a guide in clinical management. Hypothyroidism is not cured by the daily intake of thyroid hormone; it is a life-long regimen. Left untreated, the symptoms of hypothyroidism will usually progress. Rarely, complications can result in severe life-threatening depression, heart failure, or coma.

HYPERTHYROIDISM

While hypofunction of the thyroid gland is relatively common, hyperfunction is an uncommon illness affecting less than 0.25% of the population. It is more prevalent among females than males (8:1) and usually occurs in middle age; it rarely occurs in children or adolescents. Hyperfunction of the thyroid gland is known as *Graves'* disease, after the Irish physician who was one of the first to fully describe the syndrome.

The leading cause of Graves' disease is a defect in the immune system that causes the production of autoantibodies to TSH receptors located on the surface of thyroid cells. These antibodies actually act as agonists to stimulate the thyroid, causing it to enlarge (goiter formation) with the overproduction of thyroid hormones (T_3 and T_4). The underlying etiology is unknown but may have a genetic or immune basis. Typical symptoms of Graves' disease are shown in Table 9.3.

The primary treatment for Graves' disease is to control the overactive thyroid gland. There are three standard regimens for treating Graves' disease, but the choice of treatment varies from country to country and physician to physician. The selection of which treatment to use is predicated on factors such as age, degree of illness, and patient/physician preference. The treatment of choice among endocrinologists is radioactive iodine (I^{131}; a β-emitter). Because the thyroid gland concentrates iodine, this nuclide is taken up, and it irradiates the thyroid tissue that produces T_3 and T_4. Its advantages include ease of administration, effectiveness, and economics. Disadvantages include delayed effect, overdose, and the fact that it cannot be used in pregnant women. Young patients with relatively small glands and mild disease can sometimes be treated with drugs.

Antithyroid drugs such as *propylthiouracil* (PTU) and *methimazole* inhibit the iodination of tyrosyl residues as well as the coupling of monoiodotyrosine and diiodotyrosine into T_3 and T_4. In addition, PTU inhibits the peripheral conversion of T_4 to T_3. Unfortunately, there is a very high relapse rate with these drugs and a cure is very infrequent, if at all. The final alternative is thyroidectomy. In this case, it is very difficult to determine exactly how much is to be excised. Not surprisingly, a consequence of surgery is the production of a hypothyroid individual who will require daily levothyroxine for the remainder of their life.

TABLE 9.3
Symptoms of Graves' Disease

Protruding eyes	Fatigue	Changes in sex drive
Weight loss	Muscle cramps	Heart palpitations
Increased appetite	Tremor	Blurred or double vision
Nervousness	Frequent bowel movements	
Restlessness	Menstrual irregularities	
Heat intolerance	Goiter	
Sweating	Rapid heart rate	

THE ADRENAL CORTEX

The adrenal glands are located anatomically above the kidneys. They are comprised of a three-layer cortex and a medulla. The medulla is the source of catecholamines such as epinephrine, the "fight or flight" hormone. The cortex is the source of aldosterone, the primary mineralocorticoid that is involved with the regulation of sodium reabsorption in the kidneys. In addition, the cortex is also the source of steroids known as glucocorticoids of which cortisol is the principle endogenous example. Synthesis and release of cortisol is under the control of adrenocorticotrophic hormone (ACTH).

Cortisol helps maintain homeostasis by regulating numerous enzymes throughout the body by affecting gene expression subsequent to binding to a cytosolic receptor and transport to the nucleus. During periods of stress, cortisol plays an important role in increasing blood glucose levels and elevating blood pressure. Clinically, cortisol and its derivatives are used for replacement theory in the management of *Addison's Disease* (hypofunctioning of the adrenal cortex) as well as for their anti-inflammatory and immunosuppressant properties.

The anti-inflammatory property of cortisol and its derivatives is probably the main pharmacological effect of this group of drugs used in therapy. The reason being that inflammation is a common denominator in tissue injury, regardless of etiology. Once the anti-inflammatory property of cortisol was discovered during the 1940s, great effort was expended in separating the anti-inflammatory potency of cortisol (the desired effect) from its inherent mineralocorticoid potency (the undesired effect). A comparison of the endogenous glucocorticoids (cortisol and cortisone) and several contemporary derivatives is shown in Table 9.4.

As can be seen, chemists have successfully achieved, over the succeeding decades, an excellent separation of anti-inflammatory effect from salt-retaining effect. In addition, compounds that possess a prolonged duration of action (short; 8–12 h biological half-life versus long; 36–72 h biological half-life) have also been developed. The increase in anti-inflammatory potency, as well as extended duration of action, is primarily the result of (1) decreased binding to plasma globulin; 30% versus 5% free and (2) decreased metabolism, respectively.

The main clinical uses of glucocorticoids are for physiological replacement therapy in adrenal insufficiency (where approximately 10–20 mg of cortisol equivalent/day is administered) as well as a wide range of nonendocrine, inflammatory disorders, as well as immunosuppression (e.g., organ transplants). In the latter cases, pharmacological doses exceeding approximately 10–20 mg of cortisol equivalent/day may be needed for prolonged periods of time. In these situations, toxicity may manifest itself in the affected patients. Side effects are basically an extension of normal physiological effects of glucocorticoids on the body (primarily involving carbohydrate, protein, and fat metabolism).

As mentioned above, endogenous glucocorticoids are stress hormones. Their job is to provide glucose from the liver, and replenish this substrate via catabolic effects on skeletal muscle and adipose tissue (this is particularly important during periods of starvation). The increased breakdown

TABLE 9.4
Comparison of Pharmacologic Properties of Glucocorticoids

Compound	Anti-inflammatory Potency	Na⁺ Retaining Potency	Duration of Action
Cortisol	1	1	Short
Cortisone	0.8	0.8	Short
Prednisone	4	0.8	Intermediate
Prednisolone	4	0.8	Intermediate
Betamethasone	25	0	Long
Dexametasone	25	0	Long

of skeletal muscle protein provides amino acids for gluconeogenesis in the liver. Blood glucose becomes elevated, a condition that can exacerbate glycemic control in diabetics. The breakdown of adipose tissue can sometimes cause a redistribution of fat to certain areas of the body such as the upper middle back, producing a "buffalo hump." Chronic administration of glucocorticoids can also produce a potentially life-threatening condition resulting from adrenal insufficiency. Pharmacologic doses will cause the hypothalamus and, hence the anterior pituitary, to cease production of ACTH via feedback inhibition.

Chronic suppression of the pituitary-adrenal axis presents a condition that must be managed properly on withdrawal of therapy in order to avoid *acute adrenal insufficiency*. There have been several strategies developed to meet this scenario including (1) the use of glucocorticoids with less than a long duration of action (to allow the pituitary to periodically "escape") and (2) gradual tapering off of the glucocorticoids to allow the pituitary–adrenal axis to recover its normal production of cortisol.

While work was being carried out in France during the 1970s on discovering glucocoticoid antagonists, a compound that proved to be a very potent antagonist to *progesterone* was discovered. It was given the developmental code identification of RU-486. The potential application of a potent progesterone antagonist was readily apparent. Progesterone is necessary for the maintenance of the decidualized uterine endometrium (i.e., keeping the implanted fertilized egg alive). The subsequent administration of RU-486 to women in their first trimester of pregnancy proved it to be a powerful abortifacent. When used in conjunction with a prostaglandin (PGF $_{2\alpha}$), expulsion of the developing fetus generally occurs within 4 h in 95% of cases. Obviously, this type of drug is surrounded by considerable controversy. Acceptance as an abortifacent in Europe still exceeds that in the United States.

CUSHING'S DISEASE

Cushing's syndrome is a hormonal disorder caused by prolonged exposure of the body's tissues to high levels of the adrenal hormone, cortisol. Dr. Henry Cushing first described a woman with signs and symptoms of this disease in 1912. In 1932, he was able to link the adrenal overproduction of cortisol to an abnormality in the pituitary. It is a relatively rare disorder with a frequency estimated at 1–5/100,000 people per year, primarily in the 20- to –50-year age range. It is caused primarily by pituitary adenomas that secrete increased amounts of ACTH. ACTH can also be produced outside the pituitary. This is called ectopic ACTH production. In addition, noncancerous tumors of the adrenal glands, called adrenal adenomas, can release excess cortisol into the blood. When the source of excess cortisol production is a tumor of the adrenal gland itself, then it is not dependent on ACTH.

Symptoms vary, but they are usually the same as glucocorticoid overdose (see above). Most people have upper body obesity, rounded face, increased fat around the neck, and thinning arms and legs. Children tend to be obese with slowed growth rates. Other characteristic symptoms include severe fatigue, weak muscles, high blood pressure, and high blood sugar (exacerbating diabetes). Irritability, anxiety, and depression are common.

Treatment of Cushing's disease depends on its etiology and can include surgery, radiation therapy, or drugs. Drugs such as *mitotane* (o,p'-DDD) are used to treat adrenal carcinoma when surgery is not possible. It causes adrenal inhibition by an unknown mechanism. Mitotane was discovered when it was observed that the o,p' isomer of the insecticide DDD caused severe damage to the adrenal cortex in dogs.

BIRTH CONTROL HORMONES

Probably the most widely used hormone preparations in the world are those used in healthy women who are not suffering from a disease. These are, of course, birth control pills that usually contain *derivatives of estrogen and/or progesterone.* While they can be used in certain gynecologic disorders with efficacy, the vast majority of prescriptions are written to prevent pregnancy. Their development introduced a new era in society (coinciding with the emergence of the "women's movement"); virtually 100% effectiveness replacing IUDs, condoms, creams, jellies, and diaphragms as well as dependence on men.

It had been known for a long time that alteration of the normal endocrine status in female experimental animals could disrupt their ability to become pregnant. During the normal monthly reproductive cycle in the human female, there is a sequential elaboration of estrogen and progesterone by the ovaries. This prepares the endometrial lining of the uterus for implantation of a fertilized egg and nourishment of it. Successful implantation and continuation of pregnancy therefore depends not only on the presence of appropriate hormones but also on exquisite timing between preparation of the endometrium and arrival of the fertilized egg. Alteration of the hormonal *milieu* out of the norm can result in failed pregnancy.

As mentioned above, physiologists had noted that altering either estrogen or progesterone levels in experimental animals could impact on pregnancy. However, this was little more than a laboratory curiosity, since there was no practical way to take advantage of the situation because pure estrogen and progesterone were of limited supply, extremely expensive, and had ultra-short half-lives (>90% first-pass metabolism). What was needed was some type of breakthrough in the extremely difficult synthetic processes for the formation of these steroids.

The breakthrough occurred when a species of *Mexican yam* was discovered that normally produced a compound that could be used as a precursor in steroid synthesis. Many laborious steps were thereby circumvented, allowing the synthesis of relatively large amounts of estrogen and progesterone at significantly reduced cost. The availability of the final product also allowed chemists to study structure–activity relationships aimed at developing new derivatives. One of these was a progesterone derivative called *norethynodrel.*

Norethynodrel was first used in clinical studies to treat *female infertility.* Ironically, initial studies demonstrated that, in fact, fertility was *decreased by virtue of blocked ovulation.* Analysis of the early batches of Norethynodrel revealed the presence of a contaminant with estrogenic potency, namely, *mestranol.* When mestranol was removed in subsequent batches, treatment with pure norethynodrel led to more breakthrough bleeding and less consistent inhibition of ovulation. Mestranol was thus intentionally reincorporated into the preparation, and this *combination* was employed in the first large-scale clinical trial of combination oral contraceptives.

In late 1959, Enovid® (norethynodrel and mestranol) was the first "Pill" approved by the FDA for use as a contraceptive agent in the United States. Today's combination preparations have an effectiveness of approximately 99.9% with *perfect use* and can contain various progestins other than norethynodrel, as well as the estrogen *ethinyl estradiol* that has largely replaced mestranol. Ethinyl estradiol differs from endogenous estrogen only in the presence of an ethinyl group on carbon 17 of the steroid nucleus. Table 9.5 shows a comparison of the relative effectiveness of various contraceptive methods when *typically used.*

Early combination preparations contained relatively high doses of the progestin and estrogenic components. *Side effects* of early hormonal contraceptives fell into several major categories: adverse cardiovascular effects, including hypertension, myocardial infarction, hemorrhagic or ischemic stroke, and venous thrombosis and embolism; breast, hepatocellular, and cervical cancers; and a number of endocrine and metabolic effects. Once a dose relationship was realized (particularly with the estrogenic component) with the side effects, doses were decreased. Today's preparations contain approximately 90% less of the progestin and 80% less of the estrogen than in the early preparations marketed, while still maintaining effectiveness. They are available in a variety of fixed-dose, biphasic, and triphasic combinations that vary in their estrogen and progestin content throughout the cycle. The goal is to use the smallest total hormone content possible, which is still effective.

The current consensus is that the contemporary low-dose preparations pose minimal risks in women who have no predisposing risk factors and, in fact, may provide certain beneficial health

TABLE 9.5
Percent of Accidental Pregnancies
in First Year of Typical Use

Progesterone implants	0.09
Vasectomy	0.15
Depo-Provera	0.30
Tubal sterilization	0.40
Copper IUD	0.80
The Pill	2.00
MiniPill	3.00
Condoms	12.00
Diaphragm and spermicidal	18.00
Spermacide alone	21.0
Withdrawal	21.0

effects (e.g., protection against endometrial and ovarian cancer). Oral contraceptive pills have been associated with increased risk for myocardial infarction, stroke, and venous thromboembolism. However, studies that suggest that these risks are minimal in appropriately chosen low-risk women have been published.

Stroke is a very uncommon event in childbearing women, occurring in approximately 11 per 100,000 women over a 1-year period of time. Therefore, even a doubling of this risk with oral contraceptive pills would have minimal effect on attributable risk. The estimated risk of *myocardial infarction* associated with oral contraceptive pill use in nonsmokers is 3 per million women over 1 year. The estimated risk of *venous thromboembolism* attributable to oral contraceptive pills is less than 3 per 10,000 women per year. However, the risk may be increased in women who smoke or have other predisposing factors to thrombosis or thromboembolism. In fact, it should be emphasized that the risk of serious cardiovascular side effects is particularly marked in women over 35 years of age, who are heavy smokers (e.g., more than 15 cigarettes per day). In addition, the literature suggests that there may be an increased risk of breast cancer associated with long-term oral contraceptive pill use in women under the age of 35. However, because the incidence of breast cancer is so relatively low in this population, the attributable risk of breast cancer from birth control pill use is small.

Following the recognition that combination birth control pills were associated with adverse thrombolic events, alternatives to combination contraceptives were developed in order to avoid or minimize side effects. For example, the *"Mini" pill* was developed in the 1970s. This product is a pro-gestin-only product taken daily. Its contraceptive effectiveness is approximately 97%. Its mechanism of action is apparently due to (1) changing the motility of the oviduct, (2) putting the endometrium out-of-phase, and (3) increasing the thickness of vaginal mucus (the vast majority of women continue to ovulate). Variations on progestin-only preparations include silastic implants (effective up to 5 years), depo-deposition intramuscularly (effective 2–3 months), and a progestin-containing intrauterine device (IUD).

Ortho Evra® (OE) is a relatively new combination contraceptive containing the most commonly prescribed progestin in oral contraceptives in the United States, together with ethinyl estradiol. Unlike typical combination oral contraceptives, OE maintains steady state hormone levels throughout the 7-day application period. This is achieved by delivering the product in a thin, soft, square patch that can be worn on any of four application sites. A new patch is applied each week for three consecutive weeks—a patch should not be applied during the fourth week. The patient's menstrual period should begin during this patch-free interval.

One of the practical disadvantages of birth control pills has been the requirement of a prescription. However, on August 24, 2006 the FDA announced the approval of the emergency contraceptive drug *Plan B as an over-the-counter option for women aged 18 and older*. Plan B is emergency contraception. It comes in the form of two levonorgestrel (a progestin) pills (0.75 mg each) that are taken orally after a contraceptive fails or after unprotected sex. Plan B acts primarily by stopping the release of an egg from the ovary (ovulation).

Plan B should be taken orally as soon as possible and within 72 h of unprotected sex. The second tablet should be taken 12 h after the first tablet.

ESTROGEN RECEPTOR

One of the earliest identified and best understood examples of eukaryotic transcriptional regulation is the estrogen receptor system, which mediates the response to the female's hormone estrogen. Estrogen acts as a hormonal master switch that induces a large number of genes during mammalian development. Estrogen is a high-affinity ligand for a transcriptional factor, the estrogen receptor, which is a prototype of a large protein class, *the nuclear receptor superfamily*. Other members include the glucocoticoid, androgen, and progesterone receptors. Although nuclear receptor proteins are present at very low concentrations (e.g., on the order of picomoles of estrogen receptor per milligram mammary tissue protein), they bind to their physiological hormones (e.g., estrogen) with very high affinities (K_d on the order of 1 nM).

PARKINSON'S DISEASE

Although replacement therapy is classically exemplified by the treatment of hypofunctioning endocrine glands, there is an important neurological disorder that can be successfully treated with a replacement strategy. Parkinson's disease (PD) is a clinical syndrome characterized by slowness of movement, muscular rigidity, resting tremor, and an impairment of postural balance. In the absence of therapy, death frequently results from complications of immobility.

In the early 1960s, researchers discovered that Parkinsonian symptoms appeared when brain levels of *dopamine* (DA) were reduced. The syndrome is the result of an 80–90% loss of *dopaminergic neurons*, and the attendant neurotransmitter (dopamine), in the *substantia nigra* region of the brain. Neurons from the substantia nigra normally project into a region of the basal ganglia where they *inhibit firing of cholinergic neurons*. These cholinergic neurons, in turn, form excitatory synapses onto other neurons that project out of the basal ganglia. The net result is that the *cholinergic neurons are without their normal inhibition*. The loss of dopaminergic neurons and their dopamine suggested to researchers that replacement of the neurotransmitter could restore function. However, dopamine itself is highly polar and does not cross the blood-brain barrier. So a different strategy had to be devised.

Dopamine is endogenously synthesized in the terminals of dopaminergic fibers originating with the amino acid tyrosine and, subsequently, l-dihydroxyphenylalanine (L-DOPA), the rate-limiting metabolic precursor of dopamine. Fortunately, L-DOPA is significantly less polar than dopamine and can gain entry into the brain via an active process mediated by a carrier of aromatic amino acids. Administration of L-DOPA was initially found to dramatically alleviate the slowness of movement, increased muscle tone, and tremor that are typical of PD. Although L-DOPA reduces many of the motor symptoms of PD, it does not affect nonmotor symptoms and does not halt the progression of the degeneration of DA-containing neurons.

In clinical practice, L-DOPA (levodopa) is conventionally administered in combination with a peripherally acting *inhibitor* of aromatic L-amino acid decarboxylase (e.g., *carbidopa*). If L-DOPA is administered alone, the drug is largely decarboxylated by enzymes in the intestinal mucosa and other peripheral sites. Inhibition of peripheral decarboxylase by carbidopa markedly increases the fraction of orally administered L-DOPA that remains unmetabolized and available to enter the brain (i.e., its bioavailability).

Dopamine receptor agonists are also available for therapy in Parkinson's disease. The strategy of using dopamine agonists early as monotherapy or in combination with levodopa to delay long-term levodopa complications is gaining wider acceptance. It has also been reported that dopamine produced from L-DOPA in the body has a larger number of actions compared with dopamine receptor agonists alone, which might contribute to L-DOPA's efficacy.

Although replacement therapy is basically limited to endocrine disorders, it still plays an important therapeutic role in clinical pharmacology. The number of people requiring replacement therapy for diabetes and hypothyroidism, alone, makes insulin and thyroid hormone among the most commonly prescribed drugs in the United States. For example, the drug Synthroid® is taken daily by 8 million people to correct hypothyroidism, and its share of the market is worth $600 million per year. As more information is discovered about the role of other endogenous substances in the body, new examples of replacement therapy will occur.

SELECTED BIBLIOGRAPHY

Diabetes Information. U.S. Food and Drug Administration: http://www.fda.gov/diabetes. 2004

QUESTIONS

1. Which of the following is/are true regarding the endocrine system?
   a. Comprised of specialized tissues or glands
   b. Hormones are released into the blood stream activity of the beta-cells of the pancreas
   c. Transmission is rapid throughout the body
   d. All of the above
   e. a and b

2. In normal replacement therapy of a hypofunctioning gland, which of the following will apply?
   a. A pharmacological dose is most advantageous
   b. A physiological dose will not be sufficient to compensate
   c. A pharmacological dose is the only way to cure the disease
   d. A physiological dose is generally most appropriate
   e. A physiological dose is the only way to cure a disease

3. Which of the following occurs with insulin-dependent, juvenile-onset, type 1 diabetes?
   a. Overactivity of the beta cells of the pancreas
   b. Elevated blood insulin levels
   c. Increase in body weight
   d. Reduced blood glucose levels
   e. Decrease in body weight

4. Which of the following is/are the cause of death in untreated insulin-dependent, juvenile-onset, type 1 diabetes?
   a. Excess blood glucose
   b. Excess urine formation
   c. Kidney failure
   d. Ketoacidosis
   e. None of the above

5. Which of the following is/are true regarding insulin?
   a. It is a low molecular weight steroid
   b. It is produced in the alpha cells of the pancreas
   c. It is used in type 1 diabetes
   d. It is always used in type 2 diabetes
   e. a and c

6. The first commercial insulin preparations were obtained from which of the following?
   a. Slaughtered pigs
   b. Human cadavers
   c. Slaughtered cows
   d. Slaughtered sheep
   e. a and c

7. Which of the following is/are true of today's insulin preparations?
   a. Differ in onset and duration of action
   b. Are primarily produced by recombinant technology
   c. Are less antigenic since they are based on human insulin
   d. Offer no advantage over bovine or porcine insulin
   e. a, b, and c

8. Hypofunctioning of which gland is particularly significant in neonates?
   a. Adrenal
   b. Ovary
   c. Testes
   d. Liver
   e. Thyroid

9. The principle mechanism of action of combination oral contraceptive agents is which of the following?
   a. Altered oviduct motility
   b. Induction of preovulation
   c. Inhibition of ovulation
   d. Direct inhibitory effect on the ovaries
   e. None of the above

10. Which of the following is/are true regarding prednisone versus cortisol?
   a. Has shorter duration of action
   b. Has greater anti-inflammatory potency
   c. Has greater salt-retaining potency
   d. Is an endogenous mineralocorticoid
   e. Is a precursor of cortisone

10 Chemotherapeutic Agents: Antibiotics and Anticancer Drugs

There have been at least four so-called revolutions in pharmacology. These include (1) the development of *vaccines* in the nineteenth century; (2) the discovery of *antibiotics* during the first half of the twentieth century; (3) the therapeutic introduction of *psychopharmacological drugs* for the treatment of mental disorders during the 1950s; and (4) the development of *genetic engineering* for drug production during the 1970s and 1980s. This chapter will deal with the discovery and therapeutic principles underlying the use of chemotherapeutic agents, primarily antibiotics and anticancer drugs.

ANTIBIOTICS

Antibiotics (i.e., anti-infective or antimicrobial drugs) may be directed at one of several disease-producing organisms including bacteria, viruses, fungi, helminthes, and so forth. The vast majority of antibiotics are bacteria fighters; although there are millions of viruses, there are only about half-a-dozen antiviral drugs. Bacteria are more complex than viruses (while viruses must "live" in a host [us], bacteria can live independently) and so are easier to kill.

The impact of antibiotics on human health is not difficult to assess. Since 1900, the overall death rate from diseases like pneumonia and tuberculosis has declined from 797 per 100,000 to 59 per 100,000 in 1996, according to the *Centers for Disease Control and Prevention.* As a result, life expectancy during that period increased from 47.3 to 76.1 years. A further correlation between antibiotic introduction and declining death rate can be appreciated by comparing the decline in death rate in the United States with the introduction of antibiotics following World War II (Table 10.1). While the decline in death rate is undoubtedly multifactorial (nutrition, sanitation, etc.), antibiotics have clearly made a great contribution to humanity. Infections such as pneumonia, tuberculosis, and diarrhea/enteritis were the three leading causes of death in 1900. Today, the leading causes are heart disease, cancer, and stroke.

HISTORY

In 1546, Girolamo Fracastro of Verona proposed the then remarkable theory that diseases were transmitted by minute particles of *living* matter with the properties of multiplication and airborne dissemination. He considered that particles with great penetrating power caused diseases such as

---

TABLE 10.1
Correlation of Antibiotic Introduction on Death Rate in the United States

Year	Antibiotic	Death Rate (per 100,000)
1945	Introduction of penicillin	40
1946	General distribution of penicillin	37
1947	General distribution of streptomycin	34
1951	Introduction of isoniazid	15
1956	Introduction of paraaminosalicylic acid	9
1964	Introduction of myambutol	5
1972	Introduction of rifampin	2.5

---

plague and smallpox. Fracastro's living particles have, of course, been equated with *microorganisms*, although he did not suggest that they were disease specific. Unfortunately, lack of convincing scientific evidence led to Fracastro's ideas being largely ignored.

Credit for the actual discovery of microorganisms is given to *Antonie van Leeuwenhoek* in Holland, in 1676. Using a microscope of his own invention, he reported seeing *"animalcules"* in various specimens, including scrapings from his own teeth. Although his discovery was important, it nevertheless did little to counteract the prevailing theory of *spontaneous generation*.

As late as the mid-nineteenth century, most medical practitioners and scientists believed that diseases were caused by poisonous miasmas or imbalanced bodily "humors." It was the well-known work of Pasteur, Koch, Semmelweis, and other "microbe hunters" that led the way to the modern belief that a wide variety of microbial agents cause infectious disease. But surprisingly, the origin of the germ theory of disease traces itself not to these well-known figures but to *Agostino Bassi*, an Italian lawyer-turned-farmer, who in 1835 was the first to demonstrate that a microorganism, a *fungal mold*, could cause disease in an animal (muscadine in silkworms).

This observation was quickly applied to human disease in the late 1830s, when the *fungal agents of tinea infections of the beard and scalp* were first described by Remak and Schonlein. Similar studies of fungal blights in plants would help to establish the idea that microorganisms could cause disease (e.g., great Irish potato blight).

Knowledge of fungal diseases did not immediately lead to cures, however. It was not until 1939 that the first modern *antifungal agent, griseofulvin—a product of Penicillium griseofulvum—* (Figure 10.1), was discovered, almost inadvertently, during research for penicillin-like antibiotics; it was ignored because of its lack of antibacterial activity.

Fortunately, in 1958, it was tested in guinea pigs and shown effective in treating infections of *Microsporum canis* and subsequently developed for use in the treatment of human *ringworm*. In 1956, the first systemically effective drug for fungal infections, *amphotericin B*, was isolated from a bacterium. Amphotericin had the disadvantage of having to be given intravenously, however. In the 1970s, a systemically effective drug, *ketoconazole*, was introduced, which not only had low toxicity but could also be taken *orally*.

Enhancements in modern medicine have inadvertently increased the likelihood of serious opportunistic fungal infection. Since the last quarter of the twentieth century, the rise of tissue and organ transplants involving immunosuppressive drugs and temporarily debilitating medical treatments has created new opportunities for fungi. Therefore, the search for more and better antifungal agents goes on, from new treatments for athlete's foot to improved therapeutics for fungal infections in AIDS patients. The human body is normally an inimical environment for opportunistic fungi, but when the body is immunocompromised, it can become simply nourishing and a place for fungi to thrive.

The concept of spontaneous generation in relation to microorganisms persisted until *Louis Pasteur's* classical experiments on *fermentation* in 1861. Pasteur demonstrated that when organisms from the air were excluded from heat-sterilized liquids, such as sugar solutions and urine, fermentation *failed* to take place. Although the debate regarding spontaneous generation would last into the 1870s, a commission of the *Academie des Sciences* officially accepted Pasteur's results in 1864.

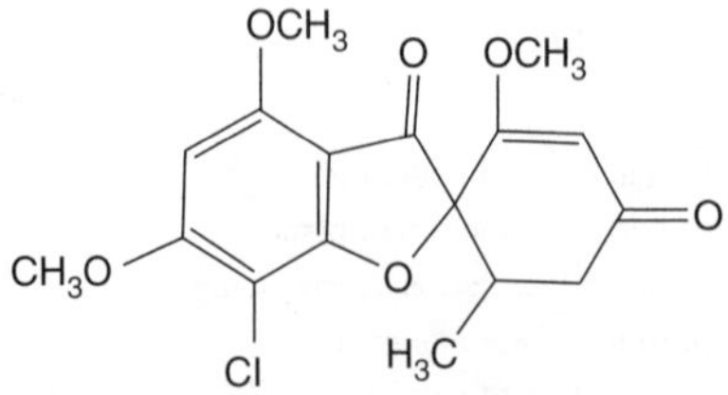

Griseofulvin

FIGURE 10.1 Griseofulvin, the modern antifungal agent.

Despite Pasteur's critical demonstrations, and his conceptualization of the *"germ theory of disease,"* Robert Koch did not establish the actual disease role of microorganisms in causing infections, plagues, and epidemics until the late nineteenth century through his work on *anthrax, tuberculosis,* and *cholera.*

Robert Koch was a German scientist who is credited for the founding of modern medical microbiology. Koch's first major breakthrough in bacteriology occurred in the 1870s, when he demonstrated that the infectious disease *anthrax* developed in mice *only* when the disease-bearing material injected into a mouse's bloodstream contained *viable rods or spores* of *Bacillus anthracis.* Koch's isolation of the anthrax bacillus was a momentous achievement, since this was the *first* time that the causative agent of an infectious disease had been demonstrated beyond a reasonable doubt.

In 1891, the Russian *Romanovsky* made a significant observation with pharmacological implications when he suggested that *quinine cured* malaria by *damaging the parasite more than the host* and suggested that similar situations might also occur with other drugs. The important therapeutic implications of this prediction were most fully developed by Paul Ehrlich (1854–1915), discussed previously, who coined the term *chemotherapy*. Ehrlich defined chemotherapy as *the use of drugs to injure an invading organism without injury to the host*. The essence of chemotherapy is that, ideally, there is some qualitative or quantitative difference between the infecting pathogen and host that can be selectively exploited therapeutically.

Ehrlich's first chemotherapeutic experiments, beginning in 1904, were performed with organic dyes obtained from the prolific German synthetic chemical industry, the most advanced in the world at the time. During 1904, Ehrlich successfully demonstrated the curative properties of the substance *trypan red* against trypanosome-infected *mice*; thereby, it became the first *man-made* chemotherapeutic agent. Unfortunately, the drug proved inactive in man. For the remainder of his life, Ehrlich concentrated his efforts in studying *aromatic arsenicals* that had also shown promise in the treatment of trypanosomiasis.

In 1910, his labors paid-off when he made an historic discovery while investigating one of these arsenicals, the *antisyphilitic* drug *arsphenamine*. This particular drug, with the laboratory code designation *"606,"* was so effective in laboratory tests that it was announced as a *cure* for the dreaded disease and was referred to as a *"magic bullet."* It worked because the arsenic-based compound is a *bit* more poisonous to syphilis bacteria than it is to humans. The treatment made people dreadfully ill (requiring 20–40 treatments over the course of a year to cure the disease), but it did not kill them, which syphilis would eventually do. Although the marketed form of the chemical, *Salvarsan*, ultimately proved to be too toxic for widespread human use, arsphenamine was the opening event in the chemotherapeutic revolution for the treatment of human infections.

Ehrlich's contribution to societal health did not meet with universal favor, however. Far-right fundamentalists of the day threw rocks at his window proclaiming that syphilis was God's punishment for fornicators and that Ehrlich was interfering with divine will.Antibiotics are unique in two significant respects. First, they include members of the only class of drugs that actually *cure* a disease. As indicated previously, most drugs merely provide symptomatic relief while the disease or condition runs its course, or replace an endogenous chemical that is being produced in inadequate amounts. In either case, the drug has not altered the basic etiologic factor that produced the disorder. Antibiotics, on the other hand, can contribute to an authentic cure by irreversibly eradicating the cause of the disease, namely the pathogen. Secondly, the utility of antibiotics is intimately related to their ability to produce toxicity, albeit selectively. The selective toxicity of an antibiotic refers to the degree to which the substance is able to perturb the life processes of the pathogen without simultaneously affecting similar functions in the host.

As mentioned above, the basis for selective toxicity resides in some uniquely important difference in the biochemistry between host and microbe. Antimicrobial drugs exploit this difference and are able to selectively damage the target cell. For example, the drug may (1) inhibit a reaction vital only to the microbe and not the host. The target reaction may, in fact, have no counterpart in the host. For example, penicillin inhibits the cross-linking of microbial peptidoglycan and thereby prevents microbial cell wall synthesis. Animal cells have membranes of a different composition; (2) inhibit a reaction that yields a product vital to both microbe and host. However, the host has an alternative mechanism of obtaining the substance. For example, sulfa drugs inhibit intracellular folic acid synthesis by microbes. Human cells can utilize preformed folic acid and are not susceptible to this antimetabolic effect; (3) undergo biochemical activation to a toxic form in the microbe. For example, acyclovir is used to treat herpes infections. In order to be active, it must undergo *triple phosphorylation* before it is able to inhibit herpes virus *DNA polymerase*; (4) selectively accumulate in the microbe because of a more active cell membrane transport mechanism. For example, quinine accumulates more readily in the malarial plasmodium cell than in the host cell; and (5) has a higher affinity for a critical site of action in the microbe. For example, chloramphenicol binds to a fragment of the 70S ribosome of bacterial cells thereby inhibiting synthesis of bacterial proteins. The drug has a much lower affinity for human ribosomes that are 80S.

Antibiotics can be either *bactericidal* or *bacteriostatic*. That is, they can either kill the pathogen directly or arrest its replication until the body's immune system can be mobilized. Generally, bactericidal drugs are more desirable, especially in the immunocompromised patient. However, when a microbe is killed by a cidal drug and immediately cleared from the body, the antigenic stimulus is greatly reduced. In some cases, it is so reduced that no immune response is triggered. Therefore, sometimes it may be more advantageous to use a static drug that will permit the body sufficient time to develop an appropriate immune response. Theoretically, it is not usually a good idea to combine cidal and static antibiotics, since cidal drugs depend on active bacterial growth in order to be effective. For example, during the 1950s, it was found that the human mortality rate for pneumococcal meningitis was higher when chlortetracycline (static) was administered with penicillin (cidal) than penicillin alone.

PENICILLIN

One of the most important events in the history of antibiotics is the discovery and production of penicillin. In 1928, while investigating staphylococcus variants at St. Mary's Hospital in London, *Alexander Fleming* observed that when a particular strain of mold, *Penicillium notatum* (named because the cells were pencil-shaped when viewed under a microscope), contaminated these cultures, they underwent lysis. Fleming named the active substance penicillin. Unfortunately, because Fleming was such a poor public speaker, his public presentation of his seminal discovery went unheeded, and it took an additional 12 years before the potential of penicillin was realized.

Fortunately, the production of relatively large quantities of penicillin was achieved by a group of researchers at Oxford University under the direction of *Howard Florey*, since no pharmaceutical company could be persuaded to take up the challenge. Florey's group experimented with treating both humans and animals during this period. By May 1940, crude preparations that were found to produce dramatic therapeutic effects when administered parenterally to mice with experimentally produced streptococcal infections were available. In 1941, the group accumulated enough material to conduct trials in several patients desperately ill with staphylococcal and streptococcal infections refractive to all other therapy. Their work culminated with publication of a paper in the journal *Lancet* and concluded with the statement: "*Enough evidence, we consider, has now been assembled to show that penicillin is a new and effective type of chemotherapeutic agent, and possesses some properties unknown in any antibacterial substance hitherto described.*" With classic British understatement, the dawn of the antibiotic era had begun.

As an interesting historical footnote, in March of 1996, the drug company Pfizer paid $35,160 at auction for a small culture of the original mold used by Fleming. The specimen is one of two that Fleming gave to his laboratory assistant, Dan Stratful, and contains a handwritten inscription ("The mold that makes penicillin." Alexander Fleming). Pfizer was one of the U.S. companies that finally participated in the commercial mass production of penicillin during World War II. The first marketable penicillin cost several dollars per 100,000 units; today, the same dose costs only a few cents. Commercial production results in more than 100,000,000 pounds of penicillin per year.

Several natural penicillins can be produced, depending on the chemical composition of the fermentation medium used to culture penicillium. *Penicillin G* (benzylpenicillin) has the greatest antimicrobial activity of these natural penicillins and is the only *natural* penicillin used clinically. However, penicillin G is not stable. It is extremely acid-labile. Only about one third of an oral dose is absorbed under the most ideal conditions. Therefore, it is generally *not given orally. It is for this reason that it must be administered by intramuscular injection.* Several newer derivatives of penicillin G that do have good to excellent oral absorption (e.g., cloxacillin, ampicillin, and amoxicillin) have been developed.

The selective toxicity of penicillin can be dramatically illustrated by the fact that a person, with normal renal function, can receive approximately 12.5–15 g of penicillin per day with no ill effects; however, as little as 0.002 μg/ml may kill some bacteria such as pneumococous. Therefore, the toxic to therapeutic ratio is extremely high. Unfortunately, this is not always achieved with antibiotics. This can be illustrated with the antifungal drug amphotericin B. For treatment of fungal infections, daily dosages of 0.5–0.6 mg/kg (35–42 mg for a 70 kg person) are needed. However, a dose of 1 mg can cause fever, chills, and low blood pressure in some patients. Chronic use can lead to fatal kidney damage. Therefore, although antibiotics are often associated with a relatively high margin of safety, there are important exceptions.

During the 1930s, another significant class of antibiotics was discovered. The *sulfa drug Prontosil*, with its *active metabolite sulfanilamide*, was found to be effective against streptococcal infections, first in mice and then in humans. Sulfonamides were actually the *first* effective chemotherapeutic agents to be employed systemically for the prevention and cure of bacterial infections in humans, since penicillin was really not widely available until the early 1940s. In fact, the individual credited with discovery of this class of drugs, and recipient of the Nobel Prize for his work, *Gerhard Domagk*, allowed it to be administered successfully to his daughter who was suffering from streptococcal septicemia at the time.

MECHANISM OF ACTION OF ANTIBIOTICS

As discussed above, there are a number of ways by which an antibiotic can selectively interfere with biochemical processes in a microbe. This portion of the chapter will deal in more detail with the respective mechanisms. These will include the cell wall and membrane, nucleic acid and protein synthesis, and intermediary metabolism.

Penicillins, cephalosporins, and related drugs are known as *β-lactams*, since they share a four-membered *β*-lactam ring. The mechanism of action of *β*-lactam type drugs is more complex than originally thought. Penicillin and cephaloporin appear to be analogs of a natural structural unit (D-alanyl-D-alanine) in the *cell walls* of gram-positive bacteria. These antibiotics become covalently bound to a family of enzymes known as *penicillin-binding proteins* (PBPs) that are responsible for constructing the peptidoglycan lattice of bacterial cell walls. Failure to achieve adequate synthesis of the cell wall results in *increased cell permeability, leakage, and death.* Penicillin will not harm any cell wall already made but will interfere with *new* cell wall formation.

Microbes also have a *plasma membrane* that resides adjacent to their cell wall. *Polymyxins* are amphipathic agents (containing both nonpolar, lipophilic; and polar, lipophobic groups) that interact with phospholipids in microbial *cell membranes*. The result is disruption of the membrane and increased permeability. However, because microbial and mammalian cell membranes are not exceedingly dissimilar, polymixins can produce significant toxicity in humans (i.e., they have low selective toxicity). This is also true for the related drug nystatin. This is why these particular antibiotics are not generally used systemically and are usually *restricted* to topical application.

Some antibiotics are known to interfere with microbial *nucleic acid* function. *Rifampin,* for example, inhibits *DNA-dependent RNA polymerase*, leading to suppression of the initiation of RNA chain formation. Nuclear RNA polymerase from a variety of eukaryotic cells does not bind rifampin, and RNA synthesis is correspondingly unaffected. Drugs belonging to the quinolone group interfere with *DNA gyrase*, the enzyme responsible for "super coiling" microbial DNA into a compact form while retaining its functionality. Eukaryotic cells do not contain DNA gyrase (type II DNA topoisomerase is the equivalent but is several orders of magnitude less sensitive).

There are a number of sites within the sequence of *protein synthesis* where antibiotics can act. These include (1) inhibition of the attachment of mRNA to 30S ribosomes by aminoglycosides; (2) inhibition of tRNA binding to 30S ribosomes by tetracyclines; (3) inhibition of the attachment of mRNA to the 50S ribosome by chloramphenicol; and (4) erythromycin inhibition of the translocation step by binding to 50S ribosomes thus preventing newly synthesized peptidyl tRNA moving from the acceptor to the donor site.

Finally, *sulfonamides* can interfere with *intermediary metabolism*. Because of their structural similarity to (para-aminobenzoic acid, PABA), they can function as *competitive inhibitors for dihydropteroate synthase*. The result is interruption of microbial synthesis of *folic acid* by blocking formation of the folic acid precursor, dihydropteroic acid. Sensitive microorganisms are those that must synthesize their own folic acid. Conversely, resistant bacteria and normal mammalian cells are unaffected, since they do not synthesize folic acid but use the preformed vitamin.

RESISTANCE TO ANTIMICROBIAL AGENTS

One of the unfortunate realities of antimicrobial therapy has been the sobering realization that pathogens can develop drug resistance. Once on the verge of defeat, thanks to medicine's arsenal of approximately 160 antibiotics, bacteria began a resurgence a number of years ago. With each passing decade, bacteria that defy not only single but also multiple antibiotics—and therefore are extremely difficult to control—have become increasingly common. The emergence of antibacterial resistance in pathogenic strains is a worldwide problem. For example, during the past 50 years, the development of penicillin-resistant strains of pneumococci has exceeded 50% in isolates from some European countries. In 1997, in three geographically separate patients, a new strain of *Staphylococcus aureus* was encountered. Previously, this bacterium, already resistant to all antibiotics, save vancomycin, showed resistance to *vancomycin*. The emergence of *vancomycin-resistant organisms* has been one of the greatest fears among public health professionals. For many infections, vancomycin is the antibiotic of last resort. *S. aureus* causes 260,000 infections each year in the United States, which, if left untreated, can be fatal. There are now strains of entercocci, pseudomonas, and enterobacters that are resistant to all known drugs.

The remarkable capacity of *S. aureus* to develop resistance to antibiotics is no more clearly illustrated than its recently reported success against linezolid (Zyvox®). Linezoid is the first entirely new type of antibiotic (oxazolidinones) introduced in 35 years. The FDA approved it in April 2000 for the treatment of several infections including *resistant strains of S. aureus*. However, it took only slightly more than a year for resistance to manifest itself. In the summer of 2001, the first report of staph resistance to the new antibiotic was observed in an 85-year-old man undergoing dialysis.

In recent years, strains of multi *drug-resistant tuberculosis* (TB) have spread around the world, killing thousands. In fact, the death rates for some communicable diseases such as tuberculosis have started to rise in industrialized countries. The number of TB cases worldwide has reached epidemic proportions. The World Health Organization reports that one third of the world's population is infected, projecting 1 billion new infections and 35 million deaths in the next 20 years. In the United States alone, according to a 1995 report from the former Office of Technology Assessment, 19,000 hospital patients die each year due to hospital-acquired bacterial infections. Until recently, infections caused by *Staphylococcus epidermidis* and *Enterococcus faecium* were treatable with antibiotics. This is no longer the case. Up to 30% of the pneumonia found in some areas of the United States no longer responds to penicillin. Heavily used, antibiotics have become an evolutionary force, selecting for and enhancing the survival of bacterial strains that can resist them. According to the *Centers for Disease Control* (CDC), antibiotics are used excessively in 20–50% of cases.

The speed with which bacteria "acquire" resistance to antibiotics cautions against prescribing them too frequently. Between 1983 and 1993, the *percentage* of patients receiving antibiotics rose from 1.4 to 45. During those years, researchers isolated *Eschericia coli* annually from patients, and tested the microbes for resistance to 5 types of *fluroquinolones*. Between 1983 and 1990, the antibiotics easily killed all 92 *E. coli* strains tested. However, in the interval from 1991 to 1993, 11 of 40 tested strains (28%) were resistant to all five drugs.

While the plea to more closely regulate the clinical use of antibiotics in humans is an obvious admonition to the medical community (humans take an estimated 3 million pounds yearly), there are other sources of concern. For example, the American Medical Association estimates that more than half of the total mass of antibiotics used in the United States is *fed to animals*, not to cure them of illness, but as *growth promoters* or to *prevent illness*. The Animal Health Institute, which represents makers of animal drugs, indicates that more than 20 million pounds of antibiotics are used yearly in the United States. The Union of Concerned Scientists estimates that as little as 2 million pounds go to sick animals. This is exactly the type of profligate usage that promotes the emergence of resistance.

In a study published in 2001, researchers at the University of Maryland collected 200 samples of ground beef, ground chicken, ground turkey, and ground pork from three supermarkets in the Washington, DC area. Twenty percent of the samples were contaminated with *salmonella*, a bacterium blamed for approximately 1.4 million cases of food poisoning a year in the United States. Of the salmonella strains isolated, 84% were resistant to at least one antibiotic and 53% to three or more.

In another study published in the same year, researchers at the CDC found that half of 407 supermarket chickens bought from 26 stores in four states—Georgia, Maryland, Minnesota, and Oregon—carried the sometimes fatal germ *E. faecium* in a form resistant to Synercid®, one of the few drugs of last resort against the infection.

In a similar study reported in 2003, colleagues at the Swiss Federal Veterinary Office and the University of Zurich isolated *antibiotic-resistant thermophilic Campylobacter* (CB) from poultry products sold at 122 retail stores in Switzerland and Liehtenstein. *CB* is a major cause of foodborne gastrointestinal infections in many developed countries, and poultry is the most common source of the bacteria. Antibiotic resistance is of particular interest because the same antibiotics are used to treat animals and humans infected by the bacteria.

The researchers collected 415 raw poultry samples and found that 91 contained CB strains. From these, 87 strains were isolated and 51 were killed by all the antibiotics tested. Of the remaining 36 strains, all were resistant to 1 antibiotic, 19 were resistant to 2 antibiotics, 4 were resistant to 3 antibiotics, 2 were resistant to 4 antibiotics, and 2 were resistant to 5 antibiotics. The bacteria were most often resistant, in order of most resistant to least resistant, to ciprofloxacin, tetracycline, sulfonamide, and ampicillin. One strain was resistant to 5 antibiotics, including 3 frequently used to treat CB in humans: ciprofloxacin, tetracycline, and *erythromycin*. A previous study in the United States found that 90% of CB was resistant to at least one antibiotic.

The researchers also reported that the number of samples with bacteria did not depend on the way the poultry was raised. The country of origin (all in the EU) also had little significance for the presence of bacteria. However, frozen products showed much *lower* rates of bacterial presence than fresh products.

Antibiotics do not usually induce adaptive mutations; instead, they act as fierce agents of selection, killing off all bacteria except a favored few that, by chance, are immune to the antibiotic—a strain that earlier, for other reasons, might not have competed successfully with its fellows. The fact that bacteria quickly evolve resistance to antibiotics reflects the enormous diversity of forms and biochemical capacity at work in the microbial world. In that world, there is a continuing conflict of measure and countermeasure, raging between host and parasite—in this case, between the pharmaceutical companies, generating new antibiotics, and the microbes, generating new resistant strains to replace their more vulnerable ancestors.

In order for an antimicrobial agent to be efficacious, it must reach the target pathogen and bind to it in sufficient concentration to express its effect. Bacteria can develop resistance by: a number of mechanisms including (1) preventing the drug from *reaching the target*. For example, the "porin" channel proteins in gram-negative bacteria can become altered, thereby preventing certain antibiotics from gaining entrance; (2) certain bacteria can increase their ability to *metabolize* antibiotics. For example, gram-positive bacteria (which do not have an outer cell membrane) such as staphylococci export beta-lactamases into their immediate environment and destroy β-lactam antibiotics such as penicillins and cephalosporins. This is a major problem with *Haemophilus* and gonococci. In an attempt to circumvent this problem, β-lactamase inhibitors are sometimes simultaneously given in order to protect the antibiotic. Gram-negative bacteria may also export β-lactamases as well as have them in their periplasmic space between the inner and outer membrane; (3) changes can occur at the *drug-binding site*. For example, a common cause of resistance to protease inhibitors used in the treatment of AIDS is that a phenyl group in the active site "flips" out of reach of the tightly binding inhibitor. This creates a gap where van der Waals contacts, once formed by the inhibitor, are lost; and (4) some microbes can increase the transport of antibiotics out of the cell.

Mutations in HIV accumulate and interact with each other and cause resistance to one drug and then others, one of the pivotal problems in treatment. In the past, the complexity of HIV drug-resistance testing and the limited information on its clinical utility made routine application impractical. Recent advances in automated assay technology have allowed rapid characterization of HIV in blood samples, so an increasing number of commercial laboratories now offer phenotypic and genotypic testing. This comes at a time when, globally, HIV infections are increasing at a rate of more than 5 million per year. At this rate, by 2010, there will be 45 million new infections. Most of these cases will be in the third world.

Perhaps the greatest problem in developing countries is that of HIV resistance. Evolution is the enemy. As with bacterial diseases and antibiotics, different HIV strains are resistant to at least one of the major reverse transcription inhibitors or protease inhibitors. And these strains are spreading throughout the HIV-infected population, with multiple-strain infections being ever more common. The AIDS community is also faced with the dilemma that opportunistic diseases that flourish in the absence of a functional immune system are the ultimate cause of death. Chief among these, especially in the developing world, is tuberculosis (TB). According to the *Bill and Melinda Gates Foundation*, one out of every three people with HIV/AIDS will die of TB (www.gatesfoundation.org). With the rapid rise of antibiotic-resistant strains of TB, the potential for a catastrophic epidemic is ever present.

GENETICS OF BACTERIAL RESISTANCE

Many bacteria possessed resistance genes even before commercial antibiotics came into use. Scientists do not know exactly why these genes evolved and were maintained. One argument is that natural antibiotics were initially elaborated as the result of chance mutations; the bacteria so endowed were more likely to survive and proliferate.

Bacteria can obtain the various types of resistance mechanisms described above by undergoing modifications in their genetic constitution. Many bacteria simply *inherit* their resistance genes from their forerunners. In addition, *genetic mutations* that can confer a new trait can occur. For example, it has been estimated that bacteria undergo spontaneous *mutation* at a frequency of approximately one in ten cells. These mutations can confer resistant traits to the subsequent progeny. Mutations are believed to be responsible for the development of resistance to *streptomycin* (ribosomal mutation), *quinolones* (gyrase gene mutation), and *rifampin* (RNA polymerase gene mutation), the end result being that the drug does not bind. It is this vertical, Darwinian process, whereby a few existing members of a heterogeneous population that happen to have a genetic advantage, reproduce in the presence of the antimicrobial drug and become the dominant surviving strain. However, although mutation of the microbe's genome can occur, the major mechanism of resistance development in pathogenic bacteria is *plasmid* mediated.

Plasmids are autonomously replicating pieces of *extrachromosomal DNA* present in bacteria. They are encoded with subtle, yet vital changes for the synthesis of important cellular proteins. Because they are relatively large, they can contain information pertaining to several genes. One of these genes codes for *β-lactamase*, an enzyme that can hydrolyze the four-member heterocyclic *β*-lactam ring present in *penicillins* and *cephalosporins*.

There are several mechanisms by which plasmids can serve as the vehicle to transfer resistance determinants to sensitive bacteria. These include *transduction, transformation*, and *conjugation*. Resistance that is acquired by this type of horizontal transfer can become rapidly and widely disseminated.

Transduction involves the introduction of new genetic information via a *bacteriophage* (a virus that infects bacteria). In this situation, the bacteriophage contains DNA that can carry a gene for drug resistance. Transductive transfer of phage DNA is particularly important for the development of resistance among strains of *S. aureus* that become endowed with the ability to synthesize penicillinase.

Transformation is a process whereby *fragments of free DNA* in the environment of the microbe become incorporated into its own genome. For example, penicillin-resistant pneumococci produce altered PBPs that have low affinity binding sites for penicillin. Nucleotide sequence analysis of the genes encoding these altered PBPs indicates that the *insertion* of foreign genetic material has taken place. Presumably, these DNA fragments (transposons) originate in closely related streptococcal strains and become incorporated into resident PBP genes by homologous recombination.

The process by which the passage of genes occurs directly from bacterium to bacterium by direct contact is referred to as *conjugation*. A pilus or tube, which joins the donor and recipient organisms and through which genetic material is passed, is temporarily formed. The donor must possess two genetic factors in order to participate in conjugation: an *R-factor* that codes for the resistance trait and an *RT-factor* that codes for the synthesis of the pilus. Conjugation occurs largely in gram-negative bacteria. The clinical significance of conjugation was first demonstrated in Japan in 1959, after an outbreak of bacillary dysentery. The responsible pathogen, *Shigella flexneri*, was found to be resistant to not just one but four different classes of antibiotics (tetracycline, sulfonamide, streptomycin, and chloramphenicol).

SELECTION OF APPROPRIATE ANTIBIOTIC

Ideally, biological specimens containing the infectious agent would be obtained and identification of the pathogen carried out. In addition, *in vitro* antimicrobial susceptibility studies might then be determined. In practice, this is generally not done, since clinical decisions are often based on the presentation of patient symptoms. In this manner, therapy can be started immediately with a minimum of expense. The drawback to this expeditious prescribing is that antibiotics are subject to inappropriate use, which has contributed to the development of *resistance*.

After the September 11, 2001, attacks on the World Trade Center and Pentagon, the Washington, DC and New York city anthrax incidents heightened the awareness of not only the public but also the scientific community to the threat of homeland terrorism and biological warfare. These events emphasized the importance of rapid microbiologic diagnosis for the timely and adequate implementation of preventive and control measures.

According to experts in the field, the future of biological warfare detection will rely on four technological principles: measuring particles by shining light to illuminate samples, detecting specific agents or toxins by various immunoassays, amplifying DNA by polymerase chain reaction (PCR) and detecting the results with specific gene probes, and using mass spectrometry to detect biological warfare agents.

Similarly, the *Singapore Defense Medical Research Institute* is applying *real-time* PCR diagnostics to develop methods of detecting and identifying infectious pathogens. Its Biomedical Sciences Laboratory is developing diagnostic assays that select gene targets unique to the bacterium or virus in question, designing PCR primers against the gene target, testing the PCR assay against reference strains of the virus or bacterium, and validating the procedure using clinical samples.

This process consists of extracting nucleic acids from the "raw" sample, followed by PCR analysis to detect the pathogen in question. Conventional PCR methods would take at least 2 h and be followed by gel electrophoresis analysis, which could take another 3–4 h. However, with real-time PCR coupled to a capillary thermocycler, the whole process can be completed in less than 40 min. Therefore, through the application of molecular diagnostics, researchers can process crude specimens and detect and identify causative pathogens in less than a day, compared with 4 days previously.

Until recently, few people outside the agriculture and microbiology communities had heard of *anthrax*. Anthrax is primarily a disease of livestock, particularly cattle and sheep, but it can affect all mammals, including humans, who come in contact with infected animals or their by-products. Only recently has anthrax achieved widespread notoriety, because of its potential use as a biological weapon.

Almost all naturally occurring cases of anthrax are cutaneous or gastrointestinal. Blackish sores on the skin characterize cutaneous anthrax. Anthrax was actually named from a Greek word that refers to coal or charcoal. After entering the body by skin lesions, ingestion, or inhalation anthrax spores germinate in macrophages, causing septicemia and toxemia. Anthrax toxin is comprised of three proteins: lethal factor (LF), which is a protease that causes cell death; edema factor (EF), which is an adenylate cyclase that impairs host defense; and protective antigen (PA), which is required for the entry of both LF and EF into cells. Together, LF and PA constitute the *lethal toxin*; likewise, EF and PA collaborate to form the edema toxin. Recent evidence has shown that lethal toxin represses the transcriptional activity of the glucocorticoid receptor, which is a crucial component of the body's defenses against inflammation. The study reports that lethal toxin blocks the glucocorticoid receptor by inhibiting the p38 mitogen-activated protein kinase pathway. These findings suggest that glucocoticoid receptor inactivation contributes to anthrax toxicity and raise the possibility of developing new strategies to combat this deadly disease.

Inhalation anthrax is an extremely rare disease that normally results from exposure to contaminated animal hides and hairs, with most transmissions occurring in an industrial setting. Anthrax is a biowarfare threat because its spores can be made into an aerosol form that can resist environmental degradation, and can be milled into an ideal size for reaching the lower respiratory tract (1–6 μm). Although the exact number of inhaled spores required to produce death in humans is unknown, most estimates put the level in the 8,000–10,000 range.

As soon as the first case was confirmed in Florida, a relatively new drug gained notoriety—Cipro®. This fluoroquinolone (ciprofloxacin) became the mode of therapy for those people exposed to the anthrax bacillus (approved by the FDA for anthrax on July 28, 2000). Despite appeals for restraint in the use of Cipro®, pharmacies in Mexican border towns reported being cleaned out of the antibiotic by Americans searching for readily available and relatively cheap drug. Only time will tell if inappropriate, irrational use of Cipro® results in loss of effectiveness in treating anthrax infection. However, the CDC did determine that 19% of 490 people in Florida experienced side effects 1–2 weeks after beginning therapy with Cipro®.

The use of Cipro® to treat anthrax infection emanated from research carried out in 1990 at Ft. Detrick, Maryland (see below). The army was concerned that Saddam Hussein could introduce germ warfare in the Gulf War in the form of anthrax. Sixty monkeys were infected with a strain of Bacillus anthracis by aerosol and were divided into six groups. One group received a vaccine alone; another received the vaccine and antibiotics; and 3 groups were treated for 30 days with 1 of 3 different classes of antibiotics: penicillin, doxycycline, or Cipro®. A control group received saline injections.

By day 8, 9 of 10 control monkeys had perished. By day 10, 8 of 10 monkeys who received vaccine alone were dead. By contrast, the monkeys treated daily with antibiotics survived into the fourth week. The combination of vaccine and doxycycline performed best. Nevertheless, Pentagon officials recommended using a combination of Cipro® and vaccine since Cipro® was a newer drug and, presumably, more effective against a conceivably genetically engineered anthrax. However, in October 2001, the FDA issued a health advisory update reminding all health professionals that doxycycline is approved for the treatment of anthrax in all its forms (inhalation, cutaneous, and ingested).

BIOTERRORISM

Microorganisms and warfare go back more than two millennia. Scythian archers are known to have dipped their arrowheads in manure and rotting corpses in order to increase the deadliness of their weapons. In the fourteenth century, Tartar forces, in what is now Ukraine, threw plague-laden bodies over the walls of enemy cities. During the French and Indian War in North America, during the eighteenth century, British troops under the command of Sir Jeffrey Amherst gave unfriendly Native Americans blankets known to be contaminated with *smallpox*. In 1797, Napoleon tried to infect residents of a besieged city in Italy with *malaria*.

During World War I, a German agent grew *anthrax* and other bacteria in his Washington, DC home. The anthrax was used to infect some 3000 horses and mules destined for Allied troops in Europe. Many of the animals died and hundreds of soldiers were infected.

In 1942, the British began testing "*anthrax bombs*" on Gruinard Island, a 500-acre island off the northwestern coast of Scotland. The Gruinard experiments established the environmental consequences of using anthrax as a weapon of mass destruction; a lesson Soviet scientists would discover for themselves decades later. Instead of the spores dying or being dissipated by the wind, they remained to the point that Gruinard became known as "*Anthrax Island.*"

During World War II, the Japanese dropped fleas infected with *plague* (*Yersinia pestis*) on Chinese cities, killing hundreds and possibly thousands. Thousands of documents captured from the Japanese following the war further attest to the Japanese use of anthrax, typhoid, and plague on Manchurian towns and cities. This information proved to be a stimulus for the United States to seriously begin to study the area of germ warfare.

By the early 1950s, the government had established its own germ warfare laboratory at an army base located at *Ft. Detrick, Maryland*. Over time, the scientists identified approximately 50 different viruses and rickettsiae that were good candidates for germ warfare; a number that was nearly three times the number of suitable bacteria. Viruses were considered to be particularly ideal agents, since they were basically unaffected by antibiotics and they could be selected to primarily *debilitate,* rather than kill, the victim. Incapacitation ties up more resources of the enemy and is more humane. President Eisenhower was briefed at a National Security Council meeting on February 18, 1960, to the effect that controlled *incapacitation* promised to "open up a new dimension of warfare."

Despite the allure of incapacitating viruses, the scientists at Ft. Detrick continued their research on more virulent viral strains. Among them was an old nemesis—*smallpox.* Smallpox was an ancient foe, highly contagious, and killed approximately one-third of those infected. It has been estimated that smallpox has killed more people over the ages than any other infectious disease, including the plague. In the twentieth century alone, it has been estimated that smallpox was responsible for the death of a half billion people worldwide, exceeding all of the wars, epidemics, and pandemics combined. Smallpox has been considered an excellent choice for bioterrorism, since it has a consistent, long incubation period that allows the operatives responsible for the attacks to leave the country prior to outbreak.

America's participation in germ warfare research took an abrupt turn when, on November 25, 1965, President Richard Nixon proclaimed "*… the U.S. shall renounce the use of lethal biological agents and weapons, and all other methods of biological warfare. The U.S. will confine its biological research to defensive measures.*" In 1972, the United States, the Soviet Union, and more than one hundred nations signed the *Biological and Toxin Weapons Convention*. This document prohibits the possession of deadly biological agents except for research into selective defensive measures. It was the world's first treaty banning an entire class of weapons. Unfortunately, the treaty was filled with loopholes and ambiguities ad nauseum, as well as a lack of enforcement, therefore achieving virtually nothing.

At the same time that the 1972 treaty was being created, two scientists in Northern California began a collaboration that transformed the world of microbiology. Stanley Cohen and Herbert Boyer applied existing technology to the creation of recombinant life forms that provided the foundation for *genetic engineering*. The concept was deceptively straightforward. Snip a gene from one organism and insert it into another. By using certain enzymes that break DNA at certain points, Cohen and Boyer's team was able to remove the gene for resistance to penicillin from a microbe, for example, splice the gene into plasmid DNA, and allow *E. coli* to take up the plasmid. The result was a new microbe resistant to penicillin. Subsequently, gene expression of other substances such as insulin and human growth hormone has created a novel area of drug production. Unfortunately, this technology can also be utilized to convert normally harmless bacteria, such as *E. coli* to higher levels of pathogenicity, as well as highly pathogenic microbes, such as anthrax, to "super" bugs.

Congressional investigations have shown that even after Nixon's ban on offensive germ warfare studies, and inventories, the central intelligence agency (CIA) had retained a small arsenal (at least 16 pathogens; usually in the mg to gram range) stored at Ft. Detrick. In comparison, the Soviet Union had not only continued to research germ warfare (e.g., the development of "Superplague," and the capacity to produce 300 tons of anthrax spores in 220 days.), but also flagrantly violated the treaty for 20 years. It had produced an industry that created disease by the ton. The Soviet Union's plan for World War III had included hundreds of tons of anthrax bacteria and scores of tons of small-pox and plague viruses. A comparison of germ warfare production between the United States and the Soviet Union during its maximum is shown in Table 10.2.

According to data collected by the Center for Nonproliferation Studies at the Monterey Institute of International Studies, there have been 285 incidents throughout the world during the past 25 years in which terrorists have used chemical or biological weapons. One of these attacks occurred in the United States almost 17 years to the day prior to the World Trade Center's catastrophe. On September 9, 1984, citizens who had dined in a restaurant in The Dalles, Oregon began to complain of stomach cramps. Symptoms worsened over the next several days with hospitalization being sometimes necessary. Some customers threatened to sue the local owner for food poisoning. Over the next few days, the local health department received complaints regarding two other restaurants.

On September 21, a second wave of reports occurred involving people who had fallen ill at ten different restaurants in the small town. For the first time in the history of the community's only

TABLE 10.2

Comparison of Dry Agent Production (Metric Tons per Year) in the United States and the Soviet Union

	United States	Soviet Union
Staphylococcal enterotoxin B	1.8	0
F. tularensis (tularemia)	1.6	1,500
Coxiella burnetii (Q fever)	1.1	0
B. anthracis (anthrax)	0.9	4,500
Venezuelan equine encephalitis virus	0.8	150
Botulinum	0.2	0
Yersinia pestis (bubonic plague)	0	1,500
Variola virus (smallpox)	0	100
Actinobacillus mallei (glanders)	0	2,000
Marburg virus	0	250

Source: J. Miller, S. Engelberg, and W. Broad (2001) *Germs: Biological Weapons and Americas Secret War*. New York: Simon & Schuster.

hospital, all 125 beds were filled. By the end of the outbreak, nearly a thousand people had reported symptoms. The offending agent was identified as *Salmonella typhimurium*. Extensive investigations of employees, water sources, septic-tank malfunctions, as well as suspect food items, did not produce an explanation. In addition, the deputy state epidemiologist proclaimed that there was no evidence to support deliberate contamination. It would take another year before an explanation occurred.

On September 16, 1985, the Bhagwan of the Rajneeshees cult ended a 4-year vow of silence by holding a press conference at his ranch/cult center. The Bhagwan leveled numerous charges at his recently departed personal secretary and the commune's *de facto* leader. Among the most revealing allegations was that his secretary was responsible for the poisoning. Federal and state police then formed a joint task force to investigate the situation. Analysis of "bactrol discs" revealed that the salmonella in the growth discs was identical to that which had sickened people in The Dalles, the previous year. The smoking gun had been found.

The reason for the poisoning of patrons in local diners was related to politics. Since the cult and its followers had arrived in this sparsely populated Oregon area, they had begun to make attempts to take the town over. Numerous strategies had failed. Finally, it was decided that perhaps control of the town could be taken over at the ballot box. In theory, if enough of the locals came down with a sickness during an election then, perhaps, the candidates supported by the cult could win. Such was not to be the case. Although little media attention was generated at the time, the incident is still significant, since it represents the first large-scale use of bioterrorism on American soil. A comparison of deaths from selected causes is shown in Table 10.3 and can be used to put anthrax fatalities into perspective.

ANTICANCER DRUGS

Cancer involves the uncontrolled proliferation of cells that can produce the growth of tumors or alter the formation of blood cells. Numerous factors can influence the development of neoplasia, but the major causes appear to be environmental and genetic. While most environmental carcinogens appear to be mutagens, normal regulatory control of cell growth in the body apparently can be perturbed by either (1) the expression of oncogenes or (2) the loss of tumor suppressor genes. In a human cell, there are 30–50,000 different genes that can become defective to produce cancer. In any event, the result is malignant transformation.

Therapeutic modalities in cancer treatment may involve surgery, radiation, and/or chemotherapy. The objectives of cancer chemotherapy include (1) cure, (2) reduction in tumor size, and

TABLE 10.3
Deaths from Selected Causes in the United States*

Cause of Death	Number
Smoking-related	23,077
Flu-related	3,674
Auto accidents	2,448
Alcohol-induced	1,101
Murders	971
AIDS	847
Prescription drug errors	404

* Deaths are for an average 3-week period not adjusted for seasonal fluctuations. Sources include American Cancer Society, Institute of Medicine, National Transportation Safety Board, and National Center for Health Statistics.

(3) prolongation of life. At the present time, approximately 50% of patients with cancer can be cured, with drug treatment estimated to contribute in 17% of cases. Cancer chemotherapy can be curative in testicular cancer, diffuse large cell lymphoma, Hodgkin's disease, choriocarcinoma, and certain childhood tumors (acute lymphoblastic leukemia, Burkett's lymphoma, Wilms' tumor, and embryonal rhabdomyosarcoma). Certain cancers are more resistant to chemotherapy than others (e.g., lung and colon).

The objective of cancer chemotherapy is to kill 100% of the tumor stem cells. This is always a challenge for the attending oncologist. In certain cases of disseminated cancer, there may be a total body cell burden of 10^{12} cancerous cells (1 trillion). Even with a kill percentage of 99.9%, there will still be 10^9 cells remaining; the result of a "three log kill." Some of these remaining cells may be resistant or not be accessible to the drug. In comparison, a "three log kill" may be curative for bacterial infections since host resistance factors can eliminate residual disease, unlike the situation in treating cancer. Strategies to maximize the probability of obtaining total cell death with chemotherapy include the following:

- Combination therapy
- Drugs with differing toxicity profiles
- Drugs with differing mechanisms of action
- Drugs with synergistic actions
- Combine with surgical and radiation intervention

Historically, anticancer drugs have been discovered through large-scale screening of synthetic chemicals and natural products against animal tumor systems. The drugs discovered in the first two decades of cancer chemotherapy (1950–1970) primarily interacted with DNA or its precursors, inhibiting the synthesis of new genetic material or causing irreparable damage to DNA itself. This strategy was based on the quantitative difference between tumor cells and most normal cells, that is, a *high mitotic index*. In other words, because tumor cells divide at a higher rate, their genetic machinery is more prone to be affected by drugs that influence mitosis. Unfortunately, the same can be said for certain normal cells such as hair follicles, explaining why alopecia is a common side effect to drugs that interfere with nucleic acid synthesis. Table 10.4 below shows the mechanism of action of major classes of anticancer drugs:

Because anticancer drugs do not affect qualitatively different sites within cancer cells, such as penicillin does in prokaryotic bacteria, they are more prone to produce side effects. As mentioned above, organs with active cell division are typically affected. Table 10.5 presents some common side effects of anticancer drugs. It should be noted that certain drugs are associated with certain side effects.

TABLE 10.4
Overview of Major Anticancer Drugs

- *Alkylating agents*: cross-link two strands of DNA, leading to impairment of DNA replication and RNA transcription (e.g., cyclophosphamide)
- *Antimetabolites*: folic acid (e.g., methotrexate), purine (e.g., 2-chlorodeoxyadenosine) and pyrimidine (e.g., 5-fluorouracil) analogs that interfere with synthesis of DNA precursors
- *Natural products/antibiotics*: anthracyclines (e.g., doxorubicin) damage DNA by intercalating DNA and inhibiting topoisomerase II
- *Antimitotics*: Inhibit microtubule synthesis; inhibit cell division (e.g., paclitaxel)
- *Hormones*: glucocorticoids, estrogen antagonist (e.g., tamoxifen), and leuteinizing
- Hormone-releasing hormone analogs (e.g., leuprolide)

TABLE 10.5
Common Toxicities of Cancer Chemotherapeutics

- *Bone marrow*: suppression of bone marrow function can lead to significant reduction in white blood cells, platelets, anemia, and neutrophils; caused by *almost* all anticancer drugs
- *Gastrointestinal tract*: nausea, vomiting, and diarrhea
- *Alopecia*
- *Renal damage*
- *Pulmonary injury:* pulmonary fibrosis can be produced by bleomycin
- *Peripheral neuropathy*

Note: Long-term complications such as cardiomyopathy (e.g., doxorubicin), leukemia (i.e., mechlorethamine), and infertility (alkylating agents) can also occur. Amelioration of certain side effects can be achieved with the judicious use of antiemetics and blood transfusions (or erythropoietin).

ALKYLATING AGENTS

Alkylation refers to the attachment of an alkyl group to a lone pair of electrons on a C, N, O, S, or any other atom in an organic molecule. Mustard gas, bis(2-chloroethyl) sulfide is an alkylating agent and is the first known chemical mutagen; it was an acutely toxic poison gas having ravaged the fields of combatants in Europe during World War I. It was subsequently studied as a chemotherapeutic agent against experimental rat tumors in the 1930s, but its acute toxicity precluded clinical use.

The systematic development of mustard analogs as cancer chemotherapeutic agents began with the studies of Louis Goodman and Alfred Gilman (the original coauthors of the textbook *The Pharmacological Basis of Therapeutics*, reverently referred to as "The Bible" of Pharmacology).

During World War II, their research was funded by the military, which wanted antidotes to chemical warfare agents, but the two collaborators had sufficient latitude that they were able to explore chemotherapeutic applications as well. The nitrogen mustard methyl-bis(2-chloroethyl)amine was first tested as an anticancer agent in mice, and then administered to cancer patients, on an experimental basis, in December 1942. These efforts marked the beginning of modern chemotherapy for cancer. Many other nitrogen mustard derivatives, including melphalan, cyclophosphamide, and chloambucil were later developed as anticancer drugs.

ANTIMETABOLITES

Inhibitors of nucleotide biosynthesis are important cancer chemotherapeutic drugs. 6-Mercaptopurine and 6-thioguanine are purine antimetabolites used in the treatment of leukemias. Azathioprine is a derivative of 6-mercaptopurine. Its bone marrow toxicity, an undesirable side effect, has been turned to advantage for suppression of the immune system in organ transplantation.

SELECTED BIBLIOGRAPHY

Albert, A. (1979) *Selective Toxicity*, London: Chapman & Hall.

Hardman, J.G., Limbird, L.L., and Gilman, A.G. (Eds.) (2001) *Goodman and Gillman's: The Pharmacological Basis of Therapeutics*, 10th ed., New York: McGraw-Hill.

Miller, J., Engelberg, S., and Broad, W. (2001) *Germs: Biological Weapons and America's Secret War*, New York: Simon & Schuster.

Moellering, R.C. (1985) Principles of Anti-infective therapy, in *Mandell, Douglas, and Bennett's Principles and Practice of Infectious Diseases*, 2nd ed., Mandell, G.L., Douglas, R.G., Jr., and Bennett, J.E. (Eds.), New York: John Wiley & Sons.

Pratt, W.B. and Fekety, F.R. (Eds.) (1986) *The Antimicrobial Drugs*, New York: Oxford University Press.

QUESTIONS

1. Credit for the actual discovery of microorganisms is given to which of the following?
   a. Paul Ehrlich
   b. Robert Koch
   c. Louis Pasteur
   d. Alexander Fleming
   e. Antonie van Leeuwenhoek

2. Which of the following is credited with conceptualizing the "germ theory of disease"?
   a. Paul Ehrlich
   b. Robert Koch
   c. Louis Pasteur
   d. Alexander Fleming
   e. Antonie van Leeuwenhoek

3. Which of the following is credited with demonstrating the actual disease role of microorganisms.
   a. Paul Ehrlich
   b. Robert Koch
   c. Louis Pasteur
   d. Alexander Fleming
   e. Antonie van Leeuwenhoek

4. Which of the following drugs was first referred to as a "magic bullet"?
   a. Penicillin
   b. Arsphenamine
   c. Cipro
   d. Sulfanilamide
   e. Ampicillin

5. The mechanism of action of penicillin involves which of the following?
   a. Inhibition of DNA-dependent RNA polymerase
   b. Inhibition of DNA gyrase
   c. Inhibition of mRNA attachment to 30S ribosomes
   d. Inhibition of peptidoglycan formation in cell walls
   e. Inhibition of mRNA attachment to 50S ribosomes

6. Microbial resistance to antibiotics can develop by which of the following mechanisms?
   a. Uptake of plasmids
   b. Inheritance
   c. Mutation
   d. All of the above
   e. None of the above

7. Which of the following is/are true regarding cancer chemotherapy versus microbe chemotherapy?
   a. The therapeutic index is generally lower
   b. The therapeutic index is generally higher
   c. A higher cell "kill rate" is required to affect a cure
   d. Cures are virtually never really achieved
   e. a and c

8. Which of the following is/are not used in cancer chemotherapy?
   a. Drugs that cross-link DNA
   b. Inhibitors of folic acid synthesis
   c. Drugs that damage DNA
   d. Drugs that inhibit microtubule synthesis
   e. None of the above

9. Which of the following is/are true regarding side effects of anticancer drugs?
   a. Primarily affect the central nervous system
   b. Primarily affect rapidly dividing tissues
   c. Are generally unpredictable
   d. Gastrointestinal problems are common
   e. b and d

10. Which of the following is/are most likely used to treat side effects from anticancer drugs?
    a. Aspirin
    b. Antiemetics
    c. Emetics
    d. Blood transfusion
    e. b and d

11 Drug Treatment of Symptoms: Neuropharmacology and Substance Abuse

NEUROPHARMACOLOGY

BACKGROUND

Neuropharmacology is the study and evaluation of the effects of drugs on the nervous system. As mentioned previously, humans have known that chemicals found in plants and animals can cause profound changes in the function of the nervous system and have used natural products such as opium, cannabis, belladonna, and alcohol for thousands of years. As people developed the capacity to extract, purify, and finally synthesize new chemical substances, the number of chemicals that can modify nervous system function has grown rapidly.

To manage the complex tasks involved in behavior, the central nervous system (CNS) employs large numbers of neurons and synapses. Underneath each square millimeter of cortex are some 100,000 neurons, each of which has approximately 6000 synapses. In view of the fact that the surface area of the human brain is on the order of 100,000 mm^2, a single brain will contain 10 billion neurons interconnected by 60 trillion synapses. It is because of this complexity, and because of the inherent function of the nervous system, that ample sites for drug action exist. Although some drugs can provide physiological replacement, and others can actually cure a disease state, the majority of drugs are taken to relieve symptoms often relating to nervous system function/dysfunction. Because of the significant role that neuropharmacological agents play in our lives, a significant amount of space will be devoted to them.

The methods by which the neuropharmacological effects of drugs can be studied are numerous. The surest, but the most dangerous, is to study the effects directly in the human population. Obviously, this is normally only done under highly regulated circumstances as discussed in Chapter 15. Unfortunately, however, there do occur periodic unregulated episodes within the general population that do provide significant neuropharmacological information. For example, such an event occurred during the 1980s in northern California with a substance known as 1-methyl-4-phenyl-1,2,3, 5-tetrahydropyridine (MPTP).

MPTP is a chemical widely employed in various organic synthesis reactions. However, the general public is not normally exposed to it. Nevertheless, its potential for neurotoxicity was sensationalized after a number of *young* individuals began to appear in California clinics in 1982, with symptoms of advanced Parkinson's disease. These individuals exhibited the characteristic symptoms of Parkinson's disease, including an inability to walk, a mask-like facial expression, impairment of speech and skilled acts such as writing and eating, and in the most severe cases, a rigid immobility that was life threatening.

Because Parkinson's disease is usually a progressive neurological disease that develops in older people, 1 out of 100 persons over the age of 60 can present with motor deficiencies such as tremors, bradykinesia, and rigidity. Therefore, its sudden, full-blown development in young adults was immediately recognized as a highly unusual situation. Questioning soon revealed that the affected people had taken an illicit street "designer" drug that had properties similar to heroin and was, therefore, popular. The drug, unfortunately, contained a small amount of MPTP as a contaminant introduced during its clandestine synthesis. The mechanism, whereby MPTP produced its deleterious effect, will be described later in this chapter, since it has contributed to our understanding of neurochemistry.

Animal testing is the traditional, more controlled means of discovering both desired neuropharmacological effects as well as undesired neurotoxicity. Fortunately, neurons and basic neuronal circuitry are very similar between mammalian species. Neurons from rats, cats, dogs, and humans share similar critical macromolecules with high conservation of structure and function through evolution. The enhanced intellectual capacity of humans results more from quantitative than from qualitative differences in the structure and function of neurons. It is the increase in size and complexity of the nervous system in humans that accounts for this, not the presence of a new type of neuron or other cellular element. For this reason, neuropharmacological responses in humans and animals are usually quite similar. Thus, animals can serve as valid models for most, though not all, neuropharmacological responses in humans.

As mentioned above, there are several reasons why the nervous system is frequently involved in response to drugs and chemical substances. Despite the existence of a blood–brain barrier (BBB), the morphological and biochemical complexity of the nervous system make it a sensitive and selective target for drug attack. For example, the weight of the average adult human brain is approximately 2% of the whole body, yet the blood flow to the adult brain is about 20% of the cardiac output. The adult human brain relies almost entirely on the metabolism of glucose to meet its energy demands, and most (>90%) of this carbohydrate is oxidized to CO_2. Very little brain glucose (a few percent) is normally converted to lactate and released to the venous blood. The very high capacity of the brain to oxidize glucose suggests that this organ may be vulnerable to oxidative stress from drugs, toxins, and ischemia.

Another point of interest is that the brain expresses more of the total genetic information in its DNA than does any other organ, perhaps 10–20 times as much. Thus, in addition to the metabolic and maintenance machinery shared by most cell types, neurons contain many unique macromolecules including enzymes, ion channels, neurotransmitters, and receptors that are not found in other cells. Drugs that target these sites produce selective changes in nervous system activities that are directly related to altered behavior. In some cases, the effect is desired while in others this is obviously not the case.

With exposures to drugs severe enough to kill nerve cells or parts of cells, long-term, often permanent, deficits in sensory processes, motor function, behavior, learning capacity, and memory can occur. Since neurons do not reproduce, recovery of lost function occurs only if the remaining nervous system can "take over" the functions of the cells that were killed. Less severe exposures will modify function, often profoundly, until the drug is eliminated from the body. In most cases, normal behavior returns, and there may be no evidence of chronic consequences. With repeated exposures to some substances, however, the consequences may take on an irreversible quality.

A BRIEF HISTORY OF NEUROPHARMACOLOGY

Man's earliest notions with regard to the nervous system were that nerves contained ethereal and nonquantifiable *spirits*. It was the Frenchman Rene Descartes, in the 1600s, who suggested that the spirits were, in fact, composed of minute physical entities. The key discoveries during the first half of the twentieth century include the demonstration that the vagus nerve liberates a chemical (i.e., acetylcholine; see below) that controls heart rate (neurotransmission) and that nerve action potentials could be recorded and analyzed using the squid giant axon as a model.

In 1920, an Austrian scientist named Otto Löewi discovered the first neurotransmitter. In his classic experiment (which came to him in a dream), he used two frog hearts. One heart (heart #1) was placed in a chamber that was filled with saline. This chamber was connected to a second chamber that contained heart #2. So, fluid from chamber #1 was allowed to flow into chamber #2. Electrical stimulation of the vagus nerve (which was attached to heart #1) caused the heart rate of heart #1 to slow down. Löewi also observed that after a delay, heart #2 also slowed down. From this experiment, Löewi hypothesized that electrical stimulation of the vagus nerve released a chemical into the fluid of chamber #1 that flowed into chamber #2. He called this chemical "*Vagusstoff*." We now know this chemical as the neurotransmitter *acetylcholine*. A diagram of Löewi's classic experiment is shown in Figure 11.1.

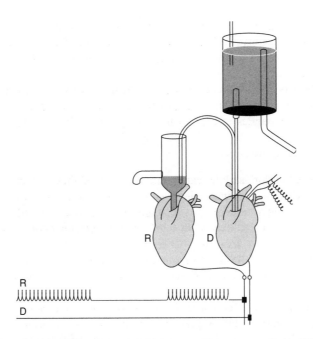

FIGURE 11.1   Loewi's demonstration of the chemical nature of neurotransmission. Heart D (donor) represents heart #1 while heart R (recipient) represents heart #2. Tracings R and D represent the respective heart beats of the two hearts. When fluid from the stimulated donor heart was allowed to interact with the recipient heart (middle of tracing R) heart rate was obviously abbreviated.

It was also during this period that Henry Dale assigned a variety of names to characterize different classes of pharmacological agents based on their action on receptors. Thus, receptors at the postganglionic nerve endings of parasympathetic nerves (which were stimulated by muscarine and acetylcholine, and blocked by atropine) were classified as *"muscarinic."* Those agents that blocked the responses of muscarine, thereby resembling atropine, were designated as antimuscarinic or *atropine-like*. In contrast to the muscarinic sites, the sites stimulated by small doses of nicotine (and acetylcholine) and blocked by large doses of nicotine were called *"nicotinic"*. Otto Löewi and Sir Henry Dale shared the Nobel Prize in medicine for 1936 for their discoveries regarding chemical transmission of nerve impulses.

In the 1950s and 1960s, a model was developed for the ionic basis of the *"action potential"* largely based on the work of Sir John Eccles, in England. It defined the voltage-dependence and time course of activation for the sodium and potassium currents that underlie the sudden *reversal of membrane potential* (going from −70 mv resting to +30 mv). During this same time frame, (1) the *synapse* was visualized utilizing the electron microscope and (2) calcium ions were demonstrated to be essential for neurotransmitter release at the neuromuscular junction.

During the 1970s, electron micrographs of active zones from freeze-fractured *neuromuscular junctions* confirmed earlier electrophysiological evidence that vesicles fuse to the presynaptic membrane to release neurotransmitter into the synaptic cleft. In addition, acetylcholine-generated electrophysiological "noise" was correlated with opening and closing of acetylcholine-activated ion channels, and successful recordings were made from single acetylcholine receptor–channel complexes.

These collective data led to a general view of neurotransmission. The transmission of messages from one nerve cell to another takes place in several steps. Packages of a neurotransmitter held in special vesicles are moved up to an active zone in the sending—or presynaptic—cell and dock at their release sites. Then, when an *electrical signal* arrives at the synapse, some of the vesicles fuse to the membrane, burst, and release their neurotransmitter. The *chemical messenger* diffuses across the gap to the receiving cell, *attaches to receptors* on the *postsynaptic neuron*, and, depending on the nature of the neurotransmitter, stimulates or inhibits electrical activity in this second neuron. Changes in synaptic strength are largely attributed to changes in the probability of any vesicle fusing and releasing its contents.

During the 1980s and 1990s, sequencing of individual subunits of receptor proteins (e.g., nicotinic), as well as their cloning, was achieved. Researchers have identified more than 20 classes of proteins that function in synaptic-vesicle fusion and recycling at the presynaptic membrane.

BASIC ANATOMY OF THE NERVOUS SYSTEM

During the course of evolution, an efficient system has evolved that enables the functions of individual organs to be orchestrated in increasingly complex life forms and permits rapid adaptation to alterations in a changing environment. This regulatory system is composed of a number of major anatomical divisions. These include the CNS (*CNS—brain and spinal cord*) and two separate pathways within the *peripheral nervous system* (PNS) for two-way communication with the peripheral organs outside the CNS. The PNS subdivisions are the *somatic and autonomic nervous systems* (ANSs) (Figure 11.2). The ANS is further divided into *sympathetic and parasympathetic divisions* (Figure 11.3).

The *somatic nervous system* is composed of *sensory afferents* and *motor efferents* and serves to perceive external states and to modulate appropriate body responses. Sensory nerves enter the spinal cord via the dorsal route; their cell bodies are in ganglia outside the spinal cord (dorsal root ganglia). Motor nerves leave the spinal cord via the ventral root. White matter consists of the myelinated axons of nerves, usually going up and down. Gray matter contains the cell bodies (containing the nucleus), dendrites with synapses and blood vessels. In both the spinal cord and brain, cell bodies are clustered into ganglia and nuclei.

The ANS, together with the endocrine system, controls the *milieu interieur*. It adjusts internal organ functions to the changing needs of the organism. The ANS operates largely *autonomously*,

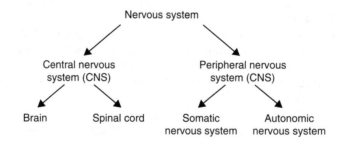

FIGURE 11.2   Subdivisions of the nervous system.

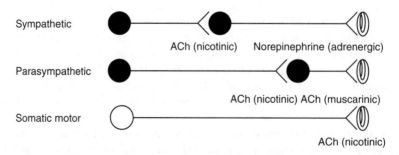

FIGURE 11.3   Diagram of autonomic and somatic motor neurons. Presynaptic neurons are depicted with solid cell bodies. Postsynaptic neurons are speckled. The neurotransmistter released by the presynaptic neuron and the type of receptor it activates are listed below each synapse.

beyond voluntary control, at the subconscious level. Its central components reside in the hypothalamus, brain stem, and spinal cord. The ANS has *sympathetic* and *parasympathetic* branches. Both are made up of afferent, mainly in the vagus nerve, and efferent fibers.

The sympathetic and parasympathetic branches usually work in opposition to each other. In simplistic terms, *activation of the sympathetic division* can be considered a means by which the body achieves a state of maximal work capacity as required in *"fight or flight"* situations. For example, blood flow to skeletal muscle is increased (for running or fighting) and cardiac rate and contractility are enhanced (to provide more oxygen for muscle exertion). Parasympathetic nerves regulate processes connected with energy assimilation (food intake, digestion, and absorption) and storage. These processes become quiescent when the sympathetic system becomes activated and operate when the body is at rest, allowing decreased respiration and cardiac activity and enhanced peristaltic activity.

The various components of the nervous system can be further differentiated into three basic cellular elements: (1) neurons; (2) interstitial cells; and (3) connective tissue, blood vessels, and microglia. The neuron is the only cell type in the nervous system involved in information processing. Each neuron is, in its own right, a receiver, an integrator, and a transmitter of information. Neurons are always in contact with other neurons so that they create simple or complex channels through which many different responses can be transmitted. All behavior, no matter how complex, results from the interactive function of the billions of neurons.

NEURONS

Neurons vary tremendously in form and size, but they all share in common the ability to respond to stimuli and to create new stimuli to affect other cells. Regardless of their structural diversity, all neurons are bounded by a plasma membrane and possess a cell body (soma), one or more axons, and, with very few exceptions, dendrites (Figure 11.4).

The bounding membrane of the neuron is typical of all cells. It is a continuous lipid bilayer sheet of some 60–80 Å thickness. Embedded in it, or passing through it, are numerous proteins and glycoproteins, many of which are found only in nerve cells. These have many functions. Some provide

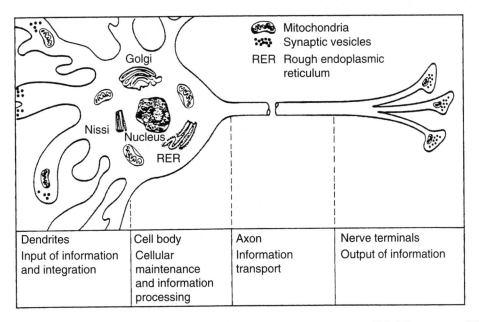

FIGURE 11.4   Structural components of nerve cells. (From T.M. Brody, J. Larner, K. P. Minneman, and H. C. Neu, (Eds.), (1994) *Human Pharmacology: Molecular to Clinical*, 2nd ed. St Louis, MO: Mosby. Reprinted with permission.)

structural support to the membrane, but *most form ion channels and receptor sites* that are absolutely essential to nerve function.

The membrane of the neuron is differentially specialized. The membrane of the *soma* and dendrites is designed to react to *chemical stimuli* and contains both neurotransmitter-gated ion channels and neurotransmitter-gated receptors associated with various G-proteins. The former evoke rapid changes in the cell's membrane potential, while the latter initiate slower, more persisting changes in neuronal excitability via the second messengers cyclic adenosine monophosphate (cAMP) and inositol triphosphate (IP$_3$).

The *axon* is specialized to react to changes in *membrane potential*. When the cell's *membrane potential* reaches a certain "threshold," the axon responds with an *action potential* that rapidly transmits an *electrical signal* from the cell body to its terminals. Finally, the *nerve terminal* is specialized to *convert* the electrical signal of the action potential back into a *chemical signal*. It responds to depolarization by releasing a neurotransmitter that acts on the soma or dendritic membranes of the next neuron or, in the PNS, to an effector site (Figure 11.5). The specialized membrane is absolutely essential to the electrochemical properties of neurons.

The cell body contains many structures of importance. The *nucleus* is usually located in the center of the cell body. It contains widely dispersed, fine chromatin material. The chromatin is composed of deoxyribonucleic acid (DNA) and its associated histone proteins. The nucleolus contains the specific portion of DNA encoding the ribonucleic acid (RNA) of future ribosomes.

In the neuroplasm of the neuron are located *mitochondria*, Nissl substance, and the Golgi apparatus. Mitochondria contain their own DNA and function as the major oxidative organelles, providing energy through the production of adenosine triphosphate (ATP). The Nissl substance, which is absent from the axon, represents the nodal points of the endoplasmic reticulum that exists throughout the soma. The *endoplasmic reticulum* is the major protein synthesizing organelle and manufactures in 1–3 days an amount of protein equal to the total protein content of the cell. The *Golgi apparatus* is primarily responsible for synthesis of membrane and the incorporation of membrane bound proteins into it. It pinches off the membrane with its associated proteins as "vesicles." Some of these vesicles contain protein needed to maintain the neurolemma, while others become secretory vesicles destined to contain neurotransmitter.

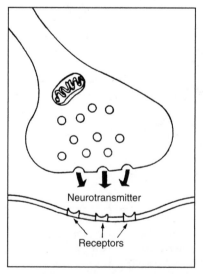

Chemical synapse

FIGURE 11.5   Simplified representation of the relationship between a nerve terminal and its effector site. From T. M. Brody, J. Larner, K. P. Minneman, and H. C. Neu, (Eds.), (1994) *Human Pharmacology: Molecular to Clinical*, 2nd ed. St Louis, MO: Mosby. Reprinted with permission.)

The dendrites represent all the processes of the cell body except for the specialized axonal process (axon). They are usually numerous and serve to increase the surface area of the neuron available for receiving synaptic input. Neurons will have one or more main dendrites that successively branch and arborize to form many smaller processes.

The axon of the typical neuron arises from a cone-shaped region of the cell body, the axon hillock. The initial segment of the axon is both the smallest region in diameter and the region with the lowest threshold to electrical activation. Distal to the initial segment, the axonal diameter enlarges and the diameter remains constant out to the terminal ending or until the axon branches. *Myelinated neurons* (see below) have their axons ensheathed by myelin segments, each segment provided by an oligodendrocyte or neurolemma cell. Between segments, the axonal membrane is exposed. These regions are termed the "nodes of Ranvier." Unmyelinated axons do not possess such a segmented sheath. Rather, they tend to collect in bundles that are loosely enclosed in troughs formed by neurolemmal cells or oligodendrocytes. The terminal end of an axon most often is profusely branching, each branch ultimately terminating in a synaptic ending.

Transport mechanisms are available within the neurons, which allow the passage of substances from the soma to axon terminal and vice versa. Most of the vesicles formed by the Golgi apparatus are transported through the axon to the nerve terminal by fast *anterograde transport*. Within the terminal, the secretory vesicles recycle many times, binding and fusing with the terminal membrane, then being "pinched off" via endocytosis and returned to the vesicle pool. The terminal membrane is constantly being replaced by newly arriving vesicles. Old membrane and proteins are returned to the cell body for degradation by way of a fast *retrograde transport* system.

Fast anterograde transport can reach rates as high as 400 mm/day. It is dependent on microtubules that provide a track along which the vesicles move. The movement is energy dependent and is mediated by a specific "motor" protein, *kinesin*. A similar process is responsible for fast retrograde transport. A second motor protein, *dynein*, is needed for movement in that direction. A third type of transport process is termed slow axoplasmic transport. It ranges from 0.2 to 5 mm/day and is responsible for the transport of cytoskeletal proteins, the neurofilaments, and microtubules, as well as an assortment of cytoplasmic proteins.

GLIAL CELLS

Approximately 50% of the weight of the brain is composed of glial cells. Glial cells do not conduct nerve impulses but support the brain in other ways. Some glial cells produce the myelin sheaths of nerves (oligodendroglia, Schwann cells), while others secrete cerebrospinal fluid (CSF). The brain has four interconnected fluid-filled reservoirs (ventricles) filled with CSF (total volume ~150 mL). CSF is not static; it circulates. It is secreted into the ventricles by the choroid plexus (~500 mL per day) then passes from the fourth ventricle into the subarachnoid space and subsequently absorbed into veins. The CSF acts as a cushion for the brain and reduces injury.

There are three types of glial cells in the CNS: astroglia (astrocytes), oligodendroglia (oligodendrocytes), and microglia. There are corresponding neurolemma cells (Schwann cells) in the PNS. Glial cells in the CNS perform a wide variety of "support" functions; while these cells are absolutely integral to neuronal function, they do play more of a support and modulatory than an information transmission role. For example, *astrocytes* are known to function in the removal of degenerative debris as well as in maintaining ion homeostasis and in metabolism of putative and acknowledged neurotransmitters. In response to virtually any form of neural insult, astrocytes become hypertrophic, displaying a response that includes enlargement of the cell body and increases in both the number and length of astrocytic processes. These are the cells, in fact, that form glial scars after brain or spinal cord injury. Astrocytes also contribute importantly to the BBB by forming an additional layer of cells around brain capillary endothelial cells.

Oligodendroglia provide the insulating *myelin sheath* for many CNS axons and are responsible for maintaining this sheath, as well as for control of the local ionic environment of the axon.

In addition, oligodendroglias provide a loose covering through which unmyelinated fibers course. The functions of microglia are not well understood but are believed to be of mesodermal origin and related to macrophage/monocyte lineage. Some microglia are resident within the brain, while additional cells of this class may be attracted to the brain during periods of inflammation following either microbial infection or other postinjury inflammatory reactions. They are *phagocytic* and remove debris throughout the CNS.

In addition to neurons and glial cells, the nervous system contains blood vessels, fibroblasts, and other connective tissue elements. In the *PNS*, processes from Schwann cells that form the multilayered myelin sheaths characteristic of peripheral myelinated nerves, surround most neuronal elements.

MORPHOLOGICAL CONSIDERATIONS

Neurons assume a vast array of forms in accordance with the functions they serve. In most neurons, the cell body and dendrites are separated from the axonal terminal by a very long tube, the axon. This creates problems unique to nerve cells. In the motor neurons that innervate hands and feet, for example, more than 90% of the mass of the neuron is in the cell processes. An often-given example of this relationship is that if the cell body of a motor neuron was enlarged to the size of a baseball, the corresponding axon would be about 1 mile long, and the dendrites and their branches would arborize throughout a large amphitheater.

The neuron is put at a metabolic disadvantage because of this relatively large size. The cell body is the only part of the neuron that can synthesize proteins, but it may make up less than 5% of the total cell mass. Because of this, very high rates of protein synthesis are required. As all proteins are synthesized in the cell body, most have to be transported long distances to their eventual target. For proteins destined for the distal portions of the axon and for the axon terminal, the specialized transport systems mentioned above must function continuously to get them to their targets in a reasonable length of time. These transport systems require a large, complex cytoskeleton to maintain them. Anything that compromises protein synthesis, axonal transport, or cytoskeletal integrity may reduce new functional and structural protein arrival to a point where structure and function of the neuron have been damaged. Neurotoxicity associated with the anticancer drug vincristine, for example, may be related to such a site of action, since this alkaloid is known to damage microtubules.

NUTRITIONAL AND BIOCHEMICAL ASPECTS

The brain is covered by three tough membranes known as meninges. These are (1) dura mater: outermost—firmly attached to the skull; (2) arachnoid: middle layer; (3) pia mater: bottom layer, firmly attached to the brain, and contains many blood vessels. Inflammation of these membranes results in meningitis.

While the meninges protect the brain primarily against external trauma, the CNS is also protected from internal threats, certain chemicals, and bacteria by the BBB. This barrier is primarily created by the capillary endothelial cells that form tight, high resistance junctions that line the blood vessels that run through the brain. They act as a continuous lipid blockade, preventing the free diffusion through extracellular pathways that occurs regularly at most other organs. For a molecule to diffuse through the BBB, it must have a sufficient amount of lipid solubility to pass directly through the endothelial cells. However, highly polar, nonlipid soluble compounds do not penetrate well, if at all. This can prove to be a problem, since the BBB prevents the brain uptake of >98% of all potential neurotherapeutics including chemotherapeutics for brain tumors. Conversely, erosion of the BBB, as occurs with inflammation, is of special concern because increased permeability permits the entry into the brain of blood-borne toxic or infectious agents.

Because the BBB is less developed in immature brains, children are more susceptible to CNS toxicity from certain toxic substances, such as lead salts, than are adults. The patency of the BBB may also become increased under conditions of disease and dehydration. Although the CNS is generally well protected from certain drugs by the BBB, the PNS does not have a comparable structure. Therefore, it is possible to have drug effects restricted to peripheral structures only, if their entry into the CNS is excluded.

The metabolic requirements of neurons often make them more susceptible than other types of cells to drug actions. Neurons are highly active metabolically in order to support their unusual demands, and are very sensitive to drug actions that interfere with normal nutrient utilization. The brain functions at ~10 watts (i.e., a "dim bulb"). However, 10 watts is a fairly high proportion of the total body energy consumption rate of 80 watts; the brain is 2% of body weight but uses 12% of body energy; 14% of total blood flow goes to the brain; and blood flow to the brain per kilogram is equal to that of a muscle doing heavy exercise.

The high metabolic activity results in part from the high rates of protein synthesis needed to maintain the specialized nerve cell and from the fact that a neuron constantly generates action potentials as part of its information processing function. Each action potential, in turn, erodes the ionic gradients existing across the nerve cell membrane, which are critical to normal function. Large amounts of energy are expended by the nerve cell in restoring and maintaining these gradients. This requires the continuous formation of large amounts of ATP, which requires aerobic metabolism.

It should also be remembered that even neurons *"at rest"* are highly electrically charged by virtue of uneven distributions of ions across the cellular membrane. Ionic pumps and carriers are continually maintaining the ionic gradients with the expenditure of energy. Therefore, given an adequate supply of energy, the concentrations of Na^+, K^+, Cl^-, Ca^{2+}, HCO^-, and H^+ ions are maintained inside the cells at levels to support the metabolic processes of the cell. It follows that even at rest, the nerve cells are in a state of dynamic homeostasis that is essential for life. The homeostasis is self-adjusting; that is, enzymes that produce energy and pump the ions require an appropriate ionic milieu to function. A *brief* disruption of this steady-state situation can be tolerated by nerve cells because of an elaborate system of "buffers" that can *temporarily* compensate for disruption, such as change in concentration of an ion, but in the long-term there is a limit beyond which the homeostasis cannot be perturbed without fatal results.

As mentioned above, neurons are almost entirely dependent on glucose as an energy supply. The neuron has little capacity for anaerobic metabolism, and is, therefore, highly susceptible to a lack of *oxygen or glucose* (thus the susceptibility of insulin-dependent diabetics to insulin overdose and loss of consciousness.). The oxygen consumption of neurons is nearly ten times higher than adjacent glial cells, and, therefore, is more often damaged by anoxic or hypoglycemic conditions. Certain *large neurons*, such as *pyramidal cells* in the cerebral cortex, cerebellum, and hippocampus or *motorneurons* in the spinal cord, have a particularly high metabolic rate. Damage is often seen first at these sites when oxygen or glucose levels are not sufficiently maintained. Neuronal damage can start within minutes and becomes irreversible within 5–6 min after oxygen or glucose delivery is stopped.

Role of Myelin

Schwann cells, a type of glial cell, differentiate to form the protective *myelin sheath* that surrounds the nerve axon and promotes long-distance propagation of the action potential in the ANS. The myelin sheath is a greatly extended and modified plasma membrane that is wrapped around the nerve axon in a spiral fashion. Each myelin-generating cell furnishes myelin for only one segment of any given axon. The axon and its myelin sheath are important to each other metabolically as well as functionally. Axons direct the formation of myelin and can provide a mitogenic stimulus for Schwann cell or oligodendrocyte cell proliferation. The myelin-forming cells can influence axonal diameter and play a role in determining the composition of the axonal membrane.

Whereas in nonmyelinated fibers sodium and potassium channels are distributed uniformly across the axonal membrane, in myelinated fibers sodium channels are concentrated at the nodes of Ranvier and potassium channels in the internodal regions. This greatly improves the efficiency of action potential propagation. A nerve signal can travel from your spinal cord to the tip of your toe in less than 25 ms. Such rapid nerve transmission is only possible because the axons have very good insulation. Layers of glial cells (astrocytes) wrap axons much like gauze wrapped around an injured finger, forming an insulating myelin sheath.

As an example of the advantages imparted by myelin, we can compare two different nerve fibers, one myelinated and the other nonmyelinated, that both conduct action potentials at 25 m/s. In the case of a nonmyelinated axon (e.g., squid giant axon), a diameter of 500 μm is required, while a corresponding myelinated human axon would only be 12 μm in diameter. The nonmyelinated axon requires 5000 times as much energy to conduct an action potential, and occupies approximately 1500 times as much space as a myelinated fiber. If the human spinal cord contained only nonmyelinated axons, it would need to be as large as a good-sized tree trunk to conduct action potentials at the same speed as it does at present.

When myelin is lost, axonal function is rapidly affected. Conduction velocity slows in proportion to the degree of demyelination and, in extreme situations, conduction can be blocked. Loss of the myelin may also lead to loss of the axon. Axons can generally survive some demyelination, but extensive loss of myelin can result in axonal degeneration. Because myelin-forming cells can proliferate, they generally reestablish a myelin sheath around an axon once the demyelinating stimulus is removed.

THE SYNAPSE

The *synapse* is a critical structure in the nervous system and serves as the communication link between neurons (Figure 11.6). Synapses in the mammalian CNS are chemical in nature. They possess three components: (1) a presynaptic element, (2) a postsynaptic element, and (3) a synaptic cleft. At a typical synapse, neurotransmission requires four steps: (1) synthesis and storage of neurotransmitter; (2) transmitter release; (3) receptor activation; and (4) transmitter inactivation.

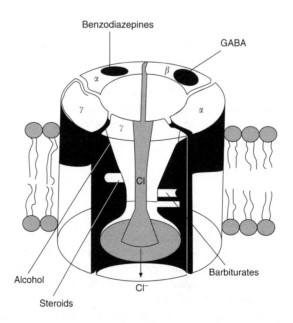

FIGURE 11.6 Schematic three-dimensional representation of the GABA$_A$ receptor complex with the recognition sites for GABA, benzodiazepines, alcohol, steroids, and barbiturates. (From G. Zernig, A. Saria, M. Kurtz, and S. S. O'Malley, (Eds.) (2000), *Handbook of Alcoholism*. With permission.)

Most neurotransmitters are synthesized within the presynaptic terminal by enzymes made in the cell body and transported to the ending by axoplasmic transport. They are subsequently stored in vesicles in the terminal. These vesicles, as well as the presynaptic terminal membrane, contain specific proteins that play essential roles in the docking and fusing of vesicles to the membrane during the process of neurotransmitter release. The release of neurotransmitter is triggered by a sequence of events that begins with the propagation of an action potential that ultimately arrives at the terminal region.

The depolarization that accompanies the action potential induces an *increase in membrane permeability to calcium ions*. A large inward electrochemical gradient exists for calcium and it moves into the terminal. The calcium that enters the terminal activates enzymes that cause the attachment of some of the vesicles to releasing sites on the terminal membrane, membrane fusion, and the release of the vesicular contents into the synaptic cleft. Transmitter release is terminated by the removal of calcium from the terminal cytoplasm, either via a calcium pump, which pumps it out of the cell, or by uptake into the endoplasmic reticulum or into mitochondria.

Once the neurotransmitter is released from the presynaptic terminal, it diffuses across the synaptic cleft. On the postsynaptic side, it complexes with a membrane bound macromolecule, its receptor. In synapses that have to generate action potentials within microseconds of neurotransmitter release, the receptors must be clustered in the postsynaptic membrane at high density, close to where the neurotransmitter is released. Such a synapse exists at the *neuromuscular junction* where acetylcholine is the neurotransmitter. Acetylcholine is released from the presynaptic nerve terminal within 50 nm of the postsynaptic muscle membrane that contains densely arrayed acetylcholine receptors ($\sim$10,000 acetylcholine receptors/μm^2). There is a steady turnover of receptors, with newly synthesized receptors replacing those that are periodically degraded or not being utilized.

Binding leads to one of two consequences. If the receptor is coupled to an ion channel, the channel is opened, ions move down electrochemical gradients, and the membrane potential is changed. If the receptor is linked to a G-protein, the binding initiates a sequence of biochemical events that result in the production of a second messenger such as cAMP or IP$_3$. These evoke long-term changes that alter excitability of the postsynaptic cell. The complexation process is usually rapidly reversible with an occupancy half-life of 1–20 ms.

Action of the neurotransmitter is terminated by several means. For many neurotransmitters, the bulk is recycled back into the presynaptic terminal via an *active uptake* process, to be reused. Alternatively, some of the neurotransmitter may simply *diffuse away* and be *enzymatically destroyed* elsewhere. In other cases, enzymes may actually be located on the postsynaptic side of the cleft, in the vicinity of the receptor, which serve to rapidly break the transmitter down into inactive metabolites.

Clearly, there are many components involved in the process of neurotransmission. These can be the targets of useful drugs as well as neurotoxicants. Examples include the local anesthetics, which target sodium channels in nerve axons; neuromuscular blocking drugs, which target the nicotinic receptor at the motor end plates; and some tranquilizers, such as diazepam, which target the GABA receptor on neurons in the CNS (see below).

SPECIFIC NEUROTRANSMITTER SYSTEMS

Certain neurotransmitter systems are more frequently involved in neuropharmacological and toxicological responses than others. We have briefly discussed the importance of the dopaminergic system previously with regard to Parkinson's disease. Additional systems for drug targeting include the cholinergic, adrenergic, glutamanergic, GABAergic, and glycinergic neurotransmitter systems (Table 11.1). To understand their significance, a more comprehensive description of their function will be given.

TABLE 11.1
Representative Receptors and Their Actions

Receptor Type	Location, Effect, and Mechanism of Action
Cholinergic	Postsynaptic and presynaptic, variable
Muscarinic	Effects, some increase IP_3, others inhibit adenylate cyclase
Nicotinic	Postsynaptic, excitatory, opens a Na^+, K^+
Adrenergic	Selective ion channel
α_1	Postsynaptic, excitatory, linked to formation of IP_3
α_2	Presynaptic, reduce transmitter release, reduce calcium entry
β_1	Postsynaptic, depressive?
β_2	Postsynaptic, excitatory, activates adenylate cyclase
Dopaminergic	Postsynaptic, depressive, activates adenylate cyclase
D_1 family (D_1, D_5)	Postsynaptic, variable effects, stimulates adenylate cyclase
D_2 family (D_2, D_3, and D_4)	Postsynaptic and presynaptic, variable effects, inhibits adenylate cyclase
GABAergic	Postsynaptic, inhibitory, opens a Cl^- selective ion channel
$GABA_A$	Presynaptic, inhibitory, reduces calcium entry
$GABA_B$	Postsynaptic, inhibitory, increases K^+ conductance
Glycinergic	Postsynaptic, inhibitory, opens Cl^- selective ion channel
Glutamatergic	Postsynaptic, excitatory, opens a Na^+, K^+ selective ion channel
AMPA	Postsynaptic, excitatory, opens a Na^+, K^+ selective ion channel
Kainate	Postsynaptic, excitatory, opens a Na^+, K^+, Ca^{++} selective ion channel
NMDA	

ACETYLCHOLINE

Acetylcholine was the first identified neurotransmitter. Acetylcholine is the neurotransmitter released by the motorneurons that innervate skeletal muscle, all preganglionic and many postganglionic autonomic neurons in the PNS, which innervate smooth muscle, cardiac muscle and glands, and many neurons within the CNS. Extensive loss of cholinergic neurons in the CNS has been found in patients having Alzheimer's disease. The structure of acetylcholine is shown in the following figure.

$$(CH_2)_2 \overset{+}{N} CH_2CH_2O\overset{\overset{\displaystyle O}{\|}}{C}CH_2$$

Two distinct receptor groups have been identified for acetylcholine, the *nicotinic* and the *muscarinic* groups (Table 11.1). Furthermore, there are at least four subtypes of nicotinic and five subtypes of muscarinic receptors. Nicotinic receptors are ubiquitous and exist at the neuromuscular junctions of skeletal muscles and on ganglion cells in the ANS. Nicotinic receptors located on cation-specific ion channels, when opened, evoke *fast*, transient depolarizations of the recipient cell. Muscarinic receptors are found in smooth muscle receiving parasympathetic innervation and elsewhere, and can be blocked by atropine. Muscarinic receptors are coupled indirectly to *slow and fast* ion channels via G-proteins.

Acetylcholine is synthesized from acetyl-CoA and choline within the presynaptic terminal by the enzyme choline acetylase. The acetylcholine formed is stored in small, lightly staining synaptic vesicles that are concentrated around the synaptic contact area. The release of acetylcholine is *calcium dependent*. The entire content of a synaptic vesicle is released into the cleft in an all-or-none manner, where it interacts with its receptors and then is rapidly destroyed by acetylcholinesterase. Under normal circumstances, the half-life for acetylcholine in the synaptic cleft is about 1 msec. The acetylcholine is hydrolyzed to choline and acetate, and the choline is actively pumped back into the presynaptic terminal, to be used to synthesize more acetylcholine.

GLUTAMATE

Glutamate is the primary *excitatory* neurotransmitter in the brain. Glutamate is formed by the Krebs's cycle and is found free and stored in vesicles in synaptic terminals. Its release is calcium dependent, and an uptake system exists in presynaptic terminals and in glia to terminate its action after release. It is possible that glial cells metabolize glutamate to glutamine and return it to the neuron for reuse. An excessive release of glutamate can be lethal to cells in the immediate vicinity.

Three subtypes of glutamate receptors are known (Table 11.1). Two of these, the AMPA and kainate receptors, are part of a cation-selective ion channel that is permeable to sodium and potassium. These channels are responsible for the fast, transient excitatory postsynaptic potentials (EPSPs) evoked by glutamate release. The third, the *N*-methyl-D-aspartate (NMDA) receptor, is part of a cation channel permeable to sodium, potassium, and calcium. Activation of this channel leads to calcium entry into the cell that can act as a second messenger in its own right to modulate cellular processes. This receptor is critical to the development of neuronal plasticity in experimental model systems and is thought to be essential to higher processes of the brain, including memory and learning.

Inhibitory modulation of neurotransmission in the CNS is carried out by two substances, gamma-aminobutyric acid (GABA) and glycine. They are differentially distributed, GABA being found primarily in the brain and glycine primarily in the spinal cord.

GAMMA-AMINOBUTYRIC ACID

Gamma-aminobutyric acid is formed from glutamate that is derived from the Krebs's cycle, by the enzyme glutamic acid dehydrogenase. In GABAergic neurons, about 10% of glutamate is converted to GABA rather than being processed further by the Krebs's cycle enzymes. Synthesis occurs in the terminal cytoplasm, and GABA is found free and bound in vesicles. Once released, GABA is taken up into the presynaptic terminal via a high-affinity, sodium-dependent transport system. It is also rapidly taken up into glia by a similar process, where it is metabolized.

Two major subtypes of GABA receptors are known: $GABA_A$ and $GABA_B$. The $GABA_A$ receptor is part of a chloride channel. It mediates *postsynaptic inhibition* and gives rise to fast transient inhibitory postsynaptic potentials (IPSPs). $GABA_B$ receptors are found both pre- and post-synaptically. Presynaptically they act via a G-protein to reduce calcium entry. Postsynaptically they act via a G-protein to increase potassium conductance. In either case, they mediate inhibition. A representation of the $GABA_A$ receptor is shown in Figure 11.6.

GLYCINE

Glycine is an important inhibitory transmitter in the *spinal cord*. The postsynaptic receptor for glycine is very similar to the $GABA_A$ receptor and forms part of a chloride channel complex. When it is activated by glycine, the channel opens transiently to produce IPSPs in spinal neurons. Both gaseous anesthetics and alcohol are believed to activate glycine receptors. Strychnine reversibly antagonizes the effects of glycine on spinal neurons, and this is thought to be responsible for its convulsant properties.

MECHANISM OF ACTION OF SELECTED NEUROPHARMACOLOGICAL AGENTS

As mentioned previously, there are many potential targets available in nerve cells for interaction with a drug. Some targets are general to all nerve cells, and drugs that affect them will produce widely dispersed effects. Other targets are found only in a subset of nerve cells, and in these cases drug effects will be restricted to them. The most common reason specific interactions occur is that neurons differ in the *transmitter system they possess*.

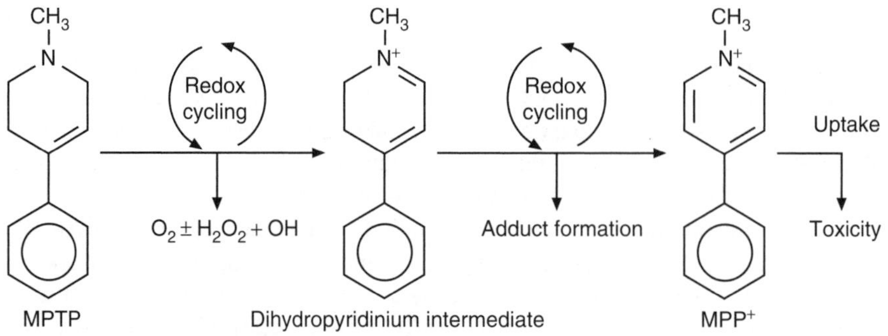

FIGURE 11.7 Conversion of MTPT to MPP$^+$.

In the first part of this chapter, the unfortunate experience of young adults with MPTP was briefly discussed. It might be instructive at this point to complete the story. As soon as it was recognized that MPTP was the neurotoxicant, a number of laboratories began to investigate its mechanism of action. It was eventually demonstrated that MPTP readily diffused into neurons and glial cells and that it served as a *substrate* for the "B" isozyme of *monoamine oxidase* (MAO) found predominantly in astrocytes. In the glial cell, the MPTP was oxidized to the primary neurotoxicant, the *pyridium ion, MPP$^+$*. Because of its structural similarity to dopamine, the MPP$^+$ was selectively taken up by dopaminergic neurons of the substantia nigra via the dopamine uptake system. Within these dopaminergic cells, the MPP$^+$ acted as a general *cellular poison*, ultimately blocking oxidative phosphorylation and killing the neuron (Figure 11.7).

A chilling follow-up to this acute development of Parkinson's disease/syndrome was subsequently found. Some of the individuals, who had taken small amounts of the illicit street drug, and therefore small amounts of MPTP, did not develop Parkinsonism within the short term following its ingestion. It was observed subsequently, however, that some of these individuals began to show delayed, early signs of the disease, years after the drug's ingestion. The basis for this delayed effect is not known with certainty, but it is likely that the initial exposure killed too few dopaminergic cells to result immediately in Parkinson's disease. However, the progression of the disease via natural degeneration of the dopaminergic cells may have been accelerated by MPTP exposure. An excess of 200 people who used MPTP one or more times, under the impression that it was a synthetic heroin, were subsequently identified.

We now know that the appearance of MPTP in the northern California drug market was part of the advent of *"designer drugs."* The term was coined to reflect the increasing sophistication of street-drug suppliers, who were beginning to tailor their products to individual preferences regarding the nature and duration of the drug effect. By slightly changing the molecular structure of a drug, its potency, length of action, euphoric effects, and toxicity can be modified.

DESIGNER DRUGS

A designer drug is an analog, a chemical compound that is similar in structure and effect to another drug of abuse but differs slightly in structure. Designer drugs are produced in clandestine laboratories to mimic the psychoactive effects of controlled drugs. The most commonly known types of synthetic analog drugs available through the illicit drug market include analogs of fentanyl and meperidine (both synthetic opioids), phencyclidine (PCP), and amphetamine and methamphetamine (which have hallucinogenic and stimulant properties).

Designer drugs came into vogue to circumvent the Controlled Substances Act of 1970. Many designer drugs when introduced in the 1970s in the United States *were initially legal*, but the Federal Drug Enforcement Administration quickly invoked its emergency authority to place an immediate ban on them, by declaring them federally scheduled drugs under the *Comprehensive Crime Control Act of 1984*. Subsequent federal legislation (1986) has prohibited the illicit manufacture of all forms of designer drugs.

The first designer drug that rapidly became part of the drug scene was methylenedioxymethamphetamine (MDMA), known by the street names of *"Ecstacy,"* "Adam," and "Essence." The drug was first invented in Germany, in 1912, by Merck Pharmaceuticals in its search for an anti-bleeding drug. MDMA can be synthesized from molecular components of methamphetamine or from safrole. Ecstasy has been one of the most controversial drugs to take center stage in society.

The drug first burst into the drug scene in the eighties, when it became the drug of choice by "rave" enthusiasts. Its popularity reached such a degree that anecdotal rumors began to circulate of the drug's neurotoxicity. Governmental concern led to the drug being outlawed in the United States in 1985. According to an annual federal survey, almost 10 million Americans have tried Ecstasy.

One of the most infamous events associated with Ecstasy was the use of PET scans of the brains of Ecstasy users on a postcard from the National Drug Institute in 1998, labeled "Plain Brain/Brain after Ecstasy." The postcards were distributed to thousands of teenagers and implied that Ecstasy users had shrunken brains with holes in them.

This strategy continued in a primate study published in 2002 with great fanfare warning that the amount of the drug consumed by the typical user at a "rave" might cause permanent brain damage. However, a retraction published a year later revealed that Ecstasy had, in fact, *not* been used. Instead, the squirrel monkeys and baboons had inadvertently been injected with overdoses of methamphetamine. This situation was significant since the principle investigator (P.I.) involved was a leading critic of recreational drug use and whose research had contributed to a government campaign suggesting that Ecstasy made "holes in the brain."

It is hard to find impartial observers in the highly polarized debate. One prominent clinician at Harvard and M.I.T. was moved to accuse the P.I. of "running a cottage industry showing that everything under the sun is neurotoxic." In 2003, a review of all Ecstasy research by a scientist from the *Center for Addiction and Mental Health* in Toronto concluded that there was no evidence that Ecstasy caused brain damage "with the possible (but as yet unproven) exception of mild memory loss."

The ease with which drugs can be modified is illustrated by the identification of at least 35 variants or analogs that have been synthesized from phencyclidine (PCP, "Angel dust"); several dozen analogs of methamphetamine have also been produced. Such drugs proved to be exceptionally potent and presented significant health hazards.

This situation became particularly acute with respect to the development of illicit analogs of fentanyl to derive heroin substitutes. Fentanyl is a synthetic opioid, a μ-receptor agonist and is about 100–200 times more potent than morphine as an analgesic. As with other narcotic analgesics, respiratory depression is the most significant acute toxic effect of the fentanyl derivatives. Fentanyl analogs can be 80–1000 more potent than heroin in causing respiratory depression. Fentanyl analogs are responsible for the overdose deaths of more than 150 in the United States. In July 2005, the FDA issued a health advisory regarding the safe use of fentanyl skin patches (brand name Duragesic) in response to reports of deaths in patients using fentanyl for pain management.

One of the more relatively new designer drugs was identified in 1994, when U.S. Drug Enforcement Agents reported that a very potent drug, methacathinone ("cat"), was introduced to the streets as a cocaine-like drug, whose effects could last up to 5–7 days. At least three deaths have been associated with the drug.

ALCOHOL

Ethyl alcohol is one of the most widely consumed drugs in the world. It is a good example of a drug that is a *general CNS depressant*. Ingestion of even small amounts diminishes performance, particularly performance dependent on training and previous experience. Mood is affected and can range from euphoria to deep depression. Memory, concentration, insight, and motor function are impaired in a dose-dependent fashion. With large ingestions, a state similar to general anesthesia develops. The doses that produce death are not much higher than those inducing anesthesia.

For many years, it was thought that alcohol and other lipophilic solvents exerted their depressant effects on the CNS by virtue of "nonspecific" membrane fluidizing properties, causing neuronal swelling. This swelling was believed responsible for perturbing the functions of key macromolecules embedded in the membrane, including the ion channels and various receptors. However, the discovery that *alcohol acts on receptor-gated ion channels (GABA$_A$, NMDA, and 5HT$_3$)* in a saturable and specific manner has now led to the belief that the behavioral and neurochemical properties of alcohol are the consequence of a number of specific receptor interactions of this chemical in the brain.

An important finding relating to alcohol's mechanism of action is that ethanol interacts with the GABA$_A$ receptor-channel complex in the CNS (see above), and *augments GABA$_A$-mediated synaptic inhibition.* This occurs at concentrations that do not produce comparable effects on other types of neurotransmitter receptors. Normally, activation of the GABA$_A$ receptor–channel complex increases the permeability of the nerve cell to chloride ions for approximately 10–20 msec. Inebriating amounts of ethanol prolongs the time that the channel remains open by two- to three-fold, when alcohol binds to the receptor. At higher concentrations, neurotransmitter release is reduced from all nerve terminals, probably due to reductions in calcium entry.

The effects of alcohol on the GABA$_A$ receptor may be important to the development of tolerance and physical dependence that occurs to individuals who drink large amounts of alcohol on a chronic basis. There is evidence that chronic alcohol ingestion leads to a reduction in the number of GABA$_A$ receptors in the brain as a compensatory response to the continual presence of the drug (i.e., down-regulation). After this process occurs, when alcohol levels in the CNS fall, and its potentiating effect on GABA$_A$ receptors is lost, the brain becomes hyperexcitable and the dependent individual experiences anxiety, general malaise, and tremors. This acts as a powerful stimulus for the alcoholic to ingest more. During a prolonged withdrawal, the lack of alcohol to potentiate inhibition causes increasing hyperexcitability and frank signs of withdrawal including tremors, hyperreflexia, and convulsions.

Many important pharmaceutical agents produce CNS depression and have been extensively studied to determine their mechanism of action. One group of drugs, exemplified by the barbiturates, affects the nervous system much like alcohol does, whereas a second group, the benzodiazepines, are remarkably selective potentiators of GABA$_A$-mediated inhibition. Since they are commonly found in the home and are responsible for a number of suicides and alcohol-related deaths, they merit consideration.

BARBITURATES

The barbiturates, such as phenobarbital, were at one time extensively used as sleeping pills and as sedative agents to reduce stress and anxiety in people. They, like alcohol, produce a spectrum of depressant effects that are dose dependent. Small doses promote tiredness and sleep, while higher doses can produce a general anesthetic state and death. The barbiturates can also produce tolerance and physical dependence after chronic ingestion of high doses. The withdrawal complications are very similar to those seen with alcohol. Although not prescribed to a great extent today, barbiturates continue to be readily available on the street.

Barbiturates probably interact more specifically with hydrophobic domains of membrane proteins than does alcohol. Interestingly, they produce opposite effects on the GABA$_A$ receptor that mediates inhibition in the CNS, and the glutamate receptors that mediate excitation. Barbiturates enhance GABA$_A$ receptor-mediated inhibition by binding to a site *within the chloride channel part* of the complex. Barbiturates are more effective channel stabilizers than alcohol and can maintain the channel in its open state 2–10 times longer than normal. The same levels of barbiturates depress

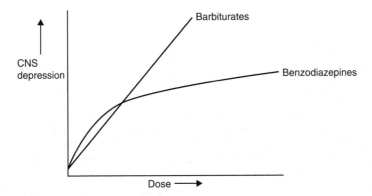

FIGURE 11.8   Comparison of dose–response curves in producing CNS depression.

excitatory transmission mediated by glutamate. Why the function of one receptor complex should be enhanced while another is attenuated remains unknown.

BENZODIAZEPINES

The benzodiazepines, of which *valium* is a prototype, are very selective drugs that target only the $GABA_A$ receptor–chloride channel complex. First discovered in the 1960s, this class of drugs was soon observed to produce marked changes in animal behavior and aggressiveness, and eventually was marketed for use in humans. Most produce modest sedation and quite effectively alleviate anxiety resulting from any cause. Some produce a greater degree of sedation (e.g., halcion) and have become the modern "sleeping pills." They are remarkably good at what they do, and the benzodiazepines are among the most widely prescribed drugs in medicine today.

The advantages benzodiazepines possess over barbiturates are due to their *relatively selective* interaction with the $GABA_A$ receptor. They bind to a location on the receptor complex distinct from the binding site for the neurotransmitter GABA (an allosteric site). When they bind, they alter the structure in a way that *increases the affinity* of the GABA binding site for GABA. This increase in affinity for GABA results in a potentiation of GABA's effects when it is released from GABAergic nerve terminals. The benzodiazepines do not affect the $GABA_B$ receptor, any other receptor, or transmitter release. Figure 11.8 illustrates the major difference in the dose–response properties of barbiturates and benzodiazepines. For drugs with a dose-dependent plateau, such as the benzodiazepines, this translates into a significant improvement in safety profile.

CANNABINOIDS

Marijuana (Δ^9-tetrahydrocannibinol; THC) is unusual among drugs of abuse in that there is *little* evidence that it serves as a reinforcer in animal models of self-administration. It has also been difficult to demonstrate physical dependence.

During the 1990s, the brain receptors for THC in brain GB_1 and immune system GB_2 were isolated and cloned. These cannabinoid receptors belong to the G-protein-coupled superfamily of receptors. Since the discovery of a brain receptor implies an endogenous ligand for that binding site, the search for such a compound began immediately thereafter. In 1992, a compound that occurs naturally in the brain called *arachidonylethanolamide*, belonging to the class of endogenous compounds called eicosanoids, was shown to bind to the THC receptor and to produce pharmacological effects similar to those of THC itself. The compound has been given the name *anandamide* by its Hebrew discoverers after the Sanskrit word *ananda*, meaning bliss. Interestingly, chocolate and cocoa powders contain compounds related to anandamide that may explain the familiar phenomenon of chocolate craving. Recently, 2-sciadonoylglycerol, the first nonendogenous cannabinoid receptor agonist not isolated from *C. sativa*, was isolated from a pine tree.

Cannabinoids may share at least some common neuronal mechanisms with opioid compounds. Studies of intracellular events associated with ligand binding to either cannabinoid or opiate receptors indicate that these receptors are linked via G-proteins to the production of cAMP. Certain studies have also indicated that there may be some interaction between cannabinoid binding sites and opiate receptors in the reward pathway. In addition, there is increasing evidence that cannabinoids interact with opiate systems involved in the perception of pain. In fact, cannabinoids clearly produce analgesic effects in both experimental animals and humans and, of all the potential clinical uses of cannabinoids; the mediation of analgesia has received the most attention. Some evidence also indicates that the cannabinoid receptor system is an analgesic system.

Cannabinoids and alcohol activate the same reward pathways, and the cannabinoid CB_1 receptor system plays an important role in regulating the positive reinforcement properties of alcohol. In fact, both cannabinoids and alcohol cause the release of dopamine in the nucleus accumbens. Recent evidence suggests that ethanol preference, which is dependent on CB_1 receptor, is higher in young mice than in old mice, and higher in female mice than in male mice.

It should be apparent to the reader by this point that the release of dopamine in the nucleus accumbens is a general biochemical consequence of numerous drugs of abuse; many, if not all drugs with rewarding properties, act directly or indirectly through mechanisms that involve dopamine at the level of the nucleus accumbens.

Partly because of THC's analgesic property, efforts have been made to facilitate the availability of THC to the public. Several states have passed initiatives to decriminalize the use of "medicinal" marijuana. In 1985, THC was made available as a *pill* sold under the brand name Marinol®. The drug was found to be useful in relieving glaucoma and pain, nausea and vomiting in cancer patients, and in enhancing appetite and inducing weight gain in AIDS and cancer patients. In July of 1999, Marinol was reclassified as a Schedule III drug. Unfortunately, Marinol® lacks one of the main advantages of smoking: quick onset of effect. So the debate goes on with no clear resolution in sight.

The issue of cannabis use and the relief of pain have been argued for decades. Cannabis is listed in the Materia Medica section of the sixth edition of the *Merck Manual* in 1934 as a hypnotic; *analgesic;* and sedative used for neuralgia, migraine, and neurasthenia. The Institute of Medicine's 1999 report on medical marijuana stated, "The accumulated data indicate a potential therapeutic value for cannabinoid drugs, particularly for symptoms such as pain relief, control of nausea and vomiting, and appetite stimulation." The report went on to say that, there are no convincing data to support the concern that the medical use of marijuana would lead to a general increase of marijuana use in the general population.

In the Institute of Medicine's report, the researchers also examined the physiological risks of using marijuana and cautioned, "Marijuana is not a completely benign substance. It is a powerful drug with a variety of effects. However, except for the harms associated with smoking, the adverse effects of marijuana use are within the range of effects tolerated for other medications." In spite of the established medical value of marijuana, physicians are presently permitted to prescribe cocaine and morphine—but not marijuana.

Organizations that have endorsed medical access to marijuana include the Institute of Medicine; the American Academy of Family Physicians; American Bar Association; American Public Health Association; American Society of Addiction Medicine; AIDS Action Council; British Medical Association; California Academy of Family Physicians; California Legislative Council for Older Americans; California Medical Association; California Nurses Association; California Pharmacists Association; California Society of Addiction Medicine; California–Pacific Annual Conference of the United Methodist Church; Colorado Nurses Association; Consumers Union; Kaiser Permanente; Lymphoma Foundation of America; Multiple Sclerosis California Action Network; National Association of Attorneys General; National Association of People with AIDS; National Nurses Society on Addictions; New Mexico Nurses Association; New York Nurses Association; Massachusetts Medical Society; and Virginia Nurses Association.

The U.S. Penal Code states that any person can be imprisoned for up to 1 year for possession of *one marijuana cigarette* and imprisoned for up to 5 years for growing a single marijuana plant.

On September 6, 1988, the Drug Enforcement Administration's Chief Administrative Law Judge, Francis L. Young, ruled: "Marijuana, in its natural form, is one of the safest therapeutically active substances known….[The] provisions of the [Controlled Substances] Act permit and require the transfer of marijuana from Schedule I to Schedule II. It would be **unreasonable, arbitrary, and capricious** for the DEA to continue to stand between those sufferers and the benefits of this substance."

*In strict medical terms marijuana is far safer than many foods we commonly consume. …it is physically impossible to eat enough marijuana to induce death. …By any measure of **rational analysis** marijuana can be safely used within the supervised routine of medical care.*

Between 1978 and 1997, 35 states and the District of Columbia passed legislation recognizing marijuana's medicinal value. In 2002, California's high court approved medical marijuana. Users of medical marijuana, however, are still subject to prosecution under federal law.

The dispute over marijuana appears to be over its smoked or vaporized form. Capsules of THC can be prescribed in many states for cancer and AIDS patients suffering nausea and appetite loss. But proponents of medical marijuana argue that the inhaled form is more effective and contains additional ingredients that the capsules do not.

A novel cannabis-based medicine, initially developed to help multiple sclerosis (MS) patients, can also reduce arthritis pain, a British company reported in 2004. The drug company awaiting approval from United Kingdom and Canadian regulators to use its spray preparation to treat MS and severe neuropathic pain, said phase II clinical tests showed it could benefit rheumatoid arthritis patients. There are some 400,000 adults in the United Kingdom with rheumatoid arthritis as potential patients.

COCAINE

Cocaine is a natural product originally isolated from a bushy shrub, *Erythroxylon coca*, that grows in the Andes Mountains of Peru. Cocaine's potential for addiction was known and used with sinister intent by South American Indian chiefs hundreds of years ago. The chiefs maintained a messenger system along the spine of the Andes to control their thinly populated kingdoms, which stretched for thousands of miles along the mountains and were isolated from each other by rugged terrain. The messengers had to run at high altitude and needed stimulants for this exhausting task. Their wealthy employers provided the runners with coca leaves along their routes for this purpose and enslaved them further by paying them with more coca leaves, thus maintaining the addiction for which the runners were willing to continue their jobs. When coca leaves reached Europe with the Spanish conquistadors, its introduction led to one of the first European waves of psychoactive drug use.

Cocaine enjoyed a short popularity in human medicine as a local anesthetic, but the primary concern today is that cocaine's CNS effects appeal to many people, and cocaine is presently a major drug of abuse. Its popularity boomed in the 1980s when "free base" cocaine or "crack" became available. The ability to achieve rapid, high brain levels of cocaine by smoking crack has greatly increased its abuse potential and also its toxicity.

Although cocaine can function as a local anesthetic, most of its actions relate to a second mechanism. Cocaine increases synaptic concentrations of catecholamines (i.e., dopamine and norepinephrine) in the brain by *blocking their reuptake mechanisms*. Normally, when these transmitters are released from nerve terminals, they are rapidly removed from the synaptic cleft by specific energy-dependent *"transporter"* proteins that carry them back into the terminal. By *blocking* these transporter systems, cocaine prolongs the time the catecholamines remain in the synapse and intensifies their actions. This increase in dopamine concentration in the CNS appears to be the basis for the various euphoric and related changes that occur in people who use cocaine. A similar mechanism has been suggested for methamphetamine.

Interestingly, the breeding of a strain of "*knockout*" mice devoid of the gene for synthesis of the dopamine transporter protein results in hyperactive animals. This is probably because their neurons cannot remove released dopamine from synapses and consequently dopamine remains in the synapse 100 times longer. The animals attempt to compensate for this defect in their brain by "down-regulating" the entire dopamine system including (1) decreased synthesis of dopamine within the neurons and (2) reducing the number of postsynaptic receptor sites. Eventually, because of the absence of the dopamine transporter protein in these animals, they lose their sensitivity to cocaine.

Cocaine also blocks the reuptake of norepinephrine in the PNS; the combination of central and peripheral actions leads to a high probability of toxicity. *The cardiovascular system is particularly sensitive to the actions of cocaine*, and cardiac arrhythmia's marked increases in blood pressure, cerebral hemorrhage, myocardial ischemia, and outright heart failure are not uncommon with cocaine use. Even young, otherwise healthy, individuals with normal coronary and cerebral arteries have died suddenly after cocaine use from cerebral hemorrhage or ventricular fibrillation. There have been several deaths of famous athletes attributed to cocaine cardiotoxicity. These cardiotoxic effects may be related to increased intracellular calcium levels and involve both cardiac and vascular actions of the drug.

The cardiovascular complications of cocaine abuse now accounts for a major fraction of drug-related emergency room visits and deaths. In 1986, for example, cocaine use was the third highest drug-related cause for an emergency room visit, ranking behind only opioids and alcohol in drug-induced death. Approximately 1700 cocaine-related deaths were reported to the National Institute of Drug Abuse in 1987.

ANESTHETICS AND ANALGESICS

PAIN: the ultimate, universal symptom. It is virtually impossible to comprehend the collective pain and distress that members of our species, as well as others, have endured through the millennia. Broken bones, impacted wisdom teeth, infections, animal bites, amputations, and childbirth to name just a few. Prior to 1846, attempts to provide comfort during surgical operations were minimally effective, at best, and the development of surgery was necessarily limited. From the earliest days of medicine, surgeons had tried all manner of primitive techniques to ease their patient's pain. The Egyptians, for example, used diluted narcotics (probably the best). Other surgeons made their patients drunk with alcohol and then tied them to wooden benches that served as operating tables. In Europe, some surgeons choked their patient's unconscious before operating. Still others applied pressure to a nerve (sensory) or artery (depriving the distal area of oxygenation) to make an area "fall asleep." In the sixteenth century, the French surgeon (and barber) *Ambroise Pare* devised a novel expedient: He put a wooden bowl over the head of a patient and pounded a hammer against it to knock him/her unconscious (much like heavy-metal "music"). Today, the two principle areas of pain management with pharmacological agents include anesthetics and analgesics.

Although the analgesic properties of both nitrous oxide (NO) and diethyl ether (ether) had been known since the late 1700s (NO was synthesized by Priestly in 1776), these agents were not used for medicinal purposes at the time. However, because of their effects on the CNS, these drugs were used in carnival exhibitions to entertain the audience, by producing "highs," as well as in social gatherings ("ether frolics") to entertain the participants. It remained for the emergence of two *dentists* in the mid-1840s to usher in one of the most significant advances in the history of medicine: the successful achievement of reversible general anesthesia.

Dentists were instrumental in the introduction of gaseous anesthetics because they came in daily contact with persons suffering from excruciating pain, often of their own making. It was during a theatrical production that Horace Wells, a dentist, observed that one of the participants became injured during his performance yet felt no pain while under the influence of *nitrous oxide*. Wells was so impressed with the effect that he had one of his own teeth extracted the next day while breathing the gas. Unfortunately, Well's attempt to publicly demonstrate this remarkable effect in 1845 with a volunteer was a failure (the patient cried out during the operation).

In 1846, William T.G. Morton, a former associate of Wells, performed a demonstration using *ether* on a patient named Gilbert Abbot. Both Wells and Abbot must truly be considered heroes in this regard. In a scene reminiscent of Hollywood, Morton arrived late to the proceedings just as the surgeon was about to begin. After administering the ether to the patient, Morton turned over responsibility of the event to the surgeon. When the surgery was complete, with the absence of consciousness and pain, the surgeon declared to the audience, *"Gentlemen, this is no humbug."* Unfortunately, the subsequent lives of Wells and Morton were humbug. Wells died insane—from chloroform abuse, while Morton failed in his attempt to patent the use of ether and died an embittered man. The subsequent development of major general anesthetic agents is shown in Table 11.2.

The ideal gaseous anesthetic agent produces anesthesia while allowing the use of a high concentration of oxygen. The *minimum alveolar concentration* (MAC) of an anesthetic agent at one atmosphere that abolishes movement in response to a noxious stimulus in 50% of subjects (analogous to an LD_{50}) provides the standard definition of inhaled anesthetic potency. Table 11.3 compares the potency of seven inhalation anesthetics. In 30–60 year-old patients, MAC values for nitrous oxide, desflurane, sevoflurane, enflurane, isoflurane, halothane, and methoxyflurane are compared at 1 atmosphere, which indicates that, with the exception of nitrous oxide, they all are potent and can be given with a high concentration of oxygen, thus ensuring delivery of enough of the anesthetic while providing adequate aeration.

TABLE 11.2
Gaseous Anesthetics after 1846

- 1847—Chloroform; pleasant odor, nonflammability, hepatotoxin, cardiovascular depressant
- 1863—Nitrous oxide introduced
- 1868—Nitrous oxide with oxygen described
- 1920—Four stages of anesthesia described*
- 1929—Cyclopropane discovered
- 1956—Halothane introduced, potent, and noninflammable

* The somewhat arbitrary division is as follows: I, stage of analgesia; II, stage of delerium; III, stage of surgical anesthesia; IV, stage of medularry depression.

TABLE 11.3
Minimum Alveolar Concentration

Inhalation Anesthetic	Minimum Alveolar Concentration (%)*
Nitrous oxide	105.00
Desflurane	6.00
Sevoflurane	1.85
Enflurane	1.68
Isoflurane	1.40
Halothane	0.75
Methoxyflurane	0.16

* Minimum alveolar concentration is the anesthetic concentration at 1 atm that produces immobility in 50% of patients or animals exposed to a painful stimulus.

General anesthesia produced by inhalational agents depends on the concentration (i.e., *partial pressure* or tension) *of the agent in the brain*. Solubility of a gaseous anesthetic agent in blood is quantified as the blood:gas partition coefficient, which is the ratio of the concentration (partial pressure) of an anesthetic in the blood phase to the concentration of the anesthetic in the gas phase, when the anesthetic is in equilibrium between the two phases. For example, the partition coefficient is 0.5 if the concentration of an anesthetic in arterial blood is 3% and the concentration in the lungs is 6%. A low blood:gas partition coefficient reflects a low affinity of blood for the anesthetic, a desirable property because it predicts a more precise control over the anesthetic state and a more rapid recovery from anesthesia.

The blood:gas coefficient of solubility can range from 12 for very soluble agents such as methoxyflurane to 0.47 for a relatively insoluble gas such as nitrous oxide. Therefore, more highly blood-soluble anesthetic molecules will dissolve in the blood and body reservoirs (e.g., muscle and fat) before producing a significant change in brain partial pressure. The bottom line is that there is an *inverse relationship* between blood solubility of an anesthetic and the rate of increase of its arterial blood partial pressure.

The factors mentioned above that affect gas uptake also regulate the rate of elimination of gaseous anesthetics (i.e., pulmonary ventilation and blood flow, and solubility in blood and tissue). When ventilation with nitrous oxide is terminated, for example, lung, blood, and high-flow brain tensions of the gas decline *rapidly*. In such circumstances, the anesthetist or anesthesiologist has almost direct control of brain tension. Nitrous oxide will, of course, persist for a longer period of time in muscle and fat, because these tissues have a lower rate of blood flow. With an agent of very high solubility, a decrease of inspired tension produces only a very slow change of brain tension as a result of the "inertia" of the system.

Any volatile material, regardless of its route of administration, can be eliminated from the circulation via the lungs. The mechanism is simple diffusion, and is governed by lipid and blood solubility and partial pressure. The rate of elimination of volatile material from the circulation is directly related to pulmonary blood flow and respiratory rate. For example, in shock patients with reduced cardiac output, a decline in gaseous anesthetic-to-blood concentration to nonanesthetic levels will occur more slowly. These patients will, therefore, require more time to regain consciousness. Similarly, the use of a respiratory depressant such as an opiate analgesic for presurgical medication would be expected to prolong recovery from an anesthetic gas by reducing respiratory rate.

One of the most important discoveries in the development of gaseous anesthetics was the observation that halogenation increased potency as well as ensured nonflammability. Halothane was the first fluorinated inhaled anesthetic commercially developed; it was wildly successful, rapidly displacing all other potent inhaled anesthetics. Efforts to develop other halogenated anesthetics with more of the characteristics of the ideal inhaled anesthetic agent than halothane led to the introduction of isoflurane, desflurane, and sevoflurane.

Special factors govern the transport of gaseous anesthetic molecules from inspired gas through the lungs to blood and then to the brain, including (1) concentration of the anesthetic agent in inspired gas; (2) pulmonary ventilation rate delivering the anesthetic to the lungs; (3) transfer of the gas from the alveoli to the blood flowing through the lungs; and (4) transfer of the agent from the arterial blood to all the tissues of the body. The steady-state concentration in the brain is, of course, of greatest importance. Because the brain is well perfused, anesthetic partial pressure in brain becomes equal to the partial pressure in alveolar gas (and in blood) over the course of just several minutes.

One of the troublesome aspects of the inhalation anesthetics is their relatively low margin of safety. They have therapeutic indices in the range of 2–4, making them among the most dangerous drugs in clinical use. The toxicity of these drugs is largely a function of their side effects, and each has a unique side-effect profile. Metabolic degradation products of inhaled anesthetics can injure tissues. The type of injury depends on the extent of metabolism and the nature of the metabolites. Desflurane, halothane, and isoflurane are all metabolized to trifluoroacetate, which can cause hepatotoxicity through an immunologic mechanism involving trifluoroacetyl hapten formation and an autoimmune response. Therefore, the selection of a particular gaseous anesthetic agent is often based on matching a patient's pathophysiology with drug–effect profiles.

Although inhalation anesthetic agents have an analgesic component (stage I), in that the response to noxious stimuli can be blunted, the analgesic effect is *mild* at low doses, and is only satisfactory at dangerously high doses. Therefore, the use of most general anesthetics is accompanied by some type of analgesic *adjunct*. Nonsteroidal anti-inflammatory drugs (NSAIDs), such as cyclooxygenase-2 inhibitors or acetaminophen (Chapter 14), sometimes provide adequate analgesia for minor surgical procedures and they can be administered in a range of forms. However, because of the rapid and profound analgesia produced, opioids (e.g., fentanyl and its derivatives as well as morphine, etc.) are the *primary* analgesics used during the perioperative period. The primary analgesic activity of each of these drugs is produced by agonist activity at μ-opioid receptors.

The association of opiates with street drugs and the potential for tolerance problems make many people reluctant to use them. Opiates do cause dependence with long-term use, because the opioid receptors develop a tolerance to the drugs. But in short-term controlled use for treating pain, the risk of addiction is small.

Researchers are always seeking alternatives. One interesting lead was discovered on the back of a South American poison frog, *Epipedobates tricolor*, and named *epibatidine*. This compound was found to be 200 times as potent as morphine but has an entirely different mode of action. Derivatives of epibatidine are being screened as analgesics.

General anesthetics are rarely given alone. In addition to the analgesic agents mentioned above, benzodiazepines (midazolam, Versed®; diazepam, Valium®) are commonly used as adjuncts for the relief of anxiety, amnesia, and sedation prior to induction of anesthesia. Neuromuscular blockers (e.g., succinylcholine or pancuronium) can also be administered during the induction of anesthesia to relax skeletal muscles.

There are mainstream alternatives to pharmacotherapy that have found widespread application. *Transcutaneous electrical neural stimulation* (TENS) is an increasingly familiar approach in which two electrode pads are fixed to the skin covering an area causing pain. A pulsating electric current is fed to the electrodes and is thought to somehow block the nerve signals in that region, preventing the pain signal from reaching the brain. There appears to be some evidence that TENS stimulates the release of endorphins (the body's own painkillers). TENS is commonly used to treat acute and chronic pain, back and cervical muscle and disc syndromes, arthritis, fibromyalgia, and others. Regional anesthesia and nerve blocks are widely used methods of pain management during surgery and obstetrical procedures.

The disruption of pain pathways need not be temporary, of course. Radiofrequency current can be used to create discrete thermal lesions in a neural pathway. This deliberate nerve damage interrupts transmission, and because of its permanence, it can be used palliatively for patients with cancer pain or chronic noncancer pain that does not respond to conventional treatment.

HOW DO GASEOUS ANESTHETICS PRODUCE THEIR EFFECTS?

Perhaps the most unusual aspect regarding the structure of gaseous anesthetics is the lack of a basic chemical structure that can produce anesthesia. Table 11.4 compares the diversity of chemical classes that can produce anesthesia.

The first chemical clue relating the structure of anesthetics to their potency was discovered in 1899 by a pharmacologist, Hans Horst Meyer, and an anesthetist, Charles Ernst Overton. Working independently, Meyer and Overton noted a strong correlation between the *polarity* of a compound and its *potency* as an anesthetic. They expressed polarity as the oil/gas partition coefficient, while anesthetic potency was expressed as the partial pressure in atmospheres. Figure 11.9 is a Meyer–Overton correlation for 18 anesthetics used on mice. Note that olive oil is used, which has become the most commonly used reference solvent.

TABLE 11.4
Chemical Classes Producing Anesthesia

- *Inert gases*—xenon, argon, and krypton
- *Diatomic gases*—hydrogen and nitrogen
- *Simple organic compounds*—chloroform, cyclopropane
- *Ether and halogenated ether* (isoflurane, enflurane, methoxyflurane, desflurane, sevoflurane, and fluroxene)
- Polyhalogenated alkane—halothane

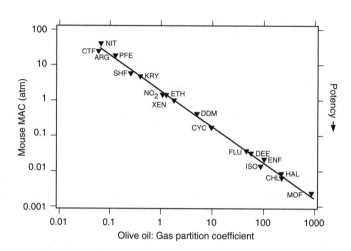

FIGURE 11.9 Meyer–Overton correlation for volatile general anesthetics in mice. The slope of the regression line is –1.02 and the correlation coefficient, $r^2 = 0.997$. CTF, carbon tetrachlorids; NIT, nitrogen; ARG, argon; PFE, perfluoroethane; SHF, sulfur hexafluoride; KRY, krypton; NO$_2$, nitrous oxide; ETH, ethylene; XEN, xenon; DDM, dichlorodifluoromethane; CYC, cyclopropane; FLU, fluroxene; DEE, diethylether; ENF, enflurane; ISO, isoflurane; HAL, halothane; CHL, chloroform; MOF, methoxyflurane. (From E. Moody and P. Skolnick, (eds.) (2001), *Molecular Basis of Anesthesia*. With permission.)

The slope of the regression line implies that MAC (minimal alveolar concentration effective in 50% of animals) is inversely proportional to partition coefficient, or potency is directly proportional to partition coefficient. The Meyer–Overton correlation suggests that the site at which anesthetics bind is primarily a hydrophobic environment. Although a wide variety of compounds lie on the Meyer–Overton correlation line, there are many compounds that do not. This suggests that the chemical properties of the anesthetic site differ from those of olive oil.

The prevailing debate among investigators in the field of volatile anesthetics mechanism of action is the *lipid/protein* controversy. The center of the debate is whether lipids or proteins are the primary targets for general anesthetics. In the fluid mosaic model of the cell membrane, proteins have been envisioned as having active functions while lipids have played a passive, supporting function. Recent advances in cell physiology, however, question a simple dichotomy between lipids and proteins. Therefore, the divisions in the lipid/protein controversy have become less clear.

Interesting calculations have been carried out by others dealing with the interaction of anesthetic molecules on lipids and proteins. For example, at MAC, the concentration of anesthetic molecules in the hydrophobic phase is approximately 50 mM. Assuming that the anesthetic molecules are uniformly distributed throughout the lipid bilayer of a 50 Å thick cell membrane, there would be only one anesthetic molecule for every 60 lipid molecules (i.e., 1.5% of the molecules in the membrane and only 0.5% of the membrane volume). Under these circumstances, the anesthetic molecules would be distributed too diffusely to have a significant effect on membrane status. If, however, anesthetic molecules became preferentially located adjacent to a protein then, conceivably, a local effect on protein function could occur.

A similar argument has been made for anesthetic–protein interactions. Halothane, for example, has a molecular weight of 197. The $GABA_A$ receptor channel (a putative receptor site for volatile anesthetics; see below) has a molecular weight of approximately 250,000. Is it possible that a single molecule of halothane could significantly affect the function of such a large protein? Some proteins are designed to undergo allosteric changes on the binding of small molecules. For example, γ-aminobutyric acid (GABA), the neurotransmitter that permits the $GABA_A$ receptor channel to undergo the closed-to-open channel transition, has a molecular weight of 103.

THE $GABA_A$ RECEPTOR

The $GABA_A$ receptor is a ligand-gated *chloride* channel that underlies synaptic *inhibition* in the brain. When the endogenous neurotransmitter, GABA, binds to the receptor, the anion channel opens and chloride enters the cell. This sequence of events *hyperpolarizes* the neuron, rendering further depolarization or transmission of impulses less likely.

The $GABA_A$ receptor has been recognized for many years as the target of alcohol, barbiturates, and benzodiazepines. More recently, it has been recognized that other drugs such as volatile anesthetics act at these receptors as well (e.g., the concentration at which these drugs enhance $GABA_A$ function correlates well with their anesthetic potencies). The suggestion that increased inhibition of the CNS might be expected to produce "anesthesia" has resulted in the identification of this receptor as a significant anesthetic target.

Studies using synaptoneurosomes (produced by homogenizing brain tissue and recovered by differential ultracentrifugation) have demonstrated that volatile anesthetics can enhance the uptake of chloride ion in a stereoselective manner. The results of these neurochemical studies have been found to correlate reasonably well with data obtained using electrophysiological techniques. Although the $GABA_A$ receptor has received the most recent attention regarding the mechanism of action of volatile anesthetics, it still appears premature to totally disregard excitatory amino acid receptors (NMDA, AMPA, or kainite), as well as calcium and potassium channels; glutamate receptors apparently can be eliminated.

INTRAVENOUS ANESTHETICS

In addition to gaseous anesthetics, there are several drugs that can achieve anesthesia when given intravenously. Intravenous anesthetics are small, hydrophobic, substituted aromatic or heterocyclic compounds. Lipophylicity is the key factor governing the pharmacokinetics of these drugs. After a single intravenous bolus, these drugs preferentially partition into the highly perfused and lipophilic brain and spinal cord tissue, where it produces anesthesia within a single circulation time. Termination of anesthesia after a single bolus dose is primarily by *redistribution* out of the nervous system rather than by metabolism.

Intravenous anesthetics include (1) etomidate, (2) midazolam, (3) propofol, (4) thiopental, (5) ketamine, and (6) opioid agonists. The first four agents act by enhancing the activity of the inhibitory neurotransmitter GABA in the CNS. Ketamine antagonizes the effect of the excitatory neurotransmitter N-methyl-D-aspartate (NMDA) on NMDA receptors, and opioid agonists stimulate opioid receptors.

The ideal intravenous anesthetic has a rapid onset of action and is quickly cleared from the bloodstream and CNS, facilitating control of the anesthetic state. The ideal agent also protects vital tissues, has other desirable pharmacologic effects (e.g., an antiemetic effect), does not affect the circulatory system or cause other adverse effects, and is inexpensive. *Propofol* is the most widely used intravenous anesthetic agent for induction. It is highly lipophilic and distributes rapidly into the CNS and other tissues, which accounts for its rapid onset of action. Propofol produces unconsciousness within the time it takes for the drug to travel from the injection site to the brain, which is referred to as one "arm-brain circulation time" and requires less than 1 min. Propofol is rapidly and extensively metabolized in the liver and at extrahepatic sites, which means it has a high rate of total body clearance. It can be euphorogenic but does not have the residual psychotic effects that ketamine has.

Several reasons suggest the use of intravenous anesthetics for anesthesia induction, but not for anesthesia maintenance. Administration of multiple doses by intravenous injection or a continuous intravenous infusion can result in drug accumulation and delays in recovery. The lack of a means for continuously measuring the depth of anesthesia is perhaps the most important reason for avoiding the use of intravenous anesthetics for anesthesia maintenance. The use of inhaled anesthetics for maintenance of anesthesia provides greater control of the depth of anesthesia, because sophisticated devices are available for monitoring the concentration of the inhaled anesthetic agent delivered to the patient.

Thiopental (an old prototype) is a derivative of barbituric acid, while propofol is a substituted propylphenol. Onset and duration of anesthetic effect for the two drugs are similar. However, recovery is more rapid following infusion with propofol (a desirable feature). The relatively rapid clearance of propofol explains its less severe hangover in patients, compared to thiopental, and may allow for a more accelerated discharge from the recovery room.

LOCAL ANESTHETICS

The development of local anesthetics and their structure–activity relationship are described in Chapter 14, in the drug screening section. Suffice it to say that the development of these drugs has opened up an entirely new era in relieving pain in the conscious patient. When applied locally to nerve tissue in appropriate concentrations, local anesthetics *reversibly* block the action potentials responsible for nerve conduction. They act on any part of the nervous system and on every type of nerve fiber. Their action is reversible at clinically relevant concentrations and nerve function recovers with no evidence of damage to nerve fibers or cells. The first local anesthetic, *cocaine*, was accidentally discovered to have anesthetic properties in the late-nineteenth century.

Cocaine was first isolated in 1860 by a chemist named Albert Niemann. Like most organic chemists before and after, Niemann had the habit of tasting compounds that he isolated. On this particular occasion Niemann noted that it caused a numbing of the tongue. Carl Köller, who used it as a topical anesthetic for ophthalmological surgery, first introduced cocaine into clinical practice in 1884. Local anesthetics are also used topically for diagnostic procedures, such as endoscopy, to depress the cough or gag reflex by blocking sensory nerve function. Subsequently, cocaine became popular for its use in infiltration and conduction block anesthesia.

Local anesthetics block nerve conduction by *decreasing or preventing* the large transient increase in the permeability of excitable membranes to Na^+ that is normally produced by depolarization of the nerve cell membrane. This effect is due to their direct interaction with voltage-gated Na^+ channels. As the anesthetic action progressively takes effect, the threshold for electrical excitability correspondingly increases, the rate of rise of the action potential declines, and impulse conduction slows. These factors decrease the probability of propagation of the action potential, and nerve conduction eventually fails. Examples of different types of local anesthesia are shown in Table 11.5.

ANALGESICS

Unfortunately, to feel pain is an absolutely essential condition for survival. Pain-initiated avoidance behavior protects the individual. Morphine, obtained from opium, from the juice of the opium poppy (*Papaver somniferum*), has been known for millennia to alleviate pain. As mentioned in Chapter 5,

TABLE 11.5

Various Types of Local Anesthesia Techniques

- *Infiltration Anesthesia*—the injection of local anesthetic directly into tissue without taking into consideration the course of cutaneous nerves; duration can be extended with the addition of epinephrine (vasoconstrictor)
- *Field Bock Anesthesia*—produced by subcutaneous injection in such a manner as to anesthetize the region distal to the injection site
- *Nerve Block*—injection of anesthetic into or about individual peripheral nerves or nerve plexuses; produces area of anesthesia greater than with the above techniques
- *Spinal Anesthesia*—injection of local anesthetic into the CSF in the lumbar space. In most adults, the spinal cord terminates above the second lumbar vertebra. Therefore, in this region there is a relatively large space to accommodate injected drug. The use of various specific gravity preparations can be used to manage the height up the spinal cord that the drug will travel

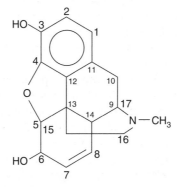

FIGURE 11.10   Structure of Morphine.

endogenous opioids have also been identified. The word "opioid" is now used to refer to all drugs with morphine-like actions. The structure of morphine is shown in Figure 11.10. Diacetylmorphine (heroin) is made by acetylation at the 3 and 6 positions.

In human beings, morphine-like drugs produce analgesia, drowsiness, changes in mood, and mental clouding. A significant feature of the analgesia is that it occurs without loss of consciousness. When therapeutic doses of morphine are given to patients in pain, they describe the pain as being less intense, less discomforting, or entirely dissipated; drowsiness can occur. An additional component can be the experience of euphoria.

Opioid analgesics function as agonists at opioid receptors widely distributed in both spinal cord and brain to produce a decrease in the perception of pain (particularly slow pain). It is well established that the analgesic effects of opioids arise from their ability to inhibit directly the *ascending* transmission of nociceptive information from the spinal cord dorsal horn and to activate pain control circuits that *descend* from the midbrain. Opioid receptors in the spinal cord may mediate various analgesic reflexes and agonists acting at these sites produce significant analgesic responses. These receptors are most concentrated in the limbic system, which regulates emotional behavior, as well as in areas such as the medial thalamus and periaqueductal gray, which mediate pain perception. A preponderance of evidence indicates that analgesic effects of opioids are mediated predominantly by μ receptors.

BOTULINUM TOXIN

Although not normally considered a drug, botulinum toxin has proved to be a useful tool in understanding neuronal function and plastic surgery. In addition, it has recently found a therapeutic use treating prolonged muscle spasm. In one study, 185 children with cerebral palsy were treated with *botulinum toxin type A* (BTX-A) to treat leg and ankle muscle contractions. A small amount of the toxin is injected directly into the muscle fiber to cause that muscle to relax. After 1 year, 46% reported improved walking after receiving injections of BTX-A into the calf muscle once every 3 months. After 2 years, up to 58% had maintained improvements in their walking ability. The toxin acts to reduce muscle contractions by *inhibiting acetylcholine release* at all cholinergic synapses, including the CNS, as discussed below. At the skeletal muscle motor end plate, reduced acetylcholine release leads to weakened muscles, decreased spasticity, and discomfort. BTX-A has also been used to treat severe muscle spasms in stroke patients and cosmetically to reduce the appearance of wrinkles.

Botox® is a trade name for BTX-A and is a nonsurgical, physician-administered aesthetic treatment for moderate to severe frown lines between the brows in people aged 18–65; it works by reducing the contractions of the muscles that cause those persistent frown lines that develop over time; in theory, if an area of the body cannot move, it cannot wrinkle.

Botulinum toxin is one of seven toxins produced by the bacterium, *Clostridium botulinum*. It is among the most lethal substances known, and it has been estimated that 1–2 ounces of the pure toxin could kill the entire population of the United States. Poisoning of man and animals occurs when food containing the toxin is ingested. The most common source is improperly prepared canned fruits and vegetables or fish products. Although only about 100 cases are reported in the United States per year, botulinum poisoning is still a world problem, particularly in Asia, where thousands of cases occur yearly. The lethality rate is 15–40%. Clinical symptoms usually develop 18–36 h after ingestion. Most are due to cholinergic blockade and include weakness, blurred vision, difficulty in swallowing and speaking, progressive weakness of skeletal muscles, and eventually respiratory paralysis. Sensation and consciousness are left unaffected.

There are seven distinct botulinum neurotoxins that differ somewhat in structure and potency. All are polypeptides of about 150 kDa molecular weight. Their amino acid homology is generally high. The mechanism of action of botulinum toxin is now well understood. The toxin is synthesized as a single polypeptide chain that is proteolytically cleaved by the bacteria to form two peptides held together by a disulfide bond. One, the heavy chain, is approximately 100 kDa in size, and the other, the light chain, is approximately 50 kDa in size. When the toxin is ingested, it is absorbed from the gastrointestinal (GI) tract and distributed via the blood stream to nerve terminals in the periphery. The toxin binds to a site on *cholinergic nerve terminals* and is subsequently internalized by endocytosis; once this occurs acetylcholine cannot be released.

The endocytotic vesicles are processed to form endosomes that normally ferry their contents to lysosomes for destruction. As part of their function, the endosomes contain enzymes that progressively render their contents more and more acidic. At a pH of approximately 4, the heavy chain of botulinum toxin undergoes a conformational change that leads to its insertion into the endosomal membrane. This insertion creates a large channel through which monovalent cations can move and through which the light chain likely leaves the endosome to gain access to the nerve terminal cytoplasm.

The *light chain*, when separated from the heavy chain, behaves as an *enzyme* that selectively cleaves a peptide associated with synaptic vesicles. This peptide, *synaptobrevin*, is required for docking and fusion of the vesicle during acetylcholine release. By enzymatically cleaving it, botulinum toxin renders vesicle docking and fusion impossible, and cholinergic neurotransmission comes to a halt. Because the light chain has enzymatic activity, just a few molecules can catalyze the destruction of synaptobrevin on thousands of vesicles. In this way, extreme potency is achieved via amplification of the process.

NICOTINE

Nicotine is an alkaloid derived from the tobacco plant *Nicotiana tabacum*. It is a liquid at room temperature and acquires a brown appearance with a characteristic odor when exposed to air. It is widely available in tobacco products and in certain pesticides (a fact smokers would be well advised to remember). Tobacco products can contain from 0.2 to 5% nicotine and if ingested, particularly by children, can be very toxic. Only a small amount of nicotine found in tobacco is volatilized and absorbed during smoking. However, the nicotine that is absorbed is done so quite rapidly through the alveoli and is detectable in the brain only 8 s after the first inhalation. Nicotine is believed to be the major component of tobacco, associated with its addictive potential and cardiovascular toxicity.

The actions of nicotine relate to its ability to activate one of the two groups of cholinergic receptors, the *nicotinic receptors*. Nicotine and a second substance, muscarine, a mushroom toxin, were known long before acetylcholine was identified as a neurotransmitter, and the receptors in the PNS were initially distinguished by whether they responded to nicotine or to muscarine. Thus, the nomenclature of nicotinic and muscarinic cholinergic neurons was established.

Nicotinic receptors are located in autonomic ganglia, at neuromuscular junctions (Figure 11.3), and within the CNS. Activation of the latter is involved in the psychoactive and addictive properties of nicotine. Like most addictive drugs, nicotine can cause dopamine to be released in a specific brain region known as the shell of the nucleus accumbens. The shell links the amygdala and the core of the nucleus accumbens. Stimulation of peripheral ganglia leads to acceleration in heart rate, increase in blood pressure, and constriction of blood vessels, particularly in the skin. At high concentrations, a pronounced tremor develops and convulsions are possible. Even higher exposure promotes a "*depolarization block*" of ganglionic and neuromuscular function. Under these conditions, heart rate drops precipitously, blood pressure plummets, and skeletal muscle paralysis can develop.

CHOLINESTERASE INHIBITORS

As mentioned in Part II of the book, there are drugs that can interfere with the inactivation of neurotransmitters. In that particular case, the *reversible* cholinesterase inhibitor neostigmine was discussed within the context of treating myasthenia gravis. Excessive blockade of acetylcholinesterase at both muscarinic and nicotinic synapses results in a sustained excess of acetylcholine that persistently activates the effector they innervate. Muscarinic stimulation results in excessive salivation, lacrimation, bronchiolar secretions, and bronchoconstriction. Nicotinic stimulation produces effects such as those described above for nicotine.

Reversible cholinesterase inhibitors actually find their greatest clinical use in the treatment of *open-angle glaucoma*. Relief is achieved by enhancing the contraction of the ciliary muscle and the iris sphincter. This contracture pulls the iris off of the lens and facilitates fluid movement through the *canal of Schlemm*. The result is decreased pressure with reduced distortion of the lens and increased movement of aqueous humor out of the anterior chamber of the eye.

There is another class of cholinesterase inhibitors known as *irreversible* organophosphates. Their mechanism of action involves phosphorylation of serine residues in the esteratic site via *covalent bonds*. These compounds are highly toxic and are not used clinically. Human exposure occurs through the use of pesticides or nerve gases. An example of a nerve gas is the infamous *sarin* that was used in the terrorist attacks in Japan during the mid-nineties. Nerve gases are among the most potent synthetic toxic agents known; they are lethal to laboratory animals in submilligram doses. Antidotal treatment in cases of this type of poisoning includes (1) general supportive measures, and (2) management with atropine for the treatment of muscarinic symptoms and pralidoxime (2-PAM) for the regeneration of the enzyme. 2-PAM exerts a nucleophilic attack on the phosphorous; the oxime-phosphate is then split off, leaving the regenerated enzyme. However, this is not a rapid process.

SCHIZOPHRENIA AND ANTIPSYCHOTIC DRUGS (NEUROLEPTICS)

Schizophrenia is a complex *psychotic* disorder affecting multiple functional modalities and is one of the two most common psychotic emotional disturbances (the other being manic-depressive illness).

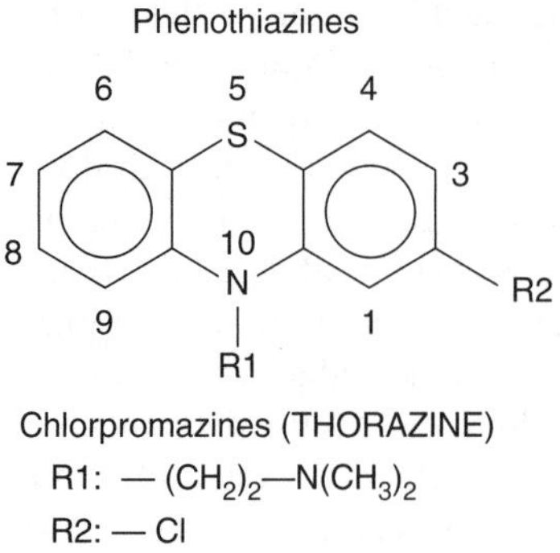

Phenothiazines

Chlorpromazines (THORAZINE)
R1: — $(CH_2)_2$—$N(CH_3)_2$
R2: — Cl

FIGURE 11.11   Chemical structure of the prototypic phenothiazine antipsychotic.

One percent of the world's population is affected by classic schizophrenia. Records show that in 1955, a patient with schizophrenia occupied one out of every four hospital beds in the United States. The symptoms of schizophrenia include virtually the complete range of abnormal phenomena that afflict the human mind. The symptoms most characteristic of schizophrenia include delusions, hallucinations, formal thought disorder, inappropriate affect, blunted affect, impoverished thought, and diminished volition.

Antipsychotic drugs (neuroleptics) may be defined as medications effective in the palliative treatments of psychotic disorders, most notably schizophrenia, although not exclusively. *Phenothiazines* are the oldest and largest class of antipsychotic drugs. They include the prototypical antipsychotic *chlorpromazine*, which in the mid-1950s initiated the present era of pharmacological treatment of psychiatric disorders. Soon after chlorpromazine was introduced in the United States, the population of the state mental hospitals—which until then had been increasing by 10–15% yearly—began to plummet. The drugs belonging to this class are three-ring heterocyclic compounds in which two aromatic rings are linked by a third ring containing sulfur and nitrogen atoms (Figure 11.11).

The antagonism of central dopamine receptors by antipsychotic drugs has been postulated as a critical determinant of the therapeutic efficacy of this class of drugs and forms a core of the "*dopamine hypothesis.*" In essence, this hypothesis postulates that schizophrenia is a manifestation of *hyperdopaminergic* activity in the CNS. In support of this theory are the facts that (1) all widely used antipsychotic drugs have a profound affinity for binding to dopamine D_2 receptors; (2) the clinical potencies of antipsychotic drugs are directly related to their affinities for the dopamine D_2 receptor; and (3) the therapeutic concentrations of antipsychotic drugs in the plasma or the spinal fluid exactly match the antipsychotic dissociation constants at the dopamine D_2 receptor.

The words "neuroleptic" and receptor "occupancy" have similar semantic connotations. The term neuroleptic originates from the Greek *leptikos* that means, "to seize" and implies that the drug seizes the neurons. The term occupancy, of course, evokes a similar meaning at a receptor level through its roots in the Latin *occupare* that also means to seize. Research has shown that the fraction of brain dopamine D_2 receptors occupied by antipsychotic drugs is consistently on the order of 75%, as calculated from the therapeutic concentration and the antipsychotic dissociation constant. The clinical potencies of neuroleptics and their blockade of dopamine receptors correlates while there is a lack of correlation with serotonin, alpha adrenergic, and histamine receptors. Additional support for the dopamine hypothesis comes from the finding that the density of dopamine D_2 receptors is elevated in postmortem brain tissue from schizophrenic patients. Furthermore, positron emission tomography reveals elevated dopamine D_2 receptors in brains of schizophrenics.

Despite the preponderance of data correlating the dopamine D_2 receptor with schizophrenia, alternative sites in the brain (serotonergic, adrenergic, glutamatergic, and GABAergic) are also being investigated to explain the actions of "atypical" neuroleptics.

ANTIDEPRESSANT DRUGS

Depressive illness constitutes one of the most frequently seen mental disorders. The morbidity and mortality associated with alteration of mood is one of the major problems facing behavioral health professionals, with the U.S. National Comorbidity Study of 1994 showing a lifetime prevalence of major depression of 12.7% in males and 21.3% in females. Most mood disorders are chronic and require long-term management. Pharmacotherapy continues to be a mainstay treatment of depression. Because depressant mood disorders are so prevalent in our society, antidepressant drugs are among the most frequently prescribed medications.

The discovery of the antidepressant effect of medications was coincidental to their use for other disorders. Initial work published in 1952 reported that iproniazid (originally used for the treatment of tuberculosis) could elevate mood. Although the use of iproniazid was discontinued due to toxicity, many other additional medications have been tested and approved for the treatment of depression. These include MAO inhibitors, tricyclics, selective serotonin reuptake inhibitors, and a heterogeneous class of atypical drugs.

The principle groups of antidepressants available today are all presumed to exert their action via alteration of brain monoamine metabolism. These amines include norepinephrine, dopamine, and serotonin. The involvement of catecholamines in the pathogenesis of depression was invoked as early as 1965. A deficiency in brain serotonin was theorized in 1967, while a role for dopamine in depression was formally proposed in 1975. The drugs that are used to treat depression basically act to increase neurotransmitter concentration in the synaptic cleft either by (1) decreasing neurotransmitter degradation or (2) inhibiting neurotransmitter reuptake.

An example of a class of drugs that interrupt *neurotransmitter degradation* is the *MAO inhibitors*. MAO is a mitochondrial enzyme that exists in two forms (A and B). Its major role is to oxidize monoamines such as norepinephrine, serotonin, and dopamine by removing the amine grouping from the neurotransmitters. Under normal circumstances, MAO acts as a "safety valve" to degrade any excess transmitter molecules that may spill out of synaptic vesicles when the neuron is in a resting state. MAO inhibitors prevent this inactivation. In their presence, any neurotransmitter molecules that leak out of the synaptic vesicles survive to enter the synapse intact. Receptors are thus exposed to a greater amount of the neurotransmitter.

Several clinically utilized MAO inhibitors such as phenylzine and tranylcypromine are irreversible inhibitors of both MAO-A and B (presumably via covalent binding). The irreversible inhibition of MAO means that neurons so affected must synthesize new enzyme before normal biological activity is reestablished. Research indicates that the antidepressant effect of these drugs is primarily due to *inhibition of MAO-A*. Relatively new MAO inhibitors are of the *reversible type and include moclobemide*.

MAO inhibitors were the first widely used antidepressants, but because of various undesirable side effects, they are employed today in only a more limited number of cases. People who are treated with MAO inhibitors, for example, must be careful of their diet. They should not eat food rich in tyramine or other biologically active amines. These foods include cheese, beer, and red wine. Individuals on MAO inhibitors are unable to inactivate tyramine present in the food. Because tyramine causes the release of endogenous norepinephrine, patients are susceptible to increased blood pressure (e.g., potential lethal cerebral hemorrhages) and cardiac arrhythmias.

Fortunately, another group of antidepressant drugs was developed to take the place of MAO inhibitors. These drugs are called *tricyclics*, because all have chemical structures resembling a three-ring chain. Imipramine was the first of the *tricyclic antidepressants* (TCAs) synthesized as a me-too follow-up to chlorpromazine. All TCAs inhibit the presynaptic reuptake of the monoamine neurotransmitters norepinephrine and serotonin. By inhibiting reuptake, more neurotransmitter is left in the synaptic cleft, thus potentiating their effects. The relative effect on serotonin or norepinephrine reuptake inhibition varies from one TCA to another. In addition to the blockade of neurotransmitter uptake, most TCAs have direct affinities for several heterogeneous receptors.

As scientists improved their techniques for detecting low levels of amines, they began to measure the amine concentrations in postmortem human brains. Several researchers measured levels of serotonin and norepinephrine in the brains of people who had committed suicide as a result of depression and compared the levels to individuals of the same age who had been killed in accidents. The suicides' brains had lower levels of serotonin. Subsequent studies also revealed that certain depressed patients had lower levels of serotonin metabolites in their CSF. These findings accelerated the effort to develop drugs that would be effective on serotonergic neurons.

This newer class of antidepressants, with relatively few side effects, is the *selective serotonin reuptake inhibitors* (SSRIs). This group of compounds has a selective effect on the presynaptic reuptake of serotonin and has assumed the role of first-line antidepressant agents in the management of depression. Most SSRIs have only modest clinically relevant effects on other brain systems. As such, their clinical profile is primarily a reflection of their effect in enhancing the synaptic availability of serotonin. The prototypic drug in this class is *prozac* that has received considerable publicity since its entry into the market in 1988. These drugs have proven to be quite popular in the management of depression since their introduction, despite claims since 1991 that these antidepressants cause patients to become acutely suicidal. But drug makers and regulators long dismissed these claims, saying that they were anecdotal reports without any basis in rigorous trials. In 2002, nearly 11 million children and teenagers were prescribed antidepressants of the SSRI class; the most popular being Zoloft, Paxil, and Prozac.

Then, in 2003, it was announced by two drug companies that teenagers and children who took Paxil and Effexor were more likely to become suicidal than those given placebos. This was followed in September of 2004, when the FDA announced that some SSRIs appeared to be linked to suicidal behavior in children and teenagers. This finding has caused a stir that has yet to be silenced. On the one hand, supporters of the drugs point out that it may be impossible to separate the suicidal tendencies related to depression (suicide is the third leading cause of death among teenagers, trailing only homicide and accidents) from a putative drug effect, and that restricting the drug's usage may prevent some patients from access to the beneficial effects of the drugs. The contrarian opinion is offered by parents who have lost their children to suicides while on the drug and want to protect other families.

One month later in October, the FDA said that all antidepressants must carry a "black box" warning, linking the drugs to increased suicidal thoughts and behavior among children and teens taking them. The acting FDA Commissioner stated "...*that these drugs provide significant benefits for pediatric patients when used appropriately,*" he said at a news conference. He went on to say that "the new labels warn of the risk of suicidality and encourages prescribers to balance this risk with clinical need." The drug labels also include details of pediatric studies that, thus far, have pointed to Prozac as the safest antidepressant for youth to take.

Preliminary results of a large drug trial in 2004, undertaken not by a pharmaceutical company but by the National Institute of Mental Health, showed that fluoxetine (Prozac) is effective in the treatment of depression in adolescents. This confirmed the belief of many that fluoxetine has a role in the treatment of adolescents.

MANIA

While neuroleptics can effectively treat the depression present in bipolar disorder, the metal ion *lithium* exerts a therapeutic effect on the other aspect; it relieves the symptoms of mania. For many years, the only treatment for mania was sedation. Before the advent of neuroleptics, manic patients typically received large doses of barbiturates that simply rendered them unconscious. When they woke up, their manic behavior would take up where it had left off. Later, psychiatrists preferred to prescribe sedating neuroleptics, such as chlorpromazine, for their manic cases because those drugs did not put the patients to sleep, but while chlorpromazine effectively hampers a manic's activity, it does not affect the underlying disorder.

In contrast to neuroleptics, the metal lithium introduced to psychiatry in the mid-1960s, truly aborts the manic condition. Lithium is the simplest drug in the modern pharmacopoeia. Although only a simple cation, lithium has the capacity to profoundly influence the lives of patients with manic depression (now called *bipolar disorder*). For 50 years, lithium has been the mainstay treatment for this disease, providing literally life-saving mood stabilization for countless patients. Many biochemical actions of lithium have been identified, but the mechanism for its therapeutic action remains an enigma. The therapeutic effects of lithium only become evident after a few weeks of treatment at a low plasma concentration (near 1 mM), and continued treatment with lithium can prevent *recurrence* of the disease symptoms. Recent studies have suggested that at least part of lithium's action may be mediated by inhibition of glycogen synthase kinase 3 (GSK-3) via competitive inhibition of Mg^{++}—leading to mood stabilization and alterations in gene expression or cell structure and function.

The widespread involvement of GSK-3 in various conditions, in which lithium might be beneficial, is growing rapidly. These include polyglutamamine toxicity, ischemia, HIV-gp 120-mediated neurotoxicity, apoptosis, and Alzheimer's disease.

Unlike the neuroleptics, lithium does not cause sedation, nor does it transform mania into depression. Instead, it actually appears to restore the patient to a normal state of mind. The calming effect of lithium was actually discovered by accident in a flawed experiment during the 1940s. While investigating whether urine from manic patients contained some toxic nitrogenous substance (uric acid), John Cade (an Australian psychiatrist) mixed uric acid with a number of metals to increase solubility. When lithium *urate* was administered to guinea pigs they appeared to be calmed. Cade then tested lithium in another salt, lithium *carbonate*, to determine whether the key factor in the "calming effect" was the uric acid or the lithium. This lithium too "calmed" the guinea pigs. Impressed with these results, he proceeded with experiments to administer lithium salts to manic patients in the clinic.

We now know that there is nothing abnormal about the urine of manic patients. In all probability, lithium appears to calm guinea pigs only because it makes them sick. Nevertheless, his clinical results were sufficiently positive that Cade published the results in an obscure Australian journal in 1949. In 1954, a Danish psychiatrist confirmed Cade's findings and the use of lithium began to spread in Europe. It was not until the mid-1960s, however, that lithium was marketed commercially in the United States, but it was not used for the treatment of mania until 1970.

METHYLPHENIDATE (RITALIN®)

One of the most controversial CNS-acting drugs in contemporary society is methylphenidate (Ritalin®). This drug is structurally related to amphetamine and is a "mild" stimulant that has abuse potential similar to amphetamine; methylphenidate is classified as a Schedule II controlled substance. Methylphenidate is effective in the treatment of narcolepsy and attention-deficit hyperactivity disorder (ADHD). Its use in ADHD has caused the greatest controversy.

ADHD is a frequently diagnosed disorder, particularly among juveniles; boys being diagnosed at 3–4 times the rate of girls. Symptoms are generally thought to include inappropriate levels of attention and concentration, inappropriate levels of distractibility and impulsivity of some sort, and a combination of the above. A psychologist, psychiatrist, or pediatrician typically diagnoses the condition; but diagnostic methods remain controversial.

Since 1990, the number of American children taking Ritalin® has more than doubled, between 1.5 and 2.5 million. There was a 77% increase in spending on behavioral medications between 2000 and 2003. Money spent on ADHD medicine saw the biggest increase over the 3 years, particularly among very young children.

Defenders of the drug give testament to the profound effect it can have in turning problem adolescents into model students. Proponents point to studies showing that 75% of children on Ritalin® experience positive effects. Opponents label the drug as "kiddie cocaine" and assert that the current state of ADHD diagnosis and treatment is tenuous at best. Undoubtedly, the truth lies somewhere in between, with the proper diagnosis being the key. It is a diagnosis that really did not exist prior to the late 1970s to early 1980s. A correct diagnosis is basically ratified when the medication works.

According to the American Academy of Pediatrics, New England Journal of Medicine, American Medical Association, and the Tucson Unified School District, the following are some statistics on ADHD:

- ADHD is the most common psychiatric disorder in children, affecting from 3 to 10% of school-age children in the United States.
- ADHD is much more common in boys, occurring at three times the rate it does in girls.
- Psychostimulant medications are effective in 70 to 95% of ADHD children, and some 1.5 million U.S. children take them.
- Prescriptions for Ritalin (methylphenidate) and other psychostimulants rose eightfold during the 1990s in the United States.
- For approximately 50% of ADHD children, symptoms persist into adulthood.
- In Tucson's largest school district, some 8% of elementary-school children are taking medications for ADHD, as are 6% in middle school, and about 5% in high school.
- The stimulant drugs used to treat ADHD do not damage the brain; they appear to enhance brain growth, helping afflicted children catch up in brain size to their more "normal" peers.

One of the unfortunate realities of Ritalin use has been its propensity for abuse. A number of studies have revealed that grade-schoolers have obtained the drug from their peers undergoing therapy for ADHD. In one study published in 2001, 651 students aged 11–18 from Wisconsin and Minnesota was focused on. The researchers found that more than a third of the students who took ADHD medication said they had been asked to sell or trade their drugs. Users have crushed the pills and snorted the powder in order to get a "cocaine-like" rush. It is hoped that newer generation products, for example, time-release medications, will be less prone to this abuse, since their formulation makes them more difficult to crush.

Concerta® is a once-a-day treatment for ADHD. It is the first *extended-release* formulation of *methylphenidate* that lasts through 12 h, conveniently providing symptom control from morning through early evening with just one dose. Although Concerta® resembles a conventional tablet in appearance, it actually uses osmotic pressure to deliver methylphenidate at a controlled rate throughout the day.

CURARE

Curare is a natural product isolated from trees and bushes of the *Strychnos* and *Chondodenron* geni. The active principle (D-tubocurarine) is a water-soluble and heat-stable alkaloid that can be extracted, heated, and concentrated to produce a pasty residue containing a high concentration of curare. This extract has been used for centuries in South America as an "arrow poison." Curare is not absorbed from the GI tract nor can it penetrate the BBB. In order for curare to produce its effects, it must be "injected" into the body.

The effects of curare develop rapidly after it enters the body. Victims develop rapid weakness of voluntary muscles followed by paralysis, respiratory failure, and death. The cause is a blockade of nicotinic cholinergic receptors at the neuromuscular junctions in skeletal muscle. Unlike botulinum toxin, release of acetylcholine by the cholinergic nerve terminals is not affected. When curare is present, however, the acetylcholine that is released cannot bind to the receptors because they are *reversibly* occupied by the curare. As a consequence, nerve–muscle communication fails and paralysis ensues.

It is critical to the use of curare by hunters as an arrow poison since it is not absorbed from the GI tract. Animals killed by curare tipped arrows can contain many lethal doses of curare in their carcasses around the point of arrow penetration. Because curare is heat stable, it is not destroyed by cooking and is normally ingested by the hunters. If it were absorbed from the GI tract to an appreciable degree, they would become paralyzed and die from systemic toxicity.

Curare has no effect on sensation, consciousness, or pain and it does not enter the CNS. Victims injected with many lethal doses of curare will survive with no apparent damage, if adequate respiration can be provided for them. Because of this, curare and its derivatives are used in medicine to produce paralysis during delicate surgical procedures, where involuntary or reflexive movement would be disastrous. The anesthetist provides artificial respiration for the patient until curare is eliminated from the body.

SUBSTANCE ABUSE

BACKGROUND

One of the unique aspects of the CNS is that it is the driving force behind the myriad of factors relating to substance abuse. Man has been "abusing" chemicals possessing pharmacological effects on the CNS for millennia. It is the specific quality of certain drugs for influencing CNS function that makes them candidates for abuse. If one examines the main types of abused drugs (Table 11.6), there is considerable diversity in chemical structure. However, they all share the single common feature of affecting brain function to the extent that certain elements of "reality," or consciousness, are altered. Within this context, they are typically taken for religious experiences, to "explore" the subconscious, or suppress anxiety in social settings. Conversely, drugs that do not affect brain function do not represent societal drug abuse problems. For example, one does not hear of insulin or penicillin "junkies."

The National Institute on Drug Abuse (NIDA) was founded in 1974, and since that time there have been significant advances in understanding the processes by which drugs cause addiction. Animal models that replicate key features of human addiction are available, and these models have made it possible to characterize the brain regions that are central for the development of addiction and other drug effects, such as physical dependence. A large number of drug-induced changes at the molecular and cellular levels have been identified in these brain areas, and rapid progress is being made in relating individual changes to specific behavioral abnormalities in animal models of addiction.

By 1974, the basic framework by which many drugs of abuse produce their immediate effects on the nervous system was known. Since that time, one of the most dramatic advances in drug-abuse research has been the identification of the molecular target of almost every major drug of abuse. This advancement occurred with the development of radioligand-binding techniques and the subsequent biochemical characterization of these drug-binding sites with the application of molecular biology to clone and isolate these targets. In view of the fact that drugs of abuse differ greatly in their chemical structure, it is not surprising that each was found to act on its own unique protein target; all drug-abuse targets identified to date are proteins that are involved in synaptic transmission, although different drugs affect different neurotransmitter systems.

TABLE 11.6
Main Types of Abused Drugs

Class	Example(s)
Opiates	Morphine
CNS stimulants	Cocaine, amphetamines
CNS depressants	Barbiturates, benzodiazepines, alcohol
Hallucinogens	LSD, mescaline, Cannabinoids
Miscellaneous	Nicotine, caffeine, phencyclidine, inhalants

There are numerous theories as to what the underlying factors are in drug abuse, whether they are psychologically or biochemically based. In essence, psychological factors driving drug abuse are believed to be based on either some "positive effect" or some "negative avoidance." Biochemical factors appear to be somewhat more complicated, since our understanding of the relevant processes are not as clearly understood. However, we do have a reasonably good understanding of a very important component of drug abuse, namely, the "*reward pathway*."

During the 1970s and 1980s, it became clear to researchers in the field that physical dependence is a largely separable phenomenon from addiction. Some drugs that are very addictive (e.g., cocaine) do not produce prominent physical dependence. In 1982, it was shown that rodents work to electrically stimulate discrete areas of the brain, indicating the presence of brain-reward regions. Subsequent work demonstrated that rodents also work to self-administer drugs of abuse (but not other drugs) and that this self-administration behavior is disrupted by lesioning these brain-reward areas.

We now appreciate the fact that the most important brain-reward region involves dopamine-containing neurons in the ventral tegmental area (VTA) of the midbrain and their target areas in the limbic forebrain, in particular, the nucleus accumbens (NAc) and frontal regions of the cerebral cortex. Of particular interest is the fact that the VTA-NAc pathway seems to be a site where virtually all drugs of abuse converge to produce their acute reward signals. The discovery that dopamine-containing neurons regulate behavioral responses to food and drugs of abuse as far back in evolution as worms and flies emphasizes the primal nature of this reward system.

Reward Pathway

Various experimental paradigms have, over the years, indicated that specific limbic structures in the brain (nucleus accumbens and the amygdala) appear to be consistently associated with what has become to be considered as a common reward pathway through the brain. At present, the reinforcing or rewarding properties of drugs, modulated by specific discriminative cues and concurrent aversive properties, are considered essential in determining the addictive potential or abuse liability of these compounds. The neuropharmacological correlates of reward are considered to be the key to our scientific understanding of drug addiction, and these neuronal mechanisms are the targets of research efforts to elucidate effective pharmacological adjuncts to drug addiction treatment programs.

Natural reward centers have developed over the course of evolution to *reinforce* useful behaviors (e.g., pleasure, sexual satisfaction, food, and drink). These reward centers are innervated by *dopaminergic* neurons. Highly addicting drugs such as cocaine and methamphetamine substitute for natural neurotransmitters to produce an artificial state of reward (*euphoria*) and a compulsion to sustain that state. We now know that cocaine and methamphetamine can increase the level of dopamine in the synapses of dopaminergic fibers, by blocking dopamine reuptake transporter proteins.

At the beginning of the 1990s, the identification of brain-reward regions and the development of increasingly sophisticated animal models of addiction made it possible to search for drug-induced changes in these regions that account for the complex behavioral abnormalities that underlie an addicted state. Much of this work has focused on the VTA-NAc pathway.

One of the earliest findings was the discovery that, like opiates, chronic administration of either cocaine or alcohol upregulates the cyclicAMP (cAMP) pathway in the NAc, as well as a less familiar pathway (cAMP response element-binding protein [CREB]). There is now considerate evidence that upregulation of these pathways represents a mechanism of "motivational tolerance and dependence." These molecular adaptations decrease an individual's sensitivity to the rewarding effects of subsequent drug exposures (tolerance) and impair the reward pathway (dependence) so that after removal of the drug, the individual is left in an amotivational, depressed-like state.

At approximately the same time that several drugs of abuse were shown to upregulate the cAMP pathways in the NAc, the occurrence of other adaptations common to drugs of abuse was reported. These included alterations in levels of G-protein subunits, tyrosine hydroxylase (the rate limiting enzyme in dopamine synthesis), neurofilament proteins, glutamate receptors, and neuropeptide systems. Although the precise functional consequences of most of these adaptations remain to be seen, this work has contributed to the consensus that drugs of abuse focus, at least in part, on common neural and molecular substrates to produce acute reward and chronic changes in reward mechanisms that contribute to addiction.

TOLERANCE

Tolerance is characterized by a diminishing drug effect following repeated administration. The result is a requirement for higher doses with subsequent use to produce the same effect. The term does not give any indication of the mechanism, however. We have already considered one type of tolerance, *pharmacokinetic tolerance*, when discussing phenobarbital. This barbiturate has the capacity to stimulate hepatic microsomal enzymes that can increase the rate of its own metabolism. Since the same enzymes metabolize many other drugs, they too are metabolized more quickly.

In other situations, *pharmacodynamic tolerance* can occur, in which there are alterations at the receptor level. This is believed to be the case with opiates such as morphine and its receptor, while barbiturates can apparently decrease the number of $GABA_A$ receptors in the brain. Possible mechanisms have been described previously.

There are several important aspects of the tolerance phenomenon. For some drugs, tolerance will develop to one effect of the drug and not to other effects. For example, with the opiates, tolerance to the euphoric and analgesic effects is routine following chronic use, but less tolerance develops to the respiratory depression that opiates can produce. This has obvious toxicological implications, since the opiate abuser is placed in greater jeopardy as the dose required to achieve euphoria becomes elevated; the margin of safety for inhibition of the respiratory center decreases. *Cross-tolerance* infers that individuals tolerant to one drug will be tolerant to other drugs in the same class, but not to drugs in other classes. For example, a person tolerant to the sedative effects of one barbiturate will likely become tolerant to this effect in other members of the same class. However, that individual will not be tolerant to the sedative effects of opiates. A schematic representation of tolerance is shown in Figure 11.12.

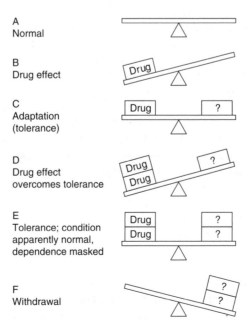

FIGURE 11.12   Representation of the body's response to an addicting drug that develops tolerance.

DRUG DEPENDENCE

Drug dependence can manifest itself as physiological and/or psychological dependence. Physiological dependence is characterized by a syndrome of signs and symptoms manifested on *withdrawal* of the drug. Dependence on drugs of abuse develops only when the drug is administered in sufficiently large doses, at a high enough frequency, and over a long enough period of time. It is believed that excessive bombardment of relevant receptors under these circumstances causes long-lived molecular adaptations in the signaling properties of neurons. Physical dependence is more marked with the opiates and barbiturates than cocaine or methamphetamine.

The mechanism of addiction and physical dependence formation is probably best understood for the opiate class of drugs. A single dose of opiate is believed to inhibit the firing of neurons in the locus ceruleus (LC) by interacting with their μ-receptors. Long-term opiate administration causes a decrease in μ-opiate receptor signaling in the LC (tolerance) without causing a decrease in the number or affinity of these receptors—thus implicating postreceptor signal transduction mechanisms as the site of adaptation. The adaptation may involve upregulation of a cAMP cascade (see above) leading to increased phosphorylation of a "slow" depolarizing Na^+ channel, producing increased neuronal excitability. This hyperactive state does not become manifested until either the drug is withdrawn or an antagonist is given. The factor believed responsible for inducing the hyperexcitable state is cyclicAMP-responsive element-binding protein (CREB).

The withdrawal syndrome for drugs within a pharmacological class is similar, but differs between various drug classes. For example, barbiturate withdrawal is different from opiate withdrawal. A withdrawal syndrome can be precipitated by abrupt cessation of drug use or the administration of a specific antagonist (e.g., nalorphine with morphine). Withdrawal syndromes vary in intensity depending on the drug class. For example, opiate withdrawal rarely constitutes a medical emergency and is considered far less dangerous than withdrawal from alcohol and barbiturates (i.e., possible death). As drugs within a certain class can produce cross-tolerance, they can also generally support physical dependence produced by other drugs in the same class (i.e., cross-dependence).

CAFFEINE

The "drug of choice" for most Americans is caffeine. In fact, caffeine (1,3,7-trimethylxanthine) is probably the world's most popular natural product, consumed in tea, coffee, and caffeinated soft drinks, as well as in nonprescription pills for combating headache and drowsiness. A cup of tea or coffee can contain 100 mg or more of caffeine. Many of caffeine's effects are believed to occur because of competitive antagonism at adenosine receptors. Adenosine is a neuromodulator that influences a number of functions in the CNS. The mild sedating effects that occur when adenosine activates particular adenosine receptor subtypes can be antagonized by caffeine. Caffeine's stimulant effect in relatively normal doses (100–500 mg) is an arousal of the cerebral cortex, resulting in greater wakefulness, mental alertness, and improved psychomotor functioning.

Caffeine qualifies as an addicting drug because it presents qualities of reinforcement and its withdrawal induces a syndrome of symptoms. These include headache, drowsiness, fatigue, decreased performance, depression, and occasionally nausea and vomiting. Symptoms appear within 12–24 h of last caffeine use, peak at 20–48 h, and last about 1 week. Although withdrawal symptoms are more common in moderate to heavy users of caffeine (in excess of three cups of coffee a day), it can also occur with low to moderate intake (235 mg/day, equivalent to 2.5 cups of coffee).

Coffee is not the only source of large doses of caffeine. Chocolate bars, for example, contain approximately 30 mg of caffeine. In addition, over the past 10–15 years, soft-drink manufacturers have produced a number of caffeinated beverages including orange juice and water. However, colas remain the principle vehicle to "Feed the Rush." A comparison of caffeine content of various colas is shown in Table 11.7.

TABLE 11.7
Approximate Amount of Caffeine (mg) in a 12-Ounce Serving

- Coffee (200)
- Jolt (72)
- Josta (59)
- Pepsi Kona (56)
- Surge (53)
- Mountain Dew (52)
- Coca-Cola (47)
- Pepsi (38)

METHADONE MAINTENANCE

One of the unique aspects of physical dependence on heroin is the legal availability of free methadone (a structurally related opiate agonist) through clinics. Methadone is a highly effective analgesic after *oral* administration. Its use is based on the principle of replacing the addict's heroin with an orally active agonist, with a *long* duration of action. This reduces drug craving in the addict and prevents withdrawal. Methadone is usually supplied on a *maintenance* basis (chronic use of the same dose) or on a *withdrawal* basis (gradually reducing the dose over 1–6 months). Because of the inherent difficulties in the withdrawal program, most recipients of methadone are in the maintenance program.

The primary objectives of the methadone maintenance programs are the prevention of progressive health deterioration and to keep in touch with drug users. This makes continuous medical supervision more possible. This is particularly important regarding the prevention of a further spread of infectious diseases such as AIDS and hepatitis. Supplying methadone may also enable addicts to live a structured life, which in turn may increase their chances of successful social integration and, possibly, in the long run, a drug-free existence.

The United States pioneered the use of methodone in the 1960s and 1970s, but now lags much behind Europe and Australia in making methadone accessible and effective. Methadone is the best available treatment in terms of reducing illicit heroin use and associated crime, disease, and death. In the early 1990s, the National Academy of Sciences Institute of Medicine stated that of all forms of drug treatment, *"methadone maintenance has been the most rigorously studied modality and has yielded the most incontrovertibly positive results ... Consumption of all illicit drugs, especially heroin, declines. Crime is reduced, fewer individuals become HIV positive, and individual functioning is improved."*

Popular misconceptions and prejudice, however, have all but prevented any expansion of methadone treatment in the United States. The 115,000 Americans receiving methadone today represent only a small increase over the number that received treatment 20 years ago. For every ten heroin addicts, there are only one or two methadone slots available. Efforts to make methadone more available in the United States run up against the many Americans who dismiss methadone treatment as substituting one addictive drug for another and are wary of any treatment that does not fulfill the single-minded, quixotic goal of leaving the patient *"drug free."*

In 1994, the Swiss carried out an interesting nationwide study to determine whether prescribing heroin, morphine, or injectable methadone could reduce crime, disease, and other drug-related ills. Some 1000 heroin addicts took part in the study. Not surprisingly, the trial quickly determined that virtually all participants preferred heroin, which was subsequently prescribed to them. In the summer of 1997, early data was reported. Criminal offenses and the number of criminal offenders declined by 60%, the percentage of income from illegal and semilegal activities fell from 69 to 10%, illegal heroin and cocaine use decreased dramatically, stable employment increased from 14 to 32%, and physical health improved significantly. There were no deaths from drug overdoses, and no prescription drugs were diverted to the black market. A cost–benefit analysis of the program found a net economic benefit of approximately $30 per patient per day (primarily due to reduced criminal justice and health care costs). The results of the Swiss study imply that given relatively unlimited availability, heroin users will voluntarily stabilize or reduce their dosage and some will even choose abstinence; that long-addicted users can lead relatively normal, stable lives if provided legal access to their drug of choice.

Because of the success achieved with methadone maintenance facilities, similar strategies are being sought to treat other forms of drug dependence. As described below, cocaine has an extremely high addiction liability. Cocaine is basically available in two forms: water soluble cocaine hydrochloride, which can be given orally, intravenously, or by nasal insufflation and cocaine free base, which is water insoluble and is usually administered by smoking. The free base is referred to as "crack" cocaine because of the popping sound it makes when the crystals are heated. Crack cocaine is highly desirable to the user because CNS effects are achieved within 1–2 min, while "snorting" requires 30–60 min to achieve peak effect.

The search for an agent to treat cocaine addiction, one that would not produce euphoria but would still prevent withdrawal, is currently underway. Unfortunately, up to the present, cocaine dependence has proved to be highly resistant to therapy, primarily because of its powerful reinforcing potency. Recently, however, animal studies have produced what may be a new direction in treating cocaine addiction. As described previously, cocaine activates the *mesolimbic dopamine system* by preventing the neuronal reuptake of dopamine. Dopamine acts at two general classes of dopamine receptors, termed D_1 and D_2. Studies in the rat indicate that selective agonists for the two receptor sites can produce different effects. Of particular interest is the observation that D_1-like receptor agonists prevent cocaine-seeking behavior while D_2 agonists do the opposite. Further evaluation of this lead may produce a possible pharmacotherapy for cocaine addiction.

An alternative strategy for the treatment of cocaine addiction involves the use of an anticocaine vaccine. Experiments in rats have demonstrated reduced desire for the drug as well as reduced uptake of cocaine into the brain. The vaccine consists of a synthetic cocaine derivative attached to proteins that trigger immune responses to cocaine. The cocaine derivative is not addictive, and brain levels of free cocaine were reduced by 40–60% in the study. There are approximately 400,000 cocaine abusers in drug-treatment programs in the United States.

ADDICTION LIABILITY

Drugs vary in their propensity to produce dependence. One way to experimentally assess this quality is to expose animals to a behavior paradigm within which the animal can *self-administer* a drug by pressing a lever attached to a drug delivery system (see Figure 11.13) and a counter.

When exposed to a variety of drugs, one can quantify that a rat or monkey prefers to self-administer certain drugs more than others by recording the number of lever presses over time. Not surprisingly, both the rat and monkey, like humans, prefer psychoactive drugs. The degree to which animals will go to self-administer drugs is illustrated by the fact that, in some cases, monkeys will self-administer cocaine until death. If the drug concentration in the administered solution is reduced, the animals will try and compensate by increasing the frequency of lever presses. Similarly, the animals will lever press more frequently if they begin to go into withdrawal. A comparison of psychoactive drugs assessed in this type of situation is shown in Table 11.8 (a liability index of 1 is the highest).

What drives addictive behavior? There are many laboratories pursuing this question with the attendant expenditure of significant resources. The rationale being that if we can understand the neurobiological factors driving this type of deleterious behavior, the scientific community may be able to develop efficacious pharmacological agents to combat the problem. At the present time, a popular model revolves around certain "*reward pathway centers*" (mentioned previously) in the brain.

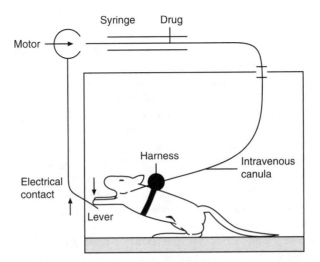

FIGURE 11.13   Apparatus for self-injection of drugs by laboratory animals. The diagram shows a rat pressing a lever to receive an intravenous injection of the drug contained in the syringe above the cage. Rats and other laboratory animals in this situation will readily self-inject most of the drugs that humans regard as pleasurable, though exceptions include hallucinogens such as lysergic acid diethylamide. Because there is good agreement between animal and human data, tests such as this can be used to assess the likely "abuse potential" for new drugs.

TABLE 11.8
Addiction Risk of Major Psychoactive Drugs

Drug	Liability Index
Cocaine, amphetamine, methamphetamine	1
Nicotine	1
Opiates (e.g., morphine, heroin)	2
CNS depressants (e.g., alcohol, barbiturates,	2
benzodiazepines)	3
Cannabis	4
Caffeine	5
Hallucinogens (e.g., LSD, PCP)	5

These reward centers are dopaminergic neurons originating in the ventral tegmental area and projecting primarily to the nucleus accumbens in the forebrain and on to the prefrontal cortex, forming the mesolimbic and mesocortical systems, respectively; an area involved in learning. Data indicate that dopamine release within the brain highlights, or draws attention to, certain significant or surprising events. These include not only those that the organism finds rewarding, such as appetite, feeding, and reproduction, but also events that predict rewards. By underscoring such events by neuroadaptation, the dopamine signal helps the animal learn to recognize them.

These natural reward centers have developed over the course of evolution to reinforce useful behaviors. Virtually every drug of abuse influences dopamine-mediated neurotransmission by affecting directly or indirectly the activity of these cells. For example, amphetamine and cocaine increase the extracellular concentration of dopamine by inhibiting the reuptake of dopamine by the dopamine transporter.

Nicotine, on the other hand, reaches the brain in as little as 10–20 s, where it stimulates nicotine receptors to cause dopaminergic neurons to release large quantities of dopamine. After a few short hours, dopamine levels decline causing withdrawal symptoms to readily appear (e.g., anxiety, irritability, and inattentiveness). When cigarette smokers say they need a smoke to steady their nerves, what they really mean is they need a "fix" to contend with their nicotine withdrawal.

The development of pharmacological strategies to deal with addiction are not limited to those described above. In 1996, the FDA approved a nicotine nasal spray as a treatment for adults trying to quit smoking. The efficacy of the nicotine nasal spray is comparable to other smoking cessation products such as nicotine gum or patches (which are now available OTC). It is recommended that patients use the nasal spray for 3 months. Because nicotine is highly addictive, it is possible to become addicted to the nasal spray. Patients' chances of becoming dependent on the nasal spray increase if they use it longer than 6 months (its recommended maximum duration of usage). Not surprisingly, most people using the spray experienced nasal or sinus irritation. Approximately $500 million is spent annually in the United States alone on nicotine replacement patches and gum, yet these quitting aids do not work for most smokers. For example, about 80% return to smoking after removing the patch.

In the late 1990s, a new approach to nicotine addiction was introduced. It involves the use of an antidepressant known by its generic name as *bupropion*. Bupropion is believed to act like nicotine in that it apparently can boost brain levels of dopamine as well as norepinephrine. Some patients have successfully terminated drug therapy after a few months with no ill effects.

According to 1997 figures, 25% of the adult population in the United States cannot or would not give up the habit of smoking cigarettes. This is despite the knowledge that smoking causes cancer, heart disease, and numerous other health problems. Quite a testament to the addictive liability of nicotine. The financial cost that drug addition extracts from society is, of course, very high. For cigarettes alone, it has been estimated that the average annual excess medical costs incurred per smoker compared to nonsmoker is approaching $1000; total annual value of lost productivity and disability time related to smoking is approximately $50 billion; and total deaths in the United States per year attributed to smoking in excess of 400,000. The relationship of cigarette consumption to mortality rate in males has been known for years and is shown in Figure 11.14.

Addiction has been defined by some as a chronic, relapsing disease of the brain. If this is an accurate portrayal, then there are numerous implications for society including altering our criminal justice strategies as well as medical treatment. If we know that criminals are drug addicted, it may no longer be reasonable to simply incarcerate them. If they have a brain disease, imprisoning them

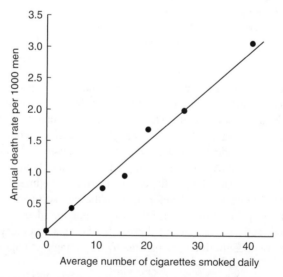

FIGURE 11.14 Number of cigarettes smoked daily and death rate from lung cancer. (From R. Doll and A.B. Hill, (1964) *British Medical Journal* 1: 1399–1410. With permission.)

without treatment would appear to be a futile expedient—if not immoral. Understanding addiction as a brain disease can also affect how society approaches and deals with addicted individuals. Society has learned to deal with people in different brain states such as schizophrenia and Alzheimer's disease. As recently as the beginning of this century, individuals with schizophrenia were institutionalized in prison-like asylums. If, in fact, the brain were the core of the addiction problem, then it would appear reasonable to approach the brain's needs as a central part of the solution.

We also need to understand what makes some individuals particularly vulnerable to addiction and others relatively resistant. Epidemiological investigations indicate that approximately 50% of the risk of drug addiction (including addiction to opiates, cocaine, nicotine, and alcohol) is genetic, but the specific genes involved have not been identified. Only with the identification of these genes will it be possible to understand how genetic and nongenetic factors interact to determine an individual's risk for an addictive disorder.

War on Drugs

A predictable consequence of the illicit use of psychoactive drugs is the imposition of societal "guidelines" as to what constitutes their licit or illicit use. In this context, a more accurate title for this section might read "*War on Some Drugs*." Those drugs, which are licit in our society, such as alcohol and tobacco that have arguably more undesirable qualities to many illicit drugs, have, of course, enjoyed a somewhat exempt status historically. While alcohol use can certainly involve legal sanctions (e.g., DUI, its use has basically been decriminalized with an emphasis placed on restriction of use. Tobacco has enjoyed even less governmental regulation of use (although this has been changing; see Appendix I). If you are "legally of age," you can buy the drug unsupervised from a vending machine. In both cases, sale of the drug occurs despite governmental health warnings either on the package itself, or in close proximity to the site of purchase and/or consumption.

If there is to be a war, of any kind, one would presume that it could be justified on some rational basis. Perhaps the three main historical reasons typically cited to justify wars are a perceived threat, some driving "moral principle;" or the desire for more geographical territory. Obviously, the latter factor is not involved in our country's war on drugs. Therefore, the energy for our government's position probably emanates from the first two and it might be instructive to examine some of the relevant issues. For example, how successful has the war on drugs been? In 1988, Congress passed a resolution proclaiming its goal of "*a drug-free America by 1995*." Despite this obviously absurd declaration, as subsequent history has shown, the beat goes on. Politicians refuse to deal with the reality of illicit drug use as a disease for fear of being labeled "soft" on drugs, and continue to increase a succession of Drug Czar's budgets since the 1960s, to ludicrous proportions; all to appease the well-intentioned conservative members of society.

So, how many people actually use illegal drugs. Obviously, this is a very difficult question to answer with certainty. Because of this, there are disparate figures in the literature. All of them are subject to a certain degree of skepticism. For example, the Federal Government's Household Survey on Drug Abuse, conducted annually, is probably the most commonly cited set of statistics (including by the Drug Enforcement Agency) on the prevalence of drug use. According to the 1994 survey, there were approximately 12.6 million people who indicated they had used some illegal drug in the last month and perhaps 30–40 million who had used some illegal drug within the last year. Of the 12.6 million who used an illegal drug within the last month, approximately 10 million were presumed to be casual drug users, and approximately 2.6 million classified as addicts.

It should be appreciated that making random phone calls to the public generates this data. Therefore, only people who have phones and answer them are included in the study. In addition, the respondents are essentially being asked if they have committed a felony. Other surveys of drug use have put the number at twice as high. Obviously, there is no highly precise, accurate data available on this important question. This lack of hard data is one of the problems associated with attempting to establish an appropriate drug policy.

TABLE 11.9
Number of Yearly Drug-Related
Deaths in the United States[a]

Drug	Number of Deaths
Tobacco	400,000
Alcohol	80,000
Cocaine	2,200
Heroin	2,000
Aspirin	2,000

[a] No reported deaths due to marijuana.
Source: NIDA research Monographs.

While the question of prevalence is an important criterion, it would also be helpful if there were some statistics relating to the dangers of illicit drug use. We mentioned previously that there are some addiction data relating to animal research models as well as rating scales devised by experts in the field. These generally result in a drug profile characterized by the following sequence, in order of decreasing addiction liability of some common drugs—heroin, methamphetamine, cocaine, alcohol, nicotine, caffeine, and marijuana, for example.

The ultimate undesirable property of a drug is, of course, its propensity to take human life. Interestingly, if we look at data published by the *National Institute of Drug Abuse* (Table 11.9), we see that tobacco and alcohol are by far associated with death with the highest frequency. It is also interesting to note that all illegal drugs *combined* are responsible for approximately 1% of the total number killed by alcohol and tobacco. It has been estimated that tobacco is responsible for killing more people each year than all the people killed by all the illegal drugs in the last century.

Often, before people die, it is necessary that they spend a considerable amount of time in the hospital with all the attendant costs. Both alcohol and tobacco play significant roles in this regard. In fact, a series of lawsuits were generated in the 1990s by several states with this in mind (see Appendix I). It is the state's contention that tobacco companies should be held liable for health costs caused by their products, and they should be required to compensate the states for this expense. The city of San Francisco has also taken this position.

How effective has the war on drugs been? Three important criteria addressing this question have to do with illicit drug availability, the prevalence of their use, and the incarceration rate of violators. With regard to availability, the Rand Corporation's 1988 analysis of drug interdiction effectiveness at the border and the General Accounting Office's 1991 report on cocaine flow, the answer is *virtually nil*. This is further substantiated by the government's survey of illicit drug use that actually demonstrates an increase in 1994. According to a 1997 General Accounting Office study, over the 7 years that began in 1988, *"farmers planted new coca [plants] faster than existing crops were eradicated."* Despite costing billions of dollars and half a dozen lives over 7 years, international drug eradication efforts have not reduced the supply of illegal drug. In fact, cost has gone down while availability has gone up (Tables 11.10 and 11.11). Obviously, if drug availability was significantly curtailed, this negative correlation would not be expected. Despite this information, government expenditures on various aspects of interdiction continue to increase.

At the present time (2006), the number one drug problem for many counties across the United States is not cocaine, heroin, or marijuana but *methamphetamine*, according to a survey conducted by the *National Association of Counties* in 2005. A synthetic drug that is easily manufactured, methamphetamine has spread from the west coast and is heading east. A form of speed that is usually smoked, snorted, or injected, methamphetamine quickly becomes addictive.

TABLE 11.10
Average Price and Purity of Cocaine in the
United States during 1981–2000

	Price per Pure Gram ($)	Purity (%)
1981	275.12	47.53
1985	212.50	55.00
1989	105.09	76.75
1993	110.45	72.01
1996	94.52	68.61
2000	51.0	58.00

Source: System to Retrieve Information from Drug Evidence, DEA, 1981–96; National Drug Control Policy, 2000.

TABLE 11.11
Average Price and Purity of Heroin in the
United States during 1981–2000

	Price per Pure Gram ($)	Purity (%)
1981	3,374.40	6.73
1985	2652.71	14.16
1989	1,457.89	30.31
1993	1,404.20	37.20
1996	1,126.57	41.48
2000	378.0	45.00

Source: System to Retrieve Information from Drug Evidence, DEA, 1981–96; National Drug Control Policy, 2000.

Methamphetamine is imported from Mexico, Canada, and Asia as well as produced in small or large labs across the United States, using household ingredients like cold medicines (ephedrine is a useful starting ingredient) and fertilizers. Methamphetamine can be manufactured in barns, garages, back rooms of businesses, apartments, hotel and motel rooms, vacant buildings, and vehicles.

The one statistic that might be referred to as indicating "success" of the war on drugs is the number of drug-related incarcerated prisoners in the United States. Between 1926 and 1970, according to the *Department of Justice*, the total prison population (state and federal) remained quite consistent at approximately 200,000 per year. However, in the 20-year period between 1974 and 1994, the corresponding prison population increased approximately sevenfold to 1.4 million (Source: Uniform Crime Reports, Federal Bureau of Investigation); driven most forcefully by the war on drugs. This era coincided with the successive administrations of Nixon, Reagan, and Bush, all proponents of the war on drugs theme. One can, of course, also conclude that this data indicates exactly the opposite. That is, because of greater market demand and availability, the number of "users" and "sellers" in their respective pools increased in a corresponding manner.

Carrying out a war is always expensive. In 1980, the federal budget for drug control was approximately $1 billion, and state and local budgets were approximately two or three times that. By 1997, the federal budget had ballooned to $16 billion, two-thirds of it for law enforcement agencies, and state and local funding to at least that. On any day in 1980, approximately 50,000 people were behind bars for violating a drug law. By 1997, the number had increased to approximately 400,000.

According to a Justice Department study, 30,099 people were charged with federal drug offenses in 1999, more than double the number 15 years earlier, and, significantly, most of those convicted were drug traffickers. The study reported that only 4% were convicted of simple possession. It also found that drug offenders are serving longer sentences. The average prison stay rose to 5½ years in 1999 from 2½ years in 1986. Drug prosecutions made up 32% of the federal criminal caseload in 1999, compared with 18% in 1984.

The above data is mirrored in the experience of the state of California. During the 1980s, California achieved the highest incarceration rate in the world-exceeding South Africa and the Soviet Union. In 1980, there were 23,726 inmates in California prisons. By 1992, the prison populations jumped to 102,554 (approximately 32% for drug law violators) as 18 new prisons were built; the population is now estimated at 162,317 in 2002. In 1994, California began spending more on its prisons than on its state universities. That pattern has continued since then. California's jailing costs have grown steadily from $200 million in 1975 to $4.8 billion in 2000—now estimated at $21,400 annually per prisoner. A corresponding effect was an increase in the total number of employees working in the Department of Corrections to 30,800 or approximately one for every three inmates.

Drug War theory holds that harsh punishments can make inner city high school students graduate and accept minimum wages rather than drop out and clear $1500 a week selling drugs. It assumes Columbians can be forced to give up $500 an acre for producing cocoa leaves and accept $5 for growing coffee beans. For the smuggler, the profits are even more attractive. One kilogram of heroin is worth $11,000 in Columbia. In Miami, it sells for $50,000 to $70,000—three times as much as a kilogram of cocaine. Drug War theory proposes that enlarging prisons and filling them to overflowing will crush a very profitable industry. Capitalism theory and the Drug War theory are mutually exclusive. One may be true and the other false, or they may both be false, but they cannot possibly both be true.

Shortly after the repeal of Prohibition, in 1936, August Vollmer, a leading expert on American policing, spoke on drugs: "Repression has driven this vice underground and produced the narcotic smugglers and supply agents who have grown wealthy…. Drug addiction is not a police problem: *it never has and never can be solved by policemen. It is first and last a medical problem* …." In June 1995, the European Parliament issued a report acknowledging that "there will always be demand for drugs in our societies… *the policies followed so far have not been able to prevent illegal drug trade from flourishing.*"

In closing, the following should be pointed out. In February 2002, President George W. Bush announced two important new aspects of his drug policy. First, instead of making an absurd, unrealistic date to win the war on drugs, his goal is to reduce illegal drug use by 10% in 2 years. This appears more realistic. Secondly, instead of the "*Just Say No*" campaign of the 1980s, the Bush administration is pushing a policy that in essence reads, "*Please get help.*" This represents a significant alteration in emphasis from punishment to assistance. As part of the $19.2 billion to fight illegal drugs in fiscal year 2002–2003, budgetary increases will go toward drug *treatment* and research. As part of Bush's historic announcement, he declared "*We must aggressively promote drug treatment because a nation that is tough on drugs must also be compassionate to those addicted to drugs.*" Serious and welcome words indeed.

Decriminalization

The United States is not the only country in the world with a drug "problem." How have other countries dealt with the situation and is there anything instructive we can gain from their experience? Probably the most interesting current situation involves the Netherlands. Like many other European countries, the Netherlands is a signatory of the *Frankfurt Accord* that adopts *decriminalization* as the primary approach to drugs. The primary objective of Dutch drug policy has always been health protection rather than incarceration. Therefore, drug legislation in the Netherlands is quite different than in the United States.

Although the harm done to society is taken into consideration, a great effort is made by the Dutch to prevent criminal prosecution from being more damaging to the individual drug user than the drug itself. Since 1976 (the *Baan Commission*), the goal of Dutch policy is to maintain a distinction between the market for "soft" drugs (i.e., cannabis products such as hashish and marijuana) and the market for "harder" substances such as heroin and cocaine. Criminal penalties for and police efforts against heroin trafficking were actually increased while those against cannabis were relaxed. The Dutch approach is part of a long tradition of "*gedoogbeleid*"—the formal, systematic application of *discretion*.

The Dutch goal is achieved by allowing some limited freedom of movement for the retail trade and possession of small quantities of soft drugs for personnel use. However, possession of even soft drugs for *commercial* purposes outside of regulated outlets is considered a serious offense. For example, in the case of *soft* drugs the *maximum* penalty for possession, selling, or production of approximately 1 ounce is a month detention and/or a fine of approximately $3125. In comparison, the maximum penalty for *hard* drugs varies from 1-year imprisonment (and/or a $6250 fine), for the possession of "consumer amounts," to 12 years of imprisonment (and/or a $62,500 fine) for import and export. The maximum penalties may be increased by one-third if the crime has been committed more than once.

Compare the Dutch approach to the sentencing of a 25-year-old convicted drug dealer in America for selling small bags of marijuana to a police informant in 2004; the drug dealer was sentenced to 55 years in prison. The judge in the case said the sentence was "unjust, cruel, and even irrational," but that the law that forced him to do so had not proved to be unconstitutional and thus had to stand. The judge also posed the following question: "Is there a rational basis for giving [the defendant] more time than the hijacker, the murderer, the rapist?" According to trial testimony, the defendant was carrying a pistol in an ankle holster while selling marijuana. He was not accused of brandishing the weapon or threatening anyone with it.

Over the years, Dutch flexibility regarding drug regulations has led to the establishment of so-called "*coffee shops*," where the *commercial sale* of soft drugs is not prosecuted if certain regulations are observed. These rules of operation include no advertising, no sales to individuals under 16 years of age, no "hard" drugs in or near the premises, no breach of "decorum," and they are permitted only in certain specified sections of the community. Interestingly, the fact that cannabis is relatively easy to obtain in the coffee shops has not resulted in a larger consumption increase than in other countries. In fact, the opposite occurs. For example, in the Netherlands, Dutch teenagers are less likely to sample marijuana than their American peers; from 1992 to 1994, only 7.2% of Dutch youths between the ages of 12 and 15 reported having tried marijuana, compared to 13.5% of Americans in the same age range.

According to Dutch police estimates, there were between 1200 and 1500 coffee shops in the Netherlands in 1991. Most of these coffee shops offer a wide range of hashish and marijuana products from various countries and of varying quality. Prices (1995) range from 10 to 15 Dutch guilders per gram (approximately $175–270/oz) compared with a street price of approximately $400/oz in the United States.

The trend toward decriminalization of cannabis has accelerated in Europe. Across much of Western Europe, possession and even minor sales of the drug are effectively decriminalized. Spain decriminalized private use of cannabis in 1983. In Germany, the Federal Constitutional Court effectively sanctioned a cautious liberalization of cannabis in a 1994 decision. In Australia, cannabis has been decriminalized in several states. By contrast, in 1996 in the United States, 641,642 people were arrested for marijuana, 85% of them for possession, not sale, of the drug. Add to this the discrepancy in sentences for crack use and for powdered cocaine use. In the United States, a person caught with just 5 g of crack gets a *mandatory* prison sentence of 5 years, with *no* chance of parole. It takes 500 g of powder-cocaine to trigger the same response. Is a 100 to 1 ratio the result of rational thinking or discretion?

America's *"drug-free"* mentality can also be seen in its myopic approach to needle exchange *vis-a-vis* the Europeans. The spread of HIV among people who inject drugs illegally was what prompted governments in Europe to experiment with harm-reduction policies. During the 1980s, health officials realized that infected users were spreading HIV by sharing needles. Having already experienced a hepatitis epidemic attributed to the same mode of transmission, the Dutch were the first to tell drug users about the risks of needle sharing and to make sterile syringes available and collect dirty needles through pharmacies and other facilities. Governments elsewhere in Europe soon followed suit. Local authorities in Germany, Switzerland, and other countries authorized *needle exchange machines* to ensure 24-h access. In some European cities, addicts can actually exchange used syringes for clean ones at local *police stations* without fear of prosecution or harassment.

Despite the logic of the needle exchange program, the United States had refused to adopt it; this even after AIDS being the leading killer of Americans aged 25–44 for most of the 1990s. In 1991, the National AIDS Commission appointed by President Bush called the lack of federal support for such programs *"bewildering and tragic."* In 1993, a CDC-sponsored review of research on needle exchange recommended federal funding, but officials in the Clinton administration de-emphasized a favorable evaluation of the report within the Department of Health and Human Services. In July 1996, President Clinton's Advisory Council on HIV/AIDS criticized the administration for its failure to heed the *National Academy of Sciences'* recommendation that it authorize the use of federal money to support needle exchange programs. An independent panel convened by the *National Institute of Health* reached the same conclusion in 1997. In 1998, the American Medical Association, the American Bar Association, the World Bank, and the U.S. Conference of Mayors endorsed the concept of needle exchange. America's failure to adopt needle exchange programs as national policy has resulted in the infection of an estimated 10,000 people with AIDS.

DRUGS IN SPORTS

BACKGROUND

In addition to the "recreational" use of illegal drugs, one of the more "creative" uses of drugs is to improve athletic performance. While the use of performance enhancing drugs in the world of sports is not really drug abuse in the common use of the term, it does, however, involve the illicit use of "banned" substances. Therefore, it is appropriate to include a discussion of this topical subject in this particular section. It is an issue that constantly appears in the headlines.

Viewed objectively, we seem to have a somewhat schizophrenic attitude toward the various components that can make up an athletic event. Lets examine the situation. Basically, an athletic event is composed of athlete + equipment + conditions = performance. Humans have constantly striven to improve athletic performance. Which of the factors have people attempted to modify in order to improve athletic performance? First, how about conditions? One of the most significant developments in the history of sprinting is the rubberized track. Ask any runner if their times are faster on a rubberized track and he/she will laugh. Why was the rubber track developed? How about equipment? The world record in the pole vault jumped 9 in. the year the fiberglass pole was introduced. You either used the fiberglass pole or you were finished in the pole vault event. No amount of training by human pole-vaulters could have achieved the same unprecedented increase in height. You need only watch the fiberglass pole flex as vaulters are catapulted into the air. Has there been any outcry from purists yearning for a return of the bamboo pole and 15-ft jumps? There are other numerous examples of equipment changes including starting blocks, lighter shoes with sharper spikes, electrical timing, and the use of "rabbits." One of the few physiological factors that some athletes are able to legally utilize is training or performing at high altitude (Bob Beamon's long jump record set in Mexico City in 1968 lasted for approximately 25 years; an unprecedented duration). Creatine monohydrate is routinely taken as an athletic performance enhancer because it is believed to restore muscle function. "Carbohydrate Loading" is also practiced in order to increase the amount of glycogen stored in the muscles, thereby increasing endurance. Why not use drugs such as erythropoietin (see below)? What about cortisone or hGH (human growth hormone) shots? Aspirin?

HISTORY

Among the earliest reported uses of drugs to enhance performance is by the ancient Scandinavian warriors called the *Berserkers*. The Berserkers were reputed to be invulnerable, of enormous strength, and filled with a wild frenzy in battle. These qualities were ascribed to the consumption of mushrooms containing muscarine and other psychoactive alkaloids before battle. The use of drugs in the Olympics is not new and dates back to before Christ when Greek Olympians attempted to elevate their performance levels by eating bread soaked in *opium*. As mentioned previously, Peruvian Indians have chewed *coca leaves* for centuries in order to sustain strenuous work and athletic ability.

After amphetamine, strychnine, and ephedrine became commercially available in the 1800s, there followed shortly reports of their abuse by canal swimmers and cyclists in Europe and the United States.

In 1886, a French cyclist became the first known athlete to die from performance enhancing drugs (e.g., cocaine plus heroin). In the 1904 Olympic Games marathon in St. Louis, an American reportedly sped to victory aided by a preparation of egg whites, brandy, and strychnine. One might wonder why an individual would use a component now used in rat poison to increase performance. At that time, however, *strychnine* was used because of its crude excitatory effect on the CNS, which we now know is due to blocking *inhibitory glycinergic fibers* in the spinal cord. Despite strychnine's crude pharmacological properties, it still appears to be used to a certain extent. As recently as 1992, the presence of strychnine metabolites in the urine of a Confederation of Independent States athlete caused her *disqualification* from the Olympic games marathon.

Stimulant abuse escalated until the mid-1960s when more rigid anti-doping and drug testing laws were introduced. In 1968, the International Olympic Committee (IOC) introduced drug testing for the first time at the Winter Games in Grenoble, France. In the same year, the Kentucky Derby winner, Dancer's Image, was disqualified for having received the anti-inflammatory drug *phenylbutazone*. During the early 1970s, the "*Sunday Syndrome*" was described in the United States referring to the use of amphetamine and anabolic steroids in the National Football League (NFL). The NFL banned the use of amphetamine in 1971.

The term *doping* is believed to have evolved from the Dutch word *doop* that denotes viscous opium juice. The word became modified to become *dope* referring to any stupefying substance, while today it has a more general meaning. The IOC's Medical Commission (established in 1967) defines its doping policy as consisting of two parts: (1) a ban on the administration of *substances* belonging to selected classes of *pharmacological agents* and (2) a ban on the use of various doping *methods*. The original concept was to ban only substances that *clearly enhanced performance*. When reports appeared that certain drugs could seriously impair performance and render competitors vulnerable to injury (e.g., narcotics), *medical safety* became a rationale. In 1998, Juan Antonio Samaranch, then president of the IOC, rocked the sports world when he stated that if a drug only improved performance and was not deleterious to health it was *not* doping. He was clearly in the minority on this point.

When some organizations added marijuana to their lists, *social acceptability* became a rationale. Although not explicitly banned by the IOC, the NCAA and various national governing bodies ban marijuana. Marijuana has no performance enhancing potential and, in fact, it has been shown that performance skills can be impaired for as long as 24–36 h after marijuana usage. The IOC's list of banned substances has now reached approximately 150 and will undoubtedly grow.

The doping classes include stimulants, narcotics, anabolic agents, diuretics, and peptide and glycopeptide hormones and analogs. Because the banning of drugs is by class, no substances belonging to the banned classes may be used even if they are *not* specifically listed. For this reason, the term "*and related substances*" is also used. With only two exceptions (caffeine and testosterone), the mere *detection* of the substance is grounds for disciplinary action. In the case of caffeine, the definition of a "positive" is when the concentration in the urine exceeds 12 μg per mL. Present technology allows routine detection of drugs at the picogram level (10^{-12} g).

In 2003, the U.S. Olympic Committee (USOC) reported to the IOC that 24 U.S. athletes won Olympic medals in the past two decades after testing positive for banned drugs. They also reported that 23 of the athletes "already served a suspension or received other appropriate discipline under the applicable rules." As for the athletes who tested positive for banned drugs, the USOC said an "overwhelming" number of them were for stimulants commonly found in nonprescription cold medications.

STIMULANTS

As indicated above, amphetamine, cocaine, and strychnine dominated early doping incidents until the introduction of testing. Amphetamines were initially commercially available for over-the-counter (OTC) use as a nasal decongestant. During World War II, amphetamines were used as a means of delaying the onset of fatigue and increasing alertness in soldiers. Subsequently, amphetamines became prominent as an appetite suppressant and as a drug to ward off sleepiness.

The first dope testing program at a major sporting event, a cycle race in France, revealed positive urinalysis tests in over 20% of the competitors. Not surprisingly, experience has shown that runners, swimmers, speed skaters, and cyclists account for most of the problems with stimulants. The efficacy of stimulants as *ergogenic* agents in these athletes is undoubtedly due to their ability to delay the onset of fatigue, primarily via CNS effects. For example, cyclists receiving 250 mg of amphetamine before and during monitored cycling achieved a 7% increase in work productivity while reporting that they were not working harder. Unfortunately, this beneficial effect does not come without a potential price. For example, the death of a Danish cyclist in 1960 is believed due to the peripheral vasoconstrictor effect of amphetamine (i.e., decreased heat loss leading to "sun stroke"). With regard to cocaine, the few studies that exist suggest that little to no performance gains are incurred from cocaine. In 1985, 17% of NCAA student-athletes reported having used cocaine; by 1997, that figure was down to 1.5%. Unlike amphetamine, cocaine is readily metabolized in the body to its major metabolite, benzoylecgonine. In fact, it is *benzoylecgonine* that is tested for in urine.

Successful detection of the "old-guard" drugs inevitably led to the use of alternative stimulant drugs such as *caffeine, phenylpropanolamine, and ephedrine*. Because these drugs are commonly found in OTC medications, this obviously presents a problem for the competitor who is taking the medication for legitimate health reasons. This conundrum still represents one of the most complicated aspects of regulating drug use among athletes. Therefore, athletes are warned not to use this type of preparations without first checking with a pharmacist or medical doctor that their medications do not contain any of the banned stimulants.

One of the most tragic episodes relating to the use of "stimulants" during the Olympics is that of Rick DeMont. In 1972, as a 16-year-old, DeMont won the 400-m freestyle in Munich. However, a urinalysis revealed the presence of ephedrine that DeMont had been taking as an asthma medication. DeMont was required to return his gold medal (his father mailed the medal to IOC headquarters paying the postage himself) and was prohibited from swimming in the 1500-m freestyle, his best event. Should he have been disqualified? According to IOC rules, yes. However, what about pharmacological rules?

The amount of ephedrine that DeMont had taken was equivalent to 10 mg of amphetamine. Studies during the 1950s, supported by the *American Medical Association*, had indicated that as much as 20 mg of amphetamine failed to improve swimming performance of 440 yard swimmers (the equivalent of 400 m). One report concluded that "*[the] findings do not prove that athletes performing in intercollegiate meets would be helped by amphetamine*." Even if DeMont had gained some pharmacological effect (i.e., ergogenic) from the ephedrine, the presence of an additional component normally present in the medication (hydroxyzine) would have been expected to produce a sedative effect, thus operating in the opposite direction.

The recurrence of a similar situation was avoided in 1996. An 18-year-old American swimmer about to compete in his nation's qualifying meet for the Olympic team realized that he had taken a dose of his asthma medication (prednisone) too close to the event. Knowing that it would be detected, he chose to withdraw from the meet saying he would take the courageous step of waiting four more years.

As discussed in the section on alternative medicine, the United States is in the process of banning herbal products containing *ephedra* (the herbal form of the stimulant *ephedrine*). Numerous deaths have occurred from such products including the much publicized death of Baltimore Orioles pitcher Steve Bechler in 2003 from heat stroke. Toxicology tests confirmed that "significant amounts" of an OTC-containing ephedra were in Bechler's blood. Ephedra is linked to heart attacks and strokes because it accelerates heart rate and constricts blood vessels. The FDA says at least 100 deaths have been linked to ephedra.

In July 2006, a Denver Bronco's punter reportedly tested positive for banned ephedra. If his suspension is upheld on appeal, he will miss the first four regular-season games and forfeit $328,000 of his salary. He was subsequently released by the team for this violation.

Among the stimulant class of drugs are a somewhat unusual group of drugs known as *β-2 agonists*. These are drugs commonly taken to treat asthma (they are bronchodilators; see section on pulmonary smooth muscle). Two such drugs are *salbutamol and terbutaline*. These drugs are permitted to be used by athletes by inhaler only and their use must be declared to the appropriate medical authority before competition. Presumably, the use of aerosol administration is permitted because less of the drug will be administered and it will be localized in the airways.

As new drugs appear on the market, some will possess stimulant-like activity. One such drug is Provigil® (*mondafinil*), a mild CNS stimulant (structurally unrelated to amphetamine; see Figure 11.15) that is clinically used in the treatment of fatigue and sleepiness but primarily for the management of *narcolepsy*.

In 2003, a U.S. sprinter was found to have used Mondafinil® during the World Championships in Paris. The United States was stripped of its 1600-m relay gold medal for which the sprinter had run the opening leg. As a two-time offender, the runner was suspended for 2 years. The *International Association of Athletics Federations* said the drug was covered under the category of "related substances." Ten years earlier the sprinter had tested positive for the stimulant pseudoephedrine during the 1993 U.S. junior indoor championships and served a 3-month ban.

In 2004, the American sprinter Michelle Collins, the 2003 world indoor champion at 200 m, received an 8-year suspension after an arbitration panel declared that she was guilty beyond a reasonable doubt of using banned performance-enhancing substances. Collin's never failed a drug test during her career. However, she was punished on the basis of what is called a *nonanalytical positive*. She accepted a 4-year doping ban in 2005.

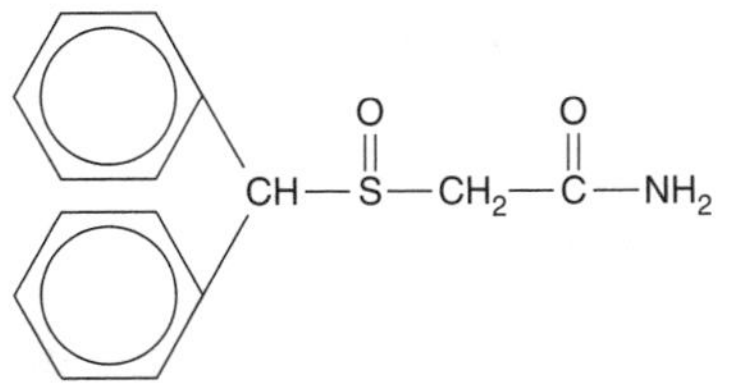

FIGURE 11.15   Chemical structure of Mondafinil.

NARCOTICS

This class of drugs, of which morphine is the prototype, includes many powerful analgesics and is mainly used medically for the management of severe pain. There is evidence that such drugs have been abused in sports creating a false sense of prowess beyond the athlete's inherent ability, particularly if injured. The IOC has banned them entirely, even their legitimate use as painkillers. A range of alternative painkillers exist, although less efficacious, including aspirin and ibuprofen. Athletes are also cautioned against some OTC preparations, including certain cough and cold remedies, which include banned substances such as the antitussive drug *dextromethorphan*.

ANABOLIC AGENTS

Stimulant and anabolic agents are the two classes of drugs most frequently used in the sport world to enhance performance. The principle group of anabolic drugs is the *anabolic androgenic steroids* (AAS). The AAS class includes the natural male hormone testosterone and structural derivatives of it. More than 40 synthetic derivatives that can be taken *orally or parenterally* have been developed. The derivatives have been developed for legitimate medical purposes to increase their anabolic/androgenic ratio for the treatment of such disorders as bone marrow failure and certain anemias. In addition, they can induce significant increases in skeletal muscle mass and strength. In a well-controlled (diet, exercise), 10-week double-blind study, published in 1996, moderately high doses of testosterone enanthate resulted in an average gain of 13 pounds of virtually pure muscle in men who could bench press an extra 48 pounds.

One of the problems with this group of drugs is that they all retain some androgenic activity that is largely responsible for their side effects. For example, in males AAS decrease the size of the testes, diminish sperm production, and produce impotence. Females experience masculinization, loss of breast tissue, clitoral hypertrophy, hirsutism, deepening of the voice, and diminished menstruation. In 1972, when the dominant East German women's swimming coach was asked about his swimmers' low voices he replied that he was concerned with *swimming, not singing*. To counteract these side effects, scientists manufactured steroids that retain their anabolic effects but have much lower androgenic effects (e.g., *androstenedione and nandrolone*).

The East German swimmers used Androstenedione in the 1980s to improve their performances. It was banned by the IOC in 1997, but is permitted by some sporting bodies such as Major League Baseball (Mark McGuire admitted using the drug in 1999 when he broke Roger Maris's home run record). Nandrolone was allegedly detected in a urine sample provided by British sprinter and Olympic gold medallist Linford Christie in 1999.

In addition to the East Germans, perhaps the widest use of AAS in swimming has been by the Chinese. During the early 1990s, their female swimmers produced remarkable results including domination of the 1992 Olympics. This continued at the World Championships in Rome in 1994, when they won 12 of 16 gold medals. However, in 1994, seven Chinese swimmers tested positive for steroid use. As a result of this, China was excluded from the Pan Pacific Games in 1995. Their overall weak performance in the sprints at the 1996 Games in Atlanta suggests that the use of AAS was eliminated.

The use of AAS by teenagers can stunt growth. This is particularly significant since surveys indicate that 5–12% of high school boys reportedly use AAS in the United States. One of the youngest athletes to fail a drug test was the 14-year-old South African runner Lisa de Villiers. She tested positive for the AAS nandrolone. In addition to the side effects listed above, AAS have been reported to be associated with a significant increase in aggressiveness both in men and women. In men, this is sometimes referred to as "*roid rage*." However, in the 1996 study alluded to above, psychological tests and questioning of the men's spouses found no evidence that steroids made them angrier or more aggressive. It should be noted that the duration of that study was only 10 weeks, however.

Although banned by the IOC in 1974, AAS have been continued to be used. Among the more notable examples is the disqualification of Ben Johnson at the 1988 Seoul Olympic Games. Johnson, whose urine contained metabolites of the anabolic steroid, *stanozolol*, had won the 100-m dash gold medal in world record time. He was disqualified and his medal returned. Johnson was subsequently banned for life following another positive test, of another nature (see below), in 1993.

Stanozolol has also been found useful by female athletes. Irina Korzhanenko of Russia lost her shot put gold medal in 2004 and was expelled from the Athens games for testing positive for stanozolol. She had previously served a 2-year suspension for steroids that ended in 2001.

In addition to being disqualified for having an AAS detected, an athlete can also be disqualified for having alterations in hormonal balances. For example, the presence of a testosterone to epitestosterone ratio (T:E) greater than *four to one* in the urine of a competitor constitutes a *prima facia* violation (unless there is evidence that the ratio is due to a physiological or pathological condition—the likelihood of which appears to be <1.0%). Floyd Landis of the United States, the "winner" of the Tour de France in 2006, turned up a T:E of 11:1 in his "A" and "B" samples.

The use of this particular test is based on the following biochemistry. Epitestosterone is a nonmetabolite, stereoisomer of testosterone with no known physiological function, normally produced in a fixed ratio to testosterone. Therefore, an elevated ratio above 6 indicates exogenous administration of an AAS. It was this parameter that led to Johnson's lifetime ban, not simply detection of an AAS, per se. In order to circumvent this testing procedure, athletes have learned to take the "epi" form in carefully calibrated doses to maintain a "normal" ratio.

The use of AAS involves high doses that exceed the medical replacement dose by 10- to 100-fold depending on the sport (swimmers use lower doses while weight and power lifters use the most). Simultaneous use of several AAS is common. Most users begin with one oral drug and then add others either orally or by injection. This regimen, known as *"stacking"* can include as many as 14 drugs or more. Another strategy involves *"cycling"* when the drugs are taken for 14–18 weeks, followed by a break. The former East Germans were the acknowledged experts on the use of AAS and actually developed a testosterone nasal spray under their State Plan 14.25. Unlike earlier oil-based injectable forms of testosterone, newer *water-soluble* oral AAS can wash out of an athlete's system *in days* making detection more problematic.

In 2003, the FDA drew attention to a new AAS called tetrahydrogestrinone (THG), or *"the clear,"* which is used by athletes to improve their performance. Although purveyors of THG may represent it as a dietary supplement, in fact, it does not meet the government's dietary supplement definition. To the contrary, it is considered a purely synthetic "designer" steroid derived by simple chemical modification of another AAS that is explicitly banned by the U.S. Anti-Doping Agency (USADA). It is structurally related to two other synthetic anabolic steroids, *gestrinone* and *trenbolone*.

THG was unveiled to the government when a track coach sent a syringe containing the substance to the USADA. The coach claimed the syringe came from the founder of a Bay Area nutritional lab in Northern California, who has denied the allegation. The founder was one of four men named in a 42-count indictment that alleges they were part of a steroid-distribution ring that provided drugs to numerous top athletes.

In the wake of the FDA's announcement, the NFL announced later in the fall of 2003 that it would begin retesting player's drug tests for THG. The new test would strike others even sooner. British sprinter Dwain Chambers was suspended in November 2003 after testing positive for THG. The governing body, U.K. Athletics, said the ban would last until November 7, 2005. Perhaps more disquieting for Chambers is being barred for life from ever competing in the Olympics.

Another type of drug classified as an anabolic agent is actually a β_2-agonist (that's right, the same type of drug used to treat asthma discussed above). *Clenbuterol* is the prototypic drug. Its use by athletes emanates from use of the drug in the livestock industry to promote growth. Its efficacy in humans is highly questionable. However, the innocent consumption of *clenbuterol*-treated meat could conceivably lead to disqualification, if detected, since it is banned. This is a conceivable situation since one study has shown that the urine of four of eight men who consumed chicken injected with an AAS tested positive 24 h later. In a somewhat more domestic situation, a Russian weightlifter, Aleksey Petrov, won the 1995 world championship but tested positive for a banned

LIVERPOOL JOHN MOORES UNIVERSITY
LEARNING SERVICES

substance and received a lifetime suspension. Fortunately, a former girlfriend later confessed in writing that she had slipped the substance into his food. Petrov was reinstated and won a gold medal in Atlanta.

Clenbuterol remains a favorite with certain athletes, sometimes with little evidence of an effect. High jumper Aleksey Lesnichyi of Belarus tested positive for clenbuterol in Athens in 2004 and failed to clear a height in a qualifying round. A female shot putter, Uzbekistan's Olga Shchukina, tested positive for clenbuterol in a pre-Athens screening. She finished 19th and last in her qualifying group and was expelled from the games.

Although not within the AAS class, female hormones have also been used to feminize males so that they can compete in women's events. A "female" gold medal sprinter in the 1964 Olympics was shown by chromosome testing to be a male; she/he was required to return the medal. *Cyproterone*, an antiandrogenic agent, is suspected of having been used to delay puberty in females. This is particularly important in female gymnastics since puberty shifts the center of gravity lower in the body and changes body proportions. The top three Soviet gymnasts in international competition in 1978 were 17 or 18 years old, but their height and weight were: 53 in., 63 pounds; 60 in., 92 pounds; and 57 in., 79 pounds.

No sport appears immune from drug testing. *Golf*, with a code of conduct calling for players to police themselves, lags behind the other sports when it comes to a formal doping policy. That could change, however. In July 2006, it was announced that testing will be done at the World Amateur Team Championship at Stellenbosch, South Africa, in October, 2006.

Cyclists have been under scrutiny for years; most notably Lance Armstrong, who won the Tour de France. His continual denials have been borne out by testing continually negative for banned drugs. The 2006 winner, Floyd Landis, has not faired as well. After having his initial urine test positive for higher than allowable testosterone, his second sample was found to contain synthetic testosterone, indicating that it came from an outside source. The test was considered "foolproof." He was immediately fired from his team and the Tour de France no longer considered him its champion.

In September of 2006, two of Lance Armstrong's former teammates admitted they used a performance-enhancing drug when they were preparing for the 1999 Tour de France. Frankie Andreau, a former team captain, and the other rider, told the *New York Times* they used EPO in preparation for the 1999 race. Neither of the riders ever had a positive test for a performance-enhancing drug.

DIURETICS

This class of drugs has been creatively used by athletes for two reasons. First, diuretics promote rapid urine excretion, thus increasing the *urinary clearance* of drugs primarily eliminated via this mechanism. In this way, they can be used in an attempt to conceal evidence of the misuse of other drugs in subsequent urinalysis tests. Second, diuretics can be used to achieve *rapid weight loss*. In sports in which competitions are in weight classes, such as boxing and wrestling, this can give an unfair advantage if taken before weigh-in. For this reason, the IOC reserves the right to take urine samples from competitors in these sports at the time of weigh-in.

Other drugs affecting renal function are also banned. For example, *"masking agents"* such as *probenecid* have been used to *prevent the tubular secretion* of AAS in order to minimize their urinary detection. On February 17, 1998, an Australian National Swimming Team member tested positive for probenecid. He had medically received the drug 3 days previously to prolong the action of penicillin for the treatment of a respiratory infection. Probenecid was a banned substance because it had been used in the past to prolong the effects of AAS. Neither the swimmer nor the physician involved knew the drug was banned. After an Australian Swimming Inc. Disciplinary Committee hearing on March 28, 1998, it was decided that the swimmer had taken probenecid *inadvertently* and solely for therapeutic purposes. Nevertheless, on May 5, 1998, the Australian Olympic Committee remarkably imposed its own ban of 3 months and a fine of $6500. This had happened in a country with a relatively rational view of drugs.

Because the original use of probenecid by athletes was in amounts that far exceeded therapeutic doses, it was extremely easy to detect. Because of its ease of detection, however, dishonest athletes no longer use it. Detection of small amounts, as occurred with the Australian swimmer, only indicates therapeutic use. Once again, the pharmacological voice of reason was muted.

Another substance classified as a masking agent is *epitestosterone* (mentioned above). Once athletes and/or their trainers realized that a T:E ratio in excess of 6 could be grounds for disqualification, they attacked the problem in a straightforward manner by simply administering more epitestosterone. The counter response of the regulatory agencies to this cat and mouse game has been to consider an *absolute* epitestosterone level of greater than 200 ng/mL grounds for further investigation.

MISCELLANEOUS DRUGS

It has been mentioned previously that certain types of *β-agonists* have been taken to enhance performance. *β-Blockers* were originally developed to reduce blood pressure and heart rate in cardiac patients (see Chapter 12). They have been widely used clinically to control hypertension, cardiac arrhymias, and angina. Some competitors in sports, where physical activity is of little or no importance, have also used *β-blockers*. For example, they have found use in shooting and archery where their calming effect can be advantageous. Even a slight reduction in heart rate can be beneficial in maintaining a bead on a target. Though they are unlikely to be of benefit to athletes in sports where physical exertion and endurance are required, the IOC reserves the right to test for these substances in those events it deems appropriate. However, beta-blockers would be expected to limit performance in aerobic endurance events.

It is well known that the administration of human *chorionic gonadotrophin* and other compounds with related activity to males leads to an increased production of endogenous androgenic steroids and is considered equivalent to the exogenous administration of testosterone. *Corticotropin* (the adrenal stimulatory trophic hormone) has been misused in an attempt to increase the blood level of endogenous corticosteroids in order to achieve their euphoric effect. The utilization of corticotropin is considered to be equivalent to the oral, intramuscular, or intravenous administration of corticosteroids. According to the Council for Prevention of Drug Use, 45% of riders in the 2000 *Tour De France* tested positive for drug use. Of the positive tests, 28 were for corticosteroids.

The misuse of *human growth hormone* (hGH) in sports is unethical and dangerous because of various adverse effects. For example, cardiomyopathy, hypertension, diabetes mellitus, and acromegaly can occur when hGH is given in high doses for a long period of time. In addition, whether hGH can enhance athletic performance is highly speculative. Substances that act as releasing factors for corticotropin and hGH are also banned.

In 1996, the IOC launched a $2 million effort with European drug firms to develop a test for hGH in time for the Sydney Olympics. This apparently did not come to fruition since up to 50% of the athletes participating at the Sydney Olympics were suspected of taking recombinant GH. It should be pointed out, however, that this estimate may very well be based on questionable data. The estimate was reached by counting the number of syringes and needles being discarded by the athletes. The reader should be able to come up with criticisms of this "method."

There is a growing group, however, touting injectable hGH for its therapeutic properties.

From 1993 to 2002, the FDA's Office of Criminal Investigations (OCI) averaged 7 hGH cases per year. In 2003, it jumped to 17. The next year it was 32, and in 2005, the OCI had 55 hGH-related cases.

In 2006, Arizona relief pitcher Jason Grimsley was caught in possession of $3200 worth of hGH—illegal to use except in specific medical cases. Even though hGH is not classified as a controlled substance like anabolic steroids, it remains illegal to possess and use in all but three cases: short stature in children, wasting diseases such as AIDS, and GH deficiency in adults. Grimsley asserts that he began using hGH for its healing abilities, which is supported by his fast return from Tommy John surgery. Former New York Yankees catcher Jim Leyritz told the New York Post that he tried hGH to recover from shoulder surgery.

Monitoring for hGH does not appear straightforward, however. On the basis of the views and technical knowledge of international experts working on research projects for hGH, urine testing for hGH does not currently appear very promising in comparison with detection of hGH in blood. Experts estimate that less than 1% of hGH can be detected in urine.

The list of proscribed drugs is constantly growing as more performance-enhancing substances come into use and the analytical methods to detect them are developed or improved. At the Lillehamer Winter Olympics in 1994, competitors were, for the first time, tested for *erythropoietin* (EPO). This naturally occurring hormone is produced by the kidney and regulates red blood cell production and, hence, the oxygen carrying capacity of the blood. This is useful for athletes, since red blood cells shuttle oxygen to the cells, including muscle cells, enabling them to operate aerobically. Contemporary assay for EPO requires, for the first time, the taking of *blood samples* from athletes. Disqualification can occur not only for its presence in the body but also simply for its mere possession. For example, in 1998, the Festina-sponsored bicycle team was disqualified from the *Tour De France* after being caught with large quantities of EPO.

Synthetic EPO is currently available and has been demonstrated to induce changes similar to a procedure known as "*blood doping*." A similar substance known as *darbepoetin* stimulates the bone marrow to produce red blood cells by the same mechanism as endogenous erythropoietin. *Lance Armstrong* was plagued for years by unsubstantiated charges of blood doping. Cyclists are not the only athletes to have found EPO to be attractive. Olympic relay gold medalist and world 400-m champion Jerome Young tested positive for EPO in 2004 and was given a lifetime ban from the USADA.

On March 11, 2004, the FDA announced a crackdown on products containing *androstenedione*, commonly know as "andro." The products are marketed OTC as dietary supplements that enhance athletic performance. In the body, androstenedione is converted into testosterone. While advertisements claim that andro-containing supplements promote muscle mass, research has not shown this to be true. In addition, studies have shown side effects and potential long-term risks; androstenedione poses the same kinds of health risks as anabolic steroids. Given the lack of proven benefits and the risks, the FDA is requesting companies to stop distributing dietary supplements containing androstenedione; failure to do so may result in enforcement action if they do not take appropriate actions. Under the Dietary Supplement Health and Education Act of 1994, the dietary supplement manufacturer is responsible for ensuring that a dietary supplement is safe before it is marketed. The FDA is responsible for taking action against any unsafe dietary supplement product after it reaches the market. The FDA is also encouraging Congress to consider legislation to classify these products as controlled substances.

BLOOD DOPING

An efficient way to increase the oxygen-carrying capacity of the blood is the technique of "*blood doping*" (mentioned above). This process basically consists of withdrawing approximately 1 L of an athlete's blood and storing it under frozen conditions for 9–12 weeks. During this period of time, the individual's hemoglobin levels will return to normal by compensatory erythropoietin in the body. The withdrawn blood is then reintroduced into the athlete just before competition. In this way, a higher hemoglobin level is achieved. Blood doping is difficult to detect because of normal variations in hemoglobin levels and the effect of training at high altitude.

Regardless of what type of doping, the USOC created a stiff anti-doping program prior to the Atlanta games. The drug program mandated a no-notice, out of competition testing for steroids and other performance boosters for all 41 Olympic and Pan American Games sports in the United States. One drug that is not presently banned is creatine, an endogenous compound involved in the production of ATP by muscle. It is normally infused just before an event with the hope of increasing energy production.

HERBAL AND NUTRITIONAL SUPPLEMENTS

Vitamin and mineral supplements, herbal preparations, and homeopathic remedies are becoming increasingly popular and are being used more and more by athletes. Competitors are continually striving to achieve an edge over their opponents; many look to these alternatives to gain the advantage. A great number of manufacturers sell their products to the sporting community as a way of gaining increased performance. The marketing of these types of products often relies on personal endorsements by well-known athletes or anecdotal evidence, neither of which may be based on scientific studies nor reliable evidence. These types of products are not licensed. Unlicensed products are not subject to strict regulatory requirements regarding the manufacturing and labeling of constituent substances that licensed pharmaceutical products are. Therefore, it is very difficult to determine the purity of the product or whether the manufacturer has varied the constituents without notice. Some unlicensed products have been found to contain prohibited substances, such as *ephedrine and caffeine*, although neither item appeared on the label.

There are more than 20 different varieties of *Ginseng* plants. Some of them have a stimulant effect in that they reduce tiredness. It is also claimed that the root of the plant improves concentration and has anti-ageing properties as well. However, there has never been any scientific support for these claims or the alleged enhancement of sporting performance. Pure Ginseng is not a banned substance but frequently products claiming to be "Pure Ginseng" include banned substances such as ephedrine, pseudoephedrine, and steroids. A related product known as Chinese ephedra or Ma huang is converted into ephedrine.

Creatine is an amino acid found in meat and fish. It is also produced in the human body by the liver, kidneys, and pancreas. Most of it is stored in skeletal muscle. Of the creatine stored, more than half of it is stored as creatine phosphate, which is involved in the production of energy (by cleavage of the high-energy phosphate bond) for high intensity activity. It is the lack of creatine phosphate that causes fatigue during high intensity activity. Additional, exogenous creatine is taken by competitors in an attempt to increase the body's natural store of the phosphate form in the belief that it will ultimately improve performance. It is thought that this supplementation will assist sporting performance by speeding up the resynthesis of intermediary substances to provide energy for short, high intensity activity and offset lactic acid production. Lactic acid contributes to muscle fatigue in such activity. Although there have been many studies about the effects of creatine, published papers from *large-scale*, *well-controlled* studies are noticeable by their absence.

There is little information on the short- or long-term side effects on the safety of creatine supplementation. However, there have been reports of some athletes suffering side effects with the alleged overdosing of creatine (e.g., the natural production of creatine being curtailed in the athlete's body). The European Commission's Scientific Committee on Food (European Commission, Opinion of the Scientific Committee on Food on Safety Aspects of Creatine Supplementation, September 7, 2000) has concluded that high doses of creatine supplementation should be avoided (i.e., >3 g per day).

Chromium picolonate is alleged to improve muscle gain. This enhancement has yet to be proven scientifically and there is considered to be a very real potential of serious side effects if chromium is taken in large doses over a period of time.

In conclusion, a new global code against drugs in sports was approved in July 2003 in Prague, Czech Republic. The World Anti-Doping Code, adopted in March by sports bodies and governments, establishes uniform rules and sanctions for all sports and countries. Significantly, the IOC changed its charter to replace its own medical code with the global version. The code calls for 2-year suspensions for steroid other serious drug offences.

Sports organizations are required to enact the code before the Athens Olympics in 2004, while Governments have until the 2006 Winter Games in Turin, Italy.

SELECTED BIBLIOGRAPHY

Baskys, A. and Remington, G. (Eds.) (1996) *Brain Mechanisms and Psychotropic Drugs*, Boca Raton, FL: CRC Press.

Brody, T.M., Larner, J., Minneman, K.P., and Neu, H.C. (Eds.) (1994) *Human Pharmacology Molecular to Clinical,* 2nd ed., St. Louis: Mosby.

The Controlled Substances Act of 1970, 21 U.S.C. §§ 801 et seq.; *Common Sense for Drug Policy, Compendium of Reports, Research and Articles Demonstrating the Effectiveness of Medical Marijuana*, Vol. I & II (Falls Church, VA: Common Sense for Drug Policy, March 1997).

Goldberg, R. (1994) *Drugs Across the Spectrum*, Minneapolis, MN: West Publishing Co.

Goldstein, A. (1994) *Addiction from Biology to Drug Policy*, New York: W.H. Freeman and Co.

Hardman, J.G. and Limbird, L.E. (Eds.) (2001) *Goodman and Gilman's The Pharmacological Basis of Therapeutics,* 10th ed., New York: McGraw-Hill.

Karch, S. (1993) *The Pathology of Drug Abuse*, Boca Raton, FL: CRC Press.

Lidow, M.S. (Ed.) (2000) *Neurotransmitter Receptors in Actions of Antipsychotic Medications*, Boca Raton, FL: CRC Press.

Moody, E. and Skolnich, P. (Eds.) (2001) *Molecular Basis of Anesthesia*, Boca Raton, FL: CRC Press.

Rothman, S.M. and Rothman, D.J. (2003) *The Pursuit of Perfection: The Promise and Perils of Medical Enhancement*, New York: Pantheon Books.

Smith, C. M. and Reynard, A.M. (Eds.) (1995) *Essentials of Pharmacology*, Philadelphia: Saunders.

Snyder, S.H. (1996) *Drugs and the Brain*, New York: Scientific American Library.

Tulp, M. and Bohlin, L. (2002) Functional versus chemical diversity: Is biodiversity important for drug discovery? *Trends Pharmacol.*, 23: 225–231.

U.S. Department of Justice, Drug Enforcement Agency, "*In the Matter of Marijuana's Resccheduling Petition*," [Docket #86-22] (September 6, 1988), p.57.

QUESTIONS

1. Which of the following produced symptoms of Parkinson's disease in the early 1980s?
   a. MOA
   b. DMA
   c. PNS
   d. NMDA
   e. MPTP

2. Which of the following was/were responsible for demonstrating the chemical nature of neurotransmission?
   a. Rene Descarte
   b. Henry Dale
   c. Claude Bernard
   d. Otto Löewi
   e. b and d

3. Which of the following is the primary excitatory neurotransmitter in the brain?
   a. Epinephrine
   b. Chloride ion
   c. Acetylcholine
   d. Dopamine
   e. Glutamate

4. Which of the following is responsible for inhibitory modulation of neurotransmission in the brain?
    a. Norepinephrine
    b. Acetylcholine
    c. γ-aminobutyric acid (GABA)
    d. Dopamine
    e. None of the above

5. The GABA$_A$ receptor complex has recognition sites for which of the following?
    a. Barbiturates
    b. Steroids
    c. Alcohol
    d. Benzodiazepines
    e. All of the above

6. Cocaine's principle mechanism of action in the CNS involves which of the following?
    a. Increased release of epinephrine
    b. Inhibition of monoamine oxidase
    c. Increased release of serotonin
    d. Blockade of dopamine reuptake
    e. None of the above

7. Which of the following is credited with the discovery of the anesthetic action of nitrous oxide in 1845?
    a. Joseph Priestly
    b. William Morton
    c. Horace Wells
    d. Otto Löewi
    e. Henry Dale

8. Which of the following receptors is presently the leading candidate to interact with gaseous anesthetics?
    a. Epinephrine (β_1)
    b. Acetylcholine (muscarinic)
    c. Glycine
    d. GABA$_A$
    e. Serotonin

9. Botulinum toxin acts in the CNS by which of the following?
    a. Preventing the reuptake of acetylcholine
    b. Preventing the reuptake of serotonin
    c. Preventing the release of epinephrine
    d. Preventing the release of acetylcholine
    e. None of the above

10. Neuroleptic efficacy in schizophrenia correlates with which of the following?
    a. Blockade of histamine receptors
    b. Blockade of serotonin receptors
    c. Blockade of adrenergic receptors
    d. Blockade of dopamine receptors.
    e. a and d

12 Cardiovascular Drugs

CORONARY HEART DISEASE

Coronary heart disease (CHD) is the single largest killer of both men and women in the world. The World Health Organization estimates that more than 16 million adults per year die of cardiovascular disease. Furthermore, an estimated 32 million adults per year have a new or recurrent myocardial infarction. In the United States, the estimated direct and indirect costs associated with cardiovascular disease exceed $100 billion per year. Risk factors include the following:

- High blood pressure
- High blood cholesterol
- Smoking
- Obesity
- Physical inactivity
- Diabetes
- Gender
- Heredity
- Age
- Stress

Like any muscle, the heart requires a constant supply of oxygen and nutrients that are carried to it by the blood in the *coronary arteries*. In CHD, plaques or fatty substances (e.g., cholesterol) build up inside the walls of the arteries for some reason(s), probably an injury of some sort. These plaques also attract blood components (e.g., platelets) that stick to the artery wall lining and are reparative, but obstructive in the process. Called *atherosclerosis*, the process develops gradually, over many years. It often begins early in life, even in childhood. The fatty accumulation can eventually break open and lead to the formation of a blood clot. If the blood clot is large enough it can occlude the vessel and critically reduce blood flow.

If not enough oxygen-carrying blood reaches the heart, the heart may respond adversely, producing chest pain (*angina pectoris*) or simply angina, for short. The pain often radiates to the left shoulder, neck, and arm. Anginal pain can vary in occurrence and be mild and intermittent, or more pronounced and steady. It can be severe enough to make everyday activities extremely uncomfortable, particularly if they are strenuous (i.e., aerobic) in nature. Nausea and breathlessness often occur simultaneously with the angina. If a blood clot suddenly occludes most or all blood supply to a distal region of the heart, a *heart attack* occurs. The location of the occlusion within the coronary arterial network is a major determinant of how much heart tissue is deprived of oxygen and, therefore, the extent of heart tissue death. If a major coronary vessel is involved, the result can be death.

If the symptoms of CHD give a warning (i.e., angina) and are not life threatening, then steps can be taken to reduce symptoms and retard progression of the disease. For many people, CHD is managed with life-style changes and medications. Others with severe CHD may require surgery (i.e., *coronary bypass*) or other procedures such as *angioplasty* or *stent implantation*. In any event, once CHD is diagnosed, it requires lifelong management.

Medications are prescribed according to the nature of the patient's CHD and other health problems that the patient may have. The *symptoms of angina* are usually addressed with three major classes of drugs: β-adrenergic receptor blockers, calcium channel blockers, and nitrites/nitrates. The tendency to produce clots is routinely treated with daily aspirin or by other platelet inhibitory and anticoagulant drugs depending on the situation (e.g., warfarin, heparin, or Plavix® ,an antiplatelet drug). For those with elevated blood cholesterol that is unresponsive to dietary and weight loss measures, cholesterol-lowering drugs may be used (i.e., the "statins") or cholestyramine and niacin (see below), or a combination of ezetimibe and simvastatin may be used.

BETA-ADRENERGIC BLOCKERS

β-Blockers competitively *attenuate* the effects of catecholamines at β-adrenergic receptors. Normally, norepinephrine, for example, produces an increase in the movement of calcium into heart cells leading to increased heart rate and contractility. β-Antagonists block this sympathetic-mediated increase in heart rate and contractility. By doing so, they decrease myocardial oxygen demand primarily during activity (i.e., aerobic) or excitement (i.e., stress, adrenal discharge). Blockers with β_1 selectivity (atenolol, metoprolol, and acebutolol) are most likely to decrease myocardial oxygen demand without producing β_2 blockade and, thus, fewer side effects.

CALCIUM CHANNEL BLOCKERS

The essential property of all cells is the control over permeability of the membrane to ions. Cells recruit different types of transmembrane ion channels to perform this function. Ca^{2+} channels are closed at negative resting membrane potentials. Membrane depolarization "gates" them into the open, ion-permeable state that is usually rapidly terminated by spontaneous closing ("inactivation"). Voltage-gated, transient, inward Ca^{2+} current is a common mechanism of initiation of Ca^{2+} and is associated with a variety of cellular responses. Rapid and complete inactivation of the Ca^{2+} current is a crucial step in terminating the Ca^{2+} influx and cellular response of tissues such as cardiac.

There are four types of calcium channels in the body (L, T, N, and P). The main type of *voltage-dependent* calcium channel in the heart and vascular smooth muscle is the *L type* ("long lasting"). Depolarization of cardiac muscle and vascular smooth muscle leads to contraction that is dependent on increased cytosolic concentrations of calcium. This occurs via two mechanisms: (1) slight depolarization of the cell activates the L-type voltage-dependent calcium channels, thereby increasing calcium influx into the cell and (2) phosphorylation of the L-type calcium channel. Endogenous β-receptor agonists such as norepinephrine activate membrane bound-adenyl cyclase on cardiac cells, which catalyzes the production of cAMP from ATP in the presence of calcium. cAMP activates cAMP-dependent protein kinases that in turn phosphorylate proteins near sarcolemmal stores thereby further increasing intracellular calcium and facilitating contraction—SA/AV node conduction and contraction.

Voltage-dependent L-type calcium receptors have four distinct binding sites near the pore for calcium flux. By binding to these receptor sites, calcium channel antagonists block the inward calcium current through the L-type channels and antagonize increases in heart rate, SA/AV node conduction, as well as heart contraction. Calcium channel blockers act on cardiac and vascular smooth muscle cells; therefore, they are used in the treatment of angina as well as hypertension, as well as certain types of arrhythmias. Calcium blockers affect bronchial, gastrointestinal, and uterine smooth muscle to a lesser extent. Calcium blockers do not affect skeletal muscle because skeletal muscle utilizes primarily pools of *intracellular* calcium.

The principle calcium channel blockers are nifedipine, verapamil, and diltiazem. Of the three, nifedipine is the more potent vasodilator. Calcium channel antagonists are effective in the treatment of *exertional* or exercise-induced angina. The utility of these agents may result from an increase in blood flow due to coronary arterial dilation, from a decrease in myocardial oxygen demand (secondary to a decrease in arterial blood pressure, heart rate, or contractility), or from both. Concurrent therapy with nifedipine and a β-adrenergic receptor blocker has proven more effective than either drug given alone in exertional angina, presumably because the beta-adrenergic blocker suppresses reflex tachycardia produced by the calcium channel blockers reduction in peripheral resistance. There is no evidence that calcium channel blockers are of benefit in the early treatment or secondary prevention of acute myocardial infarction.

NITRITES AND NITRATES

Nitroglycerin (NTG) is the prototypic nitrate that relaxes vascular smooth muscle via the formation of an active intermediate *nitric oxide* (NO), which activates guanylate cyclase to increase cGMP. NO is thought to act either directly or indirectly, via endothelium-derived relaxing factor (EDRF) to produce smooth muscle *relaxation*. The increased cGMP activates cGMP-dependent protein kinase that phosphorylates various proteins in the vascular smooth muscle. Ultimately, one of these activated proteins dephosphorylates myosin light chain to cause smooth muscle relaxation. By this general cellular mechanism, NTG relaxes vascular smooth muscle, but not skeletal or cardiac muscle.

Nitrates such as NTG dilate large capacitance, peripheral veins, thereby decreasing left ventricular and diastolic volume (less resistance to work against) as well as left ventricular and diastolic pressure (once again the heart has to do less work to move blood out of it). Therefore, nitrates and nitrites improve angina by decreasing oxygen demand of the myocardium. Nitrates and nitrites do not increase total coronary blood flow, when given orally or sublingually. In fact, by decreasing myocardial oxygen demand, NTG may actually decrease coronary blood flow. Since coronary blood flow is exquisitely sensitive to myocardial oxygen demand, if demand decreases by any mechanism, coronary blood flow will also decrease. This is part of the proof that the nitrates relieve angina primarily by reducing demand rather than supply of oxygen.

Organic nitrates are extensively metabolized by a hepatic nitrate reductase that inactivates the drug. If given orally, first-pass metabolism results in >90% degradation. Therefore, NTG is primarily administered sublingually or topically as an ointment or patch. Following sublingual administration, the onset of action occurs within 2 min, but the effect declines within 30 min. The rapid onset of sublingual NTG is why it is used to treat *acute* angina attacks. Ointment application results in effects within 60 min and they persist for up to 6 h.

Side effects from the nitrates are usually exaggerations of their therapeutic effects, particularly vasodilatation. For example, facial flushing and *particularly headaches* frequently occur. The latter can make patient compliance a problem. In addition, peripheral resistance can decrease to the point where orthostatic hypotension can be produced, leading to *syncope* (loss of consciousness). The reduction in blood pressure can also lead to baroreceptor-mediated compensatory increase in heart rate and contractility.

ASPIRIN

In response to vessel wall injury, platelets aggregate and release granular contents, leading to further aggregation, vasoconstriction, and thrombus formation. However, platelets exposed to aspirin have diminished aggregation in response to various thrombogenic stimuli. Aspirin is able to diminish platelet aggregation by blocking the synthesis of the arachidonic breakdown product thromboxane (a potent vasoconstrictor and promoter of platelet aggregation). It blocks thromboxane formation by irreversibly inhibiting *cyclooxygenase* by covalently binding to a serine residue on the enzyme. While endothelial cells can synthesize new cyclooxygenase, anucleated platelets cannot synthesize new cyclooxygenase in their ~10 day lifetime.

In unstable angina, disruption of atheroschlerotic plaques exposes the subendothelium to circulating blood elements. This initiates platelet aggregation and formation of thrombi, as well as local vasoconstriction, release of growth factors, chemotactic factors, and mitogenic factors. These events lead to repetitive reductions in coronary blood flow. In such patients with unstable angina, aspirin reduces the frequency and severity of these episodes. Aspirin results in a 50% reduction in subsequent myocardial infarctions and in mortality. One baby aspirin (81 mg) is usually sufficient to inhibit platelet aggregation. However, recent evidence indicates that the concomitant administration of *ibuprofen* can partially negate the beneficial effect of aspirin on platelets by antagonizing aspirins effect on cyclooxygenase (particularly if given before aspirin.)

Certain surgical procedures such as hip-joint replacement or cardiopulmonary bypass, in which whole blood comes into contact with foreign materials, result in initiation of blood coagulation and thrombus formation. Here, prophylactic administration of anticoagulants, usually *heparin or coumarin*, is effective in diminishing unwanted thrombus formation. Commercial heparin is obtained from hog intestinal mucosa or beef lung, and is a linear polysaccharide composed of alternating residues of glucosamine and glucuronic or iduronic acid.

Heparin acts by *binding to antithrombin III*, which serves as a *major inhibitor* of serine protease *clotting enzymes*. Abruptly ending heparin treatment can be hazardous because of reduced levels of antithrombin III. Coumarins, typified by *warfarin*, are structurally similar to vitamin K, which plays an important role in blood coagulation. By interfering with the function of vitamin K, vitamin K-dependent proteins such as clotting factors VII, IX, X, and prothrombin are reduced.

PLAVIX

Clot formation is a natural defense mechanism of the body, to protect you from excessive bleeding in the case of an injury. When you cut yourself, particles in your blood called platelets stick together to form a clot. Clot formation can also be triggered by the rupture of plaque, which is a buildup of cholesterol and other materials in the walls of the arteries. When platelets clump together on or near the plaque, they can form a clot that may limit or completely stop the flow of blood to various parts of the body. If a clot forms in an artery serving the heart, heart-related chest pain or a heart attack can occur. If a clot forms in an artery leading to the brain, a stroke can occur.

Plavix is an antiplatelet medication approved by the FDA to reduce the risk of heart attack, stroke, or vascular death in patients with established peripheral arterial disease. It is recommended for people who have suffered from a recent heart attack or stroke, or who have peripheral artery disease. Plavix taken with aspirin is also recommended for people who have been hospitalized with heart-related chest pain or had a certain type of heart attack (acute coronary syndrome).

LIPID-LOWERING AGENTS

The premise for treatment of hyperlipidemia is based on the *hypothesis* that abnormalities in lipid and lipoprotein levels are risk factors for CAD and that reductions in blood lipids can result in decreased risk of disease and complications. Low-density lipoprotein (LDL) cholesterol directly correlates with the risk of CAD. Drug therapy is often initiated when LDL levels meet or exceed 190 mg%. Results from clinical trials support the hypothesis that cholesterol-lowering strategies aimed at reducing cholesterol by 20–25% produce clinically significant reductions in cardiovascular events in patients having preexisting vascular disease. The absolute magnitude of the benefits of cholesterol-lowering is greatest in those with other risk factors (i.e., family history of CAD, cigarette smoking, hypertension, and diabetes). These risk factors are the basis for recommending lower cholesterol cut-off points and goals for those who are at high risk for developing clinical CAD. The National Cholesterol Education Program, as well as recently published studies, has identified two principle groups for aggressive drug treatment: (1) those without CAD who are at high *risk* for developing CAD (primary prevention) and (2) those with *preexisting* CAD.

The relationship between elevated triglycerides (TGRs) as a risk factor for CAD is less clear. However, serum TGRs are often inversely related to high-density lipoprotein (HDL-the "good" cholesterol). Therefore, reduction in TGR levels is associated with a rise in HDL, which has a negative correlation (protective effect) with CAD.

There are four principle classes of lipid-lowering drugs used in the treatment of CAD: (1) 3-hydroxy-3-methyl-glutaryl-coenzyme A (HMG-CoA) reductase inhibitors; (2) bile acid-binding resins; (3) nicotinic acid; and (4) fibric acid derivatives.

Examples of HMG CoA reductase inhibitors include *Lovastatin, Simvastatin*, and *Pravastatin*; the so-called "statins." These drugs *inhibit the rate-limiting enzyme* in the synthesis of cholesterol in the liver. In addition, the reduction in the formation of hepatic cholesterol leads to a compensatory *increase* in the hepatic synthesis of *LDL receptors* on the surface of hepatocytes. These receptors bind plasma LDL leading to a reduction in plasma LDL; the "bad" cholesterol.

In 1994, the Scandinavian Simvastatin Survival Study demonstrated a survival benefit from lowering cholesterol in *individuals with CAD*. Interestingly, in the following year, the West of Scotland Coronary Prevention study examined 6595 men *without CAD* who had LDLs of 155–232 mg% and who received Pravastatin. They found a 33% reduction in deaths from CAD compared to the placebo group. These data indicate that aggressive, prophylactic treatment with HMG-CoA reductase inhibitors may be beneficial in men without CAD as well as those with preexistent CAD. HMG-CoA reductase inhibitors are the most effective drugs for reducing both total and LDL cholesterol and can be used in conjunction with other lipid-lowering strategies. The drug Vytorin® contains two active ingredients: *ezetimibe* to reduce intestinal absorption of cholesterol as well as simvastatin.

Approximately 2% of patients have to discontinue taking these drugs due to side effects. The most common ones include those related to the gastrointestinal tract (abdominal pain, diarrhea, constipation, and flatulence). Occasionally, patients may also develop muscle pain. Nevertheless, in summary, HMG-CoA inhibitors are the lipid-lowering drugs of first choice for treatment of most patients at risk for CAD. A long-term decrease in the rate of mortality or major coronary events has been documented with pravastatin, simvastatin, and lovastatin.

The prototype of a bile acid-binding resin is *cholestyramine*. Cholestyramine is actually the chloride salt of a basic anion-exchange resin. Its mechanism of action involves exchanging its chloride ion for bile acids in the intestinal lumen. By binding these bile acids they prevent them from being reabsorbed and, hence, are excreted, up to a tenfold increase. Normally, bile acids exert a *negative feedback* effect on the conversion of cholesterol to bile acids in the liver by inhibiting a microsomal hydroxylase. As bile-acid levels fall, therefore, more cholesterol is catabolized to bile acids. Furthermore, as the amount of cholesterol falls in the hepatocytes, these cells attempt to compensate by increasing their LDL receptors to remove cholesterol from the plasma. Like the statins, bile-acid sequestrants show a *linear relationship* between the degree of cholesterol lowering and the reduction in clinical coronary events. In view of the fact that these drugs are not absorbed from the GI tract, they are relatively nontoxic. Bloating and constipation do make patient compliance a problem, however.

Nicotinic acid (niacin) is a water-soluble B-complex vitamin that is converted in the body into nicotinamide before being subsequently modified to NAD or NADP. Nicotinic acid's mechanism of action is not clear. It is believed to reduce the secretion of very light density lipoproteins (VLDL) from the liver. VLDL is the major carrier for TGRs. Reduction in LDL, on the other hand, may be a product of lowered VLDL since VLDL is a precursor of LDL. Many people who take nicotinic acid experience cutaneous vasodilatation, resulting in skin flushing. Tachyphylaxis can also occur within a few days creating problems with patient compliance. Other commonly occurring side effects include GI disturbances and elevated blood uric acid and glucose. These side effects are so prevalent that the drug is *not recommended* in persons with peptic ulcer disease, gout, or diabetes.

Fibric acid derivatives (aryloxyisobutyric acids) include the prototypic drug *gemfibrozil*. These types of drugs are used mainly to lower triglycerides and to increase HDL. A large placebo-controlled primary prevention trial in hypercholesterolemic men showed that patients treated with gemfibrozil had a statistically lower number of myocardial infarctions, but not of deaths from all causes.

ANTIHYPERTENSIVES

The therapeutic goal of treating hypertension with drugs is to maintain systolic blood pressure <140 mm Hg and diastolic blood pressure <90 mm Hg. Blood pressure in the body is regulated on a moment-to-moment basis by the *baroreflex* system that controls sympathetic and parasympathetic innervation of the vascular smooth muscle and heart. Sympathetic fibers innervate alpha-adrenergic smooth muscle receptors in the resistance vessels (arterioles) and regulate the contractile state of the vessels. Activating the sympathetic nervous system, therefore, increases arterial vascular resistance. Under some conditions, however, sympathetic activation and consequent increased metabolic activity of the end organ (i.e., the heart) compensate for the direct vasoconstrictor effect (i.e., on the coronary arteries) to produce a metabolically induced vasodilatation.

A low level of tonic activity of the sympathetic nerves to vascular smooth muscle adrenergic receptors exists so that withdrawal of sympathetic vasomotor tone results in *vasodilatation* and reduced pressure. Conversely, enhancement of sympathetic vasomotor tone augments the level of *vasoconstriction* leading to elevated pressure. While the parasympathetic branch of the autonomic nervous system innervates some blood vessels, it does not generally play a role in regulating peripheral resistance.

The *sinoatrial (SA) node* of the heart is innervated by both the sympathetic (β_1) and parasympathetic (vagus) nervous systems. *Sympathetic activation* increases the discharge rate of the SA pacemaker cells, and thereby *increases heart rate* (a positive chronotropic effect). Sympathetic nerves also innervate adrenergic receptors (beta$_1$) on cardiac ventricular cells leading to an increase in stroke volume (a positive inotropic effect). *Vagal activation*, on the other hand, has the opposite effect and *decreases* heart rate and conduction velocity. In normal adults, cardiac *vagal innervation is functionally predominant*, so abolition of vagal activity results in a pronounced tachycardia (increased heart rate).

The baroreflex system consists of mechanosensitive receptors in the aorta and carotid sinus that detect changes in blood pressure. The receptors give rise to *afferent* nerve fibers that relay impulses to the CNS. Within the CNS, the afferent signals are processed and ultimately transmitted to efferent sympathetic and parasympathetic fibers to the vasculature and heart. Increases in blood pressure will increase baroreceptor activity leading to an *inhibition* of sympathetic impulses to the blood vessels (thereby relaxing them) and to the heart (decreasing heart rate and contractility). In addition, parasympathetic activity to the heart is increased, leading to a reduction in heart rate and possibly contractility.

In most individuals, the etiology of hypertension is unknown and is simply referred to as *essential hypertension*. Essential hypertension is probably due to a combination of several abnormalities, including genetic predisposition, stress, and environmental and dietary factors. Specific potential mechanisms are listed in Table 12.1.

Regardless of the initiating factor(s), the primary characteristic of essential hypertension is increased peripheral vascular resistance. This can be monitored with the use of a *sphygmomanometer* (you have probably had your blood pressure taken with such an instrument). As the blood pressure of the cuff is inflated, it begins to occlude the flow of arterial blood, which then becomes turbulent and noisy (*Korotkoff* sounds) as it spurts through the artery. The blood can flow past the cuff only as long as its arterial pressure exceeds that of the cuff. Therefore, in order to measure blood pressure, the cuff is inflated (and the mercury column or needle rises) until it eliminates arterial blood flow, usually in the range of 180–200 mm Hg. As the cuff pressure is slowly released, the user notes the pressure at which the Korotkoff sounds first *reappear* (the *systolic* pressure). As the pressure continues to be released, arterial blood flow becomes easier and less noisy. The pressure at which the noise *ceases* is the *diastolic* pressure.

The goal of drug therapy is to return peripheral resistance to normal. Left untreated, there is increased likelihood of incapacitating stroke or death. Table 12.2 shows the principle drug categories used in the management of essential hypertension.

TABLE 12.1

Possible Mechanisms Leading to Hypertension

- Local blood vessel effects (vascular smooth muscle hypertrophy)
- Exaggerated activity of the sympathetic nervous system
- Defect in renal excretion of sodium
- Defect in sodium or calcium transport across cell membranes
- Multiple interactive effects

TABLE 12.2
Drug Categories Used in the Treatment of
Essential Hypertension

- Diuretics
- β-Adrenergic receptor antagonists
- α_1-Adrenergic receptor antagonists
- Centrally-acting α_2 adrenergic receptor agonists
- Direct vasodilators
- Calcium channel blockers
- Agents that interact with the renin–angiotensin system

DIURETICS

Diuretic substances increase the flow of urine in various ways (see below), but they have other effects as well, many of which are quite useful for the treatment of a variety of disorders and diseases. There are different categories of diuretics, and diverse diuretic agents are used in medicine for well-defined purposes.

Diuretics are among the most commonly prescribed drugs in the United States. Some diuretics are used to remove fluid from the tissues and cavities of the body in cases of edema. Other diuretics can also promote the elimination of waste products and poisons from the blood. They can also be prescribed to maintain the action of the kidneys.

The use of diuretics for therapeutic purposes is not new. In the sixteenth century, they were used for the treatment of peripheral edema (commonly called *dropsy*). The renowned physician Paracelsus acknowledged *mercurous chloride* as a diuretic. Before the development of modern pharmaceutical research, natural substances with diuretic properties were cataloged by physicians eager to prescribe them. For example, the physician Samuel Potter included diuretics in his compendium of materials for prescription writing. Most of the diuretics listed were herbal derivatives.

Potter distinguished between "refrigerant," "hydragogue," and "stimulant" diuretics. According to Potter's definition, refrigerant diuretics, such as potassium salts, "modify rather than increase the urine, and exercise a sedative action on *the heart and circulation*," whereas hydragogue diuretics "increase the water of the urine" and raise "arterial pressure" throughout the body or in the kidneys. Examples of hydragogue diuretics were caffeine, digitalis, and cocaine.

Other nineteenth- and early-twentieth-century physicians used diuretics before pharmacology was well advanced. Until his death in 1878, William Stokes was a pioneer in the treatment of heart failure, focusing on the beneficial diuretic properties of *mercury*.

ORGANOMERCURIALS

The twentieth century's first effective diuretics were *organomercurials*. A Viennese medical student named Alfred Vogel observed that patients passed large amounts of urine after they had received injections of organomercurial compounds intended to treat syphilis (a common practice of the day.) For the next two decades, organomercurials were the most potent diuretics in clinical use, although they were effective only when injected. Unfortunately, their prolonged use resulted in toxic side effects. These disadvantages led researchers to seek alternatives that would prove equally useful but less dangerous.

By the middle of the twentieth century, *heart disease* had surpassed infectious disease as the leading cause of death in the United States. Essential hypertension was one of the most pressing cardiovascular problems. In the late 1940s, there was little in the way of treatment for essential hypertension. In response to this growing problem, federal research efforts were focused for the first time on ways to treat heart disease.

CARBONIC ANHYDRASE INHIBITORS

The first diuretics *to replace mercurials* and prove useful in treating heart patients were called *carbonic anhydrase inhibitors*. The development of these drugs in the mid-1940s was owed to the discovery that the antibacterial agent sulfanilamide inhibited the enzyme carbonic anhydrase in the kidneys and interfered with the process of *urinary acidification*. This fact was followed by the observation that when sulfanilamide was administered to heart patients, they excreted large amounts of sodium and potassium in their urine.

Newer derivatives of carbonic anhydrase inhibitors were a widely used treatment in the 1950s. But this family of diuretics had serious disadvantages; most notably the creation of metabolic acidosis by virtue of interfering with urinary acidification. Because of this, scientists hoped to develop an agent that would inhibit the reabsorption of sodium and chloride ions in the kidneys and increase urine production without disturbing the body's balance of electrolytes.

One of the earliest strategies for the management of hypertension via electrolyte management (and still is) was to alter sodium balance by restriction of table and cooking salt in the diet. Pharmacological alteration of salt balance was developed to enhance this strategy. Researchers at Merck developed an orally active compound called chlorothiazide in the 1950s thus ushering in a new era of diuretic drugs termed *thiazide* diuretics. Today, *hydrochlorothiazide* is the prototypic drug in this class—it was first sold in 1959. Thiazides and related diuretics make up the most frequently used class of antihypertensive agents in the United States. By the late 1950s, thiazide diuretics were considered superior to the organomercurials and to oral diuretics such as carbonic anhydrase inhibitors.

THIAZIDE DIURETICS

Thiazide diuretics *promote excretion of sodium and water* by inhibiting sodium and hence water reabsorption from the luminal side of epithelial cells in the distal convoluted tubule. However, their antihypertensive mechanism of action is controversial. They initially decrease cardiac output by decreasing plasma volume. However, cardiac output returns to essentially normal within 6–8 weeks while arterial pressure and vascular resistance remain lowered. Recent evidence indicates that thiazide diuretics may act as antihypertensives by decreasing intracellular sodium in resistance vessels. Increased intracellular sodium may contribute to vascular resistance by increasing vessel stiffness and/or by inhibiting sodium-calcium exchange mechanisms leading to increased intracellular calcium and increased resistance.

The thiazide diuretics are primarily used for most patients with mild or moderate hypertension. Used alone they can lower blood pressure by 10–15 mm Hg. In more severe hypertension, diuretics are used in combination with other agents. Adverse effects include Hypokalemia (lowered serum potassium), impotence, impaired glucose tolerance, hyperlipidemia, and hyperuricemia (elevated uric acid in the blood).

The increasing use of thiazide diuretics has had a measurable impact on death rates from cardiovascular disease. The American Heart Association and the National Institutes of Health reported declining death rates, as early as 1959, that were partly attributed to the new antihypertensive thiazides. The thiazide diuretics also augmented the effects of other drugs. Diuretic medications introduced between 1950 and 1965 came to dominate the treatment of hypertension.

The precise means by which a thiazide-type diuretic lowers blood pressure is undecided. The effect of a thiazide diuretic on blood pressure may be separated into three chronological phases: (1) acute; (2) subacute; and (3) chronic, which correspond to periods of approximately 1–2 weeks, several weeks, and several months, respectively. In the acute phase, the blood pressure–lowering effect of a thiazide-type diuretic results in a net sodium loss that amounts to a 1–2 L reduction in extracellular fluid reduction (both plasma and interstitial compartments). This decrease in plasma volume both reduces venous return and diminishes cardiac output; the basis for the initial blood pressure fall with a thiazide diuretic.

In due course, the effect of a thiazide-type diuretic on volume and cardiac output lessens in importance, although blood pressure remains lowered. During the subacute phase of a treatment response, plasma volume returns to slightly less than pretreatment levels, despite the continued administration of the drug. This subacute response phase is a transitional period during which both *volume and resistance* factors contribute to the *blood pressure reduction* with thiazide-type diuretics. Diuretic therapy is a vital cog in the management of hypertension; either as monotherapy or in combination with other hypertensive classes.

BETA-ADRENERGIC RECEPTOR BLOCKERS

The common characteristic of representative beta-blockers is their ability to antagonize competitively the effects of the sympathetic effectors norepinephrine and epinephrine on *cardiac β-adrenergic receptors*. Although many beta-adrenergic antagonists have other pharmacological effects, it is clear that the blockade of cardiac β_1-adrenergic receptors is largely responsible for their ability to lower blood pressure. Compounds that exhibit selectivity for the beta$_1$ subtype of adrenergic receptors (e.g., atenolol; structure shown in Figure 12.1 below) are effective antihypertensives; thus, one hypothesis is that all drugs in this class exert their effects on blood pressure through β_1-adrenergic blockade and are beyond the scope of this book. By decreasing force and rate of contraction, cardiac output is decreased with a corresponding decline in peripheral blood pressure.

ALPHA$_1$-ADRENERGIC RECEPTOR ANTAGONISTS

Prazosin (see structure given in Figure 12.2), the prototypic drug in this class, decreases peripheral vascular resistance in arterioles and veins by blocking alpha$_1$ receptors on vascular smooth muscle. It *does not* decrease cardiac output. Because of this effect, patients taking prazosin are more prone (~50%) to postural hypotension, particularly following the first dose. In some cases, the hypotension is so severe that the patient may lose consciousness. In an attempt to compensate, the baroreceptors may produce an accompanying tachycardia.

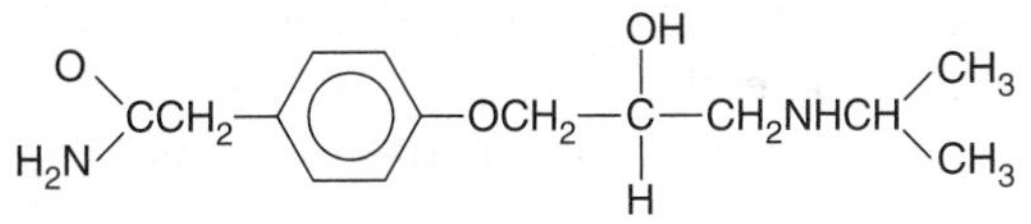

FIGURE 12.1   Structure of β_1-antagonist atenolol.

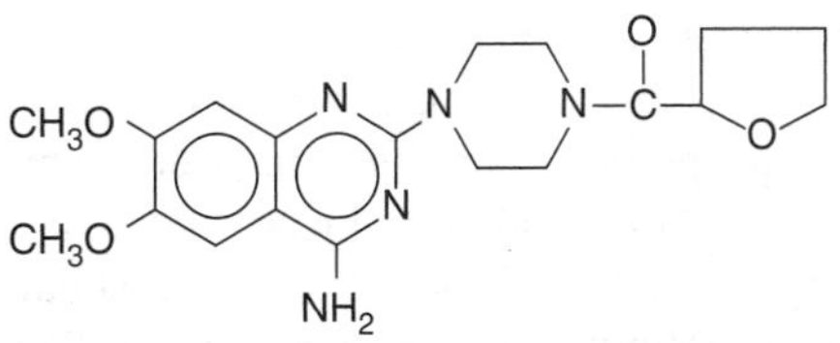

FIGURE 12.2   Structure of prazosin.

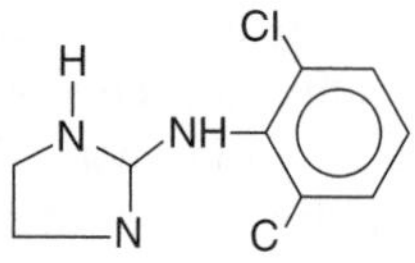

FIGURE 12.3   Structure of clonidine.

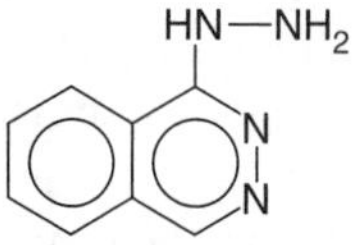

FIGURE 12.4   Structure of hydralazine.

ALPHA$_2$-ADRENERGIC RECEPTOR AGONISTS (CENTRALLY-ACTING DRUGS)

Clonidine is the prototypic drug in this class (see structure in Figure 12.3). The drug was synthesized in the early 1960s and found to produce vasoconstriction. However, during clinical testing of the drug as a topical decongestant, clonidine was found to cause hypotension, sedation, and bradycardia. The hypertensive response that follows parenteral administration of clonidine generally is not seen when the drug is given orally. The hypotensive response produced by clonidine is believed to result from decreased central outflow of impulses in the sympathetic nervous system. This central action has been demonstrated by infusing small amounts of clonidine into the vertebral arteries or by injecting it directly into the cisterna magna. However, the exact mechanism of action of clonidine is not completely understood. In view of the fact that clonidine acts in the CNS to decrease sympathetic outflow, it not only decreases peripheral vascular resistance but also heart rate and cardiac output.

Sedation and dry mouth are most common side effects. However, sudden withdrawal can result in a hypertensive crisis ("sudden withdrawal syndrome").

DIRECT VASODILATORS

Hydralazine was one of the first orally active antihypertensive drugs marketed in the United States. Its structure is shown in Figure 12.4. Initially, the drug was used infrequently because of its propensity to produce reflex tachycardia and tachyphylaxis. However, with a better understanding of the compensatory cardiovascular responses that accompany use of *arteriolar vasodilators* (the drug has little or no effect on venous smooth muscle), hydralazine was combined with sympatholytic agents and diuretics with greater therapeutic success.

Hydralazine causes *direct* relaxation of arteriolar smooth muscle. The arteriolar vasodilatation produced by hydralazine requires an intact endothelium. Therefore, one proposed mechanism of action is that hydralazine liberates *nitric oxide* from the endothelium (similar to the nitrates), which in turn *increases cGMP* to ultimately *prevent* the *phosphorylation of myosin light chain* (which is required for smooth muscle contraction), *resulting in arteriolar vasorelaxation.*

Direct vasodilators frequently produce baroreflex-induced tachycardia, but rarely orthostatic hypotension. They are usually prescribed with a β-blocker or a centrally acting antihypertensive to minimize the reflex increase in heart rate and cardiac output. It should be noted that another member of the directly acting class of antihypertensives is *minoxidil*. This potent, long-acting drug has gained considerable notoriety for its use as a topical hair restorer. Oral use can result in hirsutism (unwanted hair growth over the face as well as other parts of the body).

CALCIUM CHANNEL BLOCKERS

Depolarization of vascular smooth muscle activates the L-type calcium channels, which results in increased cytosolic concentrations of calcium and hence increased tone. Calcium channel blockers (e.g., *verapamil* and *diltiazem*) block the influx of calcium through the L-type voltage-dependent channels located on vascular smooth muscle and cardiac muscle cells as well as cardiac nodal cells. Therefore, they are used in the treatment of angina, *hypertension*, and certain arrhythmias.

The major toxicities are extensions of their therapeutic effects. Frequent or severe adverse effects include dizziness, headache, edema, constipation (especially verapamil), atrioventricular (AV) block, bradycardia, heart failure, and lupus-like rash with diltiazem. Two separate meta-analyses of 31 and 16 trials concluded that the short-acting nifedipine was associated with increased risk of reinfarction or death, in a dose-dependent manner. Therefore, it has been recommended that nifedipine should not be used for the treatment of hypertension (*Medical Letter* 1997; 39: 13).

THE RENIN-ANGIOTENSIN SYSTEM

In addition to baroreceptors, the body possesses an additional mechanism for affecting blood pressure. A *decrease in arterial pressure*, for example, causes release of the *enzyme renin* from the kidney into the blood. Renin then acts on a circulating substrate, angiotensinogen, to generate angiotensin I. Angiotensin I is then converted to Angiotensin II in the lung by angiotensin-converting enzyme (ACE) located in endothelial cells. Angiotensin II is a vasoconstrictor that constricts blood vessels, enhances sympathetic nervous system activity, and causes renal salt and water retention by direct intrarenal actions. In addition, the adrenal gland is stimulated to release the potent mineralocorticoid *aldosterone* that leads to sodium and water retention and, hence, increased plasma volume. A summary of the interrelationship between the components of the renin–angiotensin system is shown in Figure 12.5.

The main drug class derived from this scenario is *ACE inhibitors* (see Chapter 1). *Captopril* was the first ACE inhibitor developed. The hypotensive response to ACE inhibitors is the result of inhibition of angiotensin II formation, especially in hypertensive patients in whom circulating blood concentrations of this peptide are increased. ACE also metabolizes the peptide *bradykinin*. Bradykinin is a vasodilator; therefore, inhibition of its metabolism by ACE inhibitors may contribute to the hypotensive effect of these agents. Inhibition of bradykinin by ACE inhibitors may also be related to the principle side effect of these drugs, namely, *coughing*. This effect is probably due to increased levels of bradykinin, which can excite pulmonary C fiber endings and irritant receptors in the lung to reflexively cause coughing.

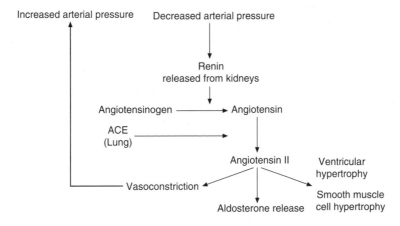

FIGURE 12.5   Renin–angiotensin system. (Courtesy of Dr. Ann Bonham, UCDavis.)

ANGIOTENSIN II-RECEPTOR ANTAGONISTS

The importance of angiotensin II in regulating cardiovascular function has led to the development of nonpeptide antagonists of the angiotensin receptor (e.g., *losartan*). By preventing effects of angiotensin II, these agents relax smooth muscle and thereby promote vasodilatation, increase renal salt and water elimination, reduce plasma volume, and decrease cellular hypertrophy. Angiotensin II-receptor antagonists also theoretically overcome some of the disadvantages of ACE inhibitors that not only prevent conversion of angiotensin I to angiotensin II but also prevent ACE-mediated degradation of bradykinin and substance P. Cough, an adverse effect of ACE inhibitors, has *not* been associated with angiotensin II-receptor antagonists.

CONGESTIVE HEART FAILURE

Congestive heart failure (also known as congestive heart disease) is the inefficacy of the heart to pump or receive sufficient blood to maintain an adequate ejection fraction (i.e., *diminished cardiac output*). Chronic heart failure occurs most commonly in the presence of long-standing hypertension or a loss of myocardial tissue, whether segmental (e.g., myocardial infarct) or diffuse (e.g., cardiomyopathy or myocarditis). The primary symptoms of congestive heart disease are the following:

- Decreased exercise tolerance
- Fatigue
- Shortness of breath
- Edema
- Tachycardia
- Sweating

The symptoms result from compensatory mechanisms in the body set in motion to try to restore cardiac output. The decrease in cardiac output from the diseased heart causes a corresponding decrease in blood pressure that leads to: (1) activation of the sympathetic nervous system with its attendant elevations in heart rate, heart contractility, arterial resistance, venous tone, and sweating; (2) activation of the rennin-angiotensin system leads to increased systemic arterial resistance, release of aldosterone (which increases sodium retention), constriction of renal vasculature, ventricular hypertrophy ("*remodeling*"), and vascular smooth muscle proliferation; and (3) remodeling leads to progressive systolic failure, wherein the myocytes become distended and "fatter" and are *less* viable. With progressive loss of viable myocytes, systolic function continues to fail with a corresponding *progressive ventricular dilation*. With progressive ventricular dilation and increases in left ventricular filling pressures, the symptoms become manifest as pulmonary congestion or fatigue caused by limited cardiac output.

The primary goals of pharmacological management of congestive heart failure are to (1) treat the *cause* of heart failure (e.g., *antihypertensives)* and (2) relieve the symptoms and delay/prevent the progression of the left ventricular dysfunction. Strategies include improving myocardial contractility (e.g., positive inotropic agents), lowering sodium retention (diuretics, ACE inhibitors), decreasing arteriolar and venous resistance in order to decrease work load (vasodilators and ACE inhibitors), and increasing exercise tolerance.

Examples of specific drugs used in the treatment of chronic heart failure include digitalis glycosides (e.g., digoxin, positive inotropic agent), diuretics (hydrochlortiazide and furosemide), and vasodilators (nitrates [nitroglycerin], ACE inhibitors [captopril], and hydralazine).

Digitalis Glycosides

As mentioned previously, digitalis was discovered by William Withering for the treatment of "dropsy" (i.e., the peripheral edema produced by congestive heart failure). Digitalis glycosides are

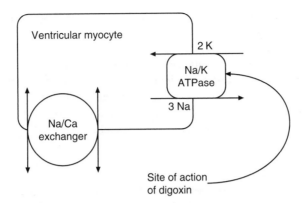

FIGURE 12.6   Mechanism of action of digoxin. (Courtesy of Dr. Ann Bonham, UCDavis.)

extracted from the foxglove plant, *Digitalis purpurea*, and other species. Among the cardiac glycosides, *digoxin* and to a lesser extent *digitoxin* are clinically used. As positive inotropic agents, they act to enhance cardiac contractility to compensate for diminished cardiac output in congestive heart disease. These drugs selectively bind to and *inhibit a membrane-bound sodium pump* (sodium, potassium ATPase). Inhibition of the sodium pump leads to an *increase in intracellular sodium* concentration, which in turn affects sodium/calcium exchange, leading to an increase in *intracellular calcium* and the *force of contraction.*

The relationship of intracellular sodium to intracellular calcium is such that a very small increase in sodium in terms of percentage increase leads to a disproportionately large increase in calcium. Therefore, a direct effect on the sodium/potassium ATPase to inhibit sodium pump activity is the *primary* mechanism of the positive inotropic effect of the cardiac glycosides, while *secondary* elevation of intracellular calcium provides the ionic "punch" to increase contractility. A diagram of the relationship between sodium/potassium ATPase and calcium is shown in Figure 12.6.

Although treatment of congestive heart failure can be palliative, cardiac output does *not* return to normal. The goal of therapy is to achieve as much restoration of cardiac function as possible. In addition to their inhibitory effect on the sodium pump, cardiac glycosides such as digoxin can also increase the effective refractory period of the *AV node* by increasing parasympathetic tone to the AV node. This will prolong the effective filling time of the ventricles. Because of digoxin's effect on AV conduction, it is sometimes used in the treatment of atrial arrhythmias (to protect the ventricles, as will be discussed below).

A moderate inhibition of sodium/potassium ATPase causes the positive inotropic (therapeutic) effect of cardiac glycosides, whereas an *excessive inhibition produces toxicity*; when the cardiac muscle is exposed to toxic concentrations of a glycoside, sodium pump inhibition and cellular calcium loading become alarmingly high. This process may lead to life-threatening ventricular tachycardia followed by ventricular fibrillation. Therefore, toxicity resulting from direct actions of the cardiac glycosides on cardiac muscle is caused by calcium overload of myocardial cells. Because the therapeutic positive inotropic effect of these drugs is also caused by enhanced calcium loading of the cells and in particular the sarcoplasmic reticulum, the therapeutic and toxic effects are inseparable. Therefore, their *low therapeutic index* is an inherent property of this class of positive inotropic drugs.

With regard to adverse effects on other organs, the primary adverse effect is on the GI tract and includes anorexia, nausea, vomiting, and diarrhea. These effects result from direct inhibition of sodium, potassium ATPase and from central stimulation of the chemoreceptor zone. The second most commonly occurring effect is in the CNS: visual disturbances (blurred or yellow vision), halos or flashing lights, and disorientation. While not lethal, these effects can be sufficient to decrease individual compliance in taking the drug. Because potassium competes with digoxin for binding sites on the sodium pump, elevations in serum potassium will diminish the effects of digoxin, while hypokalemia can augment the effects and result in toxicity at lower doses. The single most common cause of digoxin toxicity is the concurrent use of diuretics to the extent that potassium is depleted (except K-sparing diuretics, see below).

Because digitoxin has a very low therapeutic index, toxicity occurs rather routinely and can be fatal; patients must be monitored closely. Moderate overdoses can be picked up by GI or CNS complaints, however, more serious toxicity on cardiac rhythm are more difficult to distinguish from the effects of heart disease. Digitalis *antibody fragments* are available for serious toxicity, that is, when cardiac arrest is imminent. The fragments bind the drug and are excreted by the kidneys.

DIURETICS

As mentioned above, thiazide diuretics promote excretion of sodium and an osmotic equivalent of water by inhibiting sodium reabsorption in the distal convoluted tubules of the kidneys. In addition, loop diuretics (e.g., *furosemide*) inhibit sodium reabsorption in the thick ascending limb of the *loop of Henle*. Because of the large absorptive capacity of this segment, these agents are the most potent diuretics. Aldosterone antagonists such as *spironolactone* act in the collecting tubule and are *potassium-sparing* (see Figure 12.7). These drugs are used with other diuretics to prevent or correct hypokalemia.

Exaggerated pharmacological effects of diuretics to decrease sodium and water retention can result in complications relating to ion changes important in congestive heart failure; see Table 12.3.

Hypokalemia should be treated in heart failure, because either hypokalemia or heart failure can predispose individuals to experience serious arrhythmias. Therefore, potassium-sparing diuretics are sometimes used in the treatment of congestive heart failure.

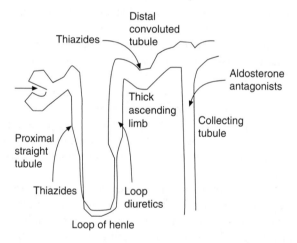

FIGURE 12.7   Sites of action of diuretics important in heart failure. (Courtesy of Dr. Ann Bonham, UCDavis.)

TABLE 12.3
Possible Adverse Effects Resulting from Diuretic Treatment of Congestive Heart Disease

- Decreased plasma volume
- Hypokalemia
- Hyponatremia (to a lesser extent)Hyperlipidemia
- Glucose intolerance
- Impotence

Vasodilators

Vasodilators such as nitrates, ACE inhibitors, and hydralazine have been discussed above. These agents are used to decrease arteriolar (afterload) or venous resistance (preload). A discussion of cardiodynamics is beyond the scope of this book. However, by decreasing preload and afterload, these drugs decrease the work that the heart has to do to increase cardiac output, which improves perfusion pressure on the arterial side and venous return on the venous side, which contributes to reducing peripheral edema.

In summary, many patients with symptoms of heart failure take a cardiac glycoside, a diuretic, and an ACE inhibitor. Diuretics and a glycoside such as digoxin improve symptoms, but have little effect on survival. ACE inhibitors improve symptoms and prolong survival, but the disease still progresses.

Antiarrhythmic Agents

In the normal heart, electrical impulses that trigger normal cardiac rhythms originate in the *SA node*, spread rapidly through the atria to the *AV node*, and then propagate over the *His-Purkinje system* to invade all parts of the ventricles. Depolarization results in contraction and repolarization results in relaxation of myocardial cells. The relationship between normal impulse conduction throughout the heart and electrical events is show in Figure 12.8. Arrhythmias may be caused by electrolyte disturbances, ischemia, trauma, drug overdoses, and so forth, but the fundamental problems are *abnormal generation of action potentials* (from nonpacemaker cells) or *abnormal conduction* (as observed with reentry arrhythmias).

Arrhythmias are characterized by abnormal formation or abnormal conductance of electrical impulses in the heart. The sodium channel is particularly important in generating action potentials and hence contraction of the ventricular myocytes. The state of the sodium channel is voltage-dependent, so the resting membrane potential of the cell influences the number of sodium channels open. The state of the sodium channels can determine whether a ventricular myocyte can generate an action potential and hence contract. The sodium channels exist in three states (Figure 12.9): (1) rest (available for activation; *m* gate closed); (2) activated (both gates open); and (3) inactivated (*h* gate closed).

The number of sodium channels available for activation determines conduction velocity of the action potential in cardiac cells. The more sodium channels available for activation, the faster the

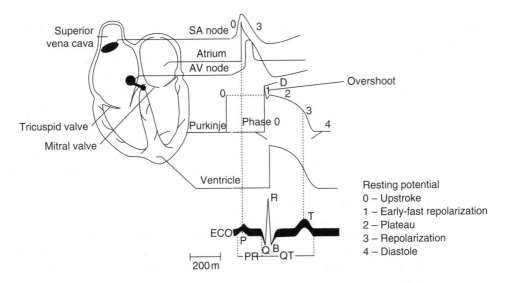

FIGURE 12.8 Normal impulse conduction throughout the heart. (Courtesy of Dr. Ann Bonham, UCDavis.)

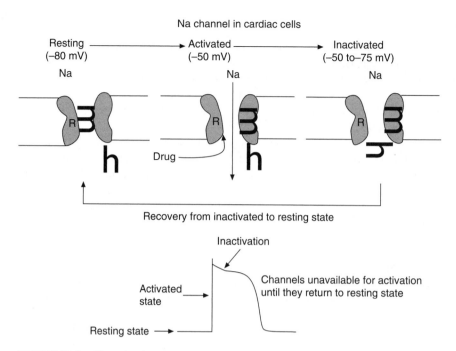

FIGURE 12.9   The role of the sodium channel. (Courtesy of Dr. Ann Bonham, UCDavis.)

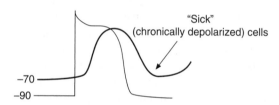

FIGURE 12.10   Comparison of healthy and diseased ventricular myocyte depolarization. (Courtesy of Dr. Ann Bonhan, UCDavis.)

conduction velocity occurs. At resting membrane potential of ventricular, atrial, and Purkinje cells (–85 mV), the *m* gate is closed, preventing any influx of sodium; therefore, no action potential develops (Resting). With an appropriate activating stimulus (slight depolarization), the *m* gate opens, sodium rushes in, and an action potential develops (Activated). A few milliseconds later and as the membrane repolarizes to –55 to –75 mV, the *h* gate closes, inactivating the channel and halting sodium influx (Inactivated). The channel must be in the resting state to be available for promulgating an action potential. During the time in which it takes the channels to go from the "inactivated" state to the "resting" state, the cell is refractory to incoming stimuli, so no action potential develops.

The state of the sodium channel varies in healthy ventricular cells and those damaged by ischemia. That variability in the state has implications for antiarrhymic therapy with sodium channel blocking agents. In "sick" or damaged ventricular cells (i.e., from ischemia or blockade of the sodium/potassium ATPase [sodium/potassium pump]), the resting membrane is *more positive* than the healthy resting membrane potential (Figure 12.10).

In healthy cardiac cells, the recovery time from inactivation of sodium channels (back to the resting state) is *quite rapid*, so that the maximum number of channels is available for activation. In contrast, in sick cells, the recovery time is *quite slow*. In these sick cells, the action potential develops from the opening of fewer sodium channels, so the action potential is a slow, sluggish upstroke as opposed to the fast upstroke in a healthy cell. A slow, sluggish upstroke results in poor

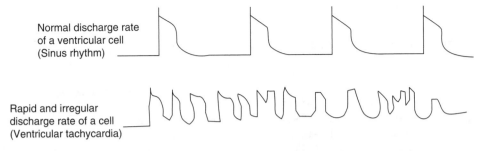

FIGURE 12.11   Example of a string of ectopic ventricular beats leading to ventricular tachycardia. (Courtesy of Dr. Ann Bonham, UCDavis.)

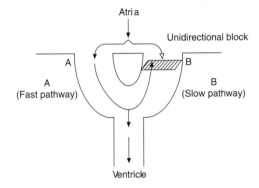

FIGURE 12.12   Example of reentry at the AV node. (Courtesy of Dr. Ann Bonham, UCDavis.)

and perhaps no propagation of the action potential. Chronically depolarized or ischemic cells may (1) fail to conduct an action potential and therefore fail to contract or to transmit the action potential to neighboring cells or (2) become an ectopic pacemaker (due to a slow sodium leak in phase 4) so that it overrides the normal pacemaker activity to cause either an occasional ectopic contraction or a string of *ectopic beats* that become a *tachyarrhythmia* (see Figure 12.11).

Electrical impulses in each cardiac cycle begin in the sinus node (SA) and continue until the entire heart has been activated. When all the cells have been discharged and are refractory, the electrical impulse dies out; it has nowhere to go. If, however, a group of cells that are not activated because of *unidirectional block* during the initial wave of depolarization recover their excitability before the impulse dies out, then those cells may serve as a *link* to re-excite areas that were just discharged but have recovered from the initial depolarization. This event is described as *reentry, reentrant tachycardia, circus movement, or echo beats*. Reentry depends on two pathways with different electrophysiological properties, that is, a refractory period longer in one pathway than in another, slower conduction, and/or decreased excitability in one pathway. The different electrophysiological properties are caused by local damage within an area of conduction. Figure 12.12 illustrates reentry.

In this example, zone B contains a unidirectional block so that it is refractory to the forward moving (*anterograde*) impulse. The impulse travels only through branch A (fast pathway) to depolarize the ventricle. As the impulse spreads back toward B, it is propagated *retrogradely* (toward the AV node) through branch B to spread depolarization through the atria (i.e., to produce an echo beat in the atria) and/or provide early reexcitation (reentry) at the AV node and through A. *A single reactivation of branch A will produce a single premature ventricular beat; continuous conduction will cause AV nodal tachycardia.* Antiarrhythmic drugs can abolish reentry activity by (1) decreasing conduction in branch B (slow pathway) to produce a *bidirectional block* and (2) increasing the refractory period in the fast pathway, so the reentrant current becomes extinct in the refractory tissue. *The goal of antiarrhythmic therapy is to suppress ectopic pacemakers or reentry pathways.*

TABLE 12.4

Comparison of Various Antiarrthymic Drugs

Class	Action	Drugs
I	Blocks Na channels	Quinidine[a], procainamide
A	Moderately depresses phase O and lengthens APD, ERP	Lidocaine, phenytoin
B	Minimally depresses phase O and shortens APD, ERP	Encainde, lorcainide, liecainide
C	Maximally depresses phase O and dose not change APD, ERP	
II	Beta-adrenergic receptor blockade	Propranolol
III	Prolong ERP, blocks K	Bratylium, sotolol[b] amiodarone[c]
IV	Calcium channel blockade	Verpamil, diltiazem

Notes:

[a] Quinidine and most class A agents also block the delayed K channels.

[b] Sotalol also has beta-adrenergic blocking properties (II).

[c] Amiodarone blocks Na channels (I) prolongs depolarization (III): noncompetitively blocks beta receptors (II), and is a weak Ca channel blocker (IV).

This table courtesy of Dr Ann Bonham, UCDavis.

Antiarrhythmic drugs have been classified by their *predominant* effects. However, drugs within a class do differ significantly. The presence of heart disease and arrhythmic states may modify their actions, and some drugs have more than one effect. Table 12.4 compares the drugs in the various classes.

Class 1 antiarrthymic drugs block sodium channels and have varying affects on action potential duration (APD) and end resting potential (ERP). *Quinidine and Procainamide* are the prototypic drugs in this class. These drugs act to (1) slow conduction velocity (phase 0) particularly in chronically depolarized cells, (2) decrease abnormal automaticity (phase 4) in ectopic foci, and (3) may also decrease normal automaticity (phase 4) in Purkinje fibers. They are frequently used for *chronic arrhythmias* owing to their oral availability and efficacy. Most common side effects are GI and CNS. As mentioned above, in some cases of AV or His-Purkinje conduction problems, quinidine can slow conduction to the extent of causing complete block. The most common problem with Procainamide is Lupus-like syndrome. Sixty five percent of patients will develop antibodies within 12 months; only 12% will show symptoms that are reversible when the drug is stopped. Procainamide can be given intravenously more safely than quinidine.

Endogenous norepinephrine stimulates cardiac β-receptors. Receptor-linked cAMP-dependent protein kinases phosphorylate calcium channels to increase intracellular calcium. Elevated intracellular calcium increases conduction velocity (phase 0) and decreases the threshold potential in normal SA and AV node cells (see Figure 12.13). *β-Blockers* slow spontaneous conduction velocity in the SA node by approximately 10–20%. In addition, β-blockers can slow conduction velocity while increasing the refractory period of the AV node. These effects control the ventricular rate in atrial fibrillation or flutter and terminate paroxysmal supraventricular tachycardias. They are also safer, although somewhat less effective, than other drugs for suppression of premature ventricular complexes (PVCs). Drugs in this class approved by the FDA for treatment of various arrhythmias include propranolol, acebutolol, and esmolol.

Problems with the β-blockers include drowsiness, fatigue, impotence, and depressed ventricular performance.

Potassium channel blockers (sotalol, amiodarone, bretylium, and dofetilide) block the outward flowing potassium channel that decreases potassium conductance, which prevents or delays *repolarization* (prolongation of APD and ERP). See Figure 12.14.

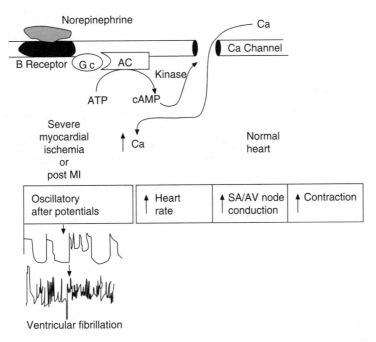

FIGURE 12.13   Role of β-receptor in affecting cardiac arrhythmias. (Courtesy of Dr. Ann Bonham, UCDavis.)

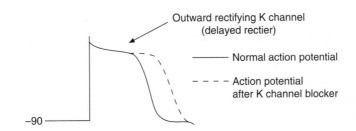

FIGURE 12.14   Effect of potassium blocker on cardiac action potential.

These drugs can be used in life-threatening ventricular tachyarrhythmias. Controlled clinical trials in patients with a history of sustained ventricular tachycardia or ventricular fibrillation indicate that amiodarone and sotalol are more effective than older drugs such as quinidine or procainamide. Both drugs, especially amiodarone, have become drugs of choice for these serious arrhythmias. In a clinical trial of sotalol, in which it was compared to six class I drugs, it was found more effective in preventing death and recurrence of arrhythmias. Orally administered amiodarone can suppress PVCs and nonsustained ventricular tachycardia or fibrillation.

Amiodarone has a higher incidence of side effects than sotalol. Seventy five percent of patients report side effects over 5 years while 15–35% require discontinuance of the drug. Severe adverse effects, including pulmonary fibrosis, can occur with usual doses of amiodarone and may be lethal or irreversible or persist for months after treatment is stopped.

Verapamil and diltiazem are prototypic calcium channel blockers. As indicated previously, these drugs influence cardiac function by blocking inward calcium movement through L channels. In so doing they block conduction velocity in SA and AV node cells. They are used therapeutically to treat reentry arrhythmias through the AV node as well as paroxysmal supraventricular tachycardias. In fact, verapamil has been reported to terminate 60–80% of paroxysmal supreventricular tachycardias within several minutes. However, because of their potent effect on AV conduction, these drugs are *contraindicated in patients with preexisting conduction problems*, since they may produce complete AV block.

SELECTED BIBLIOGRAPHY

Cardiovascular Pharmacology Lecture Notes, The University of Utah, http://lysine. Pharm. Utah. Edu/net pharm/net pharm_00/notes.html

Chobanian, A.V. Bakris, G.L., Black, H.R., et al., (2003) Seventh report of the Joint National Committee on Prevention, Detection, Evaluation, and Treatment of High Blood Pressure, *Hypertension*, 42: 1206–1252.

Hardman, J.G., Limbird, L.L., and Gilman, A.G. (Eds.) (2001) *Goodman and Gillman's: The Pharmacological Basis of Therapeutics*, 10th ed., New York: McGraw-Hill.

Katzung, B.G., (Ed.) (2001) *Basic and clinical pharmacology*, 8th ed., New York: McGraw-Hill.

QUESTIONS

1. Quinidine can produce all of the following *except*
   a. Depressed myocardial excitability
   b. Vagal stimulation
   c. Slowed myocardial conduction
   d. Decreased slope of diastolic depolarization of pacemaker cells
   e. Prolonged myocardial refractory period

2. The site responsible for the pharmacological and toxic actions of digitalis glycosides is associated with which of the following?
   a. Beta-adrenergic receptors
   b. Sodium/potassium ATPase
   c. Protein kinase C
   d. cAMP-dependent protein kinase
   e. Calcium pump

3. The system or function *not* affected by the cardiac glycosides is which of the following?
   a. The sodium channel
   b. The calcium channel
   c. The sodium pump
   d. Calcium loading of the sarcoplasmic reticulum
   e. Atrioventricular conduction

4. The following limit the clinical usefulness of digitalis *except* which of the following?
   a. Narrow margin of safety
   b. Low potency
   c. Tendency to produce arrhymias
   d. Variations in bioavailability
   e. Patient to patient variability

5. All of the following about calcium antagonists are true except
   a. They decrease peripheral vascular resistance
   b. They increase coronary blood flow
   c. They decrease cardiac afterload
   d. They decrease serum calcium concentration
   e. They may cause hypotension

6. Calcium antagonists act by inhibiting which of the following?
   a. Calcium influx through L type channels
   b. Calcium influx through T type channels
   c Calcium influx through N type channels
   d. Calcium influx through P type channels
   e. Calcium influx through M type channels

7. All of the following actions of nitrovasodilators are correct except
   a. They inhibit phosphodiesterase
   b They generate nitric oxide
   c They increase cGMP
   d They are similar to EDRF
   e. All are correct

8. The loop diuretics have their principle diuretic effect on which of the following?
   a. Ascending limb of loop of Henle
   b Distal convoluted tubule
   c Proximal convoluted tubule
   d. Collecting duct
   e b and c

9. Which of the following statements for cholesterol and cholesterol metabolism is not true?
   a. The liver is the primary organ for cholesterol uptake and degradation
   b. Most cholesterol is converted to bile acids
   c. The transport of cholesterol is primarily accomplished by binding to lipoprotein
   d. The major source of cholesterol in the body is via dietary intake
   e None of the above

10. Epidemiological studies on the incidence of atherosclerosis indicate that
    a. The greatest correlation exists for LDL cholesterol
    b. There is an inverse correlation between LDL and HDL cholesterol concentrations
    c. There is usually a consistent increase in LDL cholesterol and total cholesterol concentrations
    d. All of the above are correct
    e. None of the above is correct

13 Pulmonary Pharmacology

The basic structure of the adult human respiratory system consists of a series of bifurcating ventilatory conduits of varying length, flexibility, and diameter, which terminate in thin-walled sacs. These branches connect the external atmosphere with the internal vasculature, and are composed of conducting airways (trachea, bronchi, and bronchioles), transitory ducts, and respiratory zones (alveoli) (Figure 13.1). Each has characteristic features and functions that are not only important to normal physiology but that also significantly influence toxin and drug disposition and dynamics. Understanding the basic anatomy of the lung is central to appreciating its physiological function and the effect of drugs therein.

Examination of the human respiratory "tree" reveals that it is a structure of considerable asymmetry. Most humans, for example, have three lobes on their right lung and generally two lobes on their left. Furthermore, the right main stem bronchus angles off at 20–30° from the midline, whereas the left angles off more acutely at 45–55°. It has been determined that it is possible to reach the terminal alveoli from the trachea by traversing as few as 8 branches or as many as 20 or more, depending on which path is followed. A classic model of airway transition up to 23 generations, with associated features, is presented in Figure 13.2.

One characteristic of this branching, albeit sometimes irregular architecture, is that as air and its contents pass down the system, it travels first through a small number of high-volume tubes that connect to a larger number of smaller volume ducts. Consequences of this geometric progression are (1) an increase in the surface area-to-volume ratio (because surface area decreases by an exponent of two while volume decreases by an exponent of three and (2) a decrease in flow rate due to redistribution of the air (Table 13.1).

The 2000-fold increase in cross-sectional area, which occurs from bronchi to alveoli, also has an important clinical correlate. It implies that obstructive airway disease must be quite disseminated in the terminal region (e.g., as in diffuse fibrosis of the parenchyma) before it can be detected by measuring total airway resistance. Conversely, obstruction of higher regions (e.g., as in bronchial asthma) will have a more significant effect on airway resistance. Detailed knowledge of the geometry of the respiratory apparatus is therefore central to a comprehensive understanding of particle or gas penetration, deposition, and clearance in the lung. However, only major features will be emphasized here.

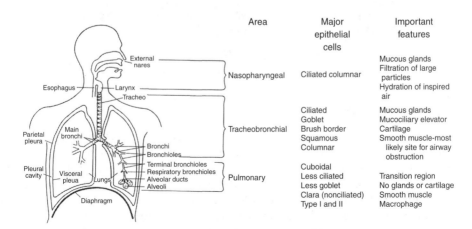

FIGURE 13.1 Relationship of major components and features of the adult human respiratory system.

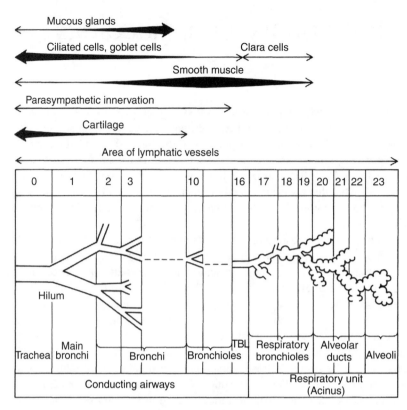

FIGURE 13.2   General architecture and associated characteristics of conducting and respiratory airways.

TABLE 13.1
Anatomic and Functional Characteristics of the Respiratory System*

Region (generation)	Number	Cross-Sectional Area	Flow Rate (cm/sec)
Main bronchi (1st)	2	3.2 cm^2	180
Bronchioles (9th)	512	9.56 cm^2	14
Respiratory bronchioles(17th)	1.3×10^5	300 cm^2	0.9
Alveoli (23rd)	300×10^6	70 m^2	0^*

* These numbers are approximations, and vary according to source.

NASOPHARYNGEAL REGION

The respiratory system is arbitrarily divided into several regions, or functional units. The first of these is the nasopharyngeal. This region extends from the external nares to the trachea. It is lined with a mucous membrane composed primarily of ciliated columnar epithelial cells that are interspersed with mucous-secreting cells and glands. Mucous secreted by these glands and cells is carried by cilia to the back of the nasal cavity, where it can be swallowed or expectorated. Several hundred milliliters of mucous may be cleared and replaced each day in this manner.

The primary function of mucous within the nasopharyngeal region is to filter large airborne particles out of the inspired air. In performing this task, mucous is quite effective, removing more than 90% of all particulate matter. Virtually all particles greater than 10 μm in diameter are affected. Therefore, particles entering the trachea are generally smaller than 10 μm in diameter. Of these, most particles larger than 2 μm in diameter are deposited on the mucous layer; only particles smaller than 2 μm are likely to reach the terminal portion of the airway.

Within the nasopharyngeal region, incoming air also becomes moistened and warmed. The temperature of inspired air is adjusted to 37°C by the air-conditioning effect of the rich vascular supply of the nasal turbinates. Humidification of inspired air is accomplished primarily in the nasal passages through an outpouring of nasal secretions. The effectiveness of this humidification function can be readily demonstrated by the discomfort that occurs when a person breathes through the mouth. This process of moisturizing incoming air serves to lessen evaporative loss of water from the terminal respiratory bed and hydrate incoming material. The latter function can have a significant effect on the subsequent deposition and transmembrane penetration of a substance (assuming it is hygroscopic).

TRACHEOBRONCHIAL REGION

The second major functional unit of the respiratory system is the *tracheobronchial.* This region encompasses the trachea, the bronchi, and the bronchioles. The tracheobronchial region serves as the *major conducting pathway* between the nasopharynx and the terminal alveoli, and regulates the regional and generalized distribution of air in the lungs. In humans, the trachea is about 2–2.5 cm in diameter and about 11 cm long, and is composed of 16–20 U-shaped semirigid cartilaginous rings. On the posterior side, there is a thin trachealis muscle that extends between the open ends of the U and is shared by the esophagus. *Contraction* of this smooth muscle—as occurs in an asthmatic attack—causes constriction of the trachea. Tracheal smooth muscle is often used as an experimental model of airway smooth muscle, because it is physiologically similar to smooth muscle (e.g., parasympathetic innervation) down to the sixth generation of bronchi.

By moving distally along the tracheobronchial region, the frequency of cartilaginous rings decreases. *Bronchi,* therefore, contain only a few terminal plates of cartilage, while bronchioles contain none. As cartilage decreases, there is an inversely proportional increase in smooth muscle. The presence of this smooth muscle further contributes to determining the control of airway diameter. Respiratory smooth muscle is under autonomic control, *principally* parasympathetic. Bronchi are nourished by the bronchial arteries that branch from the aorta, and are not part of the pulmonary circulation. Because they lack alveoli and are not exposed to pulmonary arterial blood, the bronchi cannot participate in gas exchange.

Next in line are the *bronchioles,* which lack cartilage, have limited smooth muscle, and are not held open by structural rigidity but by radial traction supplied by the elastic recoil of the surrounding parenchymal tissue. The tracheobronchial section is lined primarily with five types of epithelial cells and is coated with a thin 5 μm layer of mucous. Ciliated epithelial cells are the predominant cells in this area. Some ciliated cells have become modified into secreting goblet cells (named for their shape). These cells contain the precursor of the mucin glycoprotein, which is the principle component of the mucous that is secreted. Goblet cells are not under nervous control, but secretion can be stimulated by direct irritation.

As mentioned above, mucous secreted by goblet cells onto the surface of the airway functions to trap incoming particles and to protect the mucosa against dehydration. It also serves as the suspending vehicle for the movement of particles from the deep lung to the oral cavity. This is achieved via ciliary movement (*mucociliary escalator*) of the ciliated epithelial cells in the direction of the pharynx. In this way, undesirable particulate debris can be eliminated from the respiratory tract by expectoration from the oral cavity or by swallowing.

Mucous glands represent about 12% of the wall thickness in mainstream bronchi, gradually diminishing to 0% in bronchioles. There are approximately 6000 in the human trachea, with the greatest concentration in the second to fifth generations of human bronchi (1 gland/mm^2).

TABLE 13.2
Summary of Mucokinetic Agents

Category	Probable Mechanism of Action
Diluent	
Water	Aerosol: Decreases viscosity of gel layer; systemic: increases of sol layer hydration
Saline solution	Hypotonic aerosol: transfer of water from particles to luminal mucus; hypertonic aerosol: osmotic effect of saline, drawing water from the mucosa
Surface-active	
Propylene glycol	Altered hydration and hydrogen bonding of mucous glycoproteins
Sodium bicarbonate	Decreased mucous viscosity and adhesion, increased ciliary activity
Expectorant	
Potassium iodide	May include stimulation of glands, vagal reflex, or ciliary activity, as well as a direct mucolytic effect or potentiation of proteases
Glyceryl guaiacolate	Vagal stimulation and diredt action on bronchial glands
Ammonium chloride	Vagal stimulation and possible enhanced ciliary activity
Mycolytic	
Acetylcysteine	Destruction of disulfide bonds
Dornase	Direct digestion of DNA and indirect enhancement of mucous proteolysis

Mucous glands have been estimated to have 100 times the volume of the goblet cells, and they probably secrete the most mucous in both healthy and disease states. *They receive no sympathetic control* but are innervated by parasympathetic nerves, which promote the secretion of complex mucoproteins through duct systems that open like pores onto the airway surface.

The effective maintenance of airway mucous flow (clearance) requires healthy cilia, adequate volumes of normal viscosity secretions, and an operating cough mechanism. However, there are a number of pulmonary diseases, including chronic bronchitis, asthma, pneumonia, and cystic fibrosis, in which one or more of these factors is compromised; usually in the form of excess airway secretions. Drugs used to treat these excess secretions are called *mucokinetic agents*. A summary of mucokinetic agents and possible mechanism(s) of action is shown in Table 13.2.

MUCOLYTICS

In many types of lung disorders, there is an overproduction of mucous in the respiratory tract, which contributes to an accumulation of sputum (DNA, and cell debris). This can occur as a result of genetic predisposition (e.g., cystic fibrosis), chronic exposure to a pneumotoxin (e.g., cigarette smoking), asthma, or infections. If the excess sputum is not cleared effectively, it will tend to accumulate in smaller airways (primarily bronchioles), interfere with gas exchange, and serve as a site for infection.

The principal mucolytic drug currently available is the sulfhydryl compound, acetylcysteine. Acetylcysteine was introduced in the early 1960s and is the most popular proprietary mucolytic agent. It has been found to be beneficial after aerosol administration in certain cases of viscid mucous development (e.g., bronchitis, asthma, and emphysema). Other applications include patients with atelectasis and those with an indwelling endotracheal tube. Its use in cystic fibrosis is controversial, but may have application in selected cases.

Acetylcysteine is usually administered by inhalation; direct instillation (e.g., tracheostomy) can also be effective. The mechanism of action of acetylcysteine is dependent on its sulfhydryl group, which is thought to reduce the disulfide bonds that bridge the mucoproteins in mucin (Figure 13.3). This decrease in intermolecular binding results in a corresponding change in molecular shape and in increased flow characteristics.

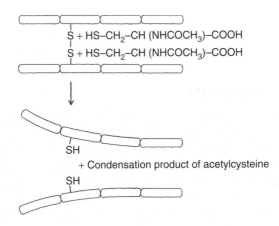

FIGURE 13.3   Mechanism of mucolytic action of acetylcysteine.

PULMONARY REGION

The final unit of the respiratory system is the pulmonary, which is composed of the terminal bronchioles, the respiratory bronchioles, the alveolar ducts, the alveolar sacs, and, finally, the alveoli themselves. With the exception of the terminal bronchioles, all these regions can exchange gas, and are collectively referred to as an *acinus*. About 200 alveoli are supplied by each respiratory bronchiole. Alveoli themselves are thin teacup-shaped, bellows-like sacs, with reported diameters ranging from 150 to 350 μm. Arranged in a line, 170 alveoli would be approximately 1 in. long. Estimates of the total number of alveoli in humans vary from 100 to 500 million. Interconnections between alveoli (the pores of Kohn) are believed to exist in the lung, and allow collateral air flow between adjacent portions.

The potential surface area of this terminal bed is quite considerable. Estimates from 35 m^2 during expiration to 140 m^2 during deep inspiration have been made. Approximately 75 m^2 is the most common figure, based on 300 million alveoli with a mean diameter of 250 μm. This surface is far larger than the skin in total area (~35-fold greater), approximating that of a tennis court. However, because only a portion of the alveolar surface is exposed to perfusing capillaries, the effective surface area for gas exchange is estimated to be 35–40 m^2. The pulmonary unit serves primarily for the exchange of gases. However, by its very nature, the respiratory system also represents a significant portal for the introduction of either noxious or therapeutic agents.

The alveoli themselves are lined with a single layer of flat epithelial cells (type I and type II), about 0.1–0.5 μm thick, that form a thin barrier between the alveolar air and the interstitial capillary lumen. Type II cells are believed to be the source of alveolar *surfactant*. Surfactant is a surface tension-lowering material that regulates surface tension-related events at the air–liquid interface, *which keeps the alveoli maximally distended for gas exchange*. If surfactant is absent, alveoli will eventually collapse, leading to decreased lung compliance, decreased functional residual capacity, and decreased total lung capacity.

Surfactant normally appears in the lung of mammals at approximately the halfway point of gestation, and its synthesis then continues throughout the remainder of the term. Premature infants often have *respiratory distress syndrome* (RDS) caused by a deficit in surfactant. RDS was originally called *hyaline membrane disease*; a term that referred to the "glassy" look of the alveoli, which was caused by the presence of plasma that had leaked in.

Each alveolus is surrounded by a dense plexus of approximately 1800 capillary segments (10 × 7 μm in area). This vascular arrangement represents the most dense capillary network in the body. In humans, lung capillaries have a diameter of approximately 6–15 μm, with a total length of approximately 1500 miles. If the 100–300 mL of blood in the pulmonary capillaries were to be spread over an alveolar surface of about 70 m^2, it would be equivalent to spreading 1 teaspoon of blood over a 1 m^2 surface. Thus, alveoli are intimately exposed to both the external and the internal environment and are, in a sense, in double jeopardy to substances therein.

CAPILLARY ENDOTHELIAL CELLS

Immediately adjacent to the alveoli and separated by a basement membrane are pulmonary capillary endothelial cells; together, they form the alveolar–capillary unit. The lungs are believed to contain as many as 50% of all the endothelial cells in the body. Endothelial cells represent a continuous series of adjoining cytoplasmic compartments lining the vasculature. Adjacent endothelial cells are held in relatively close opposition along their lateral borders by intercellular junctions.

In general, the rates at which all substances penetrate endothelial cells, with the exception of those in the brain, are far greater than those at which these same materials cross epithelial tissue. The thickness of the capillary cell surface is approximately 0.1 μm. Because this is about the same thickness as the epithelial type I cell, the total gas exchange barrier of the alveolar-capillary unit is about 0.2 μm over the major part of the air–blood contact surface.

INNERVATION

Innervation of pulmonary smooth muscle plays a particularly important role in the action of certain drugs in lung disease states. The lung receives innervation from both the parasympathetic and the sympathetic divisions of the autonomic nervous system. Importantly, parasympathetic outflow provides the excitatory innervation to airway smooth muscle and glands. This efferent nerve supply is by way of the *vagus nerve*, which uses *acetylcholine as its neurotransmitter*. The status of normal pulmonary smooth muscle tone indicates parasympathetic dominance. The vagus nerves are, therefore, responsible for the maintenance of airway tone.

Direct stimulation of the parasympathetic fibers or the administration of cholinergic agents will produce diffuse airway constriction and glandular secretion. Not surprisingly, the location of airway constriction corresponds to the distribution of cholinergic fibers. Tracheal and bronchial smooth muscles are most affected, whereas alveolar ducts and terminal bronchioles are unaffected.

In comparison to the parasympathetic pathway, the sympathetic nerve supply to the airways is not as well characterized but appears to be of relatively minor importance. It is known that postganglionic sympathetic fibers emanating from the stellate ganglia enter the lung and, in close association with postganglionic parasympathetic fibers, ramify throughout the smooth muscle from trachea to respiratory bronchioles. The presence of sympathetic fibers in lower regions is the result of innervation of blood vessels. Activation of the sympathetic innervation to lung smooth muscle results in airway dilation through the release of norepinephrine.

Most adrenergic receptors present in airway smooth muscle are of the β_2 classification. The ratio of β_2 receptors to β_1 receptors has been determined to be approximately 3:1. These β_2 receptors mediate bronchodilation and are responsive to epinephrine and other β_2 agonists. However, they do not receive direct sympathetic innervation. The mechanism that produces *bronchodilation* appears to involve the activation of membrane-bound adenylate cyclase by circulating agonists (Figure 13.4). The resultant elevation in intracellular cyclic AMP concentration is believed to decrease the availability of free calcium ions for the contractile process, thereby reducing smooth muscle tone. The mechanism may involve binding of calcium to the sarcoplasmic reticulum, uptake and sequestration of calcium by mitochondria, or actual efflux of calcium from the cell. A low level of intracellular calcium antagonizes actin–myosin interaction.

Afferent sensory fibers originate in the epithelium of airways, muscle, submucosa, and interalveolar spaces, and terminate in the vagal nuclei. There are three main types of afferents in the lung and airways: (1) irritant fibers, which play an important role in various reflexes (e.g., cough,

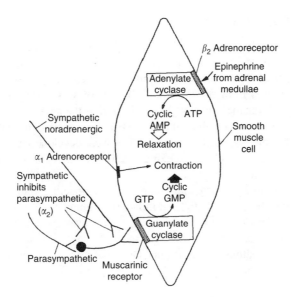

FIGURE 13.4 Hypothetic relationship between adrenergic and cholinergic "second messengers" in controlling the contractile activity of airway smooth muscle cells.

bronchoconstriction); (2) stretch receptors, which are involved with normal respiration; and (3) J receptors (juxtapulmonary capillary receptors), which are believed to lie in the alveolar walls where they are adjacent to pulmonary capillaries. These J receptors can be stimulated by factors that increase pulmonary interstitial pressure, such as pulmonary congestion, edema, microembolism, pneumonia, and chemical factors such as inhalation of irritants. Activation of J receptors produces rapid shallow breathing.

PULMONARY DRUGS

The two major lung disorders that we will consider are asthma and chronic obstructive pulmonary disease (COPD); these are two separate disorders. Asthma is characterized by the presence of *eosinophils* in bronchial lavage fluid, while in COPD *neutrophils* are paramount. This may explain why some drugs work in asthma, but do not work in COPD.

Asthma used to be a rare disease, but now it is considered an epidemic. There are about 14 million asthmatics in the United States with 4 million of them being children. Asthma is characterized by an intermittent airway narrowing and hypersecretion of airway mucous, which is associated with cough, wheezing, dyspnea, and a tightening of the chest. It is *reversible*, so if someone has asthma their symptoms can be reversed with proper management. This is an important difference between asthma and COPD—there is an *irreversible* component in COPD.

Asthma is an inflammatory disorder; so the lungs are hyperreactive, and they react to factors that they should not react to normally. Factors such as cold, exercise, dust in the air, allergens, and viral infections are a major cause of asthma exacerbation. Asthma is usually broken down into severity. In *mild asthma* there is brief intermittent difficulty in breathing—perhaps twice a week; patients are asymptomatic most of the time. Lung function is at 80% or greater of peak level. When they are symptomatic then the flow rate falls about 20%. In *moderate asthma*, the patient will have symptoms more than twice a week and may have more of the symptoms; they may require emergency care occasionally and may have more severe exacerbations, and their activity may be limited at times. In *severe asthma*, the symptoms are continuous, physical activity is limited regularly, baseline function is going to be at 60%, and they are going to require hospitalization and emergency care.

ANTI-INFLAMMATORY DRUGS

These are drugs that help with the inflammatory component of asthma. As mentioned previously (Chapter 9), the adrenal cortex produces a group of steroids known as glucocorticoids, the most notable of which is cortisol. The principal physiologic functions of cortisol involve carbohydrate, protein, and lipid regulation. During the 1930s, the observation was made that pregnant women with arthritis experienced symptomatic relief of joint pain during their pregnancy. It was believed that adrenocortical secretions were responsible, and this led to the discovery of the anti-inflammatory effect of glucocorticoids. Subsequently, derivatives of cortisol were developed, which preserved the anti-inflammatory effect of cortisol while minimizing electrolyte-related side effects. Glucocorticoids have been used to treat asthma since 1950.

Because chronic inflammation in the lung can produce remodeling of the lung, with loss of functional capacity, it is clinically desirable to keep inflammation under control. Generally, steroids are given by *inhalation* in order to avoid systemic toxicity. However, if an asthmatic patient reports to the hospital with a severe case, then they will often receive *iv methyl prednisone* or *oral prednisone*. Corticosteroids are not the treatment of choice in COPD, but they are the drugs of choice in asthmatics, in concert with β_2 agonists.

BETA$_2$ AGONISTS

The prototypical β_2 agonist is *albuterol* (Salbutamol). It is used for *acute* attacks and is usually taken by inhalation; if it is given systemically, it is prone to produce adverse effects such as *heart palpitation* and *muscle tremor* due to β_2 activation. When this activation occurs there is an increase in cyclic AMP, as described earlier, and relaxation of bronchial smooth muscle—*this drug is a true bronchodilator*. Albuterol needs to be given every 4 h; its peak effect occurs at approximately 0 min, but relief can occur within minutes.

The other main β_2 agonist that is used is *salmeterol* (Serevent). Salmeterol is a *longer acting drug than albuterol*; it is popular for asthmatics with nocturnal symptoms. Salmeterol is often given in combination with a steroid (fluticasone) under the trade name *Advair Discus*. The steroid is given to treat the inflammation and the salmeterol for bronchodilation. It is one of the top ten selling drugs in the United States.

MUSCARINIC ANTAGONISTS

At one time in the nineteenth century, extracts of the muscarinic blocker *Atropa belladonna* (atropine) found some favor in the treatment of airway disease; probably because it had some, albeit, crude efficacy in reducing bronchoconstriction and airway secretions. As mentioned previously, the principle innervation of bronchial smooth muscle is via parasympathetic fibers present in the vagus; therefore, acetylcholine is released at this muscarinic site.

The prototypic antimuscarinic drug used clinically today is *ipratropium bromide* and it is given by inhalation. *This drug is the drug of choice for COPD* because there is usually not the same involvement of inflammatory mediators as there is in asthma; the factor driving smooth muscle constriction in COPD is vagal tone.

The main side effects are dry mouth and increased mucous viscosity, due to its antimuscarinic effect. Because its usefulness is dependent on the patient's individual vagal tone, a β_2 agonist may have to be added. If the β_2 agonist fails, then a drug called *theophylline* may be added to the regimen.

THEOPHYLLINE

This drug is a xanthine derivative; its main mechanism of action is thought to be inhibition of *phosphodiesterase*—the enzyme responsible for degradation of cyclic AMP. The theory is that if levels of cyclic AMP increase we get bronchodilation. Although appealing, this model is not universally accepted. An alternative view is that theophylline is thought to *block adenosine* at adenosine receptors, activation of which causes bronchoconstriction.

Achieving the correct oral dose of theophylline is very important. One of the disadvantages of theophylline is that there is a considerable range in serum levels of the drug between patients. Treatment with theophylline preparations is associated with certain undesirable effects; it has a narrow therapeutic index. The appearance and character of these reactions is related to its serum level (Table 13.3).

Because there is a continuum of severity in asthma, theophylline is usually reserved for the more severe cases, sometimes in combination with steroids and ipratropium.

CROMOLYN SODIUM

Khellin, an extract of seeds from a Mediterranean plant, has been known for centuries to have some smooth muscle relaxing properties, and has found modest success in the treatment of bronchospasm. Unfortunately, the original preparations produced too many side effects to be of clinical value. However, studies in England during the 1960s identified a component active against allergic asthma, but with *no direct bronchodilator property*. It was introduced into the United States in 1973 under the name *cromolyn sodium*. The molecular structure of cromolyn sodium is unrelated to that of any other antiasthmatic drug (Figure 13.5).

Cromolyn has found most of its use in the treatment of *allergic rhinitis*. However, the drug may help some severe asthmatics to show improvement. Apparently, the drug acts by stabilizing mast cell membranes and preventing the release of mediators by blocking the calcium influx that triggers degranulation. One of the first studies carried out with cromolyn involved sensitized human lung tissue. In the presence of cromolyn, histamine and SRS-A (i.e., a mixture of leukotrienes C_4, D_4, and E_4) release were decreased significantly on subsequent exposure to antigen.

In some people, their asthma is exacerbated if they have constant congestion and drip, so they may find some relief with cromolyn. Cromolyn therapy has no place in the treatment of those with acute bronchospasm or of patients who suffer intermittent symptoms controllable by other means.

TABLE 13.3
Major Adverse Effect of Theophylline Therapy

Adverse Effect	Serum Level	Comments
Anorexia, nausea, vomiting	About 15 μg/ml or higher	Most common; more likely with oral preparations, suggesting effect on gastric mucosa; incidence varies with preparation
Cardiovascular	>30 μg/ml	Mainly with intravenous aminophylline; too rapid injection can lead to cardiac arrest, palpitations, tachycardia, and arrhythmias; also, hypertension or hypotension may occur
Central nervous system	>40 μg/ml	Drug-induced seizures with intravenous aminophylline, especially in children; respiratory arrest has been reported
Allergy	Not dose-related	Usually rashes, although anaphylaxis can occur; probably caused by ethylenediamine component

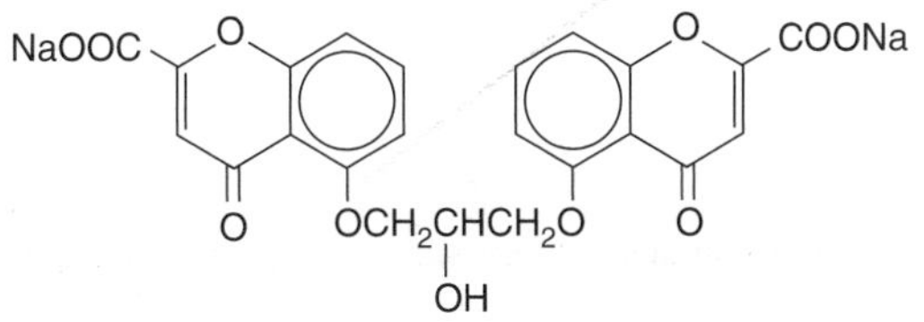

FIGURE 13.5 Molecular structure of cromolyn sodium.

LEUKOTRIENE ANTAGONISTS

Aspirin is known to block *cyclooxygenase* in the arachidonic acid (AA) cascade and shunt AA from prostaglandin formation toward *leukotrienes*. This is particularly important to the 5–10% of asthmatics who are *aspirin sensitive*. Asthmatics who are aspirin sensitive appear to be particularly sensitive to LTD_4 and LTC_4 production, which causes bronchoconstriction in these patients. On a weight-for-weight basis, leukotrienes C_4 and D_4 are at least 1000 times more potent than histamine in causing contraction of isolated human bronchi.

Montelukast is an LTD_4 receptor antagonist and is used once-a-day. It is usually given for mild asthmatics or as an additional therapy for severe asthmatics.

TREATMENT DEVICES

Most of the drugs used in treating asthma and COPD are delivered directly to the lungs. This minimizes side effects and also increases their therapeutic index. When something is taken by inhalation, particles are distributed on the basis of their aerodynamic properties. On the basis of theoretical considerations and experimental studies, it has been determined that the mass median diameter of aerosol particles corresponds to certain sites of deposition: particles that are 10 μm or more will get lodged in the mouth while particles 0.5 μm or smaller will go into the lungs and be breathed back out. Therefore, the particles that are most prone to be deposited in the alveoli are from 1–5 μm in size. So most of what we breathe in, about 90% of it, is going to get swallowed. In order to reduce *systemic absorption* of say, a steroid, it is advisable to *rinse and spit*; this will also help prevent the formation of an opportunistic infection such as *candidiasis* in the throat.

An additional development that has been devised to help prevent systemic absorption is the *spacer*. The spacer serves to collect the large particles in the aerosol before they gain access to the mouth and airway. Nebulizers are also used in small children and the elderly to facilitate drug delivery.

SELECTED BIBLIOGRAPHY

Adkinson, H.F., Schulman, E.S., and Newball, H.H. (1983) Anaphylactic release of arachidonic acid metabolites from the lung, in *Lung Biology in Health and Disease*, Newball H.H. (Ed.), Vol. 19, New York: Marcell Dekker.

Barnes, P.J. (1999) Effect of beta-agonists on inflammatory cells, *J. Allergy Clin. Immunol.*, 104: S10–S17.

Brain, J.D. and Valberg, P.A. (1979) Deposition of aerosol in the respiratory tract, *Am. Rev. Resp. Dis.*, 120: 1325–1333.

Fullmer, J.D. and Crystal, R.G. (1976) The biochemical basis of pulmonary function, in *Lung Biology in Health and Disease*, Crystal, R.G. (Ed.), Vol. 2, New York: Marcel Dekker.

Holgate, S.T. (1994) Antihistamines in the treatment of asthma, *Clin. Rev. Allergy.*, 12: 65–78.

Menzel, D.B. and McClellan, R.O. (1980) Toxic responses of the respiratory system, in *Toxicology: The Basic Sciences of Poisons*, 2nd ed., Doull, J., Klaasen, C., and Andur, M. (Eds.), New York: Macmillan.

Page, C.P. (1999) Recent advances in our understanding of the use of theophylline in the treatment of asthma, *J. Clin. Pharmacol.*, 39: 237–240.

Soderling, S.H. and Beavo, J. A. (2000) Regulation of cAMP and cGMP signalling: New phosphodiesterases and new functions, *Curr. Opin. Cell. Biol.*, 12: 174–179.

QUESTIONS

1. Mucous is most effective in clearing large particles from which airway region?
   a. Nasopharyngeal
   b. Bronchioles

    c. Alveoli
    d. a and c
    e. b and c

2. Particles of which size are likely to reach the terminal portion of the airway?
    a. All particles greater than 10 μm in diameter
    b. All particles smaller than 10 μm in diameter
    c. Particles greater than 2 μm in diameter
    d. Particles smaller than 2 μm in diameter
    e. All of the above

3. Which pulmonary region serves as the major conducting pathway between the naso-pharynx and the terminal alveoli?
    a. Larynx
    b. External nares
    c. Tracheobronchial
    d. a and b
    e. None of the above

4. Respiratory smooth muscle is principally controlled by which of the following?
    a. Autonomic nervous system
    b. Sympathetic nervous system
    c. Parasympathetic nervous system
    d. a and c
    e. All of the above

5. The tracheobronchial region of the airway is lined primarily by how many types of epithelial cells?
    a. One
    b. Two
    c. Three
    d. Five
    e. Seven

6. The mechanism of action of acetylcysteine is dependent on which of the following?
    a. The presence of a sulfhydryl group in its molecule
    b. Inhibition of mucin synthesis
    c. The reduction of disulfide bonds in mucin
    d. Destruction of goblet cells
    e. a and c

7. Which of the following is/are true regarding asthma?
    a. It has an irreversible component
    b. It has an inflammatory component
    c. It can be treated with β_2 antagonists
    d. The prototypic antimuscarinic drug used in asthma is atropine
    e. b and d

8. Which of the following is/are true regarding theophylline?
    a. Acts by stabilizing mast cells
    b. Acts by decreasing mucous production
    c. Blocks acetylcholine at sympathetic fibers in airway smooth muscle
    d. Has high therapeutic margin of safety
    e. None of the above

9. Which of the following is/are true regarding cromolyn sodium?
   a. Is a first line of defense in treating asthma
   b. Has found much of its success in treating allergic rhinitis
   c. May block release of mediators from airway mast cells
   d. Very useful in treating acute bronchospasm
   e. b and c

10. Which of the following is a leukotriene agonist used to treat mild asthmatics?
    a. Leukotriene D_4
    b. Salmeterol
    c. Albuterol
    d. Montelukast
    e. None of the above

14 Gastrointestinal Pharmacology

GASTRIC ACID

Gastric acid secretion is a complex, continuous process regulated by central neural and peripheral factors. Each factor contributes to a common final physiological event—the secretion of H^+ by parietal cells, which are located in the stomach. Acetylcholine, histamine, and gastrin all play important roles in the regulation of acid secretion (Figure 14.1).

Two major signaling pathways are present within the parietal cell: (1) the cyclic AMP-dependent pathway and (2) the Ca^{2+}-dependent pathway. Both pathways *activate* the H^+, K^+-ATPase (the proton pump). This pump reportedly generates the largest ion gradient known in vertebrates.

The stomach protects itself from damage by gastric acid through several mechanisms: (1) the presence of intercellular tight junctions between the gastric epithelial cells; (2) the presence of a mucin layer overlying the gastric epithelial cells; (3) the presence of prostaglandins E_2 and I_2 (which inhibit gastric acid secretion); and (4) secretion of bicarbonate ions into the mucin layer.

PROTON PUMP INHIBITORS

The most effective suppressors of gastric acid secretion are the gastric H^+, K^+-ATPase inhibitors. They are considered by many as the most effective drugs used in antiulcer therapy. Currently, there are several different proton pump inhibitors available for clinical use: ometrazole (Prilosec), lansoprazole (Prevacid), and rabeprazole (Aciphex). Proton pump inhibitors are *prodrugs*, requiring activation in an acid environment. The activated form reacts by covalent binding to sulfhydryl groups of

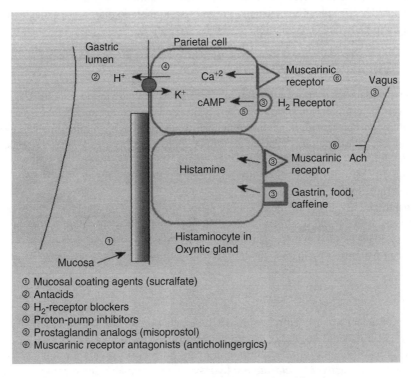

① Mucosal coating agents (sucralfate)
② Antacids
③ H_2-receptor blockers
④ Proton-pump inhibitors
⑤ Prostaglandin analogs (misoprostol)
⑥ Muscarinic receptor antagonists (anticholingergics)

FIGURE 14.1 Drugs affecting gastric acidity.

cysteines in the *ATPase*. Binding to cysteine at position 813, in particular, is essential for inhibition of acid production, which is irreversible.

Proton pump inhibitors have significant effects on acid production. When given in a sufficient dose, the daily production of acid can be diminished by more than 95%. Secretion of acid resumes only after new molecules of the ATPase enzyme are synthesized and inserted into the luminal membrane. Therefore, the acid inhibitory effect lasts longer than would be predicted from their plasma elimination half-life.

Proton pump inhibitors inhibit the activity of some hepatic cytochromes P450 enzymes and therefore may *decrease the clearance of certain drugs*. Proton pump inhibitors usually cause few side effects: nausea, abdominal pain, constipation, flatulence, and diarrhea are the most common adverse effects.

Protein pump inhibitors are used principally to promote healing of *gastric and duodenal ulcers* and to treat gastric esophageal reflux disease (GERD).

HISTAMINE H$_2$-RECEPTOR ANTAGONISTS

The description of selective histamine H$_2$-receptor blockade in 1970 was a landmark in the history of pharmacology and set the stage for the modern approach to the treatment of acid-peptic disease, which until then had relied almost entirely on acid neutralization in the stomach (see below).

There are four H$_2$-receptor antagonists currently available OTC in the United States: cimetidine (Tagamet); ranitidine (Zantac); famotidine (Pepcid); and nizatidine (Axid). H$_2$-receptor antagonists inhibit acid production by reversibly competing with histamine for binding to H$_2$ receptors on the basolateral membrane of parietal cells. The major therapeutic indications for this category of drugs are for promoting healing of gastric and duodenal ulcers, for uncomplicated gastric reflux disease, and for prophylaxis of stress ulcers. These agents are particularly effective in suppressing nocturnal acid secretion.

The overall incidence of adverse effects of these drugs is low —on the order of <3% (that is why they can be sold OTC). Side effects usually are minor and include diarrhea, headache, drowsiness, fatigue, muscular pain, and constipation.

PROSTAGLANDIN ANALOGS

PGE$_2$ and PGI$_2$ are the major prostaglandins synthesized by the gastric mucosa. Prostaglandin binding to its receptor results in inhibition of adenenylate cyclase and decreased levels of intracellular cyclic AMP. Since nonsteroidal anti-inflammatory drugs (NSAIDs) inhibit prostaglandin formation, the synthetic prostaglandins provide a rational approach to reducing NSAID-related mucosal damage. *Misoprostol* (15-deoxy-16-hydroxy-16-methyl-PGE$_1$; *Cytotec*) is a synthetic analog of prostaglandin E$_1$. Misoprostol is currently approved by the FDA for use in preventing mucosal injury caused by NSAIDs.

The most frequently reported side effect of misoprostol is diarrhea that can occur in up to 30% of patients. Misoprostol can cause clinical exacerbations in patients with inflammatory bowel disease and hence should be avoided in these patients. Misoprostal is also contraindicated during pregnancy, since it can cause abortion by increasing uterine contractility.

ANTACIDS

The function of antacids is to neutralize the HCL secreted by gastric parietal cells. Although they have been used for generations, today they are generally restricted to OTC use (see Table 14.1).

Combinations of magnesium and aluminum hydroxides also provide a relatively fast and sustained neutralizing capacity. *Magaldrate* is a hydroxymagnesium aluminate complex that is rapidly converted in gastric acid to Mg(OH)$_2$ and Al(OH)$_3$, which are poorly absorbed and thus provide a

TABLE 14.1
Components* and Neutralizing Capacities** of Some Popular Antacids

Product	Al(OH)$_3$	Mg(OH)$_2$	CaCO$_3$	Simethicone	Neutralizing Capacity
Gelusil II (T)	400	400	0	30	21
Maalox quick dissolve (T)	0	0	600	0	11
Mylanta (T)	0	150	350	0	12
Rolaids (T)	0	110	550	0	14
Tums-EX (T)	0	0	750	0	15
Gelusil II (L)	400	400	0	30	24
Kudrox (L)	500	450	0	40	28
Maalox TC(L)	600	300	0	0	28
Milk of magnesia (L)	0	400	0	0	14
Mylanta extra strength (L)	400	400	0	40	25

T = Tablet.
L = Liquid.
*Contents, mg per tablet or per 5 mL.
**Neutralizing capacity, mEq per tablet or per 5 mL.

Source: Modified from W. Hoogerwerf and Pasricha, P.J. (2001) In *Goodman and Gilman's, The Pharmacological Basis of Therapeutics,* J.G. Hardman and L. E. Limbard (Eds.), 10th ed., New York: McGraw-Hill.

sustained antacid effect. *Simethicone,* a surfactant that may decrease foaming, and hence esophageal reflux, is included in many antacid preparations.

By altering gastric and urinary pH, antacids *may* alter rates of dissolution and absorption, the bioavailability, and renal elimination of *certain drugs.* Al^{3+} and Mg^{2+} compounds are notable for their tendency to form insoluble complexes that are not absorbed.

MISCELLANEOUS DRUGS

In the presence of acid-induced damage, pepsin-mediated hydrolysis of mucosal proteins contributes to mucosal erosions and ulcerations. This process can be inhibited by sulfated polysaccharides. *Sucralfate* is one such drug. It is composed of sucrose to which aluminum hydroxide has been added. In the acid environment of the gastric lumen, sucralfate undergoes extensive cross-linking and polymerization to produce a viscous, sticky gel that forms a protective barrier for epithelial cells and ulcerative craters for several hours. The role of sucralfate in the treatment of acid-peptic disease has diminished in recent years; however, it may still be useful in the prophylaxis of stress ulcers.

Acetylcholine is released from the vagus nerve and stimulates muscarinic receptors (M$_1$) on parietal cells, leading to increased gastric acidity. Theoretically, therefore, anticholinergic compounds should be useful in suppressing gastric acid production. In fact, anticholinergic drugs such as *pirenzepine* and *telenzepine* have been used for decades around the world; they can reduce basal acid production by 40–50%. However, because of their undesirable side effects, poor efficacy, and the availability of newer more effective drugs, they have fallen out of favor in the United States.

GASTROESOPHAGEAL REFLUX DISEASE

Gastroesophageal reflux disease (GERD) is common in the United States, where it is estimated that one in five adults has symptoms of heartburn and/or regurgitation at least once a week. The incidence of GERD has been rising over the past several decades; it should be noted that GERD is a chronic disorder that requires long-term therapy.

Most of the symptoms of GERD are due to the injurious effects of the acid-peptic refluxate on the esophageal epithelium. This fact explains why the current pharmacotherapeutic approach to treating GERD is based on suppression of gastric acid. The goals of GERD therapy are complete resolution of symptoms and healing of esophagitis. Proton pump inhibitors (e.g., omeprazole, lansoprazole, rabeprazole, and pantoprazole) have been reported to be more effective than H_2-receptor antagonists (e.g., cimetidine, ranitidine, and famotidine) in achieving both of these goals; fortunately, these drugs are available OTC.

PEPTIC ULCER DISEASE

The pathophysiology of peptic ulcer disease is perhaps best understood in terms of an imbalance between mucosal defense factors and destructive factors. For example, patients with duodenal ulcer produce, on average, more acid than do control subjects; ulcers rarely, if ever, occur in the complete absence of acid (i.e., "no acid, no ulcer"). Up to 80–90% of ulcers may be associated with *Helicobacter pylori* infection of the stomach.

H. pylori has been associated with gastritis and subsequent development of gastric and duodenal ulcers. In view of its critical role in the pathogenesis of peptic ulcers, in the majority of cases, it has become routine care to eradicate this infection in patients with gastric or duodenal ulcers. However, treatment of *H. pylori* infection is not straightforward.

Single antibiotic regimens have proven to be ineffective in treating *H. pylori* and can lead to the ever present problem of resistance. On the other hand, it has been found that coadministration of a proton pump inhibitor or H_2-receptor antagonist can significantly enhance the effectiveness of regimens containing pH-dependent antibiotics such as *amoxicillin or clarithromycin*.

Because of the central role that excess gastric acid plays in the etiology of gastrointestinal ulcers, current recommendations for treatment include H_2-receptor antagonists and proton-pump inhibitors (see above).

ANTIDIARRHEAL AGENTS

Pharmacotherapy of diarrhea should be reserved for patients with significant or persistent symptoms. Among the most prevalent are bulk-forming and hydroscopic agents. Hydrophilic colloids such as *psyllium* (Metamucil) and *carboxymethylcellulose* absorb water and increase stool bulk. They are often used to treat constipation but are sometimes useful in certain cases of diarrhea and irritable bowel syndrome (IBS). A mixture of kaolin and pectin (a plant polysaccharide) is a popular OTC remedy and may provide useful symptomatic relief of mild diarrhea.

Bismuth compounds have been used to treat a variety of gastrointestinal diseases and symptoms for centuries. *Pepto-Bismol* (bismuth salicylate) is an OTC preparation estimated to be used by 60% of American households. It is also used effectively for the prevention and treatment of traveler's diarrhea.

Opioids continue to be widely used in the treatment of diarrhea and may act by interacting with μ- or δ-opioid receptors on enteric nerves. These include effects to decrease intestinal motility (μ receptors). In infants, the use of *paregoric* is a classical case of treatment of diarrhea with an opioid.

Loperamide (Imodium) is an orally acting agent present in OTC preparations. The drug is 40–50 times more potent than morphine as an antidiarreal agent and penetrates the CNS poorly. *Lomotil* is a combination of a synthetic opioid (diphenoxylate) and an anticholinergic (atropine).

TREATMENT OF CONSTIPATION

The terms laxatives, cathartics, purgatives, aperients, and evacuants often are used interchangeably. Strictly speaking, however, there is a distinction between laxation (the evacuation of formed fecal material from the rectum) and catharsis (the evacuation of unformed, usually watery fecal material from the entire colon). Most of the commonly used agents promote laxation, but some actually are cathartics, which, at low doses, are used as laxatives.

GENERAL MECHANISM OF ACTION

Laxatives are generally thought to act in one of the following ways: (1) retention of intraluminal fluid; (2) decreased net absorption of fluid, by effects on small and large bowel fluid and electrolyte transport; or (3) effects on motility by either inhibiting nonpropulsive contractions or stimulating propulsive contractions.

OSMOTICALLY ACTIVE AGENTS

Saline Laxatives (magnesium sulfate, magnesium hydroxide, magnesium citrate, and sodium phosphate). Laxatives containing magnesium cations or phosphate anions are commonly called *saline laxatives*. Their cathartic action is believed to be the result of osmotically mediated water retention, which then stimulates peristalsis.

Nondigestable sugars and alcohols (glycerin, lactulose, sorbitol, and mannitol). *Glycerin* is a trihydroxy alcohol that acts as a hygroscopic agent and lubricant when given rectally. It is for rectal use only and is given in a single daily dose. The water retention stimulates peristalsis and usually produces a bowel movement in less than an hour.

Lactulose, sorbitol, and mannitol are nonabsorbable sugars that are hydrolyzed in the intestine to organic acids, which acidify the luminal contents and osmotically draw water into the lumen, stimulating colonic propulsive motility.

Stool-wetting agents and emollients. Docusate salts (e.g., docusate calcium) are anionic surfactants that lower the surface tension of stool to allow mixing of aqueous and fatty substances. This softens the stool and permits easier defecation. Despite their widespread use, these agents have marginal, if any, efficacy in most cases of constipation.

Mineral oil is a mixture of aliphatic hydrocarbons obtained from petroleum. The oil is indigestible and absorbed only to a limited extent. When taken for 2–3 days, it penetrates and softens the stool, and may interfere with the absorption of water. Side effects of mineral oil preclude its regular usage (e.g., leakage of oil past the anal sphincter).

Stimulants. Bisacodyl is a diphenylmethane derivative similar to *phenolphthalein*; it was once among the most popular components of laxatives (e.g., Exlax). However, phenolphthalein was withdrawn from the market over concerns regarding safety. Biscodyl is available in an enteric-coated preparation given once daily. Since the drug requires hydrolysis in the bowel for activation, the laxative effects after oral ingestion are usually not produced in less than 6 h. It is therefore frequently taken at bedtime to produce its effect the next morning.

Anthraquinone laxatives are plant derivatives and are among the oldest known drugs in this group. Members of this class are activated by bacterial action in the colon. An age-old stimulant laxative derived from the castor bean is *castor oil*. It contains two well-known noxious ingredients: an extremely toxic protein, *ricin*, and an oil composed chiefly of *the triglyceride of ricinoleic acid* (the active ingredient) that acts primarily in the small intestine where it speeds intestinal transit. Despite its efficacy, castor oil is rarely used now because of its unpleasant taste.

SELECTED BIBLIOGRAPHY

American Gastroenterological Association Medical Position Statement: Evaluation of Dyspepsia. (1998) *Gastroenenterology*, 114: 579–581.

Graham, D.Y. (2000) Therapy of Helico bacter pylori: Current status and issues. *Gastroenterology*, 118: S2–S8.

Jackson, J.L., O'Malley, P.G., Tomkins, G., Balden, E., Santoro, J., and Kroenke, K. (2000) Treatment of functional gastrointestinal disorders with antidepressant medications: A meta-analysis, *Am. J. Med.*, 108: 65–72.

Kovac, A.L. (2000) Prevention and treatment of postoperative nausea and vomiting, *Drugs*, 59: 213–243.

Kuipers, E.J. and Meuwissen, S.G. (2000) The efficacy and safety of long-term omeprazole treatment for gastroesophageal relux disease, *Gastroenterology*, 118: 795–798.

Sands, B.E. (2000) Therapy of inflammatory bowel disease. *Gastroenterology*, 118: S68–S82.

Welage, L.S. and Berardi, R.R. (2000) Evaluation of omeprazole, lansoprazole, pantoprazole, and rabeprazole in the treatment of acid-related diseases, *J. Am. Pharm. Assoc. (Wash.)*, 40: 52–62.

Wolfe, M.M., and Sachs, G. (2000) Acid suppression: Optimizing therapy for gastroduodenal ulcer healing, gastroesophageal reflux disease, and stress-related erosive syndrome, *Gastroenterology*, 118: S9–S31.

QUESTIONS

1. Which of the following is/are the major signaling pathways in gastric parietal cells?
   a. cyclic GMP-dependent
   b. cyclic AMP-dependent
   c. Calcium-dependent
   d. Serotonin-dependent
   e. b and c

2. Which of the following is/are true regarding proton pump inhibitors?
   a. They are the most effective suppressors of gastric acid secretion
   b. They are prodrugs that require activation in an acid environment
   c. They bind covalently to cysteines in ATPase
   d. They are used to treat gastric ulcers and GERD
   e. All of the above

3. H$_2$ antagonists include all of the following except?
   a. Diphenhydramine (Benadryl)
   b. Cimetidine (Tagamet)
   c. Ranitidine (Zantac)
   d. Famoltidine (Pepsid)
   e. Nizatidine (Axid)

4. Which of the following is contraindicated during pregnancy, since it can cause abortion by increasing uterine contractions?
   a. Cromolyn sodium
   b. Cimetidine (Tagamet)
   c. Misoprostal (Cytotec)
   d. Ometrazole (Prilosec)
   e. None of the above

5. Which of the following is a surfactant used in many antacid preparations?
   a. Magaldrate
   b. Sucralfate
   c. Lansoprazole
   d. Simethacone
   e. None of the above

6. Which of the following is/are true regarding *H. pylori* and ulcers?
   a. Up to 80–90% of ulcers may be related to *H. pylori* infection of the stomach
   b. Single antibiotic regimens have proven to be ineffective in treating *H. pylori* infections

   c. Coadministration of Proton Pump Inhibitors and H_2 antagonists can increase effectiveness of pH-dependent antibiotics

   d. All of the above

   e. None of the above

7. Which of the following is/are bulk-forming antidiarrheal agents?
   a. Bismuth salicylate
   b. Psyllium
   c. Loperamide (Imodium)
   d. Carboxymethylcellulose
   e. b and d

8. Lomotil contains which of the following?
   a. Kaolin + pectin
   b. Diphenoxylate + atropine
   c. Loperamide (Imodium) + pectin
   d. Magnesium sulfate + mannitol
   e. None of the above

9. Which of the following was removed from the market because of concerns over safety?
   a. Bisacodyl
   b. Mineral oil
   c. Castor oil
   d. Phenolphthalein
   e. Docusate calcium

10. The active ingredient in castor oil is?
    a. Phenolphthalein
    b. Ricinoleic acid
    c. Glycerin
    d. Ricin
    e. Sorbitol

Part IV

Drug Development

15 Drug Discovery by the Pharmaceutical Industry

INTRODUCTION

Throughout history, certain plants, as well as virtually every anatomical component of animals and humans, have been ascribed some curative property: earthworms rolled in honey for the treatment of gastritis, owl brain for headache, sheep brain for insomnia, deer heart for heart disease, fox lung for tuberculosis, goat liver for jaundice, powdered human skull or the fresh blood of a dying Christian gladiator for epilepsy, rabbit testicles for bladder disease and, of course, for impotence, and cow dung for eye infections, to name but a few.

It was also during the seventeenth century that the roles of chemists and druggists began to merge, and with this amalgamation several English pharmaceutical companies had their origins. For example, Allen and Hanburys (now part of the giant GlaxoWellcome Group) began as a simple apothecary shop in 1715. Early entrepreneurs such as these imported large quantities of raw materials from around the world, which were converted into such widely used preparations as tincture of Peruvian bark (for malaria) and cod liver oil (for rheumatism and rickets).

Further significant advances in chemical knowledge occurred at the end of the eighteenth and beginning of the nineteenth centuries, among which were newer extraction procedures that allowed the isolation of purer drugs from natural sources. For example, Serturner reported the first isolation of a plant alkaloid in 1806 (morphine), which was soon followed by codeine in 1832 and papavarine in 1848. By the middle of the nineteenth century, the use of *pure* alkaloids rather than crude preparations began to spread throughout the medical world.

Starting in the mid-nineteenth century, important new synthetic drugs made their appearance: nitrous oxide (1844), ether (1846), and chloroform (1847) as anesthetics, amyl nitrite (1867) and nitroglycerin (1879) for anginal pain, chloral hydrate (1869) for sedation, and antipyrene (1883), acetanilid (1886), and acetophenetidin (1887) for the control of pain and fever. Introduction of the last three drugs marked the entry of the German chemical industry into the pharmaceutical field and changed it forever. With their vast experience in organic synthesis in the dye industry, they set the standard for pharmaceutical chemistry until World War II.

However, the development of the giant multinational drug companies of today, with their tremendous capacity for the synthesis of organic molecules, did not occur overnight. In fact, most of the early pharmaceutical companies made their profits based on the sale of *inorganic* preparations (e.g., Beecham's liver pills were bismuth salts while Boot's Epsom salts were basically magnesium sulfate).

The German company Bayer was the first to *widely commercialize* a *synthetic* drug (acetylsalicylic acid) in 1899. Germany's Bayer was not looking for a drug to relieve the pain of rheumatism 100 years ago, but a 29-year-old Bayer chemist and pharmacist named Felix Hoffman was looking for a way to relieve his father's suffering. *Sodium salicylate,* which was used to treat rheumatism victims at the time, not only had an unpleasant taste but the acid also attacked the mucosal linings of the mouth and stomach.

In the 1830s, chemists succeeded in extracting *salicin* from willow and converting it to *salicylic acid* for use in treating fevers. In the 1870s, researchers discovered that salicin derivatives also relieved pain and inflammation. Sodium salicylate became the preferred form for treating arthritis. When Felix Hoffman began experimenting with salicylic acid in the 1890s, he started with the assumption that acidity was responsible for its gut-wrecking effects. Hoping to moderate this acidity, Hoffman uncovered the long-ignored synthesis of acetylsalicylic acid in 1853 by Charles

Gerhardt, who acetylated the hydroxyl group of sodium salicylate at position 1 of the benzene ring. But Gerhardt had not pursued acetylsalicylic acid because its synthesis proved difficult. Hoffman devised a better way to synthesize acetylsalicylic acid by choosing acetic anhydride as the acetylating agent instead of Gerhardt's use of acetyl chloride.

Working in Bayer's Elberfeld, Germany, pharmaceutical laboratory, Hoffman acetylated salicylic acid in August 1897. The resultant acetylsalicylic acid powder had few of sodium salicylate's drawbacks, and besides relieving Hoffman's father's rheumatoid aches and pains, it had some additional benefits as well. Bayer scientists found aspirin helped relieve headaches and toothaches, reduced fever, and decreased inflammation.

Bayer first sold aspirin powder to the public in 1899, and introduced a water soluble tablet in 1900. The company estimates that 50 billion tablets are consumed yearly on a worldwide basis. In addition to tablets, the French prefer their aspirin in suppository form while the Italians prefer it fizzy. Aspirin is not just taken for headaches and aches and pains anymore. According to Bayer market research, palliation of heart disease is now the number one use of aspirin.

The development of acetylsalicylic acid by Bayer also began a battle of trade names that lasted well into this century. Bayer christened their new drug aspirin, the name originating from the "a" of acetyl and "spir" of *Spirea ulmania*, the plant from which salicylic acid had originally been isolated. Bayer registered the trade name and argued that if aspirin was prescribed in Germany, *their* product should be dispensed.

The analgesic *acetaminophen* is one of the world's most popular nonprescription medications. Its discovery illustrates how *serendipity* can play a role in drug discovery. In 1886, two German interns ordered some *naphthalene* from a nearby pharmacist for the treatment of intestinal parasites. The substance they received failed to kill the parasites but managed instead to reduce the patient's fever (*antipyretic*). On further review of the situation, the interns discovered that the first material was *acetanilide*, a coal-tar derivative used in the dye industry, never before given to human beings. The two doctors then approached Kalle & Company of Wiesbaden with the question who agreed to sell acetanilide under the brand name "Antifebrin."

At the same time another German company Farbenfabriken Bayer, was accumulating tons of unwanted p-aminophenol as a by-product of its synthetic dye production processes. Chemists at the company saw an opportunity to make use of this chemical waste. By using the unwanted phenol, chemists were able to produce p-ethoxy acetanilide ("phenacitin"). This product was found to be both an antipyretic and an analgesic. Phenacitin was marketed in 1888; this event was highly significant.

As stated in 1991 by Mann and Plummer (see bibliography): "For the first time, a drug had been conceived, developed, tested, and marketed, all by a private company. *It marked the creation of the modern drug industry …*"

Phenacitin was widely used during the influenza epidemic of 1889 and the Bayer company's new pharmaceutical enterprise prospered. Phenacitin remained an important analgesic (being the P in over-the-counter APCs) until concern over its nephrotoxic side effects arose in the 1960s. It was finally withdrawn from sale in 1983.

p-Acetylaminophenol (acetamoniphen) had first been synthesized in 1888 and found to be a metabolite of phenacetin in 1889, and an effective analgesic and antipyretic. However, because phenacetin was already a successful product, it was not originally developed as a commercial drug.

With the outbreak of World War I, the international pharmaceutical situation suddenly changed. England, France, and the United States, cut off from their normal supply of German drugs and other important chemicals, were pressured to create their own drug/chemical industries. Until this time, American contributions to drug development had been modest though very important. For example, the anesthetic agents nitrous oxide and ether were both developed in the United States. At the end of World War I, Bayer lost their exclusive right to the name aspirin when the allies assumed control over the company as part of the spoils of war.

In 1939, a consortium of U.S. proprietary drug manufacturers established The Institute for the Study of Analgesic and Sedative Drugs, with the intention of applying modern pharmacological science to the development and testing of analgesics. In 1951, the institute organized a symposium to evaluate the evidence surrounding acetaminophen. Researchers studied the hepatic metabolism of acetanilide *in vitro*, and discovered its metabolism to acetaminophen leading to speculation that acetaminophen might be useful in its own right. As a result, several chemical producers began selling the compound over the following years including McNeil Laboratories in Pennsylvania, which coined the brand name Tylenol®.

As mentioned previously in Chapter 10, the discovery of sulfanilamide during the 1930s ushered in a new era in drug therapy. As a result of world-wide publicity in medical journals, magazines, and newspapers, the demand for the new drug skyrocketed. Drug companies in England, France, and the United States, quick to see the potential sales in this new field, began to synthesize, test, and rush to market a vast array of sulfanilamide *derivatives* that could be patented and promoted. This approach was intensified by the relatively widespread introduction of the more effective penicillin in the mid-1940s.

It was World War II that really provided an additional "jump-start" for the involvement of American pharmaceutical companies in antibiotic production. As mentioned previously, following the discovery of penicillin, there was general apathy on the part of the drug industry to devote resources to its commercialization. However, with the obvious implications of war-time injuries and their attendant infections, Britain's Howard Florey continued his drive to develop penicillin by turning his attention to the United States. With dogged determination he succeeded in obtaining help from the Bureau of Agriculture in Peoria, Illinois—who took on the task of developing a commercial-scale fermentation process in response to America's entry into the war in 1941.

Eventually, 100,000 units of penicillin were produced by a consortium of American drug companies (Merck, Squibb, and Pfizer) by the middle of 1944. A tremendous improvement in yield was made possible by the use of a new strain of mold, as well as the use of deep fermentation tanks similar to those used in the brewery industry. Interestingly, the new strain of mold discovered was serendipitously found on a decaying cantaloupe in a Peoria food market.

It was also during the 1940s that American drug companies began a very successful relationship with steroids. The first major steroid that received attention during this period was cortisone. Cortisone is normally produced by the adrenal glands. Its interest to pharmaceutical companies emanated from several factors. The first was that it was rumored to be a secret chemical used by the Germans to assist in high-altitude flying. In addition, it was also identified as the elusive "compound E" that was responsible for ameliorating arthritis in pregnant women. By 1948, a complicated 36-stage process had been developed for its synthesis. Unfortunately, 1 g of cortisone produced in this manner cost approximately $200.

As a result of the need for more of this very effective anti-inflammatory drug, several pharmaceutical companies began major efforts to produce large quantities of the steroid, utilizing different strategies. For example, Searle attempted to extract cortisone from cattle adrenal glands while Syntex and Upjohn focused on a more straightforward chemical conversion of progesterone into cortisone. Syntex eventually reported the successful synthesis of cortisone in 1951 using hecogenin (from the agave plant) as a starting material. Although cortisone itself did not eventually prove to be particularly successful (primarily due to side effects), structural leads that have led to the development of numerous highly effective steroid drugs over the last 50 years were obtained.

Perhaps the most significant steroid-based drug developed over the past five decades was the birth control pill. It is a relatively unique drug in that it is typically taken by healthy individuals who are not suffering from an illness. In 1950, the first oral contraceptive was designed based on a regimen of progesterone for 3 weeks followed by withdrawal of the drug for 1 week to allow menstruation to occur. However, because of "breakthrough bleeding," a more potent progestin was needed.

By 1951, chemists at Syntex and Searle had produced analogs of progesterone called norethindrone and norethynodrel, respectively. Because they were more resistant to hepatic first-pass metabolism, they were able to achieve higher potency. A large-scale clinical trial began in Puerto Rico in 1956 involving 221 women who received norethynodrel *and* a synthetic estrogen (mestranol—given to minimize "breakthrough bleeding") over a 2-year period. After the results of this trial, and a subsequent larger scale study were evaluated, Searle was given permission to market the first combination oral contraceptive in 1960.

It should be clear at this point that the basic steps in drug development involve a sequence: (1) the discovery of some pharmacological effect produced by a source material (plant or animal), (2) isolation and identification of the active ingredient, (3) determination of structure–activity relationships (SAR), and (4) the synthesis of more active congeners. Once a drug can be synthesized or isolated to complete purity, then its pharmacological profile can be quantified on a mass basis in some model system. This is referred to as "forward pharmacology" or drug screening.

Drug Screening

Historically, the major source of chemical diversity for screening purposes has been natural products. In a 1997 survey, it was estimated that 39% of all 520 approved drugs between 1983 and 1994 were natural or derived from natural products, and 60–80% of antibacterial and anticancer drugs were derived from natural products. However, because there has been a decrease in the number of new drugs introduced to the world market during the 1990s, efforts are being made to improve the efficiency of the drug discovery process by using high-throughput chemistry and screening.

The discovery of new drugs has *traditionally* depended, more or less, on the *trial and error* synthesis of potential lead compounds and their bioassay for pharmacological effect in some physiological system (e.g., intact animal, isolated organ, or receptor-binding assays). Examples include drugs such as morphine, quinine, and ephedrine that have been in widespread use for some time. Lead compounds can also be suggested to the investigator through empirical knowledge of biochemical pathways or through success in the assay program itself. Examples include tubocurarine, propranolol, cimetidine, and the histamine H_2 antagonists.

One of the best examples of the successful application of traditional bioassay to the drug-discovery process is the development of the β-blocker propranolol. To this day, β-blockers are among the most widely prescribed and effective antihypertensive drugs. They were first launched in the mid-1960s, but their development can be traced back to the turn of the twentieth century. In the early 1900s (as mentioned previously), Otto Löewi noted that stimulation of the vagus nerve slowed the contractile rate in isolated hearts of frogs. Ultimately, Löewi demonstrated that applying the bathing solution from a frog heart in which the vagus nerve had been stimulated to a naive, unstimulated recipient heart, induced the same bradycardia (slowing) effect. Löewi's identification of a vagal "neurotransmitter" ("vagustoff") led to the identification of acetylcholine and, in turn, the birth of autonomic pharmacology. Characterization of the parasympathetic and sympathetic nervous systems, which culminated in the development of β-blockers, followed. All this from initial observations made in bioassays of amphibian hearts decades before terms such as "expression cloning" became an integral part of the pharmacologist's lexicon.

The development of angiotensin-converting enzyme (ACE) inhibitors also adhered to the classical paradigm of "*forward pharmacology*." In 1934, it was postulated that the kidney released a pressor substance in response to a reduction in blood flow; however, almost four decades passed before the true therapeutic significance of ACE became apparent. During the early 1970s, investigators were studying the pharmacological properties of an extract of the Brazilian pit viper, *Bothrops jararaca*; it was well-known that envenomation by *B. jararaca* resulted in severe systemic *hypotension*. It was subsequently demonstrated by scientists at Squibb that extracts of this venom lowered blood pressure by inhibiting ACE, thus attenuating angiotensin II production (see Figure 12.5). Eventually, the first orally available ACE inhibitor was developed and marketed in 1982; 50 years after pioneering work in dogs. Could the same amount of time be spent today in bringing a product to market?

Following identification of such lead compounds, the chemical structure and physical properties of the drug have been traditionally optimized in a very painstaking and time-consuming manner by synthesis of a succession of variants with subsequent testing for pharmacological activity (quantitative structure–activity relationship [QSAR]).

The QSAR is a routine tool in drug discovery that computational scientists use to analyze large sets of candidate drug molecules. Sophisticated descriptors have been developed to characterize the three-dimensional geometry and chemistry of small molecules. In rational drug design, the QSAR can help identify the features of a molecule that control activity, which is critical information for the medicinal chemist. The QSAR can also be used to select the best candidate molecules from large compound libraries, reducing testing time and costs.

Classically, the entire process has been found to be protracted, challenging, and extremely demanding of resources because a correlation between the chemical structure of a drug and its pharmacological effect is often very difficult to discern. In addition, even if success is demonstrated in some nonwhole animal system, a drug's usefulness is often compromised by side effects and transport problems revealed when the drug is administered to the whole animal. In general, the successful development of a new drug is a relatively rare event and may require the synthesis and evaluation of thousands of candidate compounds. However, once a lead compound is discovered, then structural derivatives can be evaluated and the QSAR determined.

QSAR methods date back to the 1800s, when scientists first correlated alcohol toxicity with hydrophobicity. Today's drug design efforts, however, are laboriously quantitative, incorporating molecular structure description, combinatorial mathematics, statistics, computer simulations, and database analysis. In today's data-rich environment, QSAR methods enable users to maximize their use of available data. Because they can be applied quickly and easily, the methods are useful as a screening tool, identifying drug candidates that are likely to be most effective so that more costly experimental or computational work can be focused. They also help scientists understand complex, multicomponent problems that often defy study by experiment or simulation.

QSARs identify a mathematical relationship between some property of a molecular system, such as its ability to inhibit a family of enzymes, and a series of "descriptors" representing chemical or geometric characteristics. Typical descriptors include thermodynamic properties, electronic properties, or functions related to molecular shape. A typical QSAR spreadsheet is composed of rows representing the compounds in the data set and columns representing descriptor values.

The relationship between structure and activity is derived empirically by analyzing a set of molecules for which values of the property and descriptors are known. A study may involve many descriptors, making derivation of QSARs a complex statistical exercise. But this exercise is easily automated, and its benefits are significant. QSARs identify the key structural and chemical factors that determine the property of interest. They can then be applied to predict the factors that are critical to the property that is of interest—thereby assisting in the optimized design of materials, drugs, and chemicals.

QSAR tools help explain and predict properties based on statistical correlations. Using these tools, researchers may develop predictive models based on analysis that identifies correlations in the data, or they may apply established models to predict properties.

Successful applications of QSAR technology to drug discovery research are becoming increasingly commonplace. Computational scientists and experimentalists are adding QSAR methods to their arsenal of discovery tools to complement computational methods. However, with virtual high-throughput screening comes the challenge of effectively dealing with large, noisy, and often complex data sets.

One of the earliest examples of the QSAR approach was the development of synthetic local anesthetic agents. These drugs were developed based on the structure of cocaine whose local anesthetic property was championed by Carl Köller, who introduced cocaine into clinical practice in 1884 for ophthalmologic surgery. The many local anesthetics used in clinical practice today all emanate from these early observations.

Because of cocaine's toxicity and addictive properties, a search began for synthetic substitutes for cocaine. In 1905, *procaine* was synthesized and became the prototypic local anesthetic for half a century. Newer derivatives include mepivacaine and tetracaine (Figure 15.1). Briefly, the SAR of local anesthetics revolves around their hydrophobicity. Association of the drug at hydrophobic sites, such as the sodium channel, is believed to prevent the generation and conductance of a nerve impulse by interfering with sodium permeability (i.e., elevating the threshold for electrical excitability).

Newer anti-inflammatory drugs have also been designed to combine the useful properties of the prototypic drug, aspirin, with a reduced level of gastric toxicity in derivatives. Typical of the structural modification experiments were those carried out by the Boots Company in England, which involved the synthesis and screening of numerous structural analogs of aspirin. Surprisingly, as is often the case, their "lead" or "parent" compound (Boots 7268) had originally been synthesized for use as an agricultural weed killer. In fact, it proved to be twice as potent as aspirin when tested in an anti-inflammatory screen (companies routinely test for a wide spectrum of pharmacological activity in multiscreen assays). The chemists at Boots synthesized approximately 600 similar compounds, one of which proved to be 6–10 times more potent than aspirin. Eventually, after additional structural modifications, the highly effective drug ibuprofen that possesses 30-fold greater anti-inflammatory activity than aspirin was developed (Figure 15.2).

More recent advances in anti-inflammatory drug research dealing with *nonsteroidal anti-inflamatory drugs* (NSAIDS) resulted in the development of an even newer class of compounds. Anti-inflammatory drugs such as aspirin and ibuprofen are believed to produce their effect by inhibiting an enzyme present in cell membranes (*cyclooxygenase;* COX). Aspirin inhibits COX by

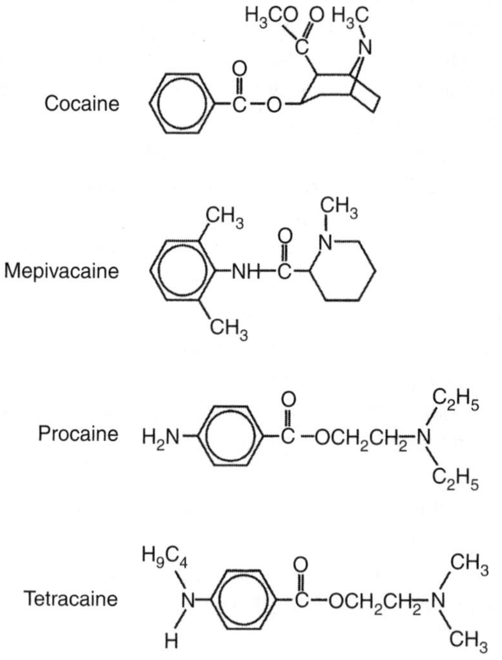

FIGURE 15.1 Structural relationship between local anesthetics.

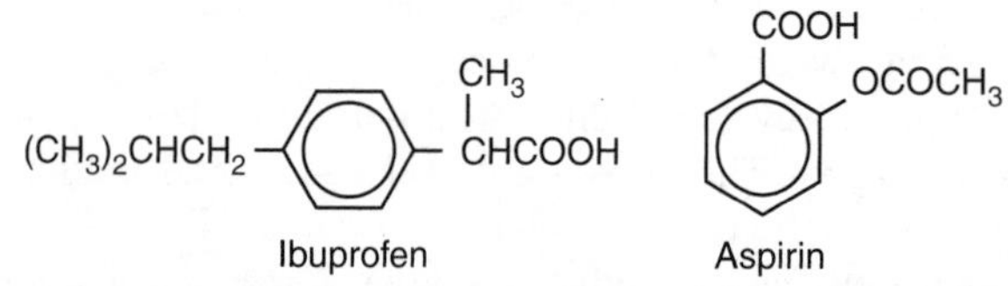

FIGURE 15.2 Structural relationship of the analgesic drugs ibuprofen and aspirin.

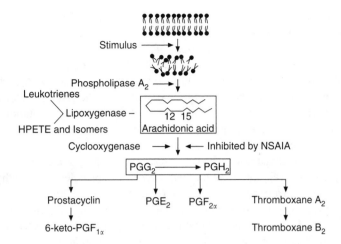

FIGURE 15.3 Arachidonic acid cascade and sites of nonsteroidal anti-inflammatory drug action.
Note: For more in-depth explanation of the cascade see J.G. Hardman, L.E. Limbird, and A. G. Gilman (Eds.)
(2001), *Goodman and Gilman's The Pharmacological Basis of Therapeutics*, 10th ed., Chapter 26. New York:
McGraw-Hill.

irreversibly (covalent) acetylating an active-site serine residue. Aspirin is distinctive among other
NSAIDs in that, the latter, function as *competitive inhibitors*. COX is a necessary enzyme involved
in the production of inflammatory mediators such as prostaglandins and leukotrienes when the
membrane is damaged (Figure 15.3). Unfortunately, these over-the-counter remedies do not possess
sufficient potency to adequately deal with the severe joint inflammation that accompanies disorders
such as arthritis. In addition, painful gastric side effects are all too common with stronger, alternative
medications such as Naproxen® (the result of COX-1 inhibition).

The introduction of recombinant DNA technology during the past 20 years has altered radically
our approach to drug discovery and has had a fundamental impact on how drug targets are selected.
On the basis of studies carried out during the early 1990s, it was discovered that there are at least
two isozymes of COX. COX-1 is apparently involved primarily in protecting the stomach lining
and performing other protective functions. COX-2, on the other hand, is the form that initiates
the arachidonic cascade producing prostaglandins and leukotrienes. Aspirin and other similar pain
relievers appear to have the capacity to inhibit both forms of the enzyme—hence their *damaging* as
well as *ameliorating* effects.

A major shortcoming of the 20 anti-inflammatory drugs that preceded the COX-2 inhibitors, the
NSAIDs, which included ibuprofen and aspirin, was that they suppressed both enzymes causing the
well-known side effect of GI damage. In fact, 7,500–15,000 deaths a year have been attributed to
NSAID's side effects. Because GI toxicity is associated with inhibition of COX-1, attempts were
made to develop drugs with more selective action on COX-2.

The power of molecular biology, which was not available 25 years ago, to impact a discipline
can be illustrated by the development of COX-2 inhibitors. Within a decade of the cloning of constitutive and inducible COX isozymes, two drug companies launched selective COX-2 inhibitors
(rofecoxib and celecoxib). Celecoxib (Celebrex®) was FDA approved in 1998 to treat osteoarthritis
and rheumatoid arthritis. Rofecoxib (Vioxx®) was approved in May 1999 to treat osteoarthritis,
acute pain, and dysmenorrhea. They were both marketed as a safer alternative to traditional pain
relievers such as Advil® and Aleve®. The 1999 sales for the two drugs were $1.5 billion and $373
million, respectively. Worldwide sales of Vioxx in 2003 rose to $2.5 billion. Clinical studies indi-
cated a significant reduction in GI perforation, ulceration, or bleeding with the COX-2 inhibitors,
as predicted. The recognition of multiple COX isoforms has had one of the greatest impacts on the
development of NSAIDs since the original synthesis of aspirin more than a century ago.

Regardless of the early enthusiasm over Vioxx® and the application of molecular biology to its development, Merck Pharmaceutical was forced to pull the drug from the market on September 30, 2004, after concerns that it *increased risk of stroke and acute myocardial infarction* were confirmed. The move came after a clinical trial linked the arthritis drug to these potentially fatal conditions. This was not the first time there was evidence linking Vioxx® to heart attack. A study earlier in 2004 showed that patients taking more than 25 mg a day had triple the risk for heart problems. These results indicate that despite the allure of molecular biology, it has its limitations. It has become apparent that the physiologic and pathophysiologic functional elements of these two isoenzymes are far more complex than comprehended.

Despite the problems associated with classical screening programs, they have, nevertheless, continued to yield numerous novel, important biologically active molecules. Among the most important recent examples is the discovery and development of drugs for the treatment of *hypercholesteremia* (see Chapter 13). In the early 1950s, scientists at Merck had begun researching the biosynthesis of cholesterol and by 1956 had demonstrated that mevalonic acid could be converted into cholesterol. In fact, the formation of mevalonic acid via 3-hydroxy-3-methylglutaryl-coenzyme A reductase was subsequently found to be the rate limiting step in cholesterol synthesis. In the 1970s, Merck scientists set up a cell culture assay in an attempt to identify substances that could inhibit the enzyme. In 1979, an inhibitor, lovastatin, was isolated from the fungus *Aspergillus terreus*. Following clinical trials, the drug was made available to selected patients with *severe* hypercholesteremia in 1982 under the trade name Mevacor. In 1987, the FDA approved its use for patients in the general population who had *high* cholesterol levels. Over the next decade, a second generation of inhibitors that had fewer GI side effects was developed.

In the past, most pharmaceutical companies maintained their own in-house facilities for screening drugs in whole animals. Today, with an emphasis on minimizing the use of experimental animals and their attendant cost, many companies "farm out" their drug leads to smaller companies that specialize in certain types of screening. Furthermore, with the advent of molecular pharmacology, companies can now screen drugs not initially in animals but, alternatively, on isolated receptors. Here again, there are companies that specialize in this service. It is only after a candidate drug has demonstrated desirable characteristics that it will undergo further evaluation in isolated tissues or organs as well as whole animals. In this manner, thousands of candidate drugs can be assessed at their target end point, without requiring the use of animals.

Increasingly, drug discovery is taking advantage of mechanistic, *in vitro* assays to broaden the search for therapeutic compounds. Examples include leukotriene B receptors, ionotropic excitatory amino acid receptors, epidermal growth factor receptors, histamine receptors, interleukin receptors, tyrosine kinase, as well as numerous others where affinity as well as inhibitory constants can be determined. An advantage of *in vitro* assays is that they are able to be adapted to allow high-throughput screening (HTS). For example, the NCI, which first began screening compounds as potential anticancer drugs back in the 1960s, used to evaluate hundreds of drugs a year; now it can do thousands. High-throughput screening facilities offer the potential to readily screen hundreds of thousands of candidate drugs per year with robotics.

The database generated from high-throughput screening, when combined with other relevant information, can provide a powerful method for the identification of trends in QSARs. In addition, this approach has had an impact on the very nature of the drug discovery process. Historically, pharmacology and drug discovery have been driven by the availability of a lead compound that suggested a specific receptor or binding site and a therapeutic potential if the activity was augmented or inhibited. Increasingly, this scenario is being *reversed*, with the discovery of the drug targets first (e.g., receptors) stimulating the search for appropriate agonists and antagonists.

Sequencing of the human genome, which was completed in April 2003, witnessed the dawn of a new era in drug discovery, one in which putative, novel members of specific classes of target proteins (e.g., receptors, enzymes, kinases, and ion channels) could be identified readily on the basis of *in silico* searches of public and proprietary DNA databases. The use of bioinformatics allows identification of putative novel target class entities before their biological significance may even be known. This "reverse pharmacology" approach to target identification has probably been applied most successfully to the identification of novel G-protein-coupled receptors (GPCR). Historically, this class of target has proved extremely predictable and it is estimated that some 45–60% of drug series in any modern day pharmacopoeia exert their actions either directly or indirectly via GPCRs. Therefore, it is not surprising that the drug industry has embraced this class so enthusiastically. Of the ~30,000 genes encoded by the human genome, ~600–1000 are estimated to be GPCRs.

Opportunities in the screening process provided by access to a "pure" supply of a drug target (e.g., receptor) include the possibility of identifying a specific drug without the prior availability of a specific lead compound. For example, the metabotropic glutamate receptor family appears to be a promising therapeutic target for which specific ligands have not been identified for any of the seven cloned receptor subtypes. However, potentially restricting the application of increasing knowledge of drug targets is the intention of some groups to patent the relevant genes, their expression systems, and their use within assays for drug discovery. Within the excitatory amino acid group of receptors alone, patents have been processed for the use of ionotropic receptors in general, as well as NMDA and metabotropic glutamate receptors.

With the capacity for high volume mass screening, the availability of new substances to screen is becoming the rate limiting factor in drug discovery. Because synthetic chemists are not able to keep up with demand, drug companies have turned to other strategies such as the vast supplies of marine and plant resources. In addition, the pharmaceutical industry has committed substantial resources of its own to an alternative strategy of drug discovery, namely *rational drug design.*

Rational drug design has been defined as "a reasoned approach to developing medicines." This involves both an understanding of the molecular pathophysiology of the disease process as well as the molecular and structural nature of the target molecule. Biological approaches to rational drug design exploits an understanding of disease pathogenesis, while structural approaches to rational drug design describes the application of the tools of structural biology to pharmaceutical development.

BIOLOGICAL APPROACHES TO DRUG DESIGN

STROKE

One area that illustrates drug development predicated on an understanding of the underlying disease pathogenesis is the treatment of stroke. Stroke is the third leading cause of death in the United States, killing approximately 150,000 people annually. In addition, another 400,000 stroke victims survive, but only a fortunate third of these are left with little or no physical or mental impairment. Approximately 80% of all strokes occur when a blood vessel becomes blocked by a clot that interrupts blood flow to a region of the brain and induces localized ischemia. The remaining 20% of strokes are caused by rupture of a blood vessel. Among the cascade of deleterious events initiated by a stroke of the first type is a deadly influx of calcium ions into nerve cells.

When a thrombotic type of stroke occurs, ischemic nerve cells rapidly deplete their energy supplies and can no longer maintain a normal resting membrane potential. As a consequence, the cells burst open their stores of "excitatory" amino acids (e.g., glutamate) that activate calcium ion channels in adjacent neurons by interacting with NMDA and AMPA receptors. The subsequent elevation of intraneuronal calcium drives a number of calcium-dependent processes into excess (e.g., calcium-dependent enzymes such as protein kinases and phosphokinases). A consequence of this hypermetabolic state is the formation of free radicals that are believed to propagate the degenerative effect.

Among the drug strategies currently being pursued to arrest this process is the development of neuroprotective drugs that, if given soon enough (within the first several hours), will hopefully prevent the inflow of calcium or reverse cell-membrane destruction. For example, in view of the fact that glutamate (as well as glycine and polyamines) can activate calcium channels, research is currently underway to develop effective antagonists of these substances that are free of significant side effects. Unfortunately, to date, clinical trials of such antagonists have been associated with patients developing hallucinations. As it turns out, this is not particularly surprising, however, since the recreational drug of abuse phencyclidine, which is also known to bind to a site within the NMDA receptor, also induces psychosis. Therefore, it may prove difficult to separate these properties.

Citicholine is a drug being developed from a somewhat different perspective. It is aimed at reversing cell-membrane destruction by supplying the membrane bilayer component choline to the brain. Phosphatidylcholine, the backbone of the cell membrane, breaks down as nerve cells are damaged, so, in theory, delivering excess choline to the brain may facilitate membrane repair. In addition, choline may also function to "mop-up" free fatty acids that could be oxidized to generate free radicals. It remains to be seen whether this approach will be successful, but it does illustrate how multiple drug strategies can be developed to attack a single medical disorder.

ANTISENSE DEOXYNUCLEOTIDES, RIBOZYMES, AND RNA INTERFERENCE

The controlled expression of genes is a cornerstone in the regulation of growth and development of cells and organisms. The transcription of DNA into RNA and its subsequent translation into a peptide is a fundamental requirement in all living beings. Interruption in the controlled progression from one step to the next can have dramatic consequences to a cell. Although numerous anticancer drugs have operated in this mode for decades, a new generation of drug candidates are being investigated, which function via significantly new mechanisms. One of the more novel means of modifying gene expression is to specifically target an RNA molecule and inactivate it, thereby preventing expression of its encoded message. Three theoretical ways of accomplishing this objective involve antisense deoxynucleotides, ribozymes, and RNA interference.

Antisense technology allows researchers to devise strategies to reduce the expression of specific proteins in cells and whole animals without having to create transgenics (see below). Using Watson and Crick base-pairing rules, it is possible to design oligonucleotides that will selectively hybridize with mRNAs for specific gene products, thus inhibiting the translation of mRNA and reducing protein expression. This specificity can be exploited for design of therapeutic agents and selective inhibitors of gene expression for research applications. The use of antisense technologies provides the scientist with a means of specifically inhibiting gene expression without having to manipulate the genome. Antisense molecules have shown activity against viral genes and may have potential use in the treatment of cancer. Several candidates are undergoing clinical trial.

The information necessary to produce proteins in cells is contained in genes. Specific genes contain information to produce specific proteins. The information required for the human body to produce all proteins is contained in the human genome and its collection of approximately 30,000 genes. Genes are composed of DNA that contains information about when and how much of which protein to produce, depending on what function is to be performed.

The DNA molecule is a "double helix," a duplex of entwined strands (see appendix for a review of its discovery by *Watson and Crick*). In each duplex, the bases or nucleotides (Adenine, Thymidine, Guanosine, and Cytosine) are weakly bound or "paired" by hydrogen bonds to complimentary nucleotides on the other strand (A to T, G to C). Such highly specific complimentary base pairing is the essence of information transfer from DNA to its intermediary, messenger RNA (mRNA, where U replaces T), that carries the information, spelled out by the specific sequences of bases, necessary for the cell to produce a specific protein.

During transcription of information from DNA into mRNA, the two complimentary strands of the DNA partly uncoil; the "sense" strand separates from the "antisense" strand. The "antisense" strand of DNA is used as a template for transcribing enzymes that assemble mRNA (transcription), which, in the process, produces a copy of the "sense" strand. Then, mRNA migrates into the cell where other cellular structures called ribosomes read the encoded information, its mRNA's base sequence, and in so doing, string together amino acids to form a specific protein. This process is called "translation."

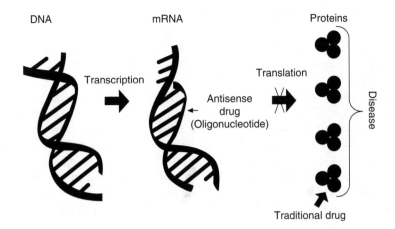

FIGURE 15.4 Mechanism of action of antisense drugs.

Antisense drugs are complimentary strands of small segments of mRNA. To create antisense drugs, nucleotides are linked together in short chains (called oligonucleotides). Each antisense drug is designed to inhibit production of the protein encoded by the target mRNA. By acting at this early stage in the disease-causing process to prevent the production of a disease-causing protein, antisense drugs have the potential to provide greater therapeutic benefit than traditional drugs that do not act until the disease-causing protein has already been produced (Figure 15.4).

Perhaps even more esoteric than antisense nucleic acids are RNA molecules that are able to specifically cleave other RNA molecules. Until several years ago, it was generally thought that all cellular processes were dictated by DNA through the structure of polypeptides that performed all the functions. During studies conducted on RNA, it was discovered that some RNA strands had catalytic properties. These nonprotein biocatalysts are referred to as *ribozymes* and *combine* the properties of antisense RNA with the ability to cleave target RNA.

An early hint of such a phenomenon occurred when the RNA "cofactor" of ribonuclease P was found capable of catalyzing the specific cleavage of pre-tRNAs in the absence of protein. However, the first real report of the ability of RNA to act as a catalyst was made from Thomas Cech's laboratory in 1982, for which he subsequently shared the Nobel Prize (1989). Cech and colleagues examined the removal of a nucleotide sequence form the preribosomal RNA of *Tetrahymena* and found that the reaction was autocatalytic for the rRNA itself. Eventually, an L 19 form of ribozyme (from the group I introns) was the first ribozyme discovered. (There are currently five classes of ribozymes: (1) the group I intron, (2) Rnase P, (3) the hammerhead ribozymes, (4) the hairpin ribozymes, and (5) the hepatitis delta virus ribozymes.) These types of studies have generated significant interest in ribozymes as potential therapeutic agents for controlling gene expression. Scientists have since discovered more than 500 ribozymes in a diverse range of organisms and have found that they share many similarities with their more widespread cousins, enzymes.

An example of the type of research that is currently being carried out deals with the *in vitro* evaluation of ribozymes on gene expression. Hammerhead ribozymes have been shown to have the ability to attack the coding region of mRNA of interleukin 6 (IL-6). In this manner, theoretically, down regulation of IL-6 may be a potential treatment of those diseases in which IL-6 overexpression is involved.

Although ribozymes have been shown to work *in vitro* in cellular assays, there are few reports demonstrating their efficacy *in vivo*. One such success utilized the rabbit model of interleukin 1 (IL-1)-induced arthritis. In this model, IL-1 is believed to generate the formation of a proteinase mediator called stromelysin that participates in the inflammatory condition. The intra-articular administration of ribozymes directed against stromelysin mRNA has been reported to produce a reduction in the message for this mediator in synovial fluid.

In 1998, researchers at the University of Florida demonstrated that a custom-made ribozyme could successfully cleave the faulty (bad) mRNA in a rat model of retinitis pigmentosa (RP). RP has a frequency of approximately 1 in 3000 Americans. As the disease progresses, night vision and peripheral vision are affected, and ultimately all sight is lost. Currently, there is no way to halt the destruction of sight.

In RP, a mutant gene codes for the formation of a protein that damages the eye's light-sensitive rod cells. Approximately 40% of people with RP have the "autosomal-dominant" form, that is, they inherited a defective gene from one parent who has the disease, but also received a normal gene copy from the other parent. The University of Florida research targets the autosomal-dominant form of the disease in their rat model. Significant protection was observed for up to 3 months.

One of the shortcomings of ribozymes is that they are short single-stranded RNA moieties with a simple secondary structure; it is possible that their use in gene therapy could be limited because they could be highly susceptible to cellular nucleases. Present research is aimed at producing ribozymes that are more resistant to degradation.

RNA Interference (RNAi)

In December of 2002, the editors of *Science* described RNAi as the "breakthrough of the year." Several companies are now exploring RNAi opportunities for drug therapy and drug target validation. The value of the drug discovery market bases on RNAi has been assessed at $650 million in 2005, increasing to $1 billion in 2010 and $1.5 billion in 2015. The hype has thus begun.

The therapeutic premise RNAi—that RNAs involved in disease can be selectively blocked with drugs—is not new. As described above, for more than 10 years, scientists have tried to develop "antisense" techniques to silence genes that contribute to disease. Antisense drugs are *single-stranded* chemically modified DNA molecules that are designed to bind directly to disease-related molecules and disable them. However, antisense technology has proven to be a problematic technology; only one antisense drug (Vitravene) to treat eye infections in AIDS patients has been approved by the FDA.

Like antisense, RNAi works by interfering with RNA, but there are important differences. The term RNAi was coined in 1998 by researchers on their discovery that naturally occurring double-stranded RNA molecules were quite potent inhibitors of a targeted gene in *C. elegans*. Their functioning is somehow related to normal endogenous pathways for development; *a natural mechanism to silence genes*. Although the technique was originally unsatisfactory in mammalian cells, the problem was overcome by trimming the RNA molecules to 21–23 nucleotides. These smaller RNAis evaded the immune system to disable mRNAs in mammalian cells. It was subsequently demonstrated that RNAis could stop HIV infections in cell cultures, thereby demonstrating the technology's clinical potential.

Membrane Fusion

A particularly timely example of biologically based drug design involves a novel strategy directed towards treating viral infections. Instead of developing an antiviral drug to attack a virus after it has infected a cell (the more traditional approach), compounds are being developed that are aimed at blocking the virus from entering the cell in the first place. Researchers are focusing on the process by which a virus fuses with the membrane of a cell permitting it to inject its genetic material. Viral proteins from influenza virus, HIV-1, and Ebola virus are composed of two distinct subunits, namely a receptor binding domain (gp120) and a fusion competent subunit (gp41).

The process of *membrane fusion* is a ubiquitous process that can occur in all eukaryotic cells but has particular significance in virally transmitted diseases such as HIV. Research in HIV-1 fusion with human lymphocytes has revealed that the virus contains an oligomeric *complex* of glycoproteins, gp120 and gp41, on its surface, which play a central role in the fusion and transference process. In its native resting state, a heterooligomer of two gp120s and two gp41s is held together by noncovalent protein–protein interactions. A portion of gp41, known as the *"fusion domain,"* is buried within this complex and mediates fusion with cells.

When an HIV-1 virus encounters a human lymphocyte displaying a CD4 receptor on its cell surface, for example, the gp120 oligomer binds to the CD4 receptor. That binding initiates a series of very important events: (1) a *conformational change* occurs within the gp120–gp41 complex, (2) that conformational change triggers an intramolecular rearrangement of domains within the gp41 that releases a "fusion protein" from its bound configuration, and (3) the formation of a *"membrane attack complex"* that permits insertion of the fusion peptide into the host cell membrane occurs.

Researchers studying the viral fusion process recognized that two coiled regions in gp41 were highly conserved among all HIVs, so they synthesized a number of peptides containing this region's respective peptide structure. Assay of these peptide fragments demonstrated that one was particularly potent in selectively inhibiting the fusion event of native, intact HIV-1 virus to lymphocytes. Apparently, the drug candidate binds to the other coiled region of gp41 and prevents the membrane attack complex from forming when gp120 binds to the CD4 receptor. The company developing this potential drug is also utilizing a proprietary computerized antiviral searching technology to identify key sequences within fusion proteins in other medically important viruses, thus also utilizing a structural approach to drug design.

STRUCTURAL APPROACHES TO DRUG DESIGN

BACKGROUND

As mentioned previously, one of the first steps in the process of drug development is the identification of lead compounds. These compounds generally have affinity for the target molecule as identified after extensive screening using receptor binding or biological assays, and are then modified to possess pharmacologically useful properties. These traditional methods of drug discovery are now being supplemented by a more direct approach made possible, in part, by increased understanding of the molecular interactions that underlie diseases.

The new approach is referred to as *structure-based* drug design, which is really a form of reverse pharmacology. The starting point is not necessarily the drug, but can be, alternatively, its molecular target in the body. If the three-dimensional structure of a substance known to be involved in a disease can be ascertained, then conceivably a chemical that interacts with a key region producing altered function could be designed. For example, the catalytic site of a viral enzyme essential for replication might be designed. In fact, many contemporary research programs are focused on the development of *inhibitors of HIV protease*, a key enzyme in HIV replication. Figure 15.5 shows a representative, computer-generated interrelationship between a candidate ligand and the binding domain of the protease. Protease inhibitors work by preventing cleavage of viral polyproteins into active proteins, which takes place during HIV's insidious and complicated replication process. The drug binds to the enzyme's active site, blocking cleavage of the polyprotein.

INHIBITORS OF PURINE NUCLEOSIDE PHOSPHORYLASE

The theoretical advantages of structure-based methodology include the creation of more lead compounds at less expense. The analogy has been made that this approach is similar to designing an effective key if the shape and arrangement of tumblers in a lock are already known. Presumably, because the final designed drug is "custom-tailored" to its target, it will be more specific and less toxic. An example of such an approach is research carried out during the 1980s dealing with the design of inhibitors of the enzyme purine nucleoside phosphorylase (PNP).

PNP normally operates in the "purine salvage pathway" of cells and is responsible for cleaving nucleosides into their respective purine and sugar components. Unfortunately, PNP can also cleave certain anticancer and antiviral drugs that are synthetic mimics of endogenous nucleosides.

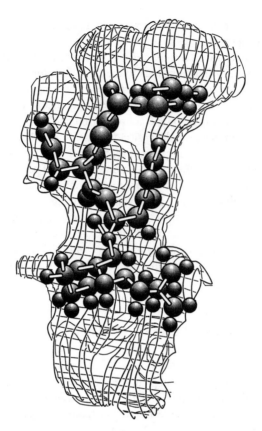

FIGURE 15.5   Computer-generated modeling of the relationship of a protease inhibitor with a binding domain.

An example is the antiviral drug 2',3'-dideoxyinosine (ddI) used in the treatment of AIDS. A successful candidate for inhibiting PNP was achieved in less than 3 years by a small group of chemists who prepared approximately 60 compounds aimed at blocking the purine binding site. The result was a PNP inhibitor 100 times more effective than the best inhibitor found by traditional methods of drug discovery. In traditional practice, the development of enzyme inhibitors often takes more than 10 years and can cost tens of millions of dollars for the screening of hundreds or thousands of candidates.

X-RAY CRYSTALLOGRAPHY

X-ray crystallography is the oldest and most widely applied technology for determining macromolecular structure to atomic resolution. Three-dimensional atomic models of proteins and nucleic acids are the basis of much of our modern understanding of biology and medicine. Until relatively recent times, receptors were hypothetical macromolecules whose existence was postulated on the basis of pharmacological experiments. However, during the 1970s and 1980s new methods became available for obtaining pure samples of many receptors as well as insight into their structure. For example, advances in molecular biology have led to the cloning and expression of many receptors. In addition, improvements in x-ray crystallography revealed more insight into their structure. In this technique, pure receptors in their crystalline form are bombarded with x-rays; the crystal defracts the x-rays according to its molecular structure, creating a pattern of spots on photographic film or on newer types of electronic detectors. While x-ray crystallography has proven to be a major technology in determining structure, newer techniques such as *nuclear magnetic resonance* (NMR) spectroscopy and neutron diffraction are also being utilized.

Enzymes are often the targets of drugs, and thus proteins are of particular interest to pharmacologists. Knowing a protein's structure gives deep insight into its function. Understanding how proteins work, and what happens when they do not, is a key to uncovering the molecular basis of disease. In the application of structure-based rational drug design, analogs of natural substrates are modeled by computer graphics to the active site of the enzyme. The structure and geometry of the protein is generally well established at the atomic level through the use of x-ray diffraction techniques. The approach of rational drug design based on knowledge of target macromolecules is made all the more powerful by the ability to actually visualize the complex that is formed between the drug and enzyme. In this situation, there is the added bonus of actually seeing conformational changes that occur by virtue of the interaction.

The first successful exploitation of x-ray crystallography in drug discovery was the development of the antihypertensive drug captopril (an ACE inhibitor) in 1975. Although the investigators at the Squibb Institute for Medical Research (now Bristol-Myers Squibb) did not know the precise architecture of their target (angiotensin-converting enzyme), they utilized the known conformation of a closely related enzyme. This type of *homology* modeling is still presently utilized. For example, many models of the various G-protein coupled receptors have been built based on homology with bacterial rhodopsin, while models of human renin and HIV protease have been built from crystal structures of aspartyl proteinases.

THREE-DIMENSIONAL DATABASES AND RECOMBINANT PROTEIN ENGINEERING

When engineering a novel protein for large-scale production *in vitro*, structure of the protein itself is of critical importance. Any significant change in protein structure may, in fact, yield a functionally inactive molecule or a protein with significantly reduced biological activity.

The primary structure of a protein is defined by its amino acid sequence, the secondary structure by the presence of alpha helixes or beta sheet (pairs of chains lying side by side), the ternary structure by covalent bonds between adjacent protein stretches, and the quaternary structure by the association of multiple subunits in a large multimodular protein complex.

A number of expression systems are used to express a recombinant protein (e.g., bacteria, yeast, insect cells, and mammalian cells), but not all yield proteins identical to their human counterpart. While most secondary and tertiary structures may be faithfully reproduced, quaternary structures and posttranslational modifications (glycosylation, acetylation) are often differentially undertaken in different cell types from different species. If any of these properties is critical for the overall activity of the recombinant protein, such characteristics have to be faithfully reproduced in the engineered protein to obtain a powerfully active molecule.

Since Christian B. Anfinson and colleagues demonstrated during the 1950s and 60s that the amino acid sequence of a protein directs its folding, significant research has focused on understanding the molecular basis of the protein folding process and on determining the inherent information in protein primary structures to predict protein tertiary structure. The importance of structural biology is illustrated by the awarding of 10 Nobel Prizes in this area since 1962. Recipients of the award include the following: the first three-dimensional structure of a biopolymer was the DNA model built by J.D. Watson and F.H.C. Crick in 1953 taking into account fiber diffraction data provided by M.H.F. Wilkins, the first three-dimensional protein structures (myoglobin and hemoglobin) were determined by M.F. Perutz and J.C. Kendrew, and the structure of the first membrane-bound protein was resolved by J. Deisenhofer, R. Haber, and H. Mechel.

Medicinal chemists have long recognized the potential of searching three-dimensional chemical databases to aid in the process of designing drugs for known, or hypothetical, receptor sites. Several databases are well-known such as the Cambridge Structural Database that contains nearly 90,000 structures of small molecules. In addition, the Protein Data Bank (PDB) and the Nucleic Acid Data Bank (NDB) contain the crystal coordinates of proteins and other large macromolecules. The IMB

Jeva Image Library of Biological Macromolecules provides access to all structures deposited at the PDB and the NDB as well as basic information on biological macromolecules.

The terms *bioinformatics* and *cheminformatics* refer to the use of computational methods in the study of biology and chemistry. Information from DNA or protein sequences, protein structure, and chemical structure is used to build models of biochemical systems or models of the interaction of a biochemical system with a small molecule (e.g., a drug). There are mathematical and statistical methods for analysis, public databases, and literature associated with each of these disciplines. However, there is substantial value in considering the interaction between these areas and in building computational models that integrate data from both sources. In the most general sense, integrating bioinformatics and cheminformatics leads to models that relate features of biological systems (sequences, protein structures, motifs) to features of the chemical structures, including small organic molecules (e.g., drugs) that interact with them. This information is useful for drug design and discovery in order to identify *pharmacophores*.

The three-dimensional orientation of the key regions of a drug that are crucially important for molecular recognition and binding are termed the pharmacophore. A pharmacophore was first defined by Paul Ehrlich in 1909 as "a molecular framework that carries (phorous) the essential features for a drug's (pharmacon's) biological activity." In 1977, this definition was updated to "a set of structural features in a molecule that is recognized at a receptor site and is responsible for that molecule's biological activity."

In modern computational chemistry, pharmacophores are used to define the essential features of one or more molecules with the same biological activity (i.e., an ensemble of interactive functional groups with a defined geometry). The game is to find structural and chemical complementaries between "the drug" and "the receptor" in the screening process.

Investigators can then search databases using a query for fragments that contain the pharmacophoric functional groups in the proper three-dimensional orientation. There are several reasons to find compounds with similar biological activity to known compounds: new compounds may have beneficial effects at different doses; they may be taken up more readily by different tissues; they may have fewer deleterious effects; they may have a different biological half-life; and they may be produced more efficiently.

For example, such a process was carried out with caffeic acid phenethyl ester, an inhibitor of HIV-1 integrase. A computer search of 200,000 compounds at the National Cancer Institute yielded 19 candidates containing this pharmacophore that demonstrated *in vitro* activity. A statistically significant correlation was found between the presence of the pharmacophore and inhibitory potency; using these fragments as building blocks, completely novel structures may be constructed through assembly and pruning. Pharmaceutical companies have developed substantial databases for their compound files to help prioritize candidates for screening.

Although observations extracted from the databases of experimentally known structures are an extremely useful empirical guide to the design of modified proteins and peptides, current biocomputational approaches to drug design are, nevertheless, limited by the relatively small subset of proteins that have been structurally characterized. Fortunately, proteins belong to a limited number of structural families whose members have very similar three-dimensional structures, thus allowing comparative modeling approaches to be used in developing databases. Various protein design software tools have been and are being developed to evaluate secondary or tertiary structures from protein sequences and to design proteins with predetermined functions and, or, physical properties.

The procedure to predict protein structure has evolved from using probability profiles on the preferential localization of residues, to relying heavily on protein structure databases to define topological organization and three-dimensional relationships among proteins. The prediction of protein structure rests on a knowledge-based approach that identifies analogies in secondary structures, motifs, domains, or ligand interactions between a protein being modeled with homologous proteins whose structures are available.

In addition to x-ray diffraction and NMR, which are direct techniques, methods based on the calculation of predicted three-dimensional structures of molecules in the range of 3–50 amino acids based on energy considerations are under rapid development. These approaches use what are commonly called *molecular dynamics and energy minimization equations* to specify the most probable conformation of polypeptides and small proteins. Often, when combined with information from other sources, such as x-ray crystallography or NMR studies, they have been demonstrated to be quite useful; however, when standing alone, their power and the accuracy of their predictive capability remains to be seen.

The multidisciplinary approach described above has been used to study protein folding phenomena and protein SAR for protein engineering endeavors, as well as protein-based and pharmacophore drug design. The validity of the predicted structure obviously depends on many factors, including the accuracy of the structures determined by the various analytical techniques, the percentage of homology in proteins used as templates, the rules used to translate amino acid alignments into geometric relationships between the template and the protein to be modeled, and the energy constraints of the resulting conformation. New discoveries regarding receptor structure, coupled with rational strategies in molecular biology and biochemical experiments, promise to speed the development of new and better drugs.

COMBINATORIAL CHEMISTRY

One of the rate-limiting steps in the drug discovery process has always been the laborious synthesis of new entities in which a chemist makes one compound at a time. If a drug company wanted to make more compounds, it had basically one option—increase its research budget and hire more chemists. Today, because of numerous economic factors, companies are discouraged from simply increasing the payroll. However, increased competition demands that medicinal chemistry departments still continue to produce new chemical entities. The problem of new lead development has, ironically, been exacerbated in recent years by developments in molecular biology and high-throughput screening, which enable companies to screen entire libraries of archived compounds in a matter of months. One solution to this bottleneck has been the development of rapid automated procedures for the synthesis of organic molecules that can be subsequently screened.

In simple terms, *combinatorial chemistry* is the process whereby thousands of compounds (a library), systematic variants of a parent chemical structure, are synthesized. Although combinatorial chemistry generally refers to a single process, in reality it comprises several integrated intellectual and technological processes: computer-aided drug design and combinatorial chemistry library design, automated solid/solution-phase organic synthesis, and high-throughput screening techniques. Applied together, the synergy of these processes has been a major leap for drug development and basic medical research.

Another advancement in sample management has been the miniaturization of assays to the point where volumes of 10 μl are routine and run in 384 wells and 1536 wells. The ability to rapidly identify high-quality lead compounds that are suitable for validation *in vitro* and *in vivo* has changed dramatically in the last decade, and it has been estimated that the frequency of leads identified from primary screens has increased by 1–2 order of magnitude.

Major advancements in compound library synthesis have contributed to streamlining the drug-discovery process by increasing vastly the number and quality of small molecule compounds available for screening. Pharmaceutical chemists can now create and test libraries of thousands, if not millions, of compounds for pharmacological properties relatively quickly. To put the results of the processes in perspective, consider that the possible number of products is defined by the number of different reagents raised to the number of synthesis steps. Therefore, for a three-step process involving ten different reagents, the theoretical yield is 10^3 or 10,000 unique chemical combinations. For a simple pentamer peptide there are 20^5 or 3,200,000 possible combinations.

These new procedures were developed during the early 1990s and have revolutionized the rate at which new compounds can be synthesized. The first stage basically involves the *random* formation of low molecular weight molecules (i.e., 500 Da) via automated technology (the search for the pharmacophore begins). This strategy is based on "the numbers game" (the belief that the more compounds that are screened the more likely it is that a "hit" will be found) based on simple chance. This approach was pioneered by scientists at Affymax (a biotechnology company). The large numbers of molecules that can be prepared in this way are providing new sources of novel compounds to be screened.

Instead of making one compound per week, 100 or more can be produced in a day. Combinatorial chemistry has expanded the size and diversity of the collections of many large pharmaceutical companies to >1 million compounds. One important advantage of making *new* pharmaceuticals is that they are not "me-too" drugs and can be protected by patent rights; *an absolute requirement of drug companies*. The utility of these techniques is being focused with the use of directional library design, particularly those designed around molecules with characteristics proven to be developable as, for example, benzodiazepine libraries.

A second key element to evolve in combinatorial chemistry is the introduction of a *rational* design or bias library. Despite the huge number of potential drug-like small molecules, with a molecular weight of less than 500, that can be synthesized, it appears unreasonable to assume that comprehensive representation with a "random" library will necessarily be achieved. Even relatively large compound libraries, designed with attention to molecular diversity, yield only a very small fraction of possible compounds. An example of a biased library would be a structure-based library developed around x-ray diffraction data of a ligand/protein complex, or based around an important protein motif. It is believed that a marriage of the above two elements is an optimal strategy for drug discovery.

An example of using the combinatorial approach to drug discovery is the attempt to produce a "*miniprotein*" version of erythropoietin (EPO). As mentioned previously, EPO stimulates the body to produce red blood cells. EPO is widely used for patients with anemias, kidney diseases, cancer, or AIDS and has annual sales of approximately $1 billion. By applying combinatorial chemistry, a new 20-amino acid molecule was discovered, which successfully mimics the 165 amino acid EPO, *in vitro*. Of particular interest is the fact that the sequence of amino acids in the small molecule is unrelated to that of the larger EPO. This research also suggests that it may be possible to make *nonprotein* versions of other important proteins such as *insulin* and avoid the need for injections.

Combinatorial libraries are generally created in the laboratory by one of two automated methods—*split synthesis* or *parallel synthesis*. In *split synthesis*, monomers of the starting structure are attached to small plastic bead-like particles. In a series of successive, repetitive steps, the initial monomer-bead complexes are randomly *mixed* and coupled with a subsequent population of monomers, creating dimers, trimers, and so forth, by employing the conditions necessary for appropriate organic reactions. This process can be continued until the desired combinatorial library has been assembled. Diversity is achieved by using separate reactions, so the components will have an equal chance to add a new building block to a site and then mixing the compounds together again. Split synthesis greatly simplifies the isolation and identification of active agents because the beads are large enough to be observed visually and separated mechanically. Combinatorial libraries can also be made by parallel synthesis, in which different compounds are synthesized in separate vessels (without remixing), often in an automated fashion. Unlike split synthesis, which requires a solid support, parallel synthesis can be done either on a solid support or in solution.

Regardless of which method is used, the large numbers of drugs developed are usually subjected to screening in automated receptor binding assays. According to one company, their high-throughput system allows two chemists to synthesize up to 1 million compounds per year. Any drug demonstrating significant affinity will proceed to the next step of evaluation. At this point in time, it is not known if the drug is an agonist or an antagonist. All that can be measured is a binding constant. It is not until the drug is assessed in some kind of "biological" system, such as isolated ion channels, that information about the nature and "effectiveness" of the drug can be determined. Success at this level may qualify the drug for evaluation in whole animal studies. Recent developments in combinatorial chemistry have been concentrated on the use of small organic building blocks, such as benzodiazepines, in order to create libraries with more drug-like qualities.

To increase the chances of finding leads, some combinatorial chemistry companies have specialized in producing very large libraries. Often, combinatorial chemistry gives small companies chemical libraries that are on the same order of magnitude as those once the domain of only the largest drug companies. With these libraries and their proprietary technologies, small companies can leverage profitable arrangements with larger companies that can include substantial up-front and milestone payments as well as long-term royalties. These arrangements, in turn, give the small companies access to biological targets and the pharmaceutical infrastructure necessary to take drug candidates through development, clinical testing, regulatory approval, and marketing.

One new wrinkle on the combinatorial strategy involves a process referred to as *combinatorial biosynthesis*. In this situation, bacterial gene expression is altered in the hope of changing the structure and function of specific enzymes. For example, one class of potential bacteria-derived drugs is the polyketides that may have antibiotic, immunosuppressant, and anticancer activity. Bacteria produce polyketides with the help of a family of enzymes known as polyketide synthases (PHSs). To this point in time, most of the normally produced polyketides screened have shown little activity.

In order to increase the likelihood of bacteria forming new, active polyketides, scientists, working like combinatorial chemists, have *mixed and matched* PKS *genes* from different organisms to create 100 different bacterial clones with unique combinations of PKS genes. Although only 25 of these clones were found to produce unique compounds, 4 of them proved to be as effective as the reference drug. Although such results are encouraging, it remains to be seen if this methodology will prove useful in the future.

Antibody-Directed Drug Design

Antibodies are part of the armamentarium that physicians can use for the treatment of a range of human conditions. A few examples include injection of antibody that recognizes tumor necrosis factor to treat rheumatoid arthritis; the experimental use of monoclonal antibodies to treat metastatic cancer; injection of antibody that recognizes the antigen OKT3 to revert organ rejection after transplantation; and the use of sheep antibodies to bind the heart medication digoxin in case of an overdose. Physicians often prefer to use human antibodies, or at least animal antibodies, in which parts of the antibody have been replaced with the human equivalent to decrease the likelihood of an allergic reaction.

A century ago, Paul Ehrlich referred to antibodies as "magic bullets" and predicted that they would evolve into multipurpose tools for the treatment of various diseases. Since that time, scientists have explored their therapeutic potential. Polyclonal antibodies, mostly in the form of sera from immunized animals, have been used since the 1890s, principally to treat infectious diseases. Although they are rather effective, the broad clinical application of these antibodies was impeded by their inherent drawbacks. Aside from the molecule of interest, sera contain a multitude of different antibodies that might interfere with the desired activity, other proteins that might be harmful to the recipient, and, possibly, infectious agents. Only with the advent of two major milestones in immunology over the past few decades could antibody-based therapies make a significant leap forward.

Historically, researchers believed that the antibody "formed" on the antigen template; but in the 1950s, a theory of natural selection for antibody formation was formulated, whereby the antibody repertoire was genetically predetermined and the antigen triggered the selection and clonal expansion of selected antibody-producing cells.

The second milestone was the development of the hybridoma technique in 1975. While working in the laboratory of Cesar Milstein, Georges Kohler developed a method of somatic cell hybridization in order to successfully generate a continuous "hybridoma" cell line capable of producing *monoclonal antibodies* (Mabs) of defined specificity *in vitro*. Briefly, hybridoma technology involves the following steps:

1. An antigen is injected into a mouse. The mouse's immune system recognizes the antigen as being foreign and directs the spleen to produce specific antibodies to attack that antigen. The spleen is then removed and the antibody-producing B lymphocytes are collected.
2. Myeloma cells are isolated from a mouse tumor. These cells have the ability to reproduce continuously in the laboratory.
3. Spleen and tumor cells are mixed together with some fusing to form "hybridomas." All the cells are transferred to a medium in which the hybridoma cells can grow while the others die. The surviving hybridomas have the spleen cell's ability to produce antibodies and the tumor cell's ability to reproduce.
4. Each hybridoma is isolated and allowed to grow into a large colony of cells that produce a single Mab.
5. Each Mab can be screened for its ability to attack the original antigen and the hybridoma colonies producing the desired antibody are kept.

Since the introduction of this methodology, a plethora of hybridoma-derived monoclonal antibodies has been developed and used as diagnostic and research reagents and a few therapeutic drugs. The need for a successful large-scale Mab production technique is indicated by the growing commercial market for antibody-based products and the increased importance of *in vivo* diagnostic as well as therapeutic applications. According to market research, total sales of *in vivo* and *in vitro* Mab-based products reached approximately $8 billion in 1993, and this volume is expected to increase in subsequent years. Therefore, significant commercial production of Mabs is being emphasized. In one procedure, Mab-producing murine hybridomas are cultured in 40 L bioreactors.

Antibody-directed drug design is based on the concept that when a monoclonal antibody is raised against an antigen, a stereochemically *negative* image of the antigen is embedded in the structure and chemistry of the antibody's *hypervariable region*, a relatively small portion of the antibody comprised of peptides contributed in part by both the heavy and light chains of the immunoglobin. Significantly, the antigen could be the active site of an enzyme, a viral component, or the recognition or combing site of a drug receptor to name but a few. Obviously, the theoretical potential use of Mabs is quite substantial.

From the Mab containing the mirror image of the target macromolecule (Mab-1), a *positive* image can also be derived. This is accomplished by raising a second antibody (Mab-2) against the hypervariable region of the Ab-1. By virtue of its stereocomplementarity to the combining region of the Ab-1, a feature it shares with the original target antigen, it must, therefore, possess common structural and electrostatic characteristics. Though it may not be perfectly homologous with the target antigen, it should incorporate at least some of the essential physical disposition of key chemical groups.

Although hybridoma technology permits the production of relatively large supplies of an antibody, only the rat and mouse myeloma lines appear to be reliably stable in long-term tissue culture. Rodent monoclonals, however, have serious limitations when used as therapeutic agents in humans, especially in diseases requiring repetitive administration. For example, they are prone to *induce immune responses* to themselves (inducing human antimouse antibody), which can neutralize their effect and damage the kidneys. In addition, murine monoclonals have a short serum half-life in humans.

After the first significant results in the 1980s, and the attendant problems described above revealed, attempts were made to "humanize" the molecules and thereby reduce the immunogenecity of the antibodies. Researchers developed new techniques such as chimerazation and humanization (complementarity-determining region, or CDR, grafting).

The first *chimeric* monoclonal was introduced into the market in 1994 (ReoPro®), which was designed to prevent complications during coronary angioplasty. In Greek mythology, the Chimera was a fire-breathing monster with a lion's head, a goat's body, and the tail of a dragon. In the lexicon of antibodies, chimeras are antibodies constructed of disparate sections. They can be constructed in various ways. For example, to reduce the immunogenicity of the rodent variable region, *humanized Mabs* have been created. In this case, a rat/human antibody has been produced in which only the hypervariable regions are of rat origin (i.e., only the antigen-binding site rather than the entire variable domain was from the rodent). This results in a decreased immune response in humans since 90% of the human immune response is directed against constant domains and 10% against the variable domain. Chimerization also produces up to a sixfold increase in half-life. An alternative method, published in 1999, involves the fusion of active antibody fragments to polyethylene glycol molecules. The resulting conjugate has a much longer *in vivo* half-life and retains its antigen-binding activity.

After the introduction of ReoPro®, three antibodies were approved in 1997 and 1998. Remicade®, used to treat rheumatoid arthritis and Crohn's disease, is so far one of the blockbusters in the antibody field, generating revenue of $1.2 billion in 2002. It is a chimeric antibody that neutralizes tumor necrosis factor α and inhibits inflammation. In rheumatoid arthritis, this reduces swelling and pain in the joints and slows down joint destruction, improving the quality of life of patients considerably. The first fully human Mab was introduced in 2003 (Humira®); annual sales are expected to exceed the billion-dollar mark for this competitor to Remicade®. The two other FDA-approved drugs of the late 1990s, Zenapax® and Simulect®, block the Interleukin-2 signaling pathway, and both have proven to be efficacious in the prevention of kidney transplant rejection.

Although most of the marketed drugs target rheumatoid arthritis and Crohn's disease, the spectrum is starting to broaden.

In view of the persistent problems in making human monoclonals by conventional fusion techniques, *recombinant DNA technology* has become an important mode of human antibody production. Successful application of genetic engineering to Mabs has produced two drugs. The FDA approved Rituxan® in 1997 for the treatment of B-cell lymphomas and Herceptin® in 1998 for certain breast cancer tumors.

Generally, when a drug only works in 25% of the target population, it will get short shrift in the market place; however, when that drug is Herceptin® and is needed to treat an otherwise lethal metastatic breast cancer, the situation changes. Herceptin®, a humanized, unconjugatedmonoclonal antibody, is an almost ideal example of a pharmacogenetic triumph—the result of a directed research plan moving from a target gene in a particular population to a therapeutic agent.

Herceptin® binds to protein produced by the human epidermal growth factor receptor 2 gene (HER-2), also known as the *neu* oncogene. The HER-2 protein was known to be overexpressed in 25–30% of breast cancers and so was considered a viable potential drug target. The protein appears to enhance cell growth and division, contributing to tumor progression. Research has shown that women with HER-2-positive metastatic breast cancer have a more aggressive disease, greater likelihood of a recurrence, poorer prognosis, and approximately half the life expectancy of women with HER-2-negative breast cancer.

In many cases, Mabs that have proved efficacious as stand-alone treatments are being tested in a variety of combination therapies. Because Mabs have a different mode of action than tradional chemotherapies, they can have a significant additive effect in attacking various cancers when used in combination with these more traditional drugs. Clinical trials have shown that Herceptin® alone, but most especially in combination with standard chemotherapeutic drugs, provided significant life extension, and in some cases remission of the cancer.

One of the most traditional cancer therapies has been the use of radiochemicals as therapeutics. Current trials of Mabs used as delivery tools for radioactive immunotherapy include those for ^{131}I-conjugated Mabs directed against primary brain tumors and ^{90}Yb-conjugated Mabs directed against cancer cells. Clinical trials of Mab-based therapeutics are moving more and more to the treatment of diseases other than cancers. Currently, researchers are conducting clinical tests to investigate the efficacy of this form of therapy against asthma, lupus, multiple sclerosis, psoriasis, and rheumatoid arthritis; in a sign of the times, work is also underway on a human monoclonal against anthrax toxin (ABthrax).

MOLECULAR PHARMACOLOGY, RECOMBINANT DNA TECHNOLOGY, AND BIOTECHNOLOGY

MOLECULAR PHARMACOLOGY

The molecular approach to drug discovery is based on the availability or understanding of a molecular target for the medicinal agent. With the development of molecular biological techniques and the advances in genomics, the majority of drug discovery is currently based on the molecular approach. Modern genomics and its offspring, proteomics and gene expression profiling, offer an almost overwhelming amount of new information.

The pharmaceutical industry has rapidly integrated genomic considerations into its research and development programs. For example, target selection, a key aspect of drug development, will greatly benefit from the identification of genes that unambiguously play a role in specific diseases processes. Likewise, pharmacogenetics (i.e., genetic profiling to predict patient response to a drug) will also be of great value in clinical care. However, the most challenging step may be target validation; that is, reliably defining candidate genes with respect to disease processes. Once a target is identified, it can be rapidly addressed through combinatorial chemistry and high-throughput screening. Lead compounds emerging from the screening process must still undergo the tedious process of pharmacodynamic and toxicological profiling, however, before being considered for clinical trials.

Pharmacogenomics, the application of genotyping (determining the genetic constitution of an organism) to patient therapy, holds great theoretical promise for solving a long-standing problem: differences in individual responses to drug treatments. The ultimate goal is to maximize drug efficacy while minimizing side effects. It has been suggested, "*to apply ... pharmacogenetic knowledge to clinical practice, specific dosage recommendations based on genotypes will have to be developed to guide the clinician ... Such development will lead to a patient-tailored drug therapy which ... will result in fewer adverse drug reactions.*"

As appealing as genetics-based therapy sounds, to date, the impact of pharmacogenetics on clinical practice has been slight. At the present time, there is only one clinical situation in which genetic testing is mandated before drug therapy: the *thioprine methyltransferase* (TPMT) polymorphism. TPMT catalyzes an important detoxication step in metabolism of thiopurine anticancer drugs such as 6-thioguanine. A thiopurine slow metabolizer phenotype is rather common. These drugs have a relatively narrow therapeutic "window," and an elevated plasma level puts the patient at increased risk of potentially fatal *myelosuppression* by virtue of life-threatening infections.

Preliminary genotyping can identify many of the high-risk patients, and doses can be adjusted accordingly. But the TPMT instance remains unique. Even in the case of isoniazid therapy for tuberculosis, where the genetic basis of increased risk of drug toxicity has been known for decades, drug administration is still performed on a "one dose fits all" basis. Research has shown that, in most cases, the genetic, environmental, and physiological determinants of drug response are so complex that it is not useful to adjust drug doses on the basis of any single variable. For most drugs, the therapeutic index is relatively high; side effects are usually controllable; and most drugs have half-lives of only a few hours.

The power of new genetic screening technologies is dramatically increasing our ability to identify gene loci that might be involved in the pathogenesis of human disease. In addition, advances in transgenic technology allow the creation of animal models that reflect particular human disease states. Therefore, we can identity the role of specific genes in particular metabolic pathways and provide models for screening novel therapeutic agents. The human genome project will identify vast numbers of genes whose functions are unknown and it will not be clear whether or not they are drug targets. Thus, ultimately, pharmacogenomics will allow the exploitation of genetic information to establish whether particular genes or gene loci are novel targets for drugs, and to develop cell lines or animal models as screening tools for identifying pharmacologically active molecules that will reverse the phenotypes (observable genetic expression) generated.

It has been known for decades that individuality in response to a drug can have a genetic basis. The ability to identify individuals who might benefit or suffer as a consequence of a particular drug therapy is of considerable medical and economic importance; if drug therapy could be tailored to individuals on the basis of their genetic makeup, it would remove some of the empiricism from current drug prescribing.

The development of pharmacogenetics has evolved from understanding how the role of particular genetic polymorphisms influences the outcome of drug therapy in genes such as glucose-6-phosphate dehydrogenase and the P450 enzymes. For example, the P450 CYP2D6 that is responsible for the metabolism of up to 25% of therapeutic drugs is highly polymorphic and inactive in 6% of the white population. Many serious drug side effects have been ascribed to this polymorphism, particularly for cardiovascular and CNS active drugs. Future research will involve the study of polymorphisms in both candidate genes and genome-wide screens, in order to identify novel genes of pharmacological significance by screening, for example, single nucleotide polymorphisms.

RECOMBINANT DNA

The development of recombinant DNA, and hybridoma technologies (mentioned previously), has revolutionized the number and kind of pharmaceutical proteins available and serve as two of the cornerstones of the biotechnology industry. This has been made possible, in large part, due to the dramatic progress made in the methods of purification of the molecules produced. To date, there have been a number of products produced by recombinant technology (see Table 15.1).

Although not listed in Table 15.1, tissue plasminogen activator (tPA) is an important recombinant product. The clotting of blood is a normal hemodynamic function required to maintain the integrity of the vascular system. It involves a complex cascade of metabolic events involving many so-called clotting factors. The end result is the formation of proteinaceous fibrin monomers that polymerize to form the matrix of the clot, which then aggregates with platelets. This hemostatic plug *normally* functions to bridge ruptures *within* the vascular wall. In this case, they are reparative. However, under certain circumstances, "abnormal" clots that *transverse* a vessel can form, thereby forming an occlusive barrier to downstream blood flow.

Several disease states can result from abnormal blood clots. For example, strokes were mentioned previously. However, the most common and deadliest thrombotic disease is myocardial infarction (MI). Atherosclerosis has long been associated with reduced cardiac function and elevated mortality due to rupture of atherosclerotic plaques. The rupture of an atherosclerotic plaque usually

TABLE 15.1
The Top Ten Bioengineered Drugs in 1998 (Sales in Millions)

1.	Epogen	Red blood cell enhancement	$1,380.0
2.	Procrit	Red blood cell enhancement	$1,363.0
3.	Neupogen	Restoration of white blood cells	$1,120.0
4.	Humulin	Diabetes mellitus	$959.2
5.	Engerix-B	Prevention of hepatitis B	$886.7
6.	Intron A	Bone marrow transplantation	$719.0
7.	Betaseron	Multiple sclerosis	$409.2
8.	Genotropin	Growth failure in children	$395.1
9.	Avonex	Relapsing multiple sclerosis	$394.9
10.	Recombivax HB	Prevention of hepatitis B	$290.0

results not only in blockage due to the plaque itself but also in the immediate formation of an occlusive blood clot, which results in an MI. Immediately after the initiation of an MI, a zone of necrosis begins to develop around the area as ischemia proceeds. It is during this early phase of ischemia (several hours) that therapeutic intervention can be not only lifesaving but also helpful in minimizing the amount of necrotic heart tissue formed.

In addition to possessing a clot-forming system, the body also has a *fibrinolytic* system that has the capacity to degrade the underlying fibrin in clots. One of the key activators of the fibrinolytic system is tPA. This protein functions to *activate plasminogen* that subsequently activates *plasmin* that is responsible for degrading fibrin. With this knowledge in mind, Genentech undertook the project of developing commercial quantities of tPA, via their recombinant technology, to be used in the acute phase immediately following an MI.

The importance of using a recombinant source is dramatized when one considers the amount of activator required for therapy. The normal concentration of tPA in the blood is approximately 2 ng/mL. Therefore, if a human dose was on the order of 100 mg, it would take 50,000 L of blood to produce a single dose of tPA, even if recovery was 100%. Obviously, blood is not an adequate commercial source for this material.

Genentech scientists chose to develop recombinant tPA by successfully cloning totide sequence for tPA into a Chinese hamster ovary cell line. Unlike bacteria (see below), this mammalian cell carried out the required glycosylation, disulfide bond formation, and proper folding of tPA in the same manner as human cells. The recombinant material was identical to the human-derived material in molecular weight, amino acid composition, sequence, immunoreactivity, and kinetic constants.

Additional, related work being carried out in this area by other biotechnology companies involves the creation of so-called "fusion proteins." In this case, the binding domain of an antibody that recognizes the major component of a clot, fibrin, is combined with the clot-dissolving portion of tPA. It is hoped that enhanced specificity in target interaction will translate into better therapeutic results. Preliminary tests have shown these combinations to actually be more potent and selective than tPA alone.

In the initial recombinant work carried out in the 1980s, bacteria were used as the recipient cell type. The underlying principle in the application of recombinant DNA is that if you insert a fragment of DNA (coded for a particular protein, e.g., insulin) into a host cell (e.g. bacteria), it will be duplicated as the cell divides, and there will be a corresponding increase in the number of copies of the fragment. In order to achieve this replication, the DNA fragment must be inserted into an appropriate section of the host cell's DNA so that it will be duplicated along with the endogenous DNA during cell division.

DNA suitable for the insertion of foreign DNA is known as a vector; the most commonly used vectors in bacteria are *plasmids*. Plasmids are small (2–3 kb) loops of DNA found in bacteria and yeast. They were first discovered when it was observed that bacteria could pass antibiotic resistance from one colony to another. This process was demonstrated to be mediated by plasmids containing genes for enzymes that inactivated the antibiotics. In addition to the work on plasmids, other research laboratories have isolated enzymes that cut DNA at specific sequences (restriction endonucleases) as well as other enzymes that can rejoin these cuts again (DNA ligases).

In cloning, the plasmid vector is incubated with a restriction endonuclease that cuts open the plasmid DNA. Exposure of the open DNA to a new DNA fragment plus a ligase reconstitutes the plasmid DNA with a new nucleotide sequence. The resulting recombinant DNA is inserted into bacterial cells that then multiply. Each cell can contain 50–100 copies of the recombinant plasmid and can duplicate every 20–30 min.

TRANSGENIC ANIMALS

Transgenic animals result from genetic engineering experiments in which genetic material is moved from one organism to another, so that the latter will exhibit a desired characteristic.

Scientists, farmers, and business corporations hope that transgenic techniques will allow more precise and cost-effective animal and plant breeding programs. They also hope to use these new methods to produce animals and plants with desirable characteristics that are not available using current breeding technology.

In traditional breeding programs, only closely related species can be crossbred, but transgenic techniques allow genetic material to be transferred between completely unrelated organisms, so that breeders can incorporate characteristics that are not normally available to them. Although the basic coding system is the same in all organisms, the fine details of gene control often differ. A gene from a bacterium, for example, will often not function correctly if it is introduced unmodified into a plant or animal cell. The genetic engineer must first construct a transgene—the gene to be introduced; this is a segment of DNA containing the gene of interest and some extra material that correctly controls the gene's function in its new organism. The transgene must then be inserted into the second organism.

In 1982, Brinster and Palmiter introduced by microinjection a cloned gene for *rat growth hormone* into the male pronucleus of fertilized mouse eggs. The gene was cloned "downstream" from an inducible promoter to increase its chances of being expressed. After insertion of the microinjected eggs into the uterus of a foster-mother mouse, a significant number of offspring expressed the gene, produced high levels of the hormone, and grew to about twice the size of normal mice. The first human drug produced by transgenics, tPA, was achieved in mice in 1987.

As mentioned above, genes are controlled by a special segment of DNA found on the chromosome next to the gene, which is called a promoter sequence. When making a transgene, scientists generally substitute the organism's own promoter sequence with a specially designed one that ensures that the gene will function in the correct tissues of the animal or plant and also allows them to turn the gene on or off as needed (see Figure 15.6). For example, a promoter sequence

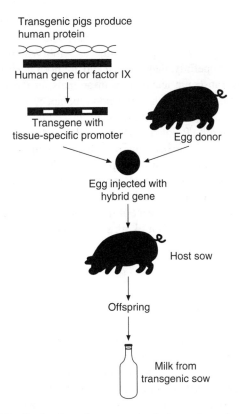

FIGURE 15.6   Production of a transgenic pig to produce a human protein.

that requires a dietary "trigger" substance can be used to turn on genes for important hormones in animals; the animal would not produce the new hormone unless fed the appropriate trigger.

Copies of the transgene are usually injected directly into a fertilized egg that is then implanted in the female's reproductive tract. However, it is difficult to control where in the chromosome the transgene will become inserted, and this sometimes causes variations in the way the gene is expressed. For this and other reasons, the process is demanding and, in general, has a low success rate. Currently, less than 5% of injected embryos result in offspring with the gene integrated into their DNA and able to be passed on consistently to successive generations. Researchers are, therefore, investigating new methods of gene transfer.

By genetic engineering, the DNA gene for a protein drug of interest can be transferred into another organism for production. Which organism to use for production is a technical and economic decision. For certain protein drugs that require complex modifications or are needed in large supply, production in transgenic animals seems most efficient. The farm animal becomes a production facility with many advantages. For example, it is reproducible, has a flexible production capacity through the number of animals bred, and maintains its own fuel supply. Perhaps most important of all, in most animal drug production, the drug is delivered from the animal in a very convenient form, the milk.

A transgenic animal for pharmaceutical production should (1) produce the desired drug at high levels without endangering its own health and (2) pass its ability to produce the drug at high levels to its offspring. The current strategy to achieve these objectives is to couple the DNA gene for the protein drug with a DNA signal directing production in the mammary gland. The new gene, while present in every cell of the animal, functions only in the mammary gland, so the protein drug is made only in the milk. Since the mammary gland and milk are essentially "outside" the main life support systems of the animal, there is virtually no danger of disease or harm to the animal in making the "foreign" protein drug.

After the DNA gene for the protein drug has been coupled with the mammary directing signal, this DNA is injected into *fertilized embryos* of the desired species with the aid of a very fine needle, called a micromanipulator, and a microscope. The injected embryos are then implanted into recipient surrogate mothers where, hopefully, they survive and are born normally.

The main aim in using transgenic technology in animals, at the present time, is to improve livestock by altering their biochemistry, their hormonal balance, or their important protein products. Several companies have designed and are testing transgenic mammals that produce important pharmaceutics in the animal's milk. Products such as insulin and growth hormone that are currently produced by fermentation of transgenic bacteria (recombinant technology), or other cell types, may soon be obtained by milking transgenic cows, sheep, or goats. The cost of these drugs may be much less than for those produced using conventional techniques. Drugs currently under study for transgenic production include α_1-antitrypsin, tPA, blood clotting factors VIII and IX, hemoglobin, and lactoferrin. An example of the potential impact of transgenics on the treatment of disease is hemophilia. It has been estimated that 300–600 milking sows could meet the world demand for clotting factor VIII.

CHIRALITY

While biological and structurally based drug designs are occupying most of the resources in contemporary drug development, there is an additional highly specialized area that is also receiving attention. This area deals with the fact that, as mentioned previously, some organic molecules contain an asymmetric carbon atom (i.e., a tetrahedral carbon atom that is bonded to four different atomic groupings). A molecule that contains such a *chiral* center can exist in two distinct mirror image-related forms called enantiomers. When both isomers are present in a 50/50 mixture the drug is in its racemic state. The word chiral comes from the Greek, which means hand like.

Chemists have known about racemates since Pasteur, at 26 years of age, told the Paris Academy of Sciences how he used tweezers to separate two types of crystals of salts of tartaric acid, which rotate polarized light clockwise (D) or counterclockwise (L). Unfortunately, this correspondence does not always hold true. In fact, the magnitude and even the direction of optical rotation are a complicated function of the electronic structure surrounding the chiral center. For example, the common enantiomer of the sugar fructose is termed D because of the stereochemical orientation about the chiral atom. But this enantiomer actually rotates the plane of polarization to the left, and its mirror image, L-fructose, rotates the plane of polarization to the right.

Accordingly, an absolute convention that allows a stereochemical designation to any compound has been developed, predicated on examination of its three-dimensional structure (essentially a rating system of groups attached to the chiral center). An example of this so-called R-S convention (where R = right and S = left) is illustrated by the anti-asthma drug albuterol (Figure 15.7). Despite its limitations, the D-L terminology is still commonly used by biochemists and pharmacologists alike.

The R and S enantiomers of a molecule will have identical physical and chemical properties under most circumstances, since they have identical energy contents and differ only at the three-dimensional level of their nonsuperimposability. However, the possibility that the two enantiomers of a chiral drug may differ in their biological effects is a phenomenon that has been recognized by pharmacologists since the beginning of the twentieth century. Table 15.2 presents some examples of chiral factors on drug disposition and toxicity that are often overlooked. In addition, it is believed that the teratogenic effect of thalidomide resides with the R form. Unfortunately, even if just the L form is given the body quickly converts it to the R form.

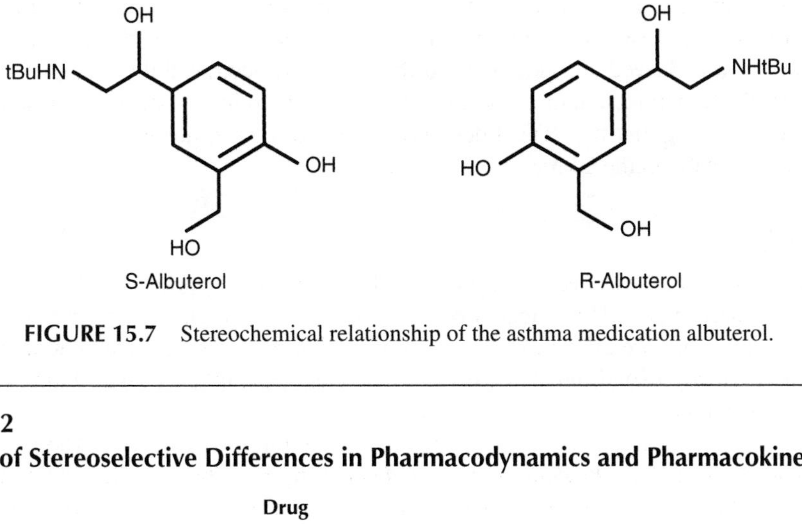

FIGURE 15.7 Stereochemical relationship of the asthma medication albuterol.

TABLE 15.2
Examples of Stereoselective Differences in Pharmacodynamics and Pharmacokinetics

Effect	Drug
Active absorption in GI tract Distribution	L-Dopa > D-dopa
	(S)-Propranolol selectively taken up by heart
	(S)-α-Methyldopa selectively accumulates in the brain
Plasma protein-binding potency	(–)-Ibuprofen > (+)-ibuprofen
	(–)-Hyoscyamine > (+)-hyoscyamine
	(S)-Warfarin > (R)-warfarin
Metabolism	(–)-Verapamil > (+)-verapamil
Drug interaction	Stereoselective inhibition of the metabolism of (S)-warfarin by sulfinpyrazone coupled to a stereoselective increase in the elimination of (R)-warfarin
Differential toxicity	(R)-2-Ethylhexaholic acid embryotoxicity > (S)-2-ethylhexaholic acid

Because of possible pharmacological differences between drug enantiomers, the science of creating single-isomer drugs is one of the fastest growing areas in pharmaceutical research and development. In 1997, the market for chiral drugs had reached $90 billion and 50% of the top 100 drugs were single enantiomers. Already, more than 80% of new drugs in the *early stages* of development are single-isomer compounds. It has been estimated that approximately 80% of prescription drugs now *sold* in the United States are single-isomer formulations. There are several reasons for this. First, regulatory pressure for chirally pure drugs has increased. Since 1992, U.S., Canadian, and European regulatory authorities have asked companies to provide information on each isomer of new racemic drugs and justify why the drug was not in its chirally pure, active form. Secondly, producing chirally pure drugs can often increase efficacy while decreasing toxicity.

Separating toxic effects from therapeutic effects is a constant challenge in drug development. In the case of our example of a chiral drug, albuterol, attempts are currently underway to achieve that goal. Apparently, the S-isomer of albuterol is actually responsible for increasing asthma patients' reactivity to stimuli, thereby leading to a paradoxical increased severity of asthma attacks. The "good-twin" R-isomer appears to be the form responsible for relaxation of bronchial smooth muscles, widening the airway, and allowing freer breathing. Clinical studies have, in fact, demonstrated that R-albuterol is four times more potent than the S form, with fewer side effects. Another example is the local anesthetic bupivicaine. The racemic form of bupivicaine has been restricted to epidural use during childbirth because it is cardiotoxic if it gains entry into the blood stream (apparently due to the R form). It is hoped that the left-handed isomer may reduce its cardiotoxicity and allow it to be used in a broader range of applications.

Research is also currently underway to investigate the possible advantages of proteins with the D stereoisomerism as drugs. One possible advantage is that they may be more resistant to proteolytic enzymes, suggesting that D-protein drugs may remain in the bloodstream for a longer time than conventional proteins. They also do not appear to be as immunogenic as conventional proteins, perhaps, because they are not cleaved and presented to the major histocompatibility complex (part of the immune system's antigen-recognition system), a process that requires proteolysis. In addition, there is some data suggesting that D-polypeptides may be able to be administered orally without being degraded enzymatically in the GI tract.

PHARMAFOODS

Over the past few years, so-called "pharmafoods" have begun to appear in both the scientific literature and the marketplace. This category of agents differs from regular drugs in that they are not found in drug stores nor are they prescribed by a physician. However, the manufacturers do claim pharmaceutical effects beyond standard nutrition. The major examples being developed in this area include benecol and olestra.

Benecol is a brand of margarine invented by a small Finnish food company (The Raisio Group.) Research published in the *New England Journal of Medicine* by Finnish researchers indicates that regular use of benecol can lower blood cholesterol levels by an average of 10% "in a randomly selected, mildly hypercholesterolemic population sample." Its active ingredient is a plant sterol from Nordic pine trees known as β-sitostanol, which apparently can block some of the body's absorption of dietary cholesterol. Presently, 5 tons of wood waste are processed to produce 1 pound of the oil that is the source of the sterol. After 20 years and more than $200 million in research and development, Proctor & Gamble received permission from the FDA in 1996 to market its fat substitute olestra in certain snack foods (e.g., potato chips, crackers, and cheese puffs). Olestra, technically a sucrose polyester, is *not* digestible, so it adds neither fat nor calories to food. However, olestra can inhibit the absorption of certain fat soluble vitamins and other nutrients. Therefore, all products containing olestra must be labeled with the following information: "*This product contains olestra. Olestra inhibits the absorption of some vitamins and other nutrients. Vitamins A, D, E, and K have been added.*" Also, as a condition of approval, Proctor & Gamble must monitor consumption and conduct studies on olestra's long-term effects.

Other products under current development in the pharmafood sector include a salt substitute for hypertension; a yogurt-like product that adds bacteria to stimulate the body's immune system; and a drink containing docosahexaenoic acid (DHA, the baby formula additive) that Japanese consumers believe boosts brain power before exams.

SELECTED BIBLIOGRAPHY

Bugg, C.E., Carson, W.M., and Montgomery, J.A. (1995) Drugs by design, in *Scientific American*, December, pp. 92–98.

Christopoulos, A. (Ed.) (2001) *Biomedical Applications of Computer Modeling*, Boca Raton: CRC Press.

Marshall, G.R. (1995) Molecular Modeling in Drug Design, in *Burger's Medicinal Chemistry and Drug Discovery*, 5th ed., Wolff, M. (Ed.), New York: Wiley.

Merchant, K.M. (Ed.) (1996) *Pharmacological Regulation of Gene Expression in the CNS*, Boca Raton: CRC Press.

Navia, M.A. and Murcko, M.A. (1992) Use of structural information in drug design, *Curr. Opin. Struct. Biolog.*, 2(2): 202–210.

Weiner, D.B. and Williams, W.V. (Eds.) (1995) *Biological Approaches to Rational Drug Design*, Boca Raton: CRC Press.

Weiner, D.B. and Williams, W.V. (Eds.) (1995) *Chemical and Structural Approaches to Rational Drug Design*, Boca Raton: CRC Press.

QUESTIONS

1. Which of the following was the first plant alkaloid isolated?
   a. Codeine
   b. Nitrous oxide
   c. Nitroglycerin
   d. Morphine
   e. Heroin

2. Which of the following was the first synthetic drug widely marketed to the public?
   a. Chloroform
   b. Ether
   c. Amyl nitrite
   d. Nitrous oxide
   e. Aspirin

3. Which of the following can be found in a birth control pill?
   a. Mestranol
   b. Cortisone
   c. Norethynodrel
   d. Testosterone
   e. a and c

4. Which of the following techniques is/are significantly increasing the number of potential lead compounds?
   a. Combinatorial chemistry
   b. Computer databases
   c. High-throughput screening
   d. Identification of pharmacophores
   e. All of the above

5. Ribozymes involve which of the following?
   a. Antisense deoxynucleotides
   b. Protein–RNA combination
   c. Catalytic RNA
   d. Catalytic DNA
   e. Mitochondrial DNA

6. Which of the following is the oldest technique for determining molecular structure to atomic resolution?
   a. Nuclear magnetic resonance
   b. Atomic fusion
   c. Differential fractionation
   d. Nuclear magnetic crystallography
   e. X-ray crystallography

7. The key region of a drug that is critical for molecular recognition and binding is which of the following?
   a. Allosteric site
   b. Affinity lattice
   c. Two-dimensional structure
   d. Amino acid sequence
   e. Pharmacophore

8. A combination rat/human antibody is known as which of the following?
   a. Chiral
   b. Chimera
   c. Enantiomers
   d. Racemate
   e. None of the above

9. Transgenic animals involve which of the following?
   a. A gene coding for a specific protein
   b. A promoter sequence of DNA
   c. Injection of the genetic material into a fertilized egg
   d. Implantation of the fertilized egg into a female's reproductive tract
   e. All of the above

10. Which of the following is/are true regarding chirality?
    a. All drugs have chiral enantiomers
    b. A symmetrical carbon atom is required
    c. The presense of a "humanized" section is required
    d. Very few drugs are sold as single chiral enantiomers
    e. None of the above

16 Pharmaceutical Development of Drugs and the FDA

INTRODUCTION

After a drug company has discovered what appears to be an active drug in their drug discovery program, regardless of which type is utilized, the candidate drug can then pass to the next stage of the drug evaluation process. This step will involve interaction of the drug company with the governmental agency that has responsibility for this area, the Food and Drug Administration (FDA). Over the years, the role of the FDA in drug evaluation has evolved into three main areas: (1) truth in labeling, (2) toxicity, and (3) determination of efficacy.

The roots of the FDA reach back to before the Civil War. The first national law came in 1848 during the Mexican War. It banned the importation of adulterated drugs; a chronic health problem that finally got Congressional attention. When Congress created the Department of Agriculture in 1862, the Patent Office's chemistry lab was transferred to the new agency and renamed the Chemical Division. The first prolonged and impassioned controversy in Congress involving a pure food issue took place in 1886, pitting butter against oleomargerine. Butter won, and oleomargerine was taxed and placed under other restraints that persisted on the Federal level until 1950.

In 1890, the division underwent another rather insignificant name change to the Division of Chemistry and, in 1901, was renamed the Bureau of Chemistry. The Bureau of Chemistry subsequently became the Food, Drug & Insecticide Administration in 1927 and, finally, officially, the FDA in 1930.

While the FDA is required to review applications from drug companies for drug approval and establish standards, the agency does not fund or conduct research to bring a drug to market. However, it does carry out highly specific applied research. In addition, the agency inspects manufacturing facilities and reviews production records. Although the agency does have responsibilities in the areas of food, cosmetics, and medical devices, it is their role in drug approval that will be the subject of this chapter. The success of the U.S. drug industry is demonstrated by sales figures for the top 12 selling drugs as of December 2005 (Table 16.1).

TABLE 16.1
Top-Selling Drugs in the United States for 2005

Product	2005 Sales ($Billions)	Disease
Lipitor	8.4	High cholesterol
Zocor	4.4	High cholesterol
Nexium	4.4	Heartburn
Prevacid	3.8	Heartburn
Advair Discus	3.6	Asthma
Plavix	3.5	Heart disease
Zoloft	3.1	Depression
Epogen	3.0	Anemia
Procrit	3.0	Anemia
Aranesp	2.8	Anemia
Enbrel	2.7	Rheumatoid arthritis
Norvasc	2.6	High blood pressure

Source: IMSHealth (2006).

DRUG LABELING

One of the first significant empowerments of the fledgling FDA was when Congress enacted the *Food and Drug Act* (also known as the Wiley Act) in 1906 directed to address unhygienic conditions in Chicago's meat packing plants (see Upton Sinclair's *The Jungle*) and the sale of "snake-oil" medicines of unknown composition. The act applied to drugs to the extent that preparations could be removed from the market if the concoctions could be shown to be *adulterated or misbranded*. As such, it dealt primarily with *truth in labeling*. Unfortunately, the law did little to control the sale of dangerous drugs and devices since there were no obligations to establish drug safety or efficacy. As is often the case, it took a catastrophic incident during the 1930s to induce further legislative action.

DRUG SAFETY

As mentioned previously, by the late 1930s, the fame of the antibiotic sulfanilamide had spread around the world and millions of *tablets* of the new wonder-drug were being used each year. Always on the look-out for a new marketing ploy, one company in Tennessee, Massengill & Co., tried a different marketing strategy to set themselves apart. On the somewhat unusual theory that most people in the South prefer to take their medicine in liquid form, the company began to experiment on how to get sulfanilamide into solution. Unfortunately, sulfanilamide does not readily dissolve in water, alcohol, or any of the other common pharmaceutical solvents. However, a chemist at the company did discover that the drug was soluble in diethylene glycol (a component of antifreeze). To the sulfanilamide/diethylene glycol solution was added some coloring matter and some raspberry flavor and the mixture marketed under the name of *Elixir Sulfanilamide*. Apparently, no one at Massengill tested the elixir for safety, in any manner whatsoever, since toxicity testing was not a requirement.

Soon after marketing of the elixir began, a physician in Oklahoma reported to the American Medical Association (AMA), not the FDA, that he had recently seen six people who had died of kidney damage and who, coincidentally, had all taken Elixir Sulfanilamide. He was curious as what the contents of the preparation were. After initial attempts to discover the ingredients in the elixir were rebuffed by the company, the presence of diethylene glycol was finally acknowledged. The situation now became clear since diethylene glycol is converted in the body to oxalic acid, a highly nephrotoxic chemical that causes a slow agonizing death from kidney failure.

Unfortunately, there were no requirements in 1937 for testing the *toxicity* or safety of drug products, and over 100 people died from diethylene glycol-induced renal failure, most of them children. All that could be done to the manufacturer under the law at the time was to penalize the company for mislabeling its product. Although the manufacturer steadfastly refused to accept responsibility for the debacle, its chief chemist committed suicide. This scandal followed closely on the heals of another drug-related tragedy during the 1930s. Dinitrophenol is a highly toxic poison with the ability to uncouple oxidative phosphorylation. In the process, the metabolic rate of the poisoned individual can increase markedly. It is this latter effect that led to its promotion for weight reduction. Unfortunately, there were numerous serious injuries and deaths.

The culmination of these episodes led Congress to enact the *Food, Drug, and Cosmetic Act of 1938*. This statute expanded consumer protection by requiring the testing of new drugs for safety *prior* to marketing. Toxicity studies were required, as well as approval of a new drug application (NDA), before a drug could be promoted and distributed. It was the requirement of toxicity testing that spared the United States from the tragedy of thalidomide that swept Europe during the 1960s. It should be noted, however, that no proof of efficacy was required in the 1938 legislation, and extravagant claims for therapeutic indications were commonly made.

Since its adoption, the 1938 law has been amended repeatedly, eventually extending FDA's regulatory powers to pesticides and food additives. In 1958, the *Delaney clause* was incorporated into the law. This now controversial provision prohibits the approval of any food additive found to induce cancer in humans or animals.

In the relatively relaxed atmosphere of pre-World War II, pharmacological research expanded rapidly in both industrial and academic settings. Many new drugs were introduced for a variety of illnesses. Because efficacy was not rigorously defined, a number of therapeutic claims that could not be supported by appropriate scientific data were made. The risk-to-benefit ratio was seldom mentioned. One advancement that was made was the Durham-Humphrey Amendment of 1951. Until this law, there was no requirement that any drug be labeled *safe by prescription* only. This amendment defined prescription drugs as those unsafe for self-medication and which should therefore be used only under a physician's supervision. Drugs initially classified as by prescription only can have their classification changed, as illustrated by antiulcer medications such as Tagamet.

Responding to widespread criticism of the government's handling of drug safety problems, the FDA announced in early 2005 that it was creating a board to advise it on drug complications and to warn patients about unsafe drugs. The acting commissioner at the time said the board would be made up of scientists drawn from throughout the federal government. The board will not have independent power to force the withdrawal of drugs but will be advisory to the FDA. In addition, the agency will soon tap into large databases, including those at the Medicare agency, to uncover dangerous side effects in drugs already on the market.

The Office of Drug Safety at the agency now has about 109 employees and tries to uncover unknown drug dangers largely by pouring over miscellaneous and haphazard injury reports sent in by doctors and drug companies. The office is part of the agency's drug review center.

DRUG EFFICACY

In 1962, the deficiency in U.S. drug laws relating to efficacy was finally remedied when Congress put in place the third cornerstone of our current public health and consumer protection legislation. Congress stated in its new enactment that before a drug product could go on the market, it had to be both safe and *efficacious*. As is traditionally the case, the official act was named after the members of Congress who introduced it in the House and Senate, respectively, and is known as the Harris-Kefauver Amendments to the Food, Drug, and Cosmetic Act.

Interestingly, the question of drug efficacy evolved in its importance at the time, since Estes Kefauver had originally begun investigating the drug industry in 1959 because of concerns over excessive pricing of prescription drugs. However, by the end of the Senate's investigative phase, Kefauver was convinced that not only were some drugs incredibly over-priced but that drugs should not be allowed on the market unless they were *both* safe and effective. After several years of acrimonious debate in the Senate, it appeared as though a weakened version of S. 1552 (known as the "double-cross bill") was the only legislation that could be hoped for. As fate would have it, it was at that time that the story of the thalidomide tragedy swept across the country, and Congress was deluged with demands for strong legislation related to drug development that included the question of efficacy.

The new regulations were long overdue. Many useless or irrational products had already been brought to market, either by outright charlatans or by overly enthusiastic individuals or companies sincerely convinced that their product was a boon to suffering mankind. For many years, the FDA had struggled hard but often unsuccessfully to keep worthless remedies off the market and to remove those already in use. The difficulty was that the companies usually had to be proven guilty of false advertising (under the 1906 law), which often required years of effort at considerable expense. The problem had been particularly notorious for the FDA in the case of proposed cancer treatments such as Laetrile, Krebiozen, and arginases.

The 1962 amendments have proven to be significant legislation in that they require appropriate pharmacological and toxicological research in animals *before* a drug can be tested in humans. The data from these *preclinical* studies must be submitted in the form of an application for an investigational new drug (IND) before *clinical* studies can be initiated. Once begun, the clinical studies involve three graduated phases (see below) of variable drug exposure to humans. The 1962

Amendments also required manufacturers to support the claims of efficacy for all drugs marketed between 1938 and 1962 (pre-1938 products were "grandfathered" in and allowed to be sold for the curious reason that they were generally recognized as safe and effective, provided no evidence to the contrary developed).

EVALUATION OF 1938–1962 DRUGS

The new law required the FDA to wait until 1964 before demanding proof of efficacy of drugs introduced between 1938 and 1962. Because of manpower constraints within the FDA, the process of independent evaluation was carried out under a contract between the FDA and the National Academy of Sciences (NAS) under its research arm, the National Research Council (NRC). Originally, some 200 experts were assembled into 30 panels to consider approximately 16,000 therapeutic claims involving more than 4,000 products marketed by nearly 300 different companies. It was eventually agreed that each product would be put in one of six different categories: (1) safe and effective; (2) probably effective; (3) possibly effective—more data required; (4) effective for limited uses; (5) ineffective as a fixed combination; and (6) ineffective. Evaluations of these drugs have been ongoing for nearly 40 years.

Occasionally, new data that can cause reclassification of a group of drugs becomes available. For example, in May, 1996, the FDA informed manufacturers that it planned to reclassify five widely used ingredients in OTC laxatives from category 1 to category 3. The five ingredients (phenolphthalein, bisacodyl, aloe, cascara sagrada, and senna) were initially marketed prior to 1962. In 1975, the NAS/NRC advisory review panel had recommended that these five ingredients be considered as safe and effective OTC stimulant laxatives, and, in 1985, the FDA did, in fact, place them in category 1.

Recent studies by the National Toxicology Program (NTP) on phenolphthalein, however, have provided new data associating the laxative with carcinogenic potential in rodents. Concern for bisacodyl arises from the fact that it is structurally related to phenolphtalein (both are members of the diphenylmethane family of laxatives). FDA concerns regarding the members of the anthraquinone family (senna, aloe, and cascara sagrada) emanate from laboratory data indicating that some of the components of senna may have mutagenic properties.

Following the release of the NTP study in December 1995, FDA's Carcinogenicity Assessment Committee met with drug manufacturers and NTP representatives to further ascertain whether this new information translated into a risk for humans. Although the FDA had never received any adverse reports linking these laxatives with cancer, the new information suggested that additional studies might be warranted. Therefore, the FDA requested that the manufacturers provide the necessary additional data to establish the safety of these five ingredients. Particular emphasis was placed on phenolphthalein.

In August 1997, the maker of Ex-Lax (which contained phenolphthalein), the nation's top-selling overnight laxative (1996 sales of $41 million), pulled three versions of the product off store shelves. The laxative had been in use since 1906. Replacement products containing senna as the active ingredient were made available several months later. The premise for forcing phenolphthalein removal was based on tests in rodents that developed a variety of tumors when fed the chemical in doses 50–100 times those recommended for humans.

PRECLINICAL TESTING

The process by which new drug candidates are discovered and developed is both time consuming and expensive. This is reflected in the high rate of attrition of drug candidates that enter clinical development, such that only approximately 10% of drug candidates that are selected for clinical development eventually become marketed drugs.

For a drug that has never been used in humans previously, the initial step that a pharmaceutical company must take is to perform preclinical toxicity studies involving appropriate *in vitro* systems or whole animals. The FDA usually requires that dose related toxicity be determined in at least two mammalian species (routinely rodents). The toxicity information obtained from these studies can then be used to make risk/benefit assessments and help determine the acceptability of the drug for testing in humans, and to estimate a safe starting dose.

Pharmacokinetic studies that document the fate of the drug including absorption, distribution, metabolism, and excretion must be provided. In addition, the company must supply information on chemistry, manufacturing, and quality control guidelines. This ensures the identity, purity, quality, and strength of both the active ingredient and the finished dosage form.

The drug company then develops a plan for testing the drug in humans and submits it to the FDA, along with its animal testing data, information about the composition of the drug, manufacturing data, qualifications of its study investigators, and assurances for the protection of the rights and safety of the people who will participate in the trial. This corpus of information comprises the IND (Investigational New Drug Application). According to the FDA's *Center for Drug Evaluation and Research Fact Book 1997*, the average length of time for a promising drug candidate to be synthesized, purified, and subjected to animal testing before IND submission is 18 months. Under normal circumstances, the IND must be evaluated within 30 days of submission. The FDA reviews the information in order to establish that the study participants will not be exposed to unreasonable risk of harm. If the FDA finds no safety problems with the plan or the drug, it permits the drug to proceed to the clinical phases of evaluation.

According to 1996 data from the FDA, drug and biotech firms filed 3522 INDs between 1984 and 1993 (approximately one per day). Since 1994, the FDA has approved year-to-year increases in the number of new candidate drugs for human testing in the United States, rising from 3350 in 1996 to 3900 in 2002; but the number of drugs that successfully negotiate the trial process and ultimately receive FDA approval is frustratingly low. Despite pharmaceutical companies' and the NIH's research budgets doubling since 1933, the number of approvals for new drugs with a *novel chemical structure* fell from 53 in 1996 to 21 in 2003 (Table 16.2).

CLINICAL TRIALS

Prior to 1962, drug trials could often be characterized as a series of uncontrolled testimonials by clinicians associated with the studies. Today, clinical trials are much more rigorous and are traditionally

TABLE 16.2
New Molecular Entities Approved

Year	Number
1993	25
1994	22
1995	28
1996	53
1997	39
1998	30
1999	35
2000	27
2001	24
2002	17
2003	21

conducted in *three* distinct phases. As each new clinical trial is started, a project manager from the drug company is assigned responsibility. The project manager in turn selects the clinical sites, guides the preparation of the protocol, and has general oversight over all aspects of the clinical study.

Clinical trials should be carried out under the highest ethical and scientific standards possible. While this is generally the case, there have been exceptions. During the period 1964–1982, for example, FDA inquiries resulted in some 45 clinical investigators being declared ineligible to receive investigational drugs, and an additional six agreed to some restrictions on their investigational work. Some of the disqualified investigators were criminally prosecuted and sentenced to fines, probation, and imprisonment for fraud, fabrication of results, felony, and so forth.

PHASE I

The first exposure of humans to the drug, the phase I study, usually takes place in a small number of *healthy volunteers*, although in the case of serious and life threatening conditions, volunteers who have the disease may be enrolled. These initial studies test the safety of the drug in humans and help to determine an appropriate dose for further investigations. In addition, pharmacokinetic data relating to absorption, distribution, metabolism, and elimination are also determined. Each year, some 40,000 ostensibly healthy individuals are used by U.S. drug companies in phase I drug tests. Volunteers, often homeless, are generally paid in the $100 to $200 per day range; about 70% of new drugs pass this stage.

As clinical studies progress, additional animal experiments continue to be carried out, in order to ensure the safety of ongoing human studies to the greatest extent possible. These include reproductive toxicity studies to examine the effects of the drug on fertility, reproduction, teratogenicity, and mutagenicity. In 1977, the FDA specifically restricted the participation by most women with childbearing potential from entering phase I and early phase II trials. However, in 1993, the FDA reversed this position because of the concern that the exclusion of women would prevent the accumulation of gender-related data.

The FDA's new guidelines strongly *encourage* inclusion of women in most early phase trials, providing that they are adequately informed of the potential risks. In fact, a characterization of drug effects by gender must now be part of all NDAs, and the agency may refuse an application that does not contain such information. The 1993 guideline identifies three specific pharmacokinetic issues in women that should be considered *when feasible*: (1) effect of the stages of the menstrual cycle, (2) effect of exogenous hormonal therapy including oral contraceptives, and (3) effect of the drug on the pharmacokinetics of oral contraceptives.

It is important to recognize, however, that the U.S. Code of Federal Regulations does not address the question of gender in clinical trials; there is no formal requirement that women make up a significant portion of a trial's patient population or even participate at all. The reality is that unless a trial specifically mandates female participation (e.g., a test for the safety and efficacy of a new birth control pill), men overwhelmingly predominate as subjects in clinical trials. For pharmaceutical companies, there is little motivation to recruit women. The first reason for this lack of motivation has to do with attempts to limit potential liabilities. Other concerns stem from this issue and focus on economic and legal realities that are stumbling blocks to expanded inclusion of women in research.

How do concerns about company liability limit the recruitment of female patients? Two issues explain this: pregnancy and infant care. No drug developer wants to be responsible if the product it is testing turns out to have an adverse effect on fetal development or harms a breast-feeding infant through milk contamination. The result, therefore, is that most trials require participating women to be either postmenopausal or nonlactating and actively using an acceptable form of birth control. Some investigators, uncertain of what constitutes an "acceptable" birth control method and fearful of patient noncompliance, simply refuse to enroll female patients of childbearing age to their trials, thereby reducing the number of women eligible to enter any given study, making recruitment that much more difficult.

From a pharmaceutical company's perspective, the costs of increasing female participation in trials are significantly greater than the odds that an approved drug, tested primarily on male subjects, will be withdrawn by the FDA because of unexpected health effects in women. Therefore, although pharmaceutical companies do not actively dissuade female participation from trials, their recruitment efforts rarely focus on women, and the lack of female participation in most research is not a point of concern.

Another issue facing clinical studies is the inclusion of *children*. In the United States, physicians who treat children often perform uncontrolled experiments. They are forced to do this because more than half of the drugs used in pediatric medicine have not been adequately studied in children and lack appropriate dosage information on the label.

The absence of pediatric testing and labeling poses significant risks. In the 1950s, many newborn babies died after receiving chloramphenicol, because their immature livers could not metabolize the antibiotic. More recent cases of adverse reactions include seizures and cardiac arrest caused by bupivacaine (a local anesthetic) toxicity, and withdrawal symptoms after prolonged administration of fentanyl (an opiate derivative and potent analgesic) in infants and small children.

In the early 1990s, the FDA encouraged pharmaceutical companies to submit pediatric labeling data. The agency's measures, which were largely voluntary, did not substantially increase the number of drugs with pediatric labeling, and the FDA concluded that additional steps were necessary.

The FDA Modernization Act (FDAMA) of 1997 addresses the desirability of pediatric research before new drug approval, when a drug is likely to be prescribed for children. In exchange for a report on the requested studies, the FDA adds 6 months of market exclusivity to any of the sponsor's formulations, dosage forms, and indications requiring the active moiety that was tested in the pediatric studies. During the pediatric exclusivity period, the FDA cannot approve another company's abbreviated NDA for a product containing this active moiety, thus delaying the entry of generics into the marketplace.

FDAMA market incentives work by attaching pediatric exclusivity to patent protection listed in the FDA's *Approved Drug Products with Therapeutic Equivalence Evaluations* (the Orange Book) for any drug product that contains the same active moiety as the drug studied and for which the party submitting the studies holds the approved NDA. Pediatric exclusivity can also be added to nonpatent, Orange Book-listed exclusivity, such as new drug product exclusivity and Orphan Drug exclusivity for rare diseases.

The FDA published its final rule in December 1998 with the proviso that pediatric assessments *must* be included in applications filed after December 2, 2000; the "Pediatric Rule." This was successfully challenged in court by a physicians' association and two public interest groups. The FDA then called upon Congress to grant the authority to require pediatric studies. Congress complied and a bipartisan group of senators introduced the *Pediatric Research Equity Act* in March 2003; the president signed the legislation on December 3; it will sunset in October 2007.

The FDA's tactics for acquiring information on pediatric drug administration have transitioned from encouraging the performance of pediatric studies to the two-pronged approach of voluntary incentives and mandatory assessments. So far, the offer of additional marketing exclusivity has been a success.

Innovator drug companies have not only complied with FDAMA-based requests but have enthusiastically sought pediatric exclusivity by submitting study proposals to expedite the FDA's issuance of a formal request. As of October 31, 2003, the FDA had issued 284 requests for pediatric studies; 228 were based on proposals from industry. Although studies meriting additional exclusivity need not result in new labeling, the FDA has added pediatric information to over 50 drug labels.

PHASE II

The subsequent phase in clinical studies, phase II, not only continues to evaluate the safety profile of the drug, identifying the most common side effects that might result from its use, but also begins to assess its activity for the particular disease that it was developed for. Phase II studies usually involve *a few dozen to a few hundred people*. By the time that phase II is completed, the drug developer knows quite a lot about the safety and activity of the drug. In fact, 80% of all drugs tested are abandoned by their sponsors after either phase I or II because of excessive toxicity or lack of significant efficacy. However, if the results are promising the sponsor may progress to phase III.

Phase III

Phase III clinical trials represent the *normal* culmination of the drug discovery/development process, and are designed to establish the safety and efficacy of the putative treatment. Large, controlled phase III studies can involve thousands of people with the targeted condition scattered among numerous research sites. Phase III studies are frequently longer in duration in order to provide additional reassurance regarding safety. Between 25 and 30% of the remaining drugs clear this hurdle. Thus, about 8% of drug submissions make it to market. The studies may also examine additional uses for a drug, or consider additional population subsets, but are primarily aimed at obtaining the necessary effectiveness data. Phase III studies also continue to generate valuable safety data, including long-term effects.

THE SCIENTIFIC EVALUATION OF DRUGS IN HUMANS

At this point, it may be useful to the reader to understand some of the background that has led to the contemporary design of human clinical trials. Although the concept of a comparative trial was known in the ninth century BC, it remained for James Lind in 1774 to perform his famous trial. Lind was concerned with comparing several different recommended treatments of the day for scurvy. Lind demonstrated that when all the proposed treatments were compared in a controlled study in human volunteers, only one proved efficacious—citrus fruit. It is important to realize that each of the treatments tested was recommended by recognized authorities of the day. It took the comparative trial to prove that citrus juice cured scurvy and the other treatments were worthless. In the process of applying this scientific method, Lind did much to destroy the credibility of testimonials.

The testimonial, someone speaking from experience, is psychologically one of the more powerful forms of persuasion. Eyewitness testimony is basic to the legal profession. However, in science, the testimonial has little evidentiary value. To illustrate this point, we need only be reminded of James Woodforde and his cat. In 1791, the parson of Weston Longville in Norfolk, England, developed a painful sty on his right eyelid. Parson Woodforde, however, knew how to treat it: "As is commonly said that the eyelid being rubbed by the tail of a black cat would do it much good, if not entirely cure it, and having a black cat, a little before dinner I made a *trial* (emphasis mine) of it, and very soon after dinner I found my eyelid much abated of the swelling and almost free of pain."

Parson Woodforde concluded that a cat's tail was of the greatest efficacy for such a malady. While the good parson's reasoning was logical, his premise was incorrect. Testimonials often involve the fallacy of *post hoc, ergo propter hoc*, that is, the assumption that because two events occur sequentially, the first is the cause of the second. (In tort law, causation must be proved.) The swelling of the eyelid may have abated of its own accord even in the absence of the tail of a black cat. Moreover, there is selection bias in testimonials; a lack of consequence rarely results in a testimonial and dead men tell no tales.

PLACEBO-CONTROLLED TRIALS

As mentioned previously in Chapter 1, the placebo effect can create havoc with clinical trials. The first placebo-controlled drug trial was published in 1933. The investigators evaluated drugs used in the treatment of angina pectoris. Among the comments made at the conclusion of their 4–26 week study was "The value of remedies in relieving anginal pain cannot be judged unless the observations are properly *controlled* (emphasis mine). The literature on the treatment of angina gives no indication that this side of the problem has been considered, although it is recognized that the disease pursues a varying course in regard to severity quite apart from any form of treatment."

OBSERVER BIAS

The importance of observer bias was addressed in 1937 when the concept of the double blind study was introduced, as also in a study of treatments of angina patients. The authors indicate in their methods that "In a further attempt to eliminate the possibility of bias, the questioner usually refrained from informing himself as to the agent that had been issued until *after* the patient's appraisal of the period had been obtained."

USE OF STATISTICAL ANALYSIS

Although the concept of patient variability had been articulated by the middle of the twentieth century, the concept that a difference between two groups could be due to chance was slow to be accepted. The first clinical trial to use a formal statistical analysis reportedly occurred in 1962. The study involved a comparison of antibody production after yellow fever vaccination by two different methods. Several years later (1966) a critique of statistical methods used in medical journal manuscripts suggested a lack of proper study design and data analysis. In this critique, the authors canonized the criterion of $P<.05$ for a difference between two groups to be considered *not* due to chance.

A problem still exists, however. Although it was established that the probability of less than 1 in 20 that a difference between two groups was due to chance as meaning that it was due to the drug, they did not establish criteria for how to properly interpret studies that failed to find this big a difference. In other words, can this lack of evidence of effect be considered to be evidence of lack of effect? Experts in the field have settled on the convention that a clinical trial must include enough patients to have at least an 80% chance of finding an effect if an effect really exists. Failure to find an effect in this large a trial is considered to be evidence of true lack of an effect. This is referred to as the *power* of the study.

How can studies that lack having this power be handled? Traditionally, one did a review of these studies, writing a narrative about them and drawing conclusions based on the subjective evaluation of this information by the reviewer. An alternative to this approach was introduced in 1988 and designated *meta-analysis*. Meta-analysis has been defined as "a systematic review of studies that uses quantitative statistical procedures to combine, synthesize, and integrate information across these studies." What this methodology does is take a group of different studies and analyze them together as if they were a single study following a single protocol.

The appeal of meta-analysis is that by combining a series of small equivocal studies into one analysis of all the patients, a more reliable result may be obtained. However, as one might appreciate, there are several issues inherent in a meta-analysis. One is whether all the small clinical trials of the drug were included or only the published "positive" trials, while the small negative trials that were done were never published. This would be like excluding the data from selected centers in a multicenter trial. Obviously this would skew the data. An additional issue is whether separate studies that do not use an identical protocol can really be combined. Obviously, there is art as well as science in meta-analysis. With these limitations in mind, meta-analysis does have its place in the clinical evaluation of drug candidates.

Once phase III is completed, the sponsor submits the test results to the FDA in the form of the NDA. At this point, FDA scientists (e.g., medical officers, pharmacologists, chemists, microbiologists, and statisticians) review the application to validate the data and determine if it does, in fact, demonstrate that the drug is both safe and effective. The manufacturing facility is also evaluated in order to ensure that a consistent and high-quality product can be produced.

The stakes in drug development are high. It takes nearly 8 years to develop a drug, almost twice as long as it did 20 years ago. The cost of failure can be mighty. In the fall of 2003, a major drug company shocked financial markets when it announced it would discontinue work on a promising new antidepressant that had already received marketing approval as an antinausea drug, after it failed in phase III trials. Shares in the company's stock fell 6.5% in a single day. Even the costs of success are staggeringly large: more than $1 billion per drug, from concept to market, according to a report by the Tufts Center for the Study of Drug Development.

After the drug company has completed testing the drug, it then submits proposed labeling for the drug, which must, in turn, be evaluated by the FDA. Labeling is generally reflective of the conditions of the trial in terms of indication and population. However, once the drug is approved, it may be employed by a physician in any manner he/she deems therapeutically appropriate, since the practice of medicine is not regulated by the FDA. Use of a drug in this manner is referred to as "off-label use."

In some cases, additional postmarketing testing may be required by the FDA, which is often referred to as "phase IV"; while spending on phases I through III has declined by 2% between 1999 and 2000, postapproval drug studies are the fastest-growing segment of the clinical trial market. It is anticipated that the proportion of postmarketing studies will increase in the future because of competitive marketing pressures on products that face expiration in the next few years. The generic drug industry's share of the prescription drug market has jumped from less than 20% to nearly 50% since 1984. Prior to 1984, only 35% of top-selling medications faced this competition.

While approval bestows a license to market a drug for commercial use, it also limits the marketing claims and recommendations for the doses, formulations, medical indications, and patient populations that were tested and approved during the phase III trials. If the study sponsor or the FDA wishes to alter any of these parameters, a postmarketing, or phase IV, study is initiated. Because most drug companies want to expand the indications for which a medication can be prescribed, almost all drugs undergo some phase IV testing.

Phase IV studies can take almost any form as long as new questions not addressed in phases I–III are answered. Postmarketing studies can be initiated by a drug company, requested by the FDA, or conducted by third parties interested in examining a drug's application for a specific population, medical condition, or use in the home or clinic. Postmarketing studies can be performed during the new drug approval process, immediately after the drug has been approved, or even years after approval, when the FDA has had the opportunity to review consumer usage data. Such studies can last for just 2 weeks for the interaction study on food or as long as several years for compound stability.

A phase IV study initiated by a drug company is often done to expand the patient population for which a drug can be marketed. For example, Pfizer's Viagra was initially approved based on clinical trials on male patients with erectile dysfunction. Soon after the drug's 1997 approval, several physicians began prescribing it to female patients suffering from sexual dysfunction. Physicians may legally prescribe any drug for any patient or indication they think might benefit from the therapy, but drug companies are not permitted to reference, market, or publicize "off-label" uses. "Off-label" drug use increases liability and provides no advice to the patient about whether and how much of a drug is safe.

Occasionally, when approved drugs enter the marketplace, unexpected, adverse effects occur. Reports of adverse drug reactions to the FDA are considered by public health officials to be the most reliable early warnings of a product's danger. The reports are filed to the FDA by health professionals, consumers, and drug manufacturers. In these cases, it is not uncommon for the FDA to rescind its approval and demand the withdrawal of the products. In fact, between 1997 and June 2005, this happened on 14 occasions involving drugs cited as *suspects* in over a 1000 deaths (see Table 16.3).

During this same period of time, defective asthma inhalers believed responsible for 17 deaths were also recalled. The FDA also has a system called MedWatch (www.fda.gov/medwatch), by which consumers and heath professionals can report adverse drug reactions directly to the agency.

TABLE 16.3
Prescription Drugs Withdrawn by the FDA
between January 1997 and June 2005

Drug	Type
Posicor	Blood pressure
Pondimin	Appetite suppressant
Duract	Analgesic
Propulsid	Heartburn
Rezulin	Diabetes
Relenza	Influenza
Baycol	Cholesterol lowering
Seldane	Antihistamine
Lotrenex	Gastrointestinal
Redux	Appetite suppressant
Raxar	Antibiotic
Hismanal	Antihistamine
Vioxx	Antiarthritis
Bextra	Antiarthritis

There are several reasons for drug toxicity to manifest itself after exposure to the public at-large. Two reasons were identified above: exposure to women and "off-label" use. In addition, the sample size of clinical trials, although statistically significant, is small when compared to the general population that will use the drug. The statistical power of phase III trials is not believed able to detect adverse reactions of 1 in 10,000 drug exposures or less.

More than 250,000 side effects linked to prescription drugs, including injuries and death, are reported each year. These adverse-event reports by doctors and others are only filed voluntarily. Experts believe the reports represent as few as 1–10% of all such events. According to the Los Angeles Times, even when deaths are reported, records and interviews show that companies consistently dispute that their product has caused a given death by pointing to other factors, including preexisting disease or use of another medicine.

The FDA is normally the federal agency that deals with drug-related deaths. However, in 2001, the DEA reported the results of extensive autopsy data and reported that the painkiller OxyContin was suspected of *playing a role* in 282 deaths between 2000 and 2001. On the basis of responses to date (October 2001), the DEA concluded that OxyContin was "*directly linked*" in 110 overdose deaths because tablets were either found in a person's stomach or a prescription for the drug was found on a body. DEA officials also classified 172 deaths as "*OxyContin possible*" cases where autopsy reports showed high blood concentrations of oxycodone (the active ingredient) without the presence of other compounds such as aspirin or acetaminophen. The review found that virtually all the deaths were of people who swallowed the pill whole or crushed rather than injected.

An example of a drug that has been subjected to essentially nonstop scrutiny after initial marketing is the sleeping pill Halcion. The FDA has examined Halcion periodically since 1982, lowering the recommended dose and adding warnings of such side effects as anxiety, behavioral changes, and abnormal thinking. Most recently the FDA has restricted the number of pills per package so that patients will not take too many. Britain banned Halcion in 1991 and said Upjohn hid safety concerns that, had the government been aware, might have blocked the drug from ever being sold there. Meanwhile, at least 100 U.S. lawsuits have been filed against Upjohn, relating to Halcion. Because of lingering questions about some Upjohn studies on Halcion's side effects, the FDA also intends to ask for outside experts to reevaluate the drug's safety.

EFFECT OF EFFICACY REQUIREMENTS ON DRUG DEVELOPMENT

Since the imposition of the 1962 amendments, both the drug industry and the FDA have endured a joint learning experience on the impact of the new requirements on drug development. This can be illustrated by the experience of one drug company over a period of 30 years. When Parke-Davis first marketed a particular epinephrine preparation in 1938, all it had to do was submit a 27-page report concerned primarily with safety. When it subsequently introduced a new expectorant in 1948, only a 73-page report was required. However, in 1962, when the same company requested FDA approval of its contraceptive, Norlestin, it had to submit a report totaling 12,370 pages. In 1968, when it sought approval for a new anesthetic, the required documents totaled slightly more than 72,000 pages in 167 volumes. Obviously, things were getting out of hand. In theory, one would expect that a report of 200 or 300 pages would suffice if the research has been properly planned and executed and all the material submitted is cogently organized. However, as recently as 1996, the drug company Serono accumulated a 40,000 page file for its growth hormone preparation intended for use in AIDS.

TIME AND COST OF DRUG DEVELOPMENT

During the past few years, the FDA has been subjected to substantial criticism because of the length of time required for the various phases of the review process as well as the attendant costs for the drug companies. According to studies carried out at Tufts University and the Center for the Study of Drug development, it can take approximately 12 years, from synthesis to regulatory clearance, to bring a prescription drug to market at a cost of approximately $231 million. In addition, for every 10,000 chemical entities synthesized, approximately 10 will enter clinical trial and 1 will gain regulatory approval. The comparative length of time normally involved in the various phases of drug development is shown in Table 16.4.

In order to expedite the FDA approval stage of the process, a Prescription Drug User Fee Act was authorized in 1992. This program has allowed the FDA to collect fees from pharmaceutical companies and use the proceeds to accelerate the review process at the Center for Drug Evaluation and Research as well as the Center for Biologics Evaluation and Research. Firms were initially charged $50,000 annually, $5,000 for each product on the market and $150,000 for an IND. This user fee is now (2000) $309,647 for each new NDA. The projected income of $75 million was to be used for new staff. The company's money now covers approximately 50% of the FDA's costs for reviewing proposed drugs. The results appear to be promising since the median approval time for new drugs in 1994 was 19 months, 21% less than in 1993. Similar improvement was also achieved with backlogged and supplemental submissions as well.

According to the FDA, drug companies are actually sending fewer novel medicines to evaluate, instead creating more "me-too" drugs similar to ones already sold. In 1999, half the drugs the FDA

TABLE 16.4
Drug Development and
Approval Process

Stage	Years
Preclinical	6.5
Phase I	1
Phase II	2
Phase III	3
FDA	1–2

Source: PharmaceuticalResearch and Manufacturers of America, Washington, DC.

approved were priority drugs, breakthroughs, or medicines deemed to advance public health. In 2000, just one-third were in these categories. One breakthrough drug in leukemia therapy (Gleevec) set a record in the spring of 2001, when it won FDA approval in less than 3 months.

Of the 78 drugs approved by the FDA in 2002, only 17 contained new active ingredients, and only 7 of these were classified by the FDA as improvements over older drugs. The other 71 drugs approved that year were variations of old drugs or deemed no better than drugs already on the market. In other words, they were "me-too" drugs.

The year 2003 saw an increase in the overall number of biologics and drugs approved and a decrease in the FDA review and approval time for most applications. The Center for Biologics Evaluation and Research and the Center for Drug Evaluation and Research approved 466 new and generic drugs and biological products. Twenty-one new molecular entities with active ingredients never before marketed in the United States, were approved, up from 17 in 2002; the average review time for standard NME applications was reduced in 2003 to 15.9 months from 23.1 in 2002.

Marcia Angell, the acting Editor-in-Chief of the *New England Journal of Medicine* has written "The me-too business is made possible by the fact that the FDA usually approves a drug only if it is better than a placebo. It needn't be better than an older drug already on the market to treat the same condition; in fact, it may be worse."

NEW FDA PROGRAMS

Over the years, the FDA has also implemented a variety of programs to make promising therapies more widely available to people with serious and life-threatening illnesses. In 1987, the FDA finalized regulations that created a "treatment IND." This was primarily in response to AIDS activists. This rule formalized the procedures that allow thousands of patients to have access to investigational drugs for treatment of serious and life-threatening diseases for which there is no satisfactory treatment *prior* to general marketing. The regulation allows for a treatment protocol, separate and distinct from the study protocols, either while clinical studies are still under way or completed, but the sponsor must actively be pursuing marketing approval. In addition, there must be sufficient data to indicate that the substance "*may be effective*," and that there are no unreasonable risks. At this point in time, the FDA was taking in excess of 2 years to review NDAs.

In the years since the *treatment IND* was created, a number of drugs have been subsequently approved for marketing including several for AIDS or AIDS-related conditions. In 1992, the Public Health Service published a policy statement permitting even more expanded availability of investigational drugs for AIDS through a "*parallel track*" mechanism. This policy outlines how promising new drugs can be made available early in the development process, once there is evidence of probable efficacy based on laboratory and available clinical data, evidence that the drug is reasonably safe, and enough data to recommend an appropriate starting dose. This policy serves people without satisfactory alternatives, who cannot tolerate or derive no benefit from the available therapies, and cannot participate in clinical trials because they do not meet the entry criteria, or are too ill to participate, or because it would cause undue hardship, such as travel, or because the trials are fully enrolled. The parallel track differs from the *treatment IND* in two important regards: (1) the parallel track applies *only* to AIDS-related therapies and (2) it makes drugs available earlier in the discovery process (i.e., late phase I or early phase II versus late phase II or phase III).

This accelerated program has already paid handsome dividends. In 1996, the protease inhibitor ritonavir was approved in 72 days, the fastest AIDS drug approved until that point and probably the fastest drug approval of any kind, to date, in FDA history. The FDA based its approval on data showing that it increases CD4 lymphocytes as well as decreases the amount of HIV in the bloodstream. In addition, the cumulative mortality rate among participants on the drug was approximately 40% of that in the control group. Also, those on ritonavir experienced a 50% greater reduction in disease progression. Other protease inhibitors have also been approved in rapid order.

In 1996, President Clinton announced a "major new initiative" giving cancer patients faster and easier access to promising treatments. The FDA immediately implemented a fast-track approval process for anticancer drugs like that begun for anti-AIDS drugs. If a drug shows effectiveness in early testing, patients will have access to it even while the drug continues to undergo tests for approval. Accelerated approval is predicted to affect approximately 100 drugs now being studied, cutting FDA review time for these drugs from 12 months to 6 months. From 1993 to 1999, the FDA approved 232 drugs regarded as new molecular entities compared with 163 during the previous 7 years (a 42% increase).

For hard-to-treat cancers, effectiveness is being redefined to include partial responses such as tumor shrinkage. Previously, before a drug was approved for marketing, it had to demonstrate such clinical benefits as increased survival or improved quality of life. Utilizing objective evidence such as tumor shrinkage will permit shorter studies for initial approval. Although abbreviated testing is not without additional risks, the risks appear acceptable for diseases such as AIDS and cancer.

In addition to expediting the availability of drugs used to treat AIDS and cancer, abbreviated new drug applications (ANDA) have been made available for the development of *generic* drugs that differ little from drugs already on the market. Market share of generic drugs more than doubled from 18.6% in 1984 to 41.6% in 1996. Another important piece of legislation affecting drug development was the *Orphan Drug Act of 1983*. "Orphans" are drugs and other products for treating rare diseases. They may offer little or no profit to the manufacturer, but may benefit people with the rare diseases. To foster orphan product development, this law allows drug companies to take a tax deduction for about three-quarters of the cost of their clinical studies. Firms are also given exclusive marketing rights for 7 years for any orphan products that are approved. An example of such a drug is interferon β-1a approved in 1996 for the treatment of multiple sclerosis, a chronic, often disabling CNS disease that affects 250,000 Americans.

INSTITUTIONAL REVIEW BOARDS

Growing out of a history of U.S. scandals and reactions to Nazi medical war crimes, the U.S. government ultimately developed strict guidelines and safeguards to protect participants in clinical trials. In 1966, the Surgeon General issued a statement on the protection of human subjects, stating no grant would be given for research involving human subjects unless the application described how the subjects would have their welfare protected, how informed consent would be obtained, and that the subjects would be protected from undue risk. This led to the formation of the Institutional Review Boards (IRB). Today, every clinical trial in the United States must be approved and monitored by an IRB to ensure that the risks are as low as possible and are worth any potential benefits.

An IRB is an independent committee of physicians, statisticians, community advocates, and others that ensures that a clinical trial is ethical and that the rights of study participants are protected. All institutions that conduct or support biomedical research involving humans must, by federal regulation, have an IRB that initially approves and periodically reviews the research. At least five people compose an IRB, and at least one member must come from a nonscientific discipline such as the law or the clergy.

To grant IRB approval, board members must jointly agree, for a specific trial and its investigator, that (1) patient risks are minimal and reasonable with respect to anticipated treatment benefits; (2) enrollment criteria are appropriate and patient eligibility is determined without regard to race, gender, economic background, and other such factors (unless appropriate and necessary for the trial, such as recruiting only females to test birth control pills); (3)informed consent documents meet all regulatory requirements; (4) patient consent will be obtained properly; (5) patient safety will be monitored continually; (6) collected data will be reviewed for completeness and accuracy; and (7) confidentiality will be maintained for all participants.

Periodically, the FDA can inspect IRB records and operations to certify that approvals, human subject safeguards (including informed consent), and conduct of business are what they should be. Occasionally, these inspections yield evidence of problems, such as in 1993, when the FDA imposed penalties on a large California university for infractions that included a failure to report deaths.

At any time in the clinical trials process, the FDA is allowed to issue a "clinical hold" if it is deemed necessary. A clinical hold is an order issued by the FDA to the sponsor to delay a proposed investigation or to suspend an ongoing investigation entirely. When a clinical hold is issued, no new subjects are allowed to enter the program, and patients already in the study must be taken off the drug unless discontinuing the treatment could interfere with patient safety. During the period of 1999–2001, the FDA temporarily halted research because of inadequate IRB review and follow-up at two locations (Duke University and the VA Medical Center of West Los Angeles). In addition, the government suspended federally funded research on human subjects at Johns Hopkins University, following the death of a healthy volunteer during an asthma experiment. Medical school officials said the patient likely died from inhaling the drug *hexamethonium*, which constricts airways. Hexamethonium was used widely as a tablet in the 1940s and 1950s to treat hypertension, but the FDA later withdrew its approval. It had never been approved as an inhalant, which was the way it was used in the Hopkins study.

SELECTED BIBLIOGRAPHY

Abramson, J., (2004). *Overdosed America. The Broken Promise of American Medicine*. New York: Harper Collins.
Avorn, J., (2004). *Powerful Medicines: The Benefits, Risks, and Costs of Prescription Drugs*. New York: Alfred A. Knopf.
Goozner, M., (2004). *The $800 Million Pill: The Truth Behind the Cost of New Drugs*. Berkeley, CA: Univ. CA. Press.
Kassirer, J.P. (2005). *On the Take: How America's Complicity with Big Business can Endanger your Health*. New York: Oxford University Press.
National Center for Policy Analysis, (1999), *Policy Report No. 230*, Washington, DC: U.S.
U.S. Department of Health and Human Services, Office of Inspector General. (1998) Institutional Review Boards: Time for Reform; Report OEI-01-97-00193. Washington, DC, U.S. Department of Health and Human Services.
Willman, D. (2000). *How a New Policy Led to Seven Deadly Drugs*? Los Angeles, CA: Los Angeles, Times.

QUESTIONS

1. Which of the following is/are true regarding phase II clinical studies?
   a. Involves patients with the disease
   b. Involves normal patients
   c. Can involve a few dozen to a few hundred people
   d. Can involve 10,000 or more subjects
   e. a and c

2. The 1906 Food and Drug Act dealt primarily with which of the following?
   a. Drug safety
   b. Drug toxicity
   c. Truth in labeling
   d. None of the above
   e. All of the above

3. Which of the following chemicals was primarily responsible for the 1938 Food, Drug, and Cosmetic Act?
   a. Sulfanilamide
   b. Dinitrophenol
   c. Thalidomide
   d. Diethylene glycol
   e. Salvarsan

4. The law requiring demonstration of efficacy for a drug occurred in which year?
   a. 1906
   b. 1938
   c. 1962
   d. 1977
   e. 1981

5. Which of the following is required before a drug can be taken to clinical trials?
   a. IND
   b. DEA
   c. NDA
   d. NAS
   e. OTC

6. The use of healthy volunteers usually only occurs in which phase of clinical studies?
   a. Phase I
   b. Phase II
   c. Phase III
   d. Phase IV
   e. All of the above

7. Which of the following groups present particular problems in clinical trials?
   a. Children
   b. The elderly
   c. Women
   d. Postpubescent males
   e. a, b, and c

8. The majority of all drugs tested are abandoned by their sponsors after which of the following?
   a. Phase I
   b. Phase II
   c. Phase III
   d. Phase IV
   e. a and b

9. How many prescription drugs were removed from the market between 1997 and 2001?
   a. 6
   b. 10
   c. 12
   d. 17
   e. 21

10. IRB's are concerned with which of the following?
   a. Clinical trial design
   b. Informed consent
   c. Proper enrollment criteria
   d. Confidentiality of participants
   e. All of the above

17 Animals in Research

The proper study of mankind is man.

Alexander Pope, 1733

I have seen numerous experiments on animals, but I have never seen an animal undergoing pain which I would not have been willing to undergo myself for the same object. Why, then, it may be asked, should not all painful experiments be done on human volunteers?

J.B.S. Haldane, 1971

Progress in the understanding and management of human disease must begin, and end, with studies of man...

Paul Beeson, M.D., 1979

INTRODUCTION

The use of animals for research purposes has been the subject of many articles and books, both in defense of and in opposition to, over the past 100–150 years. In some cases, opposition has been quite strident expressing itself in both legal and illegal acts. With regard to the latter, research establishments have been raided, animals removed, records destroyed, and equipment vandalized. In fact, the uninitiated can now become knowledgeable about pursuing this line of expression by obtaining a "handbook" for animal activists. On the other hand, a new group was formed in the United Kingdom in 2004 to represent people who have been personally targeted by animal rights activists; its name is Victims of Animal Rights Extremism (VARE).

What are the reasons for such strongly held views? One major reason, of course, is that animals can be our pets. As such, they occupy a special relationship in our lives. To a certain extent, they are like children and are dependent on our husbandry for their welfare. Most people are repulsed by the abuse of children and, hence, animals, since they are usually defenseless and are easily victimized.

Today, animals are used in scientific experiments for three general purposes: (1) biomedical and behavioral research; (2) education; and (3) drug and product testing. However, all too often, those concerned with animal welfare question whether basic biomedical research has substantial clinical value and that alternatives should be developed for teaching and testing. Scientists answer that while all research might not have immediate value, most clinical breakthroughs are based on multiple, fundamental studies carried out on experimental animals for which there are no appropriate alternatives. It is *not* the purpose of this chapter to advocate either side of the argument. Rather, the goal is to present the salient features of both sides of the issue for the reader to consider.

HISTORY

300 BC TO AD 1800

The first recorded use of *live* animals for research is generally attributed to the "*study of body humors*" by Erasistratus in Alexandria, in the third century B.C. In view of the fact that this antedates the discovery of general anesthetics by approximately 2150 years, one can only imagine the pain and suffering that "experimental" animals were subjected to in the name of science during this period. It was Galen of Pergamum, in the second century A.D., who has been credited with demonstrating the significance of animal research. Galen expounded the theory that four natural humors—blood, phlegm, yellow bile, and black bile—were responsible for health. Since dissection of the *human* body was illegal in Rome at that time, Galen based his anatomical studies on "observations" made in "apes" and pigs.

It is extremely unlikely, however, that Galen actually carried out his research on apes. In fact, apes were not widely available for examination in Europe until about the sixteenth century. In all probability, the so-called Barbary "ape" of North Africa and Gibraltar is what Galen actually used. This "ape" is, in fact, a macaque monkey that was presumably the first primate experimented on. Among Galen's discoveries was the observation, in a live animal, that cutting a particular nerve in the neck (known to come from the lower brain) abolished movement of the larynx. After the fall of Rome, learning fell into disrepute in Europe until the thirteenth century. While this may have been a dark period for civilization, it undoubtedly served as a respite for experimental animals.

One theory advanced for the historical lack of concern regarding the infliction of pain on animals during the first millennium, or so, is that life for people of this period was often little better than their pets or the beasts of the fields. Life was basically short and hard, and contained much pain and suffering. How could concern for an animal in agony be mustered when members of the family were suffering equally?

Following the Dark Ages, the Renaissance brought with it a desire for discovery in many areas including the human body. Because of this, the use of experimental animals also became popular once again. Unfortunately, influential thinkers of the day were anything but sensitive to the use of experimental animals. Francis Bacon (1561–1626), for one, championed the value of animal experimentation in his *De Augmentis Scientiarum* (The Advancement of Learning) when he asserted that "....*by the dissection of beast* **alive**, *which, not withstanding the* **dissimilitude** *of their parts to human, may with the help of a little judgment, sufficiently satisfy this inquiry.*"

The French philosopher Rene Descartes (1596–1650) was probably the most influential individual in formulating our early views regarding the status of animals in our world. According to Descartes, animals were no more than machines and were, therefore, *incapable* of thinking or feeling. Living in an age when clocks were at the cutting edge of technology, he wrote to the Marquis of Newcastle "*I know, indeed, that brutes do many things better than we do, but I am not surprised at it; for that, also, goes to prove that they act by force of nature and by springs, like a clock, which tells better what the hour is than our judgment can inform us.*" Descartes imagined insects and other creatures as elegant, miniaturized bits of clockwork "*which eat without pleasure, cry without pain, desire nothing, know nothing, and only simulate intelligence as a bee simulates a mathematician*" (in the geometry of its hexagonal honeycombs). Ants do not have souls, Descartes argued; *automatons* are owed no special moral obligations. He expressed his thoughts quite succinctly when he stated: "*The greatest of all the prejudices we have retained from our infancy is that of believing that the beasts think.*" In Descartes' world, if an animal screamed in pain it was equivalent to the mechanical squeals of an ungreased wheel.

1800–1900

While the seventeenth and eighteenth centuries saw the growth of the scientific revolution, led by such luminaries as William Harvey (1578–1657), Anthony Van Leeuwenhoek (1632–1723), and Lazzaro Spallanzani (1729–1799), it was not until the nineteenth century that organized, systematic animal research really began in earnest, and opposition to it began to develop as a consequence. By the early 1800s, the view that animals were little more than machine equivalents began to be questioned. This was particularly true in Britain where the first *Society for the Prevention of Cruelty to Animals* was formed in 1824. Despite the views of England's Francis Bacon, alluded to previously, the overriding feeling against inflicting pain on household as well as experimental animals was one of the reasons why Britain took little part in the rapid advances in physiology that took place in the early and middle decades of the nineteenth century. Notable scientists such as Boyle and Hook, as well as other Fellows of the Royal Society were often quite outspoken in their concern for the suffering of experimental animals in contrast to their continental colleagues.

As a result of this Anglo viewpoint, experimental physiology did not really begin to develop in Britain until approximately 1870, by which time the use of general anesthetics had become generally available. However, despite the availability of anesthetics, some researchers were, nevertheless, selective in their use. For example, in 1875, the physiologist Emmanuel Klein was quoted as saying he had "*no regard at all*" for the suffering of experimental animals and only used anesthetics for his own convenience. This type of insensitivity led to the appointment of a Royal commission in the same year and finally to the passing of the *Cruelty to Animal Act* of 1876. However, although this bill *regulated* painful research, it did not abolish it and, as a result, was strongly opposed by certain groups concerned with animal welfare. It was also during this period, in 1874, that *Thomas Huxley* published his critique of the Cartesian view of animals as automata. His summary conclusion was that animals were, in fact, automata but, like humans, they were *conscious* automata.

The situation was considerably different on the European continent, chiefly in France and Germany, where there was a heavy dependency on experiments involving major surgery on *unanesthetized* animals (accounts of some of these experiments have been described as "horrifying to read"). The difference in viewpoint toward the use of animals in research, particularly in France, can be ascribed to the influence of Descartes and his views on animals. Regardless of the reasons behind Descartes' position, his assertions provided the rationalization for vivisection research by the famous French experimentalists Francois Magendie (1783–1855) and his student Claude Bernard (1813–1878). Ironically, despite Bernard's reputation as an eminent experimentalist, his wife and two daughters became passionate antivivisectionists.

OPPOSITION TO ANIMAL USE IN RESEARCH

In general, the animal-cause movement can be divided into two broad groups: (1) individuals concerned with *animal welfare* who are not necessarily opposed to biomedical research using animals; however, they do want the assurance that the animals are treated as humanely as possible (pain and suffering kept to a minimum), that the number of animals used are kept to a minimum, and that the animals are used only when necessary and (2) individuals concerned with *animal rights* who insist that animals have moral rights, unlike Descartes' view, *equal* to those of humans and are *totally opposed* to biomedical research using animals. People for the Ethical Treatment of Animals (PETA) and the Animal Liberation Front (ALF) have been the most vocal and visible proponents of the animal rights movement. Early opponents of animal experimentation were termed *antivivisectionists* (derived from the Latin *vius* [living] and *sectio* [cutting]). Antivivisectionists are essentially abolitionists.

The roots of antivivisection as an organized movement are found in Britain, the birth place of anticruelty crusades of all kinds. Jeremy Bentham, a Utilitarian philosopher, composed a particularly moving passage in his *Introduction to the Principles of Morals and Legislation*. In 1789, he wrote, "… *a full grown horse or dog is beyond comparison a more rational, as well as a more conversable animal, than an infant of a day, of a week or even a month old. But suppose the cause were otherwise, what would it avail? The question is not can they reason? Nor, can they talk? But, can they suffer?*" Despite this highly relevant question, it would be 87 years before British sentiment was sufficiently galvanized to pass the 1876 Cruelty to Animal Act.

In addition to the concept of suffering introduced by Bentham, Methodist theological doctrine was also a contributing factor to the British mind-set of the day, because it held that animals also shared the potential of experiencing *immortality* with humans. This was no inconsequential tenet in a country of animal lovers. Would there be a pack of Cujos with a bad attitude at the "pearly gates?" If concern for pain and suffering in Victorian Britain, supported by arguments for the immortality of animals were not enough, the publication of Darwin's *Descent of Man* in the mid-nineteenth century also served to challenge, in a far more dramatic fashion, the premise that humans and animals were different. How could Cartesian logic be depended on if we were related in some anthropological manner to the beasts of the field?

In the second half of the nineteenth century, vivisection was actually even rarer in the United States than in Britain because of the relative paucity of experimental research. However, there were animal activists busy in North America before there was even a United States of America. In 1641, the Puritans of the Massachusetts Bay Colony drew up a list of liberties. Their formal legal code included "Liberty 92" that reads: *"No man shall exercise any Tirranny (sic) or Crueltie (sic) towards any brute Creature which are usalie (sic) kept for man's use."*

The American Anti-Vivisection Society was founded in 1883 largely as a result of events in Britain. Their attempts to ban vivisection or significantly curtail it in several states were uniformly unsuccessful. There were a number of reasons for their failures, not the least of which was the emerging public awareness of the apparent beneficial role of animal research in the successful treatment of ravaging contagious diseases such as diphtheria. By the early 1900s, the influence of experimental medicine was growing and the humane movement, which it had become known as, receded into more mundane pursuits.

Between the two world wars, the reputation and prestige of the medical scientist and the research establishment continued to grow. In the United States, antivivisectionist groups remained largely ineffective in implementing their concerns despite the support of powerful backers such as William Randolph Hearst. Such was not the case in Germany, however. Although Germany had a rich history in vivisection, there existed, nonetheless, considerable opposition to this practice. In one of histories ironies, Herman Goering made the following declaration during a broadcast on August 29, 1933: *"Experiments on animals for the purpose of defining an illness in human beings, for the preparation of serums and other experimental use, need legal regulation in detail and the keen control of the state. It is a sorry sign of science that during the past two decades, amply protected by law, materialistic scientists have wrought unbearable torture and suffering in animal experiments ... I have therefore announced the immediate prohibition of vivisection and have made the practice a punishable offense in Prussia. Until such times as punishment is pronounced the culprit shall be lodged in a concentration camp."*

It was not until after the Second World War that the humane movement in the United States became reenergized. This was due, in part, to the sudden increase in funds available for biomedical research as well as the passage of a number of state pound *seizure* laws that required release of unclaimed dogs and cats to medical research institutions to satisfy increased demand. After numerous failures to repeal these laws, humane societies turned their attention toward providing alternative shelters for homeless or lost dogs and cats. It was not until the 1980s that several states, under pressure, including New York and Massachusetts, passed laws that prohibited the release of any cat or dog from any type of shelter except for its adoption or return to its owner.

ANIMAL RIGHTS MOVEMENT

The contemporary animal rights movement had its genesis coincidental with three books published in the early 1970s. The first of these books, *Animals, Men and Morals* by Godlovitch, Godlovitch, and Harris, was published in 1971 and was an anthology that revived and presented to a new generation many long-dormant thoughts and views regarding the relationship between humans and animals. One of these was the view that animals have rights (proposed as early as 1894). This book renewed interest within the intellectual community of the relationship between human beings and animals and led to the publication in 1975 of two other important books. One of these was *Victims of Science* written by Richard Ryder who introduced the concept of *"specieism"* (an elitist term similar to racism). The other book was *Animal Liberation: A New Ethic for our Treatment of Animals* by Peter Singer. It is this latter book that is generally considered to be the progenitor of the contemporary animal rights movement. Singer's expertise in this area is reflected in his joining the Princeton faculty in 1999 as a professor of bioethics. Singer has made the controversial and provocative comment that in *some cases* animals' lives should take precedence over humans.

Singer's book revived the classic debate that has existed for centuries between Cartesian (i.e., Rene Descartes—animals are machines) and Utilitarian philosophers (e.g., Jeremy Bentham—prevention of suffering), and made it an issue of the 1970s and 1980s. Singer has also made the disquieting suggestion that raising human infants for food is morally no different from raising pigs for the same purpose. Nevertheless, one important aspect of Singer's book was that it *reintroduced* to the cause of antivivisectionism an *intellectual basis, a philosophical orientation, and a moral focus*—regardless of one's views. These foundations gave the animal rights movement a new attraction to those who had been generally indifferent to, or repelled by, the essentially emotional appeal based on love of animals that antivivisectionism had been waging for the last century. The movement now had more legitimacy and support than ever before and its goals were consistent with other contemporary societal objectives.

Despite what pro and con philosophical arguments occur at faculty cocktail parties, there are loose-knit groups that are proactive in asserting their beliefs. During the past 25 years, organizations such as the ALF and the Earth Liberation Front (ELF) have claimed responsibility for numerous acts involving public and private facilities. The groups have no formal structure, but espouse philosophies that support sabotage in defense of animal life or the environment. The Internet has facilitated their communication. An area that they have emphasized is the release of animals.

These *eco-saboteurs*, as they are sometimes referred to, are suspected of at least seven incidents since September 2001: (1) a firebombing at a federal corral for wild horses in northeastern California; (2) a fire at a primate research center in New Mexico; (3) release of more than 1000 mink from a farm in Iowa; (4) release of pigeons raised for research in Iowa; and (5, 6, and 7) fires at an Oregon tree farm, a laboratory at the University of Washington, and a fire that destroyed a McDonald's restaurant in Tucson, Arizona. In recent years, the groups have also claimed responsibility for setting fires at a Vail, Colorado ski resort, which they say impacted a lynx habitat.

The impact of antivivisectionists has been manyfold. Not the least of which has been an elevation of the consciousness of many people, including those in biomedical research, about the issue of experimental animals. As a result, a number of questions that can be justifiably directed toward those utilizing research animals have arisen. Some of these questions address scientific issues while others are more moralistic in nature. For example, questions pertaining to science include the following: Is the scientific query mundane in nature? Will the data duplicate already existing data? If animals are used will their numbers be kept to a minimum? These are not, in fact, new questions. Britain's Marshall Hall (1790–1857) promulgated four related principles of animal research over a 100 years ago

- Experiments should never be done if the necessary information could be gained by observation.
- No experiment should be performed without a clearly defined and attainable objective.
- One should avoid unwarranted repetition.
- Any justifiable experiment should be carried out with the least possible infliction of suffering.

While some type of answer might be presented relatively easily to the types of issues raised above, it is the moral dilemma that appears to be more of a conundrum. After all, an experimental animal is *not* a volunteer; animals do not have the option of consent, as their human counterparts do—they are conscripted. An animal finds itself living and/or dying within the constraints of a laboratory setting by virtue of being a "subordinate" species. As such, it is basically helpless—a prisoner, a victim if you will.

Intervention by appropriate review boards is not on the same level as an IRB for human clinical studies. It is this exploitation, or *specieism*, of sentient beings that continues to challenge our moral and ethical framework. In fact, it is this particular quandary, perhaps more than any other issue, that has contributed to the internecine conflict between members of the biomedical community as well as the general public. However, rational arguments to these and other related issues have been put forth (see the Nicoll and Russell citation in the bibliography).

CONTEMPORARY STATUS

Are animals still subjected to untoward, excessive levels of pain and suffering? The answer appears to be, unfortunately, yes. In 1952, a business meeting of the American Physiological Society included the allegation from one of its members that there was much inhumane use of animals in biological and medical research. In 1957, 58 rhesus monkeys were put inside tubes set near the drop point for a nuclear bomb test. Those set in tubes along the flashpoint of the explosion were *fried*. Researcher have shot monkeys in the head with rifles, the barrel of the gun held just an inch from their skulls; shot them in the stomach with a "cannon impactor" accelerated to 70 miles an hour to study *blunt abdominal trauma*. Monkeys have been crippled by having weights dropped on their spines.

One of the more infamous studies during the 1960s dealt with the nature of love. Briefly, the experiments involved taking away infant monkeys from their mother and measuring their response. Remarkably, this "research" found that it is not enough for monkeys to see each other through glass partitions; they need to stroke, to hold. Such experiments were not without their challenges to the investigators, however. The senior investigator in this federally funded project reported that before they began utilizing anesthetics, it sometimes took two laboratory workers to hold the struggling mother down while a third pulled the baby away. Lavish praise was bestowed on the senior investigator for this "seminal" work.

In a 1957 experiment, scientists plunged *unanesthetized* rats into boiling water in order to measure blood changes; in 1960, scientists wanting to study muscle atrophy, *immobilized the hind legs of cats with steel pins for 101 days, until the tissues withered*. In 1961, researchers studied the effect of microwave blasts on dogs. Their detailed records noted that *unanesthetized* animals began to pant rapidly as radiation increased, that their tongues swelled, that their skin crisped, and if their body temperature was allowed to climb above 107° F, the dogs died. During the early 1960s, cats were injected with acid directly into their trachea to induce mucus formation for the screening of antimucolytic drugs.

Today, most scientists and nonscientists are probably prepared to agree that standards of animal care and use have improved considerably over those of the 1950s and 1960s. However, unfortunate exceptions continue to periodically appear. In 1972, a polio researcher was credited with making the comment that "*any qualms at the 'inhumanity' of injecting viruses into the spinal cords of these 'cute' creatures, who look so much like little people, is soon dispelled by their many annoying attributes*." Does this reflect sensitivity to suffering?

Two scientific research papers published in 1976 drew considerable criticism both from within and outside the biomedical research community for their cruel design. This research involved the use of the so-called Noble-Collup drum, within which *lightly* anesthetized animals were "*tumbled*." The interior of the drum contained shelves that projected out from the surface in order to produce injury and trauma to the tumbling animal. In other words, the experiment was *designed to inevitably inflict pain*. One would hope that the submission of such a paper today would result in its rejection owing to violation of journal policy toward abuse of experimental animals. Fortunately, such editorial policies have become more commonplace in scientific journals.

In 1980, the U.S. Department of Agriculture brought a complaint against Ohio State University concerning its care of some 40 kittens used in biomedical research. The complaint enunciated that "*The kittens had lesions around their necks and many had metal tags with identification tags imbedded [emphasis mine] in the flesh of their necks. These injuries apparently resulted from chains being placed around the kittens' neck when they were young and not being replaced or lengthened as they grew older*." The fine for this deplorable act of "husbandry" was $500, which the university reluctantly paid while denying culpability.

The existence of insensitivity during the 1980s is further illustrated by a rather remarkable statement attributed to a scientist during a meeting with an NIH grant review team in 1981. This individual argued that one cannot apply "*human expectations of pain to animal surgery because pain is primarily a matter of societal conditioning to which animals are not subject*." If this is, in fact, the case, how does one justify, on scientific terms, the thousands of animals that have been used over the years in pain and analgesia research? The year 1981 was also the high-water mark, or low, depending on one's point of view, in the area of animal abuse. The alleged abuse of animals launched the precedent-setting case of the *Silver Springs Monkeys*.

Primate experiments at Silver Springs involved the procedure known as *deafferentation.* It requires opening of the spinal cord and slicing away selected sensory nerves rendering the monkey crippled. In this particular case, the procedure was carried out in order to "force recovery" of the affected limb. In order to make a crippled monkey use its bad limb, the investigator strapped on a straightjacket to bind the good arm, leaving the animal only the damaged one to use. An alternative strategy was to place animals in restraining chairs and give electric shocks if they did not move their crippled arm.

This case resulted in the first and only arrest and criminal conviction of an animal researcher in the United States on charges of cruelty to animals, the first confiscation of abused laboratory animals under a court-ordered search and seizure warrant, and the first hearing by the U.S. Supreme Court of a case involving animals in experiments. This type of event stimulated various organizations such as *The American College of Toxicology* and the *Society of Toxicology*, for example, to establish policy statements and guiding principles during the late 1980s, relating to animal experimentation.

The point here is not to list examples ad nauseum of animal abuse in the name of science, or attitudinal problems of researchers but, rather, to serve as a reminder that things are probably not perfect in our nation's laboratories despite improvement. To deny such would challenge credibility and temper continuation of necessary self-evaluation, criticism, and regulation. Constant vigilance appears to be necessary, if for no other reason than the large number of experimental animals still being used and the corresponding opportunities for negligence.

BIOMEDICAL RESEARCH

Of all the industries utilizing animal research, biomedical research undoubtedly uses the greatest number of animals and has been, therefore, a national target for animal reform. The *National Association for Biomedical Research* estimates that 23 million rats and mice were used in 1998 and made up 95% of all laboratory animals (other estimates are on the order of 30 million). In addition to rodents, dogs and cats (1–1.5%), and nonhuman primates (0.5%) make up the majority of the remainder. According to the *Institute for Laboratory Animal Resources* survey, there was a 40% decrease in the number of animals used in research between 1968 and 1978, with the largest decline occurring with nonhuman primates, dogs, cats, and birds.

The reasons for this decrease are undoubtedly multifactorial and probably include the refinement of research techniques, development of alternatives, decrease in research funding, and animal rights/ welfare activism. Funds for research have failed to increase at the same rate as costs of acquiring and carrying for laboratory animals. Researchers have also lowered the incidence of spontaneous disease among laboratory animals thus increasing their longevity. Today, the same research objectives can be obtained with fewer animals because of improved methods for breeding, rearing, genetic control, and experimental design.

As mentioned above, the vast majority of laboratory animals are rats and mice bred specifically for this purpose by licensed suppliers. Large animals, such as swine, cattle, and sheep, are supplied primarily by agricultural sources. Today, most nonhuman primates are obtained from scientific breeding centers and not from the wild, since their exportation has been prohibited by several countries. Many cats and dogs necessary for research are "purpose-bred" animals—those bred for a particular trait or whose genealogy or physiology must be known in order for the experimental results to be valid. Such animals are bred and sold by professional dealers. Other experiments can be conducted with what are known as "random source" animals whose ancestry and physiologic history are unknown. Such animals are, in fact, preferable in some experiments because their unknown and varied backgrounds more closely approximate those found among a human population. One source of such animals has been pounds.

Estimates vary widely, but of the approximately 16.2–27 million cats and dogs left in pounds and shelters each year, only about 1.1% (approximately 138,000 dogs and 50,000 cats) are used in research annually. The majority of these pound animals, between 10.1 and 16.7 million dogs and cats, are put to death by animal care and control agencies each year, according to the American Humane Association's 1989 statistics. The remaining animals are claimed by their owners or adopted. Animal rights groups have persuaded a number of state, county, and municipal legislatures to pass laws to prohibit the release of animals (primarily dogs and cats) from public pounds to researchers. The most comprehensive pound law, adopted by Massachusetts, bans the use of pound animals regardless of source. It is estimated that the additional cost of conducting experiments in Massachusetts will be $6 million a year.

BENEFITS OF ANIMAL RESEARCH

How does one determine if animal experimentation has been productive and justified? One criterion often quoted is the relationship between animal research and the Nobel Prize, which is generally considered to be an index of scientific significance. Since 1901, approximately 75% of Nobel Prizes awarded in physiology or medicine have been for discoveries and progresses made through the use of experimental animals. More specifically, many advances in medical science in the nineteenth and twentieth centuries from vaccines and antibiotics to antidepressant drugs and organ transplants, have been achieved either directly or indirectly through the use of animals in laboratory experiments. The result of these experiments has been the elimination or control of many infectious diseases—smallpox, poliomyelitis, and measles—and the development of numerous life-saving techniques—blood transfusions, burn therapy, and open-heart and brain surgery. A more extensive list of examples is shown below in Table 17.1.

TABLE 17.1
Examples of Medical Advances Made Possible Through the Use of Animals

Pre-1900	Treatment of rabbies, anthrax, and smallpox	1950s	Prevention of poliomyelitis
	Principles of infection control and pain relief		Development of cancer chemotherapy
	Management of heart failure		Open-heart surgery and cardiac pacemaker
Early 1900s	Treatment of histamine shock, pellagra, (niacin deficiency), and rickets (Vitamin D deficiency)	1960s	Prevention of rubella
			Corneal transplant and coronary bypass surgery
			Therapeutic use of cortisone
	Electrocardiography and cardiac catherization		Development of radioimmunoassay for the measurement of minute quantities of antibodies, hormones, and other substances in the body
1920s	Discovery of thyroxin		
	Intravenous feeding	1970s	Prevention of measles
	Discovery of insulin—diabetes control		Modern treatment of coronary insufficiency
1930s	Therapeutic use of sulfa drugs		Heart transplant
	Prevention of tetanus		Development of nonaddictive pain killers
	Development of anticoagulants, modern anesthesia, and neuromuscular blocking agents	1980s	Use of cyclosporin and other antirejection drugs
			Artificial heart transplantation
			Identification of psychophysiological factors in depression, anxiety, and phobias
1940s	Treatment of rheumatoid arthritis and whooping cough		Development of monocional antibodies for treating disease
	Therapeutic use of antibiotics, such as penicillin, aureomycin, and streptomycin		Discovery of HIV as causative agent for AIDS
	Discovery of Rh factor	1990s	Pancreas and liver transplantation
	Treatment of leprosy		Thrombolytic therapy for acute myocardial infarction
	Prevention of diphtheria		Human gene therapy

Behavioral research with animals has also been credited with benefit to humans. For example, fundamental information on how people learn was discovered by experiments on animals in laboratories. The behavioral modification therapies discovered or developed through such experiments are being used to treat conditions such as enuresis (bed-wetting), addictive behaviors (tobacco, alcohol, and other drugs), and compulsive behaviors such as anorexia nervosa. In addition, information gained through experiments begun 50 years ago on "imprinting" (the tendency of an animal to identify and relate to the first species it comes into contact with) has been used to train captive-born animals to relate to members of their own species.

Although improved public health and nutrition have certainly played a significant role in advancing longevity and health, for most infectious diseases this role has been minor. Despite advances in public health and nutrition, eradication of whooping cough, measles, and poliomyelitis was not achieved until the development of vaccines and drugs through research using animals. The possible development of a vaccine against AIDS is also dependent on continued studies conducted in animals, particularly primates (see below).

An example of the role(s) that primate research has played is in the development of the poliomyelitis vaccines. Although many studies on poliomyelitis in humans were conducted in the late-nineteenth century, the cause of the disease remained unknown until scientists succeeded in transmitting the virus to monkeys in 1908. There followed many years of research with primates until scientists were able, in the early 1950s, to grow the virus in human cell cultures, and development of a vaccine became possible. At that point in time, in order to ensure the safety and effectiveness of the vaccines, tests were conducted with monkeys. Furthermore, in order to produce the vaccines in pure form in great quantities, it was necessary to use kidney tissue taken from monkeys. Today, an alternative to the use of monkey kidneys has been developed for the production of the vaccine.

SCIENTIFIC CRITICISMS OF ANIMAL RESEARCH

In 1971, the *National Cancer Act* initiated a "War on Cancer" that many sponsors predicted would cure cancer by 1976. Instead, this multibillion dollar research program has not achieved its goal, and the age-adjusted total cancer mortality rate has been steadily climbing for decades. This despite the use of a 5-year survival as a "cure" even if the patient died of the cancer after the 5-year period. Why has progress against cancer not been more successful? One possible explanation is the unwarranted preoccupation with animal research. Some critics have emphasized that the crucial genetic, molecular, and immunologic differences between humans and other animals have prevented animal models from serving as effective means by which to seek a cancer cure.

Animal tests for cancer-causing substances, generally involving rodents, are notoriously unreliable. A former editor of the prestigious journal *Science* has asked, "*Are humans to be regarded as behaving biochemically like huge, obese, inbred, cancer-prone rodents?*" Of 19 known human oral carcinogens, only 7 caused cancer in nonhuman animals, using the standard National Cancer Institute (NCI) protocol. Even different rodent species produce conflicting results. When a comparison of carcinogenicity was made in rat and mouse for 214 chemicals, a correlation of only 70% was found (chance alone would have yielded 50%).

Despite extensive use, animal models have not contributed significantly to AIDS research. While monkeys, rabbits, and mice can be infected with HIV, none develops the human AIDS syndrome. Of over 100 chimpanzees infected with HIV over a 10-year period, only two became sick. Because chimpanzees turned out to be poor models for AIDS, and were expensive to maintain, all of the animals were faced with euthanasia (a euphamism for being killed). In 1997, the *National Research Council* recommended a solution. For all the chimpanzees housed in research facilities throughout the United States, a breeding moratorium was introduced and specific steps were taken toward making long-term care available for the primates. Animal rights supporters applauded the decision on the basis of moral responsibility.

Government officials have estimated that the breeding program produces approximately 25 off-spring a year at a cost of $60,000 to $100,000 per animal. Most researchers are only able to afford several animals for their studies. Statisticians have pointed out that for a study to have reliable numbers, showing that a vaccine fails 10% of the time, for example, a minimum of 29 chimpanzees would be required.

To quote Deborah Blum, author of *The Monkey Wars*, "Rhesus macaques—or any other primates—cannot just be dismissed as simple creatures. Their abilities go far beyond the basic skills of food finding and nest building. These are animals that teach each other negotiating skills, learn to operate computers, [and] recognize their kinfolk from a photograph. They are intelligent, capable, quick learners. They are, like us, complex beings. Once we recognize that, we must also recognize that the choices we make in using them are complex, too. It might once have been easy to toss a monkey into a research project, taking no particular thought. Today, the reverse is true. We should hesitate and we should think."

Numerous standard animal toxicity tests have been widely criticized by clinicians and toxi-cologists. The LD_{50} test generally requires 60–100 animals (usually rats and mice), most of whom endure substantial suffering. Because of difficulties extrapolating the results to humans, the test can be highly unreliable. Also, since such variables as an animal's age, sex, weight, and strain can have a substantial effect on the results, laboratories often obtain disparate data with the same test substances. In 2001, *The Organization for Economic Co-operation and Development* announced that it was to phase out its Test Guideline 401 (dealing with the LD_{50} test) deeming it unnecessary, inhumane, and lacking in scientific merit (*http://www.oecd.org*).

The *Draize* eye irritancy test, in which unanesthetized rabbits have irritant substances applied to their eyes, yield results that are inherently unreliable in predicting human toxicity. Humans and rabbits differ in the structure of their eyelids and corneas as well as their abilities to produce tears. When comparing rabbit to human data on the duration of inflammation after exposure to 14 house-hold products, they differed by a factor of 18–250.

Critics of animal studies contend that such studies can neither confirm nor refute hypotheses about human physiology or pathology; human clinical investigation is the only way such hypotheses can be tested. The *Medical Research Modernization Committee's* review of ten randomly chosen animal models of human diseases did not reveal any important contributions to human health. In addition, the animal models differed substantially from their human counterparts in both cause and clinical course. Furthermore, the study found that treatments effective in animals tended to have poor efficacy or excessive side effects in human patients.

In contrast to human clinical trials, vivisection involves manipulations of artificially induced conditions. Furthermore, the highly unnatural laboratory environment invariably stresses the animals, and stress affects the whole animal by altering pulse, blood pressure, hormone levels, immunological activity, as well as other functions. Unfortunately, some laboratory "discoveries" are more of an artifact than scientifically relevant. For example, during the 1980s, researchers reported 25 compounds that reduce ischemic stroke damage in nonhuman animals, but none proved effective in humans. Animal tests can also mislead in other ways. The drug *Milrinone* was reported to increase survival of rats with artificially induced heart failure, but humans taking the drug experienced a 30% increase in mortality. The drug Fialuridine appeared safe in animal tests, but it caused liver failure in 7 of 15 humans taking the drug, 5 of whom died and 2 required liver transplantation.

Animal studies also failed to predict dangerous heart valve abnormalities in humans induced by the diet drugs *fenfluramine* and *dexfenfluramine*. To this list can be added 12 drugs removed from the market in the United States. The *General Accounting Office* reviewed 198 of 209 drugs marketed from 1976 to 1985 and found that 52% had "serious postapproval risks;" not predicted by animal tests. Animal studies are reliable at only the crudest levels—such as the ability of strong acids to damage eyes. However, such effects can be assessed relatively easily with *in vitro* systems. For more subtle effects, animal models are often unreliable.

It would not be fair to state that everyone in the biomedicine community agrees with all the above conclusions, however. An article in the February 1997 issue of *Scientific American* elicited a robust debate in this area: The article was entitled, *"Animal Research is Wasteful and Misleading."* Critics of the article content that the authors skewed their analysis and included inaccuracies that could produce misconceptions and mislead, particularly, lay readers of the piece. Objections to the article can be summarized by one of its critics: "In no case…has adequate animal research led to human illness or death, as every animal study is followed by a clinical study afterwards. The statement that use of animal models has prevented illnesses and deaths by screening out toxic drugs would be truthful." More information from responsible animal use proponents can be researched at the *American Association for the Advancement of Science* (http://www.aaas.org/).

ALTERNATIVE METHODOLOGIES IN ANIMAL RESEARCH

In recent times, alternative methods in biomedical research and safety evaluation of chemicals and compounds have come under increasing scrutiny. This development represents the convergence of several factors: (1) accelerating developments in basic biologic methodology and understanding, especially *in vitro*; (2) increasing realization of the wastefulness of such tests as the classic LD_{50} and Draize, once useful but now considered archaic; and (3) increasing insistence from the public and animal rights groups that new understandings and methodologies be pressed into service of reducing animal use and alleviating animal suffering. An alternative to animal testing website may be found at http://www.sph.jhu.edu/~altweb. It also takes time to develop methods and prove that they are suitable replacements for other accepted methods. Fifteen U.S. agencies are working together as the Interagency Coordinating Committee for Validation of Alternate Methods (ICCVAM) to establish criteria for scientific validity and regulatory acceptance of new tests.

Interestingly, although never specifically required by the government, the LD_{50} test has become the standard measuring tool for FDA approval of drugs and for meeting certain toxicity requirements of the EPA. The FDA has declared that it does not require that data be based on the LD_{50} test for approval, and the EPA has established circumstances in which the test can be replaced by a "limit" test that uses fewer animals (4–10 versus 30–100) to screen for toxicity.

Animal rights organizations have been successful in changing the product testing protocols in some industries. Of particular note has been their effectiveness in the cosmetic industry. For example, an international campaign to expose the cruelty of product tests on animals led to the Benetton company's permanent ban on animal tests; a first for a major cosmetics company. Other leading companies such as Revlon, Avon, and Estee Lauder quickly followed suit. At the present time, there are more than 500 cosmetic companies that do not test products on animals. This has been particularly significant in eliminating the Draize tests for eye and skin irritancy. Companies such as General Motors (GM) have also not been immune from pressure. GM, which for a decade, had been conducting crash tests on pigs and ferrets, involving an estimated 20,000 animals, finally ceased this program.

Most research organizations and scientists follow a practice known as the "Three Rs," which stand for *replacement, reduction, and refinement* in alternatives. This concept had its roots in a book published in 1959 entitled *"The Principles of Humane Experimental Technique"* by Englishmen William Russell and Rex Burch. They wrote that scientific excellence and humane use of laboratory animals are inextricably linked. The scientific basis for the three Rs has been endorsed and reaffirmed in the 1980s and 1990s by numerous national and international agencies and scientific societies (e.g., American Society of Pharmacology and Experimental Therapeutics, Society of Toxicology, and The American College of Toxicology).

Replacement alternatives are methods that use organisms with limited sentience or do not use whole animals. They include improved information exchange to avoid unnecessary repetition of animal experiments; physiochemical techniques and structure–activity relations; mathematical and computer models; use of invertebrates, plants, and microorganisms; *in vitro* methods; and human studies, including the use of human volunteers, postmarketing surveys, and epidemiology. In the biomedical sciences, *in vitro* methods are increasingly being used, not because they provide precisely the same information as do animal studies but because they offer the best scientific approach. Such methods often use results from past animal studies as a basis for cellular and molecular investigations; unfortunately, for most basic researchers, replacement is problematic. Alternative methods such as tissue-culture systems simply cannot approximate the complexity of whole animals, especially in areas such as neuroscience and behavior. Neuroscientists point out that you cannot study learning and memory, or the effects of emotion or stress, except in a fully functioning animal.

- *Reduction* refers to areas where the number of animals used can be reduced. For example, the number of animals used in acute toxicity testing is being reduced as scientists have discovered ways to obtain accurate toxicity data using fewer animals. In addition, as mentioned in Chapter 14, scientists can now screen for the binding of some potential drugs by using isolated receptor preparations rather than using hundreds of animals.
- *Refinement* alternatives are methods that eliminate or minimize pain and distress or enhance animal well-being. Assessments of animal pain and distress are currently based on subjective evaluation of abnormal behavior or appearance. Because proper evaluation of pain relies largely on the ability to understand the behavior and needs of each species of laboratory animal, it is best for investigators to assume that a procedure that inflicts pain and distress in humans will do the same in animals. Much pain and distress can be diminished or eliminated with the proper use of anesthetics and analgesics. Researchers can enhance an animal's well-being by using environmental enrichment techniques, such as proper handling, appropriately sized cages, and group housing of social species.

Alternatives most commonly employed in biomedicine include cell, tissue, and organ cultures, computer modeling, and the use of minimally invasive procedures that produce less stress. While more toxicological research is being carried out *in vitro*, the potential of tissue and organ culture methods in toxicological protocols and hazard assessment is only in its early stages of development. Much of the emphasis in these new areas is the result of public pressure from the animal protection movement. Owing to improved cell culture techniques, experimental models have been developed to assess important biological characteristics such as

- Membrane permeability
- Active and passive transport of ions and other compounds through the membrane
- Cellular respiration and energy metabolism
- Integrity of the cytoskeleton
- Growth inhibition and cell viability
- Inhibition of cell cycle controlling factors
- Measurement of macromolecular synthesis (DNA, RNA, and proteins)
- Changes in cell morphology
- Release of mediators
- Release of specific proteins
- Release or uptake of dyes or radioactive markers
- ATP levels

Scientists have been and are continuing to search for alternative methods to the use of animals in biomedical and behavioral research for a variety of reasons, including an interest in the welfare of animals, a concern for the increasing costs of purchasing and caring for animals, and because in some areas alternative methods may be more efficient and effective research tools. However, although the search for alternatives to the use of animals in research testing remains a valid goal of researchers, the chance that alternatives will *completely* replace animals in the foreseeable future is *nil*. Nevertheless, as mentioned previously, some industries such as the cosmetic industry are making significant strides. For example, the cosmetic industry is presently involved in the organization of a database of currently available results for the evaluation of safety of cosmetic ingredients obtained or being developed with alternative methodologies. In addition, significant reduction in animal use has occurred in U.S. medical schools, drug houses, and research institutes. This is due to (1) attendant costs; as well as (2) the availability of new technological tools such as videos, computer models, improved application of statistics, improved protocol planning, increased use of tissue cultures from animals and humans, and patient simulators.

The Mario Negri Institute for Pharmacological Research of Milan (IRFMN) has been monitoring its use of experimental animals since 1968; 5 years after it started its activity. After reaching a peak number of 188,906 animals (rats, mice, and rabbits) used in experiments by the IRFMN in 1978, this number *decreased* to 24,669 in 1997 and has remained essentially unchanged since (22,333 animals in 2002). Interestingly, during the period of 1988–1998, IRFMN staff members at the institute actually *increased* by 27% while the number of published scientific articles increased by 52%; whereas the number of animals used *decreased* by 53%. In addition, the percentage of published articles during the same period that reported the results of *in vivo* and/or *ex vivo* animal experiments, was reduced from 32% to 16%.

There are also signs that significant changes are being made in how the search for new drugs is being carried out. A good example is the NCI in the United States. Over the past 35 years, 400,000 chemicals have been injected into mice deliberately bred to develop leukemia. A few drugs were found this way but not against other forms of cancer. To become more effective, the NCI has stopped using mice. They now use 60 human tumor cell lines from 7 main areas: colon, lung, melanoma, kidney, ovary, brain, and blood. By using these cell cultures they are able to screen 300 chemicals a week.

Fortunately, cell culture tests are becoming more and more common in cancer research. Some examples include

- A human leukemia cell line has been used to test 11 anticancer drugs to determine if they are more effective when used alone or in combination.
- Four human colorectal cancer cell lines have been used to test the effectiveness of seven drugs.
- Eight different human tumor cell lines have been used to find the most effective dose of the drug paclitaxel, and for what period should it be given.
- Human breast cancer tissue removed for biopsy has been tested with four different drugs.

Cell cultures have also been used to investigate differences between people. In one such study, four drugs were tested on ovarian tumors from 100 people. Because there was wide variability in response to the drugs, the patients were able to receive individual dosing regimens.

REGULATION OF RESEARCH ANIMALS

The status of laboratory animals in universities, hospitals, drug companies, and other research facilities is monitored by the U.S. Department of Agriculture (USDA) under the provisions of the Animal Welfare Act (AWA). The AWA has been amended three times since its passage in 1966. In 1985, an amendment that requires federally funded investigators to consider alternatives to animal use was added. Under the AWA, USDA officials make periodic *unannounced inspections* to ensure compliance with stringent standards for housing, feeding and watering, cleanliness, ventilation, and veterinary care. In addition, the AWA calls for the use of anesthetics and analgesics for potentially painful procedures and for postoperative care. However, the AWA excludes any other comment on how animals are used and critics characterize the AWA as a "paper tiger."

The *U.S. Public Health Service* (PHS) also has an Animal Welfare Policy that applies to all NIH-funded projects involving animals. The NIH *requires* that the institutions follow the "*Guide for the*

Care and Use of Laboratory Animals," prepared by the *Institute for Laboratory Animal Resources of the National Research Council*. Any institution that receives funding from the PHS is required by law to comply with the Guide, or else it will lose funding.

Both the AWA and the Guide mandate that each research institution establish an *Institutional Animal Care and Use Committee* that must review in detail every proposal for research involving animals and approve each proposal before the research can actually begin (in fact even before the investigator can receive funding). Among the issues covered by these requirements are standards for postoperative care and the use of anesthetics and analgesics to prevent any unnecessary discomfort to the animals.

In addition, the *American Association for Laboratory Animal Science* (AALAS) provides guidelines for animal care and use, operates a certification program for animal technicians, and develops educational materials. The AALAS also serves as a scientific forum for laboratory medicine and care. The *American Association for the Accreditation of Laboratory Animal Care* (AAALAC) offers a peer review *laboratory accreditation program* for research facilities. In addition, the FDA and the EPA have Good Laboratory Practices regulations.

HUMAN EXPERIMENTATION IN MEDICINE

The magnitude of human experimentation in the United States is quite substantial. Each year, more than 3000 clinical trials are carried out subject to FDA regulations. Thousands more trials are carried out in other countries. Each involves many volunteers, and the humans who are the first to take experimental therapies often face major risks. Yet, without human experiments we would not know with any degree of certainty whether potential new preventions, such as vaccines, drugs, and surgery are safe. Even then, these therapies can prove toxic in many ways.

Malaria is a disease caused by a parasite carried by mosquitoes, is found in 90 countries, and drug-resistant strains are spreading. For the first time, researchers have reported in 2004 that a *vaccine against malaria* can save children from infection or death. With money from the Bill and Melinda Gates Foundation, the vaccine, *tested on thousands of children* in Mozambique, was hardly perfect. It protected the children from catching the disease only about 30% of the time and prevented it from becoming life threatening only about 58% of the time. However, because malaria kills more than a million people a year, 700,000 of them children, even partial protection would be a public health victory.

In a long and continuing tradition, physicians have often chosen to become the first volunteers. Examples of some of these human guinea pigs and their remarkable commitment will be presented below. But, to set the mood, we need only look back to 1984. Dr. Barry J. Marshall, an Australian physician, had been experimenting with ulcers and, with a colleague, had identified a bacterium now known as *Helicobacter pylori* in patients with ulcers. Marshall believed that the pathogen was, in fact, the cause of the ulcers. In the next phase of his research, Marshall swallowed a tube that was used for tests to document that he had neither gastritis nor an ulcer and was not harboring *H. pylori*; then Marshall swallowed a liquid containing *H. pylori*. At 5 a.m., Marshall woke up vomiting and began suffering from gastritis. By acting as his own experimental subject he had proven to his own satisfaction that the bacteria could bring on ulcers and gastritis. The production of gastric ulcers by this strain of bacteria is now well established.

Not too long ago there was an unwritten code that if there was a scientific question asked, then the experimenter should first perform the appropriate experiment on themselves. One of history's first self-experimenters was a Viennese physician, Dr. Anton Stock (1760). Stock was particularly interested in the potential curative properties of hemlock. In his desire to experience its effects in humans, he first fed samples in meat to a little dog that was hungry. After several days, seeing no adverse effects in the animal, he began to experiment on himself. Each morning for 8 days he took several 100 mg in tea. He noted no unusual effects. Despite the failure of this crude test to do anything, Stock and other Viennese physicians prescribed hemlock for cancers, tumors, ulcers, and cataracts while it possessed no medicinal value.

In the nineteenth century, there were several dramatic demonstrations of the efficacy of the antidotal value of charcoal in poison overdoses. In 1813, the French chemist M. Bertrand, after showing that he could use charcoal to prevent arsenic poisoning in animals, gave a public demonstration of its benefits in humans. Bertrand swallowed 5 g of arsenic trioxide mixed with charcoal without ill effect. In 1852, another French chemist named Pierre-Fleurus Touery provided another demonstration. In front of a large audience of the French Academy of Medicine, he swallowed 1 g of strychnine (ten times the fatal dose) mixed with 15 g of charcoal. Other examples of nineteenth century self-experimentation have already been mentioned, including Dr. *Horace Wells* having his own teeth extracted under nitrous oxide as well as Dr. *Carl Koller* using cocaine on his own eye as a local anesthetic.

The name of Dr. *Walter Reed* is synonymous with self-experimentation. He was at the head of a U.S. military medical team (The Yellow Fever Commission) in 1900 that was established in Cuba to study yellow fever. Throughout history, *yellow fever* had been a frequent visitor to the United States. Some of its most devastating epidemics were in the eighteenth century and ranged from the Deep South to Boston. The 1793 outbreak in Philadelphia was particularly notable in that many lives were lost while internecine warfare festered among medical practitioners who disagreed about its cause.

By the mid-nineteenth century, things had changed little; the shock and surprise of a yellow-fever epidemic were still met by panic and ignorance. With the great awakening to the microbial source of the disease, the search for the causal organism reached an intensified pitch. Because the disease did not appear to be directly transmitted from patient to patient, a mosquito vector was considered as early as 1848 and seriously proposed as a mode of transmission in 1881 by Cuban physician Carlos J. Finlay.

Reed was convinced of the need for human experimentation. Under Reed's direction, Finlay's theory was tested using mosquitoes fed on infected individuals and transferred to healthy volunteers. Two theories were tested using two separate buildings: (1) infected-mosquito building and (2) infected-clothing building. In building 1, volunteers were bitten several times and placed in quarantine for monitoring. In building 2, occupants were *not bitten* but did unpack containers of soiled bed linens and clothing from yellow-fever victims in the local hospitals. Mattresses, towels, and sheets covered with black vomit and bloody discharges were also used for their bedding. Each morning these volunteers were placed in quarantine. Only the volunteers who were bitten developed the disease. Thus proving through human experiments that mosquitoes were the vectors that transmitted yellow fever (now known to be a virus; see below).

In reality, however, the team actually *confirmed findings* made almost a century previously by another self-experimenter that yellow fever was not a contagious disease. In 1800, an American, Dr. Issac Cathrall, repeatedly placed black vomit from several yellow-fever patients to his lips and tasted it. (Black vomit occurs in yellow-fever victims by virtue of bleeding in their stomachs, which is subsequently expelled.) He did not become infected. A physician named Ffirth actually went five steps more in 1802: (1) inserted black vomit into forearm; (2) dropped black vomit into eye; (3) boiled black vomit and inhaled the gas and steam; (4) swallowed black vomit taken directly from a patient; and (5) prepared pills made from black vomit.

The yellow-fever team led by Walter Reed had three other members. One of these, Dr. James Carroll, maintained until his death that he was the originator of the pact that the team test their experiments on themselves. In any event, all members agreed to the pledge. According to Carroll, while Reed was in Washington, DC, on August 27, 1900, he was exposed to mosquitoes known to be carrying the disease. Two days later, Carroll began experiencing the early symptoms of yellow fever. Four days after the bite, the symptoms had become much more severe. For three more days, Carroll's life was in the balance. Fortunately, Carroll must have had a strong constitution for he began to slowly recover and attempted to return to work on September 28. The conduct of the yellow-fever experiments was the forerunner of the current practice of informed consent, and was cited in the formulation of the *Nuremberg Code* and in many other discussions about the ethics of human experimentation.

- Yellow fever is caused by a mosquito-borne single-stranded positive-RNA *Flavivirus*. Normally endemic to the tropical regions of Africa and the Americas, the primary vector is *Aeded aegypti*. The virus is taken up when the female insect feeds on an infected animal and remains infected for life. Despite knowledge of its host and viral etiology, yellow fever is not extinct.

Scientists are a strange breed. We mentioned Dr. Marshall at the beginning of this section for his self-experimentation with bacteria. One of the most bizarre examples of self-use occurred during World War II. Dr. Claude Barlow, who had previously experimented on himself with intestinal flukes (Table 17.2), now took it on himself to determine if servicemen who had been infected with *schistosomiasis* (principally in Egypt) might pass the parasite on to previously uninfected snails in the United States. (Schistosomiasis is transmitted to humans via infected snails whose larvae have suckers that help them bore through the skin and migrate to the liver and lungs.) Table 17.2 presents selected examples of human/self-experimentation.

Barlow became fixated on determining whether the parasite could develop in a species of snail native to the United States. In order to accomplish this, he needed to have some viable parasites to carry out the research on. Unfortunately, while the parasite is quite happy living in foul canals, it was extremely fussy about living under laboratory conditions; laboratory models were a failure. To overcome this reality, attempts had been made by Barlow, and others, to infect animals in countries where the disease was common and send them to countries where the disease did not occur. The animals invariably died in transit. But Barlow had an idea to circumvent this challenge. He would transport the parasites himself in an environment he knew the parasites would not object to; his own body. By doing so, he would also avoid the necessity of an import permit.

Barlow began his self-experiment in Egypt on May 31, 1944. Over a 3-week period of time, Barlow placed specific numbers of the chosen strain of parasite to the skin over his left forearm and to his naval. On July 4, 1944, Barlow and his freeloaders flew to the United States. The first

TABLE 17.2
Selected Examples of Human/Self-Experimentation

Edward Jenner (1796)	Cowpox (8-year-old boy, with permission)
Issac Cathrall (1800)	"Black Vomit" (yellow fever, self)
Stubbins Ffirth (1802)	"Black Vomit" (yellow fever, self)
Jaime Ferran (1884)	Cholera Vaccine (self)
Louis Pasteur (1885)	Rabies Vaccine (9-year-old boy, with permission)
Edouard Brown-Sequard (1889)	Injected Testicular Extracts
Waldemar Haffkine (1892)	Cholera Vaccine (self)
Almroth E. Wright (1896)	Typhoid Vaccine (self)
Arthur Loos (1898)	Hookworm (self)
James Carroll (1900)	Yellow Fever (self)
Claude Barlow (1920)	Intestinal Flukes (self)
Maurice Brodie and William Park (1934)	Polio Vaccine (self)
John Kolmer and Anna Rule (1934)	Polio Vaccine (self)
Albert Hofmann (1943)	LSD (self)
Claude Barlow (1944)	Schistosomiasis (self)
Hilary Koprowski and Martin Kaplan (1955)	Rabies Vaccine (self)
CIA (1970s)	LSD (unspecified adults, no permission)

Note: The author would particularly emphasize reading *The Monkey Wars* and *Who Goes First?*

symptom occurred on October 31, when several itching spots that oozed serum-containing eggs of the parasite appeared. Ten days later, Barlow had a biopsy taken to look for the worms that had produced the eggs. Barlow refused to take a local anesthetic because he feared the injection might *disturb* the worms! The biopsy revealed a pair of adult worms.

By December, Barlow's condition had begun to decline. Temperatures exceeded 103° F, blood and mucus appeared regularly in his urine and stools. He could only sleep with the aid of sedatives. Being the consummate scientist, Barlow frequently examined his own specimens and kept an almost daily record of his clinical and laboratory observations. For example, in tests of his urine he found he was passing up to 12,000 eggs in each day's 24-hour sample. Barlow was a very sick man, so sick that he was subjected to extremely painful injections of antimony. Treatment with the heavy metal did clear Barlow of the infection by December 1944. In 1948, Barlow received the Medal of Merit from President Truman. He died at the ripe-old-age of 93.

One of the most remarkable examples of self-experimentation involves Dr. Werner Forssmann. Although not involving drugs or pathogens, his hubris is, nonetheless, remarkable. Forssmann obtained his medical degree in 1929 and began his internship in Eberswalde, Germany. During his studies, Forssmann had been deeply impressed by a sketch in his physiology textbook that showed French physiologists standing in front of a horse, holding a thin tube that had been put into the jugular vein in the animal's neck and then guided into the heart. Forssmann became obsessed with the potential of putting a tube into the heart of a living human. Forssmann eventually approached his mentor about introducing a tube into a human heart. His mentor refused permission even when Forssmann volunteered to perform the procedure on himself.

Forssmann decided to do the experiment anyway—in secret. By befriending a nurse, who was deeply interested in medicine, Forssmann found a kindred spirit who was sympathetic to his research idea. In fact, she volunteered to be his guinea pig. Then, in a drama befitting Hollywood, Forssmann tricked the nurse in order to obtain the necessary surgical equipment, plus a ureteral catherter, the thin tubing urologists use to drain urine from the kidneys. Realizing she was going to be the first human to have a tube placed in her heart, the nurse climbed onto a surgical table and had her arms strapped down. As the nurse adjusted her body, Forssmann dabbed iodine over *his* left elbow crease and injected novacaine to numb the skin. After the local anesthetic had taken effect, Forssmann picked up the scalpel and cut through the skin. When he reached a large vein, he put down the scalpel, picked up a hollow needle and gently pushed it into the vein. He then inserted the catheter into the needle and guided the catheter up to the level of his shoulder and left it in place.

At this point, Forssmann knew he would need documentation, as well as the nurse's cooperation. Despite her exasperation at being duped, the nurse assisted Forssman down to the basement x-ray laboratory. There, Forssmann, with guidance from the nurse, using a fluoroscopic x-ray screen, placed the catheter successfully into the right auricle. The x-ray technician snapped the picture and radiographic proof was obtained. The importance of describing the procedure in the scientific literature was obvious. However, Forssmann's mentor was concerned that it was too revolutionary to be understood by doctors. To quote the mentor, "Say that you tried it on cadavers before you did it on yourself. The reader of your paper must have the impression that it is not too revolutionary and that it was not made without a lot of forethought. Otherwise the critics will tear you to pieces." Even today, textbooks describe the fictitious, aborted first effort and the nonexistent preliminary test on a corpse.

One would have thought that self-catheterization would have been enough for Forssmann. Such was not the case. Radiopaque chemicals were just beginning to be used to help x-ray the urinary system and the stomach. Forssmann decided to investigate whether this technique could be applied to the heart. Once again, he undertook to study this question on himself. After some experiments on dogs, he eventually decided to do the experiment. At this point, he was no longer threading the catheter through the veins in his elbow crease because the most readily accessible of these blood vessels had been sewn closed after his previous catheterization experiments. Instead, he injected a local anesthetic into the skin around his groin, made an incision and inserted a catheter into the femoral vein. He then pushed it up into the abdomen, then the inferior vena cava and on into its connection with the heart. Unfortunately, this and several other attempts were unsuccessful. It remained for others to apply his revolutionary techniques to the everyday practice of medicine. Today, hundreds of thousands of cases of cardiac angiography are carried out yearly. Forssmann shared the 1956 Nobel Prize in Medicine.

During World War II, doctors in Nazi Germany invoked the name of science to justify atrocities labeled "experiments" that involved hundreds of thousands of victims. Among the 20 Nazi doctors who were tried at Nuremberg was an eminent malaria expert. This former member of the League of Nations Malaria Commission infected more than 1000 prisoners at Dachau with the parasitic disease. More than 400 died from complications arising from the use of experimental antimalarial drugs. He was hanged.

According to the U.S. chief war crimes prosecutor at Nuremberg, additional "experiments" included locking prisoners into airtight chambers and then rapidly changing the pressures to duplicate the atmospheric conditions that an aviator might encounter in falling long distances without a parachute or oxygen; and infecting individuals with cholera, diphtheria, paratyphoid A and B, smallpox, typhus, and yellow fever and then testing experimental and mostly useless vaccines on them. Some inmates were deliberately infected with typhus with the sole purpose of keeping the typhus virus alive and generally available in the bloodstream of the inmates; injecting phenol or gasoline into the veins of prisoners, who died within 60 s; and testing to determine how long humans could survive without water, after eating huge amounts of salt.

One of the most frightening cases of self-experimentation occurred at the headquarters of Burroughs Wellcome in 1944, and would make a good plot for a movie. British anesthesiologists had become impressed with the potential importance of curare in medicine. However, because of its lack of purity it was not practical to experiment with it. The giant British drug company independently prepared curare in pure form. Scientists at the drug company had carried out animal studies that indicated to them that the drug was safe. It was time for clinical tests on humans. The director of clinical research "perhaps foolishly" consented to be the human guinea pig.

For the experiment with curare, the director and his colleagues drew up a protocol. According to the protocol, the director was to lie on a table while his breathing rate, blood pressure, and pulse were being continually recorded. There would be a full tank of oxygen on hand. The experiment began with an injection of 10 mg. Although some paralysis was experienced, recovery began in approximately 15 min. A week later, the dose was increased to 20 mg. The paralysis was more widespread this time but recovery again began within 15 min. They were now ready for the third stage, and a 30 mg dose was given about 2 weeks after the first.

Within 2 min, the muscles of the director's face, neck, arms, and legs were completely paralyzed. He could not speak or open his eyes. Within 3 min his breathing muscles were paralyzed. At this point, the director was unable to communicate with his colleagues who were otherwise occupied. When they did glance at him everything appeared fine. However, they had forgotten one thing in the protocol—a means of communication.

The director could not communicate and he had the feeling he was suffocating. The back of his mouth and voice box were becoming clogged with saliva and mucus. There was nothing he could do about it. He could not move a limb, finger, or toe. He was terrified. His blood pressure and pulse rate, which had risen dramatically, showed fear, but his colleagues failed to realize how frightened he was. Once the medical team had collected the data it sought, a dose of the antidote (neostigmine) was given. But the dose was not large enough. For seven additional minutes the director received artificial respiration. Eventually his own breathing muscles took over and he was able to talk.

A less dramatic example of self-experimentation is the development of Antabuse (disulfiram), a drug that is still used today to treat alcoholics. During World War II, at a Danish company called Medicinalco, it was customary practice for pharmacologists and technicians to experiment on themselves when a new drug was being tested. The employees who did so were admitted to an unpaid group that called itself the *"Death Battalion."* The medical research director believed that pharmacologists should test a drug on themselves before doing so on another human. Although not compensated monetarily, members of the battalion were offered a glass of port if they provided a blood sample. Members were also fetted to a yearly banquet with the presentation of awards.

One of the members of the director's research team, while reading an article about the use of disulfiram against the parasitic skin disease scabies in animals, wondered if the drug might prove useful against intestinal parasites as well. The drug was first given orally to rabbits that showed no ill effects. Next the drug was given to rabbits who were infected with an intestinal parasite. There seemed to be some improvement. The inevitable question was, is the drug safe in humans? Just to be safe, they decided to take some of the tablets themselves. *Both* the scientists began taking disulfiram pills as a daily regimen, while they continued their regular tasks.

At lunchtime one day, shortly after the pill experiment had begun, one of the researchers picked up the brown paper bag that contained the sandwiches his wife had made him that morning, and removed a beer from the laboratory refrigerator. By the time lunch was over he felt groggy, his head throbbed, and he felt nauseated. By the end of the day, his symptoms had disappeared. The next day he ate an open-faced shrimp sandwich and coffee. Nothing happened.

During the next several weeks these symptoms would periodically reoccur. One day, the two collaborators met in the hall when, during the course of their discussion, they discovered that they had been having the same symptoms. Comparing notes, they realized that the only common denominator was alcohol. Subsequent studies confirmed that the problem was caused by a drug–alcohol interaction. Eventually, disulfiram was introduced clinically as aversion therapy in alcoholics. Its mechanism of action proved to be inhibition of acetaldehyde dehydrogenase that causes an accumulation of the toxic intermediate acetaldehyde during alcohol metabolism.

Out of the Nuremberg trials in 1947 came the *Nuremberg Code*, the first code to deal specifically with human experimentation. It created ethical guidelines for the conduct of medical research throughout the world. Although many researchers had customarily obtained consent from volunteers in the past, it was the Nuremberg Code that first established the practice formally. The code deals with self-experimentation in Article 5, which states: "*No experiment should be conducted where there is an a priori reason to believe that death or disabling injury will occur; except, perhaps, in those experiments where the experimental physicians also serve as subjects.*"

Following the Nuremberg trials, it was unthinkable that any such unethical human research could take place in a democratic society, much less the United States. Shockingly, in the 1960s, disclosures of glaring breaches of ethics were uncovered. Fifty unethical studies were cited. Among them, deliberately withholding penicillin from 109 servicemen who suffered streptococcal infections, thereby exposing them to the risks of rheumatic fever; administering several chemicals of no benefit to patients with advanced cirrhosis to determine their effect on the liver disease; and exposing 26 normal newborn infants to extensive x-rays so that their urinary bladder function could be studied are a few examples.

Most of the post–World War II criticism about breaches of scientific ethics involved civilian researchers working in private institutions. However, governmental researchers came under attack in 1972 when the public learned that U.S. Public Health Service officials had withheld antibiotic therapy from a group of syphilis patients whose medical histories they had carefully followed for more than 40 years. The patients, who had acquired syphilis naturally, had been asked to volunteer for what came to be known as the *Tuskegee Study*. Its aim was to observe the natural course of the infection and to further medical knowledge about the disease. In return for their cooperation, the volunteers—mostly poor and black—were to be given free medical care and free burials. Although penicillin is really only effective in curing the infection during the early stages of the disease, and most volunteers had already progressed to later stages, no volunteers were offered treatment.

SELECTED BIBLIOGRAPHY

Altman, L.K. (1998) *Who Goes First?* Berkeley, CA: The University of California Press.

Anon. (1992) *Use of Animals in Biomedical Research-The Challenge and Response*, Chicago, IL: American Medical Association.

Balcombe, J. (2000) *The Use of Animals in Higher Education: Problems, Alternatives and Recommendations*, Washington, DC: Humane Society Press.

Beeson P.B. (1979) The growth of knowledge about a disease: Hepatitis, *Am. J. Med.*, 67: 366–370.

Blom, D. (1994) *The Monkey Wars*, New York: Oxford University Press.

Fano A. (1997) *Lethal Laws: Animal Testing, Human Health and Environmental Policy*, London: Zed Books.

Fox, M.A. (1986) *Case for Animal Experimentation-An Evolutionary and Ethical Perspective*, Los Angeles: University of California Press.

General Accounting Office. (1990) *FDA Drug Review: Postapproval Risks 1976–1985*, Washington, DC: GAO.

Kaufman S.R., Czarnecki T., Haralabatos I., and Richardson M. (1991) Animal models of degenerative Neurological diseases, *Perspec Medical Res.*, 3: 9–48.

Kohn, A. (1986) *False Profits*, Oxford: Basil Blackwell.

LaFollette H. and Shanks N. (1997) *Brute Science*. New York: Routledge.

Loprieno, N. (1995) *Alternative Methodologies for the Safety Evaluation of Chemicals in the Cosmetic Industry*, Boca Raton, FL: CRC Press.

Nicoll, C.S. and Russell, S.M. (1992) Animal rights, animal research, and human obligations, *Mol. Cellular Neurosci.*, 3: 271–277.

Paton, W. (1984) *Man and Mouse*, Oxford: Oxford Press.

Rowan, A.N. (1984) *Of Mice, Models, and Men*, Albany: State University of New York Press.

Ryder, R. (1975) *Victims of Science*, London: Davis-Poynter.

Singer, P. (1977) *Animal Liberation-A New Ethics for our Treatment of Animals*, New York: Avon Books.

QUESTIONS

1. The first use of live animals for research is believed to have occurred in which century BC?
   a. First
   b. Second
   c. Third
   d. Fourth
   e. Fifth

2. Which of the following championed the value of animal experimentation and considered animals as nothing other than automatons?
   a. Francis Bacon
   b. Herman Goering
   c. Rene Descartes
   d. Jeremy Bentham
   e. a and c

3. The roots of antivivisection occurred in which country?
   a. Belgium
   b. France
   c. Germany
   d. Britain
   e. United States

4. Who is most responsible for rejecting the Cartesian viewpoint regarding the suffering of animals?
   a. Francois Magendie
   b. Claude Bernard
   c. Jeremy Bentham
   d. Peter Singer
   e. Richard Ryder

5. Which of the following authors introduced the term "specieism" in the animal rights movement?
   a. Peter Singer
   b. Jeremy Bentham
   c. Rene Descartes
   d. Francis Bacon
   e. Richard Ryder

6. Approximately how many million rodents are used yearly in biomedical research?
   a. 10
   b. 25
   c. 40
   d. 50
   e. 100

7. The "three Rs" in biomedical research stand for which of the following?
   a. Relief, regimentation, and restraint
   b. Recurrance, restraint, and redundancy
   c. Replacement, reduction, and refinement
   d. Relief, refinement, and restraint
   e. Replacement, relief, and recovery

8. Which of the following has involved human self-experimentation?
   a. Rabbies vaccine
   b. Cholera vaccine
   c. Typhoid vaccine
   d. Yellow fever
   e. All of the above

9. Which of the following performed the first heart catheterization on himself?
   a. James Carroll
   b. Walter Reed
   c. Claude Barlow
   d. Arthur Loos
   e. Joseph Forssmann

10. Which of the following infected himself with schistosomiasis in order to transport them to the United States?
    a. James Carroll
    b. Claude Barlow
    c. John Hunter
    d. Almroth Wright
    e. Edward Jenner

18 Alternative Medicine

First the word, then the plant, lastly the knife

Asclepius of Thessaly, circa 1000 BC

INTRODUCTION

If we arbitrarily designate the beginning of modern drug development to coincide with the *synthesis* of acetylsalicylic acid, then mankind has only been exposed to modern medicine for a century. During this period, a number of wonderful drugs have been developed. Most notably, perhaps, are the antibiotics during the 1930s and 1940s, and psychotropic agents during the 1950s. Antibiotics could actually cure certain infections. While the introduction of psychotropic drugs did not cure mental illness, their impact on mental health is almost incalculable. They permitted an end to institutionalization for tens of thousands of patients with the attendant reduction in hospital costs and a resumption of more normalcy of life; a legacy that remains today. Despite these successes, 80% of the world's population still uses herbs, according to the World Health Organization.

During the second half of the twentieth century the public has developed a more jaundiced view of the contemporary pharmaceutical industry and its products. High prescription costs, criminal behavior by industry officials, the cozy relationship between authors of clinical research and the sponsoring agency, inadequate testing leading to the threat of unrecognized lethal toxicity, as well as drug–drug and drug–food interactions, to name but a few. To many, each new "breakthrough" is accompanied by a new "warning" and has turned much of the population to the admonition of Hippocrates, "*Honor the healing power of nature.*" According to a 1998 study published in the Journal of the American Medical Association, people use alternative medicine not only because they are dissatisfied with conventional medicine, but because these health care alternatives mirror their own values, beliefs, and philosophical orientations toward health and life.

Alternative medicine includes (but is not limited to) the following: herbal medicine, nutraceuticals, homeopathy, aromatherapy, chiropractic, osteopathy, acupuncture, acupressure, yoga, tai chi, meditation, music or art therapy, shamanism and faith healing. In this chapter our principal focus will be on herbal medicine. The increased use of herbal medicine outside of the traditional physician-patient paradigm represents a search for other sources of health as well as an expression of assuming greater responsibility for our own health maintenance. In one sense, it is a return to an earlier period.

The shift from "traditional medicine" to "modern medicine" can be traced to the *Flexner Report* of 1910. This evaluation of medical training in the United States was highly critical of institutions of the day and resulted in the closing of 80% of the nation's medical schools, including "alternative" schools of homeopathy, herbology and naturopathy. Nevertheless, in the 1950s, academic researchers and pharmaceutical companies had programs to extract drug candidates from plants that had been selected on the basis of their herbal reputations. For example, Eli Lilly developed the leukemia drugs vinblastine and vincristine by extracting constituents of the Madagascan periwinkle, the latter having been selected not from computerized constructs or analysis of possible drug candidates, but rather on the basis of the plant's reputation as a Jamaican herbal tea.

HISTORY

As mentioned previously, in the introductory chapter of this book, interest in the treatment of disease can be found in documents as old as the existence of records. Folklore accumulated about presumed effects after the use of certain "medicines." The Ebers papyrus, written in Egypt around 1550 BC, was a compilation of some of this folklore. In India, Ayurveda (from ayur—life + veda—knowledge or science), a whole conceptual system of living is believed to have started around the same time. The codification of this system of medicine, including the concept of a formulary in which herbal remedies and recipes for them are described, was written in Sanskrit around 100 BC to AD 100 or possibly earlier. The written record of a Chinese herbal formulary comes from the Han dynasty (206 BC to AD 220).

Chinese medicinal herbs are some of our oldest alternative and complementary medicines and their ever-increasing use is a good indication of the public interest in such medicines. Although Chinese herbal medicines constitute multi-billion-dollar industries worldwide and more than 1500 herbals are sold as dietary supplements or ethnic traditional medicines, the formulations of these medicines are commonly not subjected to pre-market toxicity examinations to test their safety or efficacy.

Numerous case reports and case series of heavy metal poisoning associated with the use of traditional Chinese medicines (TCM) and Indian products have been published; lead has frequently been implicated as the cause of such poisoning but mercury, cadmium, arsenic, copper, and thallium have also been found.

Several possibilities exist to explain the presence of heavy metals in these products. First, heavy metals could be included intentionally for theoretical medicinal properties. Some Indian medical schools emphasize the importance of metals such as lead, copper, gold, iron, mercury, silver, tin, and zinc for the proper function of the human body. In TCM, mercury is part of some preparations under the terms "cinnabaris" (mercury sulfide), "calomel" (mercury chloride) or "hydrargyri oxydum rubrum" (mercury oxide). Therefore, these constituents are not strictly speaking contaminants but deliberately included for a specific curative purpose.

Heavy metals are not the only contaminants in imported herbal preparations. In 1998 California officials screened for undeclared pharmaceuticals (Table 18.1) in imported Chinese remedies on sale in herbal retail stores. Seven percent of the 251 products tested contained undeclared pharmaceuticals.

Heavy metals are not the only possible toxic ingredients in herbal remedies: Contamination with herbicides, pesticides, microorganisms or mycotoxins, insects or undeclared herbal constituents are other possibilities. Contamination with toxic herbal constituents—through misidentification of the herbal ingredients—can be a serious problem. In Belgium (in the late 1990s) the use of a TCM contaminated with plants from the *Aristolochia* species resulted in an epidemic of subacute intestinal

---

TABLE 18.1
Undeclared Pharmaceuticals that have been Found in Traditional Chinese Remedies

Acetaminophen	Fluocinolone acetonide
Paracetamol	Glibenclamide
Aminopyrine	Hydrochlorothiazide
Caffeine	Hydrocortisone
Carbemazepine	Indomethacin
Chlorzoxazone	Mefenamic acid
Clobetasol propionate	Methylsalicylate
Dexamethasone	Phenacetin
Diazepam	Phenylbutazone
Diclofenac	Phenytoin
Ethoxybenzamide	Valproate

Source: Trends Pharmacol. Sci. 23: 135–139, 2002.

nephropathy. Many of the patients required kidney transplantation. When 19 kidneys and urethras removed from ten such patients were examined histologically, there were conclusive signs of neo-plasms in 40% of the cases. In china, there were 9854 cases of adverse reactions reported in 2002: More than double the number reported during all of the 1990s. More than 90 countries sell herbal products over-the-counter.

Recent evidence suggests that consumers are beginning to become concerned about the risks of under-regulation of dietary supplements, and the majority of United States consumers now appear to support (1) the requirement that the Food and Drug Administration (FDA) review the safety of new dietary supplements before their sale; (2) increased authority to remove from sale those products shown to be unsafe; and (3) increased governmental regulation to ensure that advertising claims about health benefits of dietary supplements are true.

In North America, our country's native inhabitants relied on this continent's indigenous plants for food as well as medicines. Native Americans were using Echinacea, or purple coneflower, as a remedy for everything from snakebites and spider bites to toothaches and burns long before health food stores began to offer it in convenient capsule form. In colonial America, many settlers earned all or part of their income as "sang" hunters, searching for wild ginseng in the woods. This plant's aromatic root brought "the surprising price of seven or eight ounces of silver," according to the writings of the Swedish botanist Petr Kalm, who visited North America in the mid-eighteenth century. To colonists, the value of ginseng root lay in its reputation as a treatment for ailments ranging from asthma and bladder stones to infertility and wounds.

Perhaps the single most significant event impacting the sale of herbal drugs in the United States was the passage of the *Dietary Supplement Health and Education Act of 1994* (*DSHEA*). This was an Act of Congress (Senate Bill 784, the Hatch-Harkin bill in the Senate) to amend the *Federal, Food, Drug, and Cosmetic Act* issued in 1938 to establish standards with respect to dietary supplements, and for other purposes. The main components of the DSHEA are the following:

- To establish legal status for dietary supplements
- Protection from regulation as food additives or as drugs unless the product contains *therapeutic claims*
- Burden of proof that herbs and other supplements are *unsafe now shifts to the FDA*
- *New* ingredients introduced *after* October 15, 1994 must be shown to be safe by importer or manufacturer.

In the United States, herbal medicines exist in a regulatory limbo; they're sold as foods, food additives, or dietary supplements, though they are actually, in fact, used by the public as drugs. However, as long as no medicinal claims are made on the label, the FDA does not regulate herbal products. However, manufacturers of supplements can make "statements of nutritional support" without FDA approval, as long as the statement is true and not misleading. Such statements usually describe the supplement's effect on the "structure or function" of the human body (known as "structure/function claims") or the effect on a person's "well being."

Not surprisingly, manufacturers have taken great pains in product marketing to use statements that qualify as structure/function claims, *not as health claims*. This often requires linguistic agility. A manufacturer of saw palmetto, for example, cannot claim that its product "prevents prostate cancer," but can say instead that the product "helps maintain prostate function." Similarly, amorphous statements such as Kava kava *may* aid in relaxation or extremely general structure-function claims (e.g., "Calcium aids in the development of strong bones."). Manufacturers must also include a disclaimer that the claim has not been evaluated by the FDA and that the product is not intended to treat, cure or prevent any disease.

The 1994 Act further loosened regulatory oversight because now a product cannot be removed from the market until it has been *proved to cause harm*, and the burden of proof is on the government. Since 1994, the FDA has taken approximately 100 actions, mostly warning letters, against manufacturers that have violated labeling requirements. For example, following dozens of reports of adverse health effects and one death, the agency asked for a voluntary recall of *gamma butyrol-actone*, a supplement often promoted for body building. The agency has similarly targeted products advertised as "herbal fen-phen" because of implications that they replaced traditional pharmaceuticals. In February 2001 the FDA released a warning about the interaction of *St. John's Wort* with *indinavir* and other drugs used in combating HIV.

The government has demonstrated it's diligence in this area by regulating *ephedra* (the herbal form of the stimulant ephedrine) use in pep pills and supplements. The proposal is the FDA's first regulatory major initiative under the 1994 Act. According to the FDA, more than 800 adverse reactions, including seizures, strokes and heart attacks, have been linked to ephedra capsules, tablets and teas since 1994. The FDA puts the ephedrine-related death toll at 18 since then. Based on this and other evidence, FDA issued a rule in February 2004 declaring that dietary supplements containing ephedrine present an unreasonable risk of illness or death. Since the rule became effective in April 2004, the government has executed numerous seizures against numerous products. However, in the on-again-off again world of drugs, legislation, and vested interests, the reader should not be surprised to learn that on April 14, 2006 a federal Judge in Utah reversed the short-lived ban on ephedra.

The 1994 deregulation has fueled the explosion of consumer interest in the herbal and vitamin industry. In 1990, only 3% of the nation used herbs as medicines, according to the New England Journal of Medicine. In 1994 it was 17% according to a Gallup survey. In 1999 sales of herbs exceeded $3.3 billion, market analysts have projected an annual growth rate of 9.7% through 2004 for the herbal product market segment. According to the American Council on Science and Health, more than 40% of Americans now use some kind of "alternative therapy." Data for supermarket sales of nutritional supplements since passage of the Act are also compelling (Table 18.2).

Consumer use of herbs and medicinal plant products in the United States over the past two decades has become a mainstream phenomenon. No longer relegated to health food stores, mail order houses, and multilevel marketing organizations, herbs and phytomedicines (advanced medicinal preparations made of herbs) have become one of the fastest growing segments in retail pharmacies, supermarkets, and other mass market outlets. In addition, major health insurance companies are beginning to include herbs as covered modalities of "alternative therapies" and herb products are being considered for use by some managed care organizations.

Despite the fuzzy health claims of some neutraceutical firms, some of these products are proving their value in studies performed by academic institutions and the National Institute of Health (NIH), among others. Most of the ingredients attracting attention, such as cranberry extract and garlic, have been used as folk remedies for many years.

In one recent study, researchers found that cranberry concentrate, a common but previously unproven folk remedy for urinary tract infections (UTIs), actually did have a positive effect in preventing illness when tested in women who commonly get the infections. Researchers from

TABLE 18.2
Supermarket Sales of
Nutritional Supplements

Year	Dollars (millions)
1994	88.4
1995	106.5
1996	141.5
1997	191.0
1998	279.7

Source: ACNielsen.

the *Finnish Student Health Services* it Oulu University recruited 150 women with persistent UTIs. Fifty drank 50 mL of cranberry juice a day for 6 months. Another 50 drank a preparation of *Lactobacillus*, a "friendly" bacteria, that helps prevent yeast infections, and the final 50 women were given no treatment. After 6 months, only 8 women taking cranberry juice had experienced a UTI, compared with 19 of those taking Lactobacillus and 18 not taking anything.

In general, consumers use herbal products as therapeutic agents for treatment and cure of diseases and pathological conditions, as prophylactic agents to prevent disease over the long term, and as protective agents to maintain health and wellness. Additionally, herbs and phytomedicinals can be used as adjunct therapy, to support conventional pharmaceutical therapies. This last use is usually found in societies where phytotherapy (the use of herbal medicines in clinical practice) is considerably more integrated with conventional medicine, as in Germany.

EUROPE AND HERBAL MEDICINE

Europeans have a longer history of herbal drug use than the United States In contrast to other countries in Europe, herbal medicines have a special status in Germany, beginning with the Imperial Decree of 1901 that permitted the trade of many botanical drugs outside pharmacies. Therefore, most of the research has taken place in Germany. Because herbal medicines are usually not patentable, the profit margin on them is often much lower than for synthetic drugs. As a result, companies generally have not been willing to make the investment needed to meet the United States' stringent efficacy requirements for new drugs. However, thanks to the 1994 law many herbal products can be sold in the United States as dietary supplements, for which efficacy is essentially nonexistent. In an attempt to partially fill this void, the United States Pharmacopeia (USP) is stepping in to award its "seal of approval" to products that contain what their label claims.

This seal does not claim that the product is safe or that it works. However, quality control of ingredients is an important issue. For example, researchers at the University of California, Los Angeles (UCLA) studied 12 brands of body-building supplements and found only one contained the amount of androstenedione or related ingredients the bottle promised. One brand contained nearly double the amount listed—a potential danger, while another was a pure fraud—it contained none. Far worse, one brand contained 10 mg of testosterone, a controlled substance that is supposed to be available by prescription only. Enter the certification program by the nonprofit United States Pharmacopeia (USP) that sets standards for many pharmaceuticals. It promises that supplements that win its seal will deliver the ingredients promised.

Herbal remedies consistently rank among the top 10 in drug sales in Germany and 80% of all German physicians regularly prescribe herbal medications. Herbal drug sales represent in excess of $10 billion in sales per year. Of the 10 top-selling herbs in health care stores in the United States in 1995 six were popularized largely on the basis of European research (Table 18.3).

A partial listing of alleged natural alternatives to the top 5 OTC and prescription drug categories are shown in Tables 18.4 and 18.5, respectively. It should be emphasized that the efficacy of these products is subject to question, and consumers are advised to carry out their own research.

Germany holds the lead in the amount of high-quality research carried out on herbal medicines. In 1978 the German Ministry of Health established Commission E, a panel of experts charged with evaluating the safety and efficacy of the herbs available in pharmacies for general use. The Commission reviewed over 300 herbal drugs. Results were published by the German Federal Health Agency (now Federal Institute for Drugs and Medical Devices) in the form of monographs. A total of 380 monographs were published (254 approved; 126 unapproved), plus 81 revisions. These monographs provide guidelines for the general public, health practitioners, and companies applying for registration of herbal drugs. The process followed by Commission E resulted in what has been called the most accurate information available in the entire world on the safety and efficacy of herbs and phytomedicines (see Bibliography).

TABLE 18.3
Best Selling Herbal Products in the United States

Rank	Product
1	Echinacea (9.9)
2	Garlic (9.8)
3	Goldenseal (7.0)
4	Ginseng (5.9)
5	Gingko (4.5)
6	Saw palmetto (4.4)
7	Aloe gel (4.3)
8	Ephedra (3.5)
9	Eleuthero (3.1)
10	Cranberry (3.0)

Value in parenthesis is percent of market share.

TABLE 18.4
Natural Alternatives to the Top 5 OTC Drug Categories

OTC	Natural Alternative
Analgesics	Capsaicin, omega-3 fatty acids, vitamin E, pycnogenol
Antacids/anti gas	Licorice root, probiotics
Cold remedies	Zinc lozenges, high dose vitamin C
Allergy relief	Quercetin, pycnogenol, bee pollen
Laxatives	Fruits, vegetables, whole grain

TABLE 18.5
Natural Alternatives to the Top 5 Prescription Drug Categories

Prescription	Natural Alternative
Estrogen replacement	Isoflavones (soy foods), black cohosh
Antibiotics	probiotics, garlic, Echinacea
Antidepressants	St. John's wort, vitamin B1
Hypertension	Calcium, magnesium, potassium, garlic
Anti-ulcer (not caused by *H. pylori*)	Licorice root, bilberry

Herbal remedies hold a different place in medical practice in many European countries than in the United States. One of the most dramatic examples of the difference is in the treatment of *benign* prostate disease. This very common condition affects about 25% of men in their forties and nearly 80% of men who are over 70. In Germany, several hundred million dollars are spent annually on prostate remedies, with 80% of that spent on herbal medications. Herbal medications dominate the market for treating *nonmalignant* prostate disease. They have very few side effects and cost per dose approximately 20–35% of what synthetic drugs do. Treatment with herbal preparations typically cost under a dollar a day. Four of the most popular in Germany include: extracts from the fruit of the saw palmetto, pumpkin seeds, rye pollen extract, and nettle root.

NATIONAL CENTER FOR COMPLEMENTARY AND ALTERNATIVE MEDICINE (NCCAM)

In 1998, the Congress established the NCCAM at the NIH to stimulate, develop, and support research on complementary and alternative medicine (CAM) for the benefit of the public. Prior to 1998, the NCCAM was the Office of Alternative Medicine. The NCCAM is an advocate for quality science, rigorous and relevant research, and open and objective inquiry into which CAM practices work, which do not, and why. Its overriding mission is to give the American public reliable information about the safety and effectiveness of CAM practices. The NCCAM focuses on the following efforts:

- Evaluating the safety and efficacy of widely used natural products, such as herbal remedies and nutritional and food supplements (e.g., mega doses of vitamins)
- Supporting pharmacological studies to determine the potential interactive effects of CAM products with standard treatment medications
- Evaluating CAM practices, such as acupuncture and chiropractic.

How has deregulation worked? A meta-analysis of the herb St. John's wort (*Hypericum perforatum*) for *mild and moderately severe depression*, published in 1996 by German and American physicians, concluded that it was more effective than a placebo and was as effective as standard antidepressants but with fewer side effects. However, the authors of the analysis raised questions about the methods employed and cautioned about its efficacy in *seriously depressed* patients. The active chemical in the herb, they claimed, was not appropriately standardized. Furthermore, the study only compared St. John's wort with antidepressant drugs that were given *at or below* their lowest level of efficacy. And, finally, patients were treated for only 6 weeks. An accompanying editorial concluded that: "longer term studies are needed before it can be recommended in major depression."

The above report eventually led to the NIH's Office of Alternative Medicine (now NCCAM) to call for a trial comparing St. John's wort with the popular antidepressant Prozac. NCCAM, the National Institute of Mental Health and the Office of Dietary Supplements are collaborating on a study to evaluate the efficacy and safety of standardized extract of *Hypericum* in *major* depression.

The NCCAM is also supporting research studies on kava. However, these have been put on hold because the FDA is investigating whether the use of dietary supplements containing kava (also known as kava kava or *Piper methylsticum*) pose a health risk. The FDA's $9 million supplement division investigates problems and tries to curb use of products it can prove dangerous. Kava is a member of the pepper family. Products containing kava are sold in the United States for a variety of uses including insomnia and short-term reduction of stress and anxiety.

Recent reports from European health authorities have linked kava to at least 25 cases of liver toxicity, including hepatitis, cirrhosis, and liver failure. The FDA is currently (2002) investigating the health risks of the herbal supplement. Under review are 38 Americans, including a liver transplant recipient, with medical problems associated with kava use. As of February 2002, sales have been halted in Switzerland and are suspended in Britain; Germany is acting to make kava a prescription product; the FDA recommends avoiding kava until safety questions are answered.

It may also be of interest to the reader to know that the "War on Drugs" has come to health food stores. As of February 6, 2002 Grocery stores in the United States are no longer permitted to carry any food product containing hemp. They are subject to confiscation by the Drug Enforcement Administration (DEA). The problem with hemp is that it can contain less than 1% of tetrahydrocannabinol (THC). According to the DEA there is *no allowable limit* of THC in the United States. Unless the manufacturer can provide scientific evidence that their product contains absolutely no trace of THC, it has to go. As a result, frozen waffles, cookies, cereals, salad dressings, tortilla chips, even ice cream have been removed from the shelves. Once again, we are protected from ourselves.

VITAMINS

Vitamins were first called *accessory factors* in 1906 when it was demonstrated that normal foods contain, in addition to the nutrients then recognized—carbohydrates, proteins, fats, minerals, and water—minute traces of other substances essential to health. The curative effects of diet on scurvy, rickets, beriberi, night blindness, and so forth, had been observed and speculated upon for centuries. In 1911 the antiberiberi factor that was isolated from rice was believed to contain an amine and, hence, the term accessory factors was changed to vitamins to emphasize the fact that the factors are essential to life and not merely accessory to other nutrients. Eventually, the term vitamin*e* was replaced by vitamin when it was found that vitamin A lacks an amine group. Originally, successive letters of the alphabet were assigned to new vitamins as they were characterized and isolated, although some letters were assigned out of order; vitamin K, for example, refers to the Scandinavian word *Koagulation*. The recent trend has been towards chemical names; vitamin B_1 has become thiamin, B_2, riboflavin, and so on.

Perhaps the most controversial aspects of vitamins is do we need to take them and, if so, at what dose. Tables 18.6 and 18.7 show the recommended daily allowances (RDA) for fat and water soluble vitamins, respectively.

Opponents of emphasizing RDAs point out that these numbers are for an average person, whatever that is. And, furthermore, these numbers may be outdated and are really relevant only to avoiding deficiency states. They do not allow for the possibility of enhanced or optimal nutritional states from doses above those necessary merely to protect against scurvy, beriberi or rickets. Vitamin C is the classic example having gained notoriety from Linus Pauling. Dr. Pauling advocated mega doses (many grams per day) for the amelioration of the common cold.

Some nutritionists believe that the processing of modern foods has left us with a less wholesome diet deficient in many vitamins and minerals (refined sugar, refined flour, and fried foods).

TABLE 18.6
Comparison of RDAs for Fat Soluble Vitamins

Category	Vitamin A (μg RE)	Vitamin D (μg)	Vitamin E (mg α-TE)	Vitamin K (μg)
Infants	375	10	4	10
Children	4–700	10	6–7	15–30
Males	1000	10	10	45–80
Females	800	10	8	45–65
Pregnant	800	10	10	65

Source: Adapted from the Food and Nutrition Board, National Academy of Sciences, National Research Council, Recommended Dietary Allowances (Revised 1989).

TABLE 18.7
Comparison of RDAs for Water-Soluble Vitamins

Category	Vitamin C (mg)	Thiamin (mg)	Riboflavin (mg)	Niacin (mg NE)	B_6 (mg)	B_{12} (μg)
Infants	30–35	0.3–0.4	0.4–0.5	5–6	0.3–0.6	0.3–0.5
Children	40–45	0.7–1.0	0.8–1.2	9–13	1.0–1.4	0.7–1.4
Males	50–60	1.2–1.5	1.4–1.8	15–20	1.7–2.0	2.0
Females	50–60	1.0–1.1	1.2–1.3	13–15	1.4–1.6	2.0
Pregnant	70	1.5	1.6	17	2.2	2.0

Ibid.

Therefore, in order to regain the nutrients removed in these processes, it makes sense to supplement our diets with relatively high doses of vitamins and minerals. Fortunately, these are among the most nontoxic OTC products available; but, they are not benign. A meta-analysis of 19 randomized, placebo-controlled trials in 2004 indicate that high dosages of vitamin E increase risk of all-cause mortality, and this dose-dependent increase begins at doses of 150 IU/day. At 400 IUs, which is the most common marketed dose, the results of the study of approximately 136,000 patients indicate the risk of dying is about 10% higher than risk among people not taking the vitamin.

SELECTED BIBLIOGRAPHY

Bisset, N.G., (Ed.) (1994) *Herbal Drugs and Phytopharmaceuticals*, Boca Raton, FL: CRC Press.
Blumenthal, M., Busse, W.R., Golddberg, A., Gruenwald, J., Hall, T., Riggins, C.W., and Rister, R.S., (Eds.) (1998) *The Complete German Commission E Monographs: Therapeutic Guide to Herbal Medicine*, Austin, TX: American Botanical Council.
Duke, J.A. (1997) *The Green Pharmacy*. Emmaus, PA: Rodale Press.
Foster, S. (1996) *Herbs for Your Health*. Loveland, CO: Interweave Press.
Mowrey, D.B. (1986) *The Scientific Validation of Herbal Medicine*. New Canaan, CN: Keats Publishing, Inc.
Spreen, A.N. (1999) *Nutritionally Incorrect: Why the American Diet is Dangerous and How to Defend Yourself*. Pleasant Grove, UT: Woodland Publishing.
Stary, F. (1996) *The Natural Guide to Medicinal Herbs and Plants*. New York: Barnes and Noble.

QUESTIONS

1. Alternative medicine includes which of the following?
    a. Aromatherapy
    b. Yoga
    c. Chiropractic
    d. Herbal medicine
    e. All of the above

2. The transition from traditional medical training to modern medicine is believed to have occurred in what year?
    a. 1906
    b. 1910
    c. 1919
    d. 1921
    e. 1933

3. Perhaps the single most significant event impacting on the sale of herbal drugs in the United States was which of the following?
    a. Encouragement from Timothy Leary
    b. The "pop" culture of the 1960s
    c. The thalidomide tragedy
    d. Passage of the 1962 law requiring prescription drugs to prove efficacy
    e. Passage of the dietary supplement Act of 1994

4. Supermarket sales of nutritional supplements now exceed how many millions of dollars yearly?
    a. 275
    b. 500
    c. 750
    d. 800
    e. 900

5. Which of the following countries has had the greatest impact on herbal medicine?
    a. Spain
    b. United States
    c. Germany
    d. France
    e. Slovakia

6.   Commission E is/are which of the following?
    a. A German panel of herbal experts
    b. A British panel of herbal experts
    c. A U.S. panel of experts specializing in vitamin E
    d. All of the above
    e. None of the above

7. Which of the following has/have been linked to significant toxicity in the United States, and/or Europe?
    a. KavaKava
    b. Vitamin C
    c. Ephedrine
    d. All of the above
    e. a and C

8. Which of the following is/are true regarding vitamins?
    a. Many are lost during the processing of certain foods
    b. Some are used to treat certain sicknesses in megadoses
    c. Both water and fat soluble are important
    d. Deficiency syndromes lead to the discovery of many
    e. All of the above

9. Which of the following is/are true of vitamins?
    a. All contain an amine group
    b. All are water soluble
    c. In general they have low toxicity
    d. Recommended Daily Allowances is a highly accurate expression
    e. All of the above

10.   Which of the following was first called "accessory factor(s)"?
    a. Herbal drugs
    b. St. John's Wort
    c. Vitamins
    d. a and c
    e. All of the above

Part V

Appendices, Glossary, and Calculations

Appendix I: The History of Drug Abuse Laws in the United States

INTRODUCTION

60% of most of our violent crimes are associated with alcohol or drug use. Many times they're rob-
bing, stealing, and all of these things to get money to buy drugs, and I do feel that we would markedly
reduce our crime rate if drugs were legalized. But I don't know the ramifications of this and I do
feel that we need to do some studies. In some countries that have legalized drugs, and made it legal,
they certainly have shown that there has been a reduction in their crime rate, and there has been no
increase in their drug use rate.

—Surgeon General, Dr. Joycelyn Elders, National Press Club, December 7, 1993

The political repercussions of that unexpected statement were not fully appreciated by Dr. Elders at the time. However, on December 9, 1994, following the Republican Party's conservative-mediated victory at the polls, Dr. Elders was fired by President Clinton, ostensibly for her views on introducing the subject of masturbation into sex education classes. While this undoubtedly played a role in her political demise, it was the controversial issue of drug legalization that began her political descent.

Despite the sensational headlines that followed Elders' comments, it should be remembered that there was a time, not so long ago, when many of the drugs against which we now wage an approximately $20 billion a year "war" were perfectly legal to use. At the turn of the century, for example, opium, morphine, heroin, cocaine, and marijuana were all either legal in the United States or subject to few restrictions. They were all present in patent medicines that were nonprescription drugs of secret composition. It has been estimated that millions of people were, what we would today call, "occasional" users at that time. The factors that have contributed to the evolution of extremely restrictive contemporary American drug laws have largely resulted from common problems, real or imagined, associated with nineteenth-century use of opiates (opium, morphine, and to some extent heroin) and cocaine, on the one hand, and the twentieth-century use of marijuana.

OPIUM (NINETEENTH CENTURY)

Although fines and public whippings were imposed for alcohol abuse as early as 1645 in New England, opium probably has the oldest history of use in this country among drugs usually considered illicit. Opium was available in America before 1800 in crude extracts with or without alcohol. One of the first written reports of opium use in the United States appeared in 1842, entitled *"An opium-eater in America."* A form of drug "confession" often mimicked by subsequent drug literature. This popularizing of a European fashion by Englishman Thomas de Quincey (the Timothy Leary of the 1840s) coincided with the introduction of legislation in the same year imposing a tariff on the importation of crude opium into this country. Although the tariff legislation acknowledged, to some extent, a developing opium problem, it was designed as a *tax* not a prohibition.

For a number of reasons (discussed below), the per capita, yearly consumption of crude opium continued to rise during the remainder of the century, reaching its peak in 1896 to a level of approximately 3.1 g. In addition, the importation of opium for *smoking* was also substantial since opium dens were quite popular. Owing to growing publicity at the turn of the century disclosing the contents of patent medicines, early state regulatory laws, and public opinion regarding opium smoking, *importation* of opium ultimately became prohibited in 1909 by the *Opium Exclusion Act*. Although domestic commercial sources of opium were never developed to any great extent in the United States, opium poppies were, in fact, legally grown in the United States until 1942, when the *Opium Poppy Act* was passed.

"*Opium-eating*" was the phrase generally used throughout the latter half of the nineteenth century, which actually referred to laudanum *drinking*. *Laudanum* (from the Latin, "something to be praised") of this period often contained "*2 ounces of strained opium, 1 ounce of saffron, and a dram of cinnamon and cloves dissolved in 1 pint of Canary wine*" and was the recipe of a seventeenth-century English physician, Thomas Sydenham. A dose of this concoction produced "*-a panacea ... for all human woes*," "*-equipoise to all the faculties...*" and could be ordered by mail from Sears, Roebuck for $4 a pint. It has been estimated that no less than 1% of the population was addicted to opium at the time.

Opium also has a place in literature. Lewis Caroll, for example, made allusions to opium in "Through the Looking Glass." During her journey, Alice found a small, unlabeled bottle that she drank knowing that something *interesting* was going to happen; it did. She subsequently met a large blue caterpillar sitting with its arms folded on a large *mushroom* (interesting) quietly smoking a long *hookah* (opium pipe). Caroll is one of numerous nineteenth-century authors and notables who have been identified as chronic users of opium.

The importation of Chinese workers following the Civil War is generally associated with the introduction of *smoking* opium to Western Americans. Its practice spread widely among respectable young men and women, many of whom "*were ruined morally and otherwise*." Ironically, in 1875, the city of San Francisco, which today we associate with a liberal view towards drug use, enacted the first antidrug ordinance in America, forbidding opium smoking in opium houses or dens. This was soon followed by similar laws in New York City (1882) and the state of Ohio (1885). In addition to opium's alleged effect on the morals of America, Samuel Gompers, the industrial magnate, believed that its use by Chinese immigrants increased their productivity so substantially that whites were at a disadvantage in the labor market. As opium dens became less accessible, poorer addicts were forced to seek less expensive alternatives such as morphine, and later its derivative, heroin.

MORPHINE (NINETEENTH CENTURY)

Morphine is the most active component of crude opium (making up approximately 9%), and it was first isolated in pure form in 1806 by a German pharmacist's assistant, Frederich Sertürner. It is easy to visualize the self-testing of morphine by Sertürner, which he did frequently, nearly dying of an overdose at one point, obliging him to name the substance after Morpheus, the god of dreams. The development of morphine use in America proceeded slowly over the next half-century, although both its medicinal and psychogenic properties were noted. However, with the general availability of the hypodermic syringe during mid-century, and its use in administering morphine during the American Civil War, a new form of addiction was created.

Pennsylvania, the home of morphine manufacturers of the day (Rosengarten and Company of Philadelphia—later merged into Merck, Sharpe and Dohme), enacted an antimorphine law as early as 1860, thus anticipating the start of the Civil War by 1 year. Morphine was used regularly, and probably indiscriminately, in large doses to treat many soldiers for the reduction of pain and relief from dysentery. It would have been thought of as a wonder drug. As a consequence, a high proportion of men became addicted to morphine (*soldier's disease*). Despite the lessons learned during the Civil War, by the turn of the century morphine addiction was still quite prevalent. This fact was, in large part, due to questionable medical advocacy, such as "*Advantages of Substituting the Morphia Habit for the Incurably Alcoholic*," as well as being *available OTC for 25 cents* a day to sustain an addiction.

In 1874, C.R. Wright of St. Mary's Hospital in London carried out a series of experiments that would have far reaching repercussions in the twentieth century. Dr. Wright prepared a series of *acetylated derivatives* of morphine. One of these (diacetylmorphine) was found to be three times as potent as morphine. It was given the brand name *Heroin* (from the German for "great" or "heroic") and placed on the market in the late 1890s by Bayer Laboratories. It was originally marketed in low doses to treat patients with tuberculosis, relieve cough, and induce sleep. It was considered a nonaddicting substance and viewed as having only minor problems with tolerance and addiction. Subsequent experience would demonstrate quite dramatically, however, that heroin is, in fact, quite addicting when injected in higher doses and it was withdrawn from the market. Today, because of its potency, heroin has displaced both its forebearers, opium and morphine, as the opiate of choice for illicit use.

COCAINE (LATTER-HALF NINETEENTH CENTURY)

While opium and morphine were developing their own following into the second half of the nineteenth century, a new player was about to arrive on the scene. Although the chewing of coca leaves had been practiced for thousands of years in South America, it was not until 1859 that the purification of *cocaine*, the active ingredient, was achieved. The availability of pure cocaine allowed the creation of many innovative mixtures by patent medicine makers of the day. One of the most popular preparations that found favor in the United States during the 1870s and 1880s was imported *coca-containing wines* from Europe (a variation on Dr. Sydenham's opium in Canary wine). The most famous wine of this type was manufactured by Angelo Mariani (Vin Mariani) and contained 6 mg of cocaine per ounce. These coca wines were used "*... for fatigue of mind and body...*" and sample bottles were often "*... free to medical men and clergymen on receipt of professional card.*"

Notables of that era who were said to be fond of Mr. Mariani's coca wine included Queen Victoria, Sarah Bernhardt, Thomas Edison, Robert Louis Stevenson, Jules Verne, Alexander Dumas, and Pope Leo XIII. Probably, much the same people who indulged in opium. Robert Louis Stevenson, in fact, is believed to have used cocaine as the inspiration for the unnamed drug in *The Strange Case of Dr. Jekyl and Mr. Hyde*. Not all literary references to cocaine portrayed it in such a horrific light, however. Sir Arthur Conan Doyle's Sherlock Holmes realized that cocaine's influence was bad but could not resist its stimulating properties as illustrated in the following excerpt from "*The Sign of Four*" (1890) as described by Dr. Watson:

> Sherlock Holmes took his bottle from the corner of the mantelpiece, and his hypodermic syringe from its neat morocco case. With his long, white nervous fingers, he adjusted the delicate needle and rolled back his left shirt cuff. For some little time his eyes rested thoughtfully upon the sinewy forearm and wrist, all dotted and scarred with innumerable puncture marks. Finally, he thrust the sharp point home, pressed down the tiny piston, and sank back into the velvet-lined armchair with a long sigh of satisfaction.
>
> Three times a day for many months I had witnessed this performance, but custom had not reconciled my mind to it...
>
> "Which is it today," I asked, "Morphine or cocaine?"
>
> He raised his eyes languidly from the old black-letter volume that he had opened.
>
> "It is cocaine," he said, "a seven-per-cent solution. Would you care to try it?"
>
> "No indeed," I answered brusquely. "My constitution has not got over the Afghan campaign yet. I cannot afford to throw any extra strain on it."
>
> He smiled at my vehemence. "Perhaps you are right, Watson," he said. "I suppose that its influence is physically a bad one. I find it, however, so transcendingly stimulating and clarifying to the mind that its secondary action is a matter of small moment."
>
> "But consider!" I said earnestly. "Count the cost! Your brain may, as you say, be roused and excited, but it is a pathological and morbid process that involves increased tissue-change and may at least leave a permanent weakness. You know, too, what a black reaction comes upon you. Surely the game is hardly worth the candle. Why should you, for a mere passing pleasure, risk the loss of those great powers with which you have been endowed? Remember that I speak not only as one comrade to another but as a medical man to one whose constitution he is to some extent answerable.
>
> He did not seem offended. On the contrary, he put his fingertips together, and leaned his elbows on the arms of his chair, like someone who has a relish for conversation.

"My mind," he said, "rebels at stagnation. Give me problems, give me work, give me the most abstruse cryptogram, or the most intricate analysis, and I am in my own proper atmosphere. I can dispense then with artificial stimulants. But I abhor the dull routine of existence. I crave for mental exaltation."

During the latter decades of the 1800s, members of the medical community believed that cocaine, like opium and morphine before, was a new wonder drug. One of its original supporters was Sigmund Freud who asserted *"there is no danger of general damage to the body as is the case with the chronic use of morphine."* Freud was later to repudiate that viewpoint. Early medical uses for cocaine included use as a local anesthetic (its most significant use), antidepressant, and to relieve withdrawal symptoms of morphine addicts. It was also included in numerous tonics, elixirs, and patent medicines.

Park Davis and Company was among the first American pharmaceutical companies to market extracts of cocaine in the early 1880s. These preparations were used by physicians for a wide variety of ailments including the *"... painless cure of opium and liquor habits"* and provided the official remedy of the *Hay Fever Association*. Park Davis also appreciated the advantages of smoking cocaine by selling *coca-leaf cigarettes and coca cheroots*.

Purveyors of patent medicines were also quick to jump on the bandwagon. And, despite attempts by state regulations to curb cocaine abuse (Illinois enacted a law against cocaine sale without a prescription in 1897), patent medicine manufacturers were frequently able to obtain exemptions. In general, local laws were "chaotic," varied in severity, were difficult to enforce, and had little effect on the sale of drugs and patent medicines across state lines. In some drug stores, one could purchase a dimes or quarters worth of cocaine or morphine.

One particular patent drug manufacturer of note at the end of the eighteenth century was *John Styth Pemberton* of Atlanta, Georgia. Unfortunately, Mr. Pemberton's "French Wine Cola" version did not prove to be a successful competitor against Vin Mariani. However, when he reformulated the cocaine with caffeine and named it *"Coca-Cola,"* the rest is history. Cocaine was present as an ingredient in Coca-Cola until 1903. In retrospect, it is fortunate that the cocaine content of patent medicine formulations containing alcohol was relatively modest. Today we know that when alcohol and cocaine are combined in the body, a new compound (cocaethylene) can be formed, which is believed to contribute to cocaine's psychological and toxicological effects.

PURE FOOD AND DRUG ACT (1906)

By the beginning of the twentieth century, Americans had developed the facility to become addicted to drugs via swallowing, smoking, injecting, and snorting. Patent medicines had the broadest impact on drug use during the preceding 50 years because of their widespread distribution, extravagant claims, and popularity. Sales of patent medicines increased from $3.5 million in 1859 to $74 million in 1904. This increase in drug use occurred during a period of *laissez-faire* capitalism, when the formulation, distribution, sales, and claims of many consumer products were not regulated. However, this open market was soon to change.

By the early 1900s, there was considerable governmental concern regarding the *purity* of not only drugs, but food as well; the meat packing industry having performed just as irresponsibly as the makers of patent medicines during this era. The question of food and drug impurities received nationwide press coverage in books and periodicals of the day and led President Theodore Roosevelt to recommend in 1905 *"... that a law be enacted to regulate interstate commerce in misbranded and adulterated foods, drinks, and drugs."*

Following relatively rapid congressional hearings, the *Pure Food and Drugs Act* was passed on June 30, 1906, providing an important stepping stone toward the eventual creation of the Food and Drug Administration (FDA). The government now had the responsibility for assessing drug hazards, prohibiting the sale of dangerous drugs, and requiring drug manufacturers to report adverse reactions associated with their products. It has been estimated that within a few years of the inclusion of these labeling changes, the sale of patent medicines containing a narcotic decreased by one-third.

The Pure Food and Drugs Act, and its 1912 Sherley Amendment dealing with *false and misleading advertising*, were primarily *truth-in-labeling acts*, and were *not* intended to criminalize the purchase and use of patent medicines, regardless of their content. The government, at that time, was principally concerned that the consumer be made aware of the possible presence of alcohol, morphine, opium, cocaine, heroin, and marijuana in what they were buying and to what extent. It was hoped that with this information the consumer would be more educated in *assessing risk* when consuming the patent medicines.

SHANGHAI OPIUM COMMISSION (1909)

In addition to the issues of purity and the advertising of its foods and drugs, early-twentieth-century America, as well as other parts of the World, found itself with a *drug dependency problem*. The exact extent of the problem at that time is difficult to ascertain, since estimates of the number of addicts range from 250,000 to 1,000,000, and more, in a population of approximately 76 million. Regardless of the number of addicts, between 1898 and 1902, while the population increased by only 10%, importation of cocaine rose 40%, opium 500%, and morphine 600%. By 1900, restrictive drug laws at the state level had been enacted, and reformers began to look to the *federal government* for effective national regulation.

In response to the apparent growing problem of domestic narcotic drug abuse, as well as attempting to assist China with its own international opium struggle, the United States organized the first international meeting in 1909 to consider international *opium traffic* (*The Shanghai Opium Commission*). Thirteen nations from the Far East, or who had possessions therein, were represented. (The United States, Germany, Great Britain, the Netherlands, Portugal, Italy, France, Russia, Siam, Japan, Persia, China, and Austria-Hungary.)

Most of the participants did not share America's zeal for prohibiting the nonmedical use of opium, since they had a vested interest in protecting their profits from this commodity. England, for example, feared that the suspension of Indian opium trade would lead to an unbalanced budget. However, the attitude of the U.S. delegates at the meeting was that a worldwide prohibition of habit-forming drugs needed to be enacted and promoted. Despite the lack of enthusiasm by most of the participants, the commission did resolve that *each country should take drastic internal measures* to *control morphine and other opium derivatives*. With this admonition, the United States thus obtained a moral *imprimatur* to pursue strict federal legislation to compensate for the consistent failure of state and local laws.

Although the resolutions recommended by the Shanghai Commission were reassuring to American interests, the United States still felt that more formal *international commitments* were desired. An early American proposal for a post-Shanghai conference was, however, not accepted as a commission resolution and, nearly 3 years would pass before the desired meeting finally took place. During this interval, attempts to enact exemplary domestic legislation were made in America for several reasons. First, many other nations already had more stringent legislation than the United States and, secondly, the United States had, in fact, accepted an obligation to enact federal narcotic control at the Shanghai Commission. The most significant early attempt to establish significant narcotic control in the United States was the *Foster Bill* (the antecedent of the Harrison Act). This proposal contained sweeping regulations on narcotic use, but did not obtain the necessary congressional support to be enacted.

INTERNATIONAL OPIUM CONFERENCE (1911)

Despite delays by Germany, Great Britain, and the Netherlands, the United States succeeded in convening the first *International Opium Conference* on December 1, 1911 in The Hague. Twelve of the nations in attendance in Shanghai were represented (Austria-Hungary chose not to attend). The discussions were once again motivated by national interests resulting in the convention ultimately placing *the major burden of worldwide narcotic control on domestic legislation within each country itself.*

A mechanism was developed, however, for the signature and ratification of the convention by participants and "significant" nonparticipants alike. Although 44 nations signed, less than half of these actually ratified it and only 7 nations actually implemented it within 5 years. Ratification by the U.S. Senate was officially deposited in The Hague on December 10, 1913; however, its own domestic bill was actually deadlocked in the Senate at that time.

HARRISON NARCOTIC ACT (1914)

Following The Hague Convention, it was imperative that the United States impress other signatories with the seriousness of its intent by passing its own domestic drug legislation. A bill was introduced in 1912, which was primarily the creation of Dr. Hamilton Wright (the "Father of American Drug Laws"), who had been a representative at both the Shanghai Commission and The Hague Convention and had authored the previously defeated Foster Bill. Dr. Wright's scientific claim to fame had been "proving" that beriberi (a thiamin deficiency) was a communicable disease.

Representative Francis Burton Harrison of New York introduced the new bill to Congress. This original Harrison Bill was basically designed to eliminate narcotic use except for medical purposes. On its face, it was a simple licensing law that simply required sellers to get a license if they were going to handle opiates and cocaine.

For various reasons, groups such as the American Association of Pharmaceutical Chemists, the National Association of Medicinal Products, and the National Association of Druggists had opposed the bill in its initial form and lobbied actively for a number of modifications, resulting in submission of a "final" form in 1913. Following considerable debate between House and Senate committees over proposed amendments, the *Harrison Narcotics Act* was passed on December 14, 1914 and went into effect from March 1, 1915. Enforcement was assigned to the Bureau of Internal Revenue within the Treasury Department.

The principal features of the enacted bill required record keeping by pharmacists and physicians, registration with the Treasury Department of anyone (physicians, dentists, or veterinarians) dealing with narcotics, except the consumer, and the yearly purchase of a $1 tax stamp by retail dealers and practicing physicians. Patent medicines containing small amounts of morphine, cocaine, opium, and heroin (chloral hydrate and cannabis were omitted) could continue to be sold by mail order or by retail dealers.

The purpose of the Act was to *regulate* the use of narcotics for "legitimate medical purposes." However, as a consequence, it became *illegal* to possess narcotics without a prescription. Eventually, in the 1920s it became illegal for addicts to obtain these drugs even from physicians. The main architect of the legislation, Dr. Wright, was ironically not in government service at the time of its passage, having been summarily dismissed in June of 1914 by Secretary of State Bryan for failing to take a pledge of abstinence from alcohol.

Since addiction was not considered a legitimate disease meriting a prescription for narcotics (the medical community itself was split), an increasing number of people subsequently resorted to criminal activity in order to obtain their drugs; the cost of heroin on the streets rose from $6.50/ounce to approximately $100. The increase in crime validated the Treasury Department's fear that deprived addicts would threaten the public order. Although passage of the Harrison Act did increase the price of street narcotics, it also resulted in a reduction or complete elimination of patent medicine narcotics as well as a decline in addiction rates.

By ignoring the physiological fact of addiction, American drug policy rejected the earlier experiences of clinics in Florida and Tennessee dealing with addict maintenance (which were available during the Harrison debate) and contributed in its own way to increased urban crime, escalation in the size of police agencies, and a diminution in civil liberties. Following a number of lower court decisions dealing with loopholes, the Supreme Court subsequently authenticated the constitutionality of the Harrison Act on March 3, 1919. In a five to four decision, the court determined that maintenance of an addiction *per se* was illegal and that such use was such a perversion of the meaning of the act "*... that no discussion of the subject is required.*" So much for that.

PROHIBITION (1919–1933)

Narcotics were, of course, not the only drugs of concern during the immediate post–World War I era. If the use of narcotics could not be justified then how could that of alcohol? The temperance movement, which had been active for years, now succeeded in having the use and distribution of alcohol banned. Led by the colorful Carrie Nation, with a Bible in one hand and a hatchet in the other, public sentiment was pushed aside by her moral crusade.

The eighteenth Amendment (*National Prohibition*), also know as the *Volstead Act*, was ratified on January 29, 1919 and became law on January 16, 1920. Immediately before ratification of the Prohibition Act, a Prohibition Unit was established on December 22, 1919. The Prohibition Unit was composed of Narcotic and Alcohol Divisions. An interesting question has been asked: "*Why did the Supreme Court agree that a federal statute could outlaw narcotics, when the Constitution itself had to be amended to outlaw alcohol?*"

The strength of the temperance movement in overcoming economic realities of the day is illustrated by the effect the eightieth Amendment had on the collection of fees by the Internal Revenue Service (IRS). In 1916, gross receipts at the IRS were $513 million of which $241 million was derived from distilled spirits and fermented liquors. Thus, 47% of IRS receipts were from alcohol-related income versus 13% from personal income tax. The movements' fervor also affected the medical profession. With the cynical belief that physicians would discharge their responsibilities under prohibition no better than they had under the Harrison Act, new legislation was created. The specific law, the Willis-Campbell Act of 1921, was enacted in order to restrict the number of liquor prescriptions permitted to each physician.

The eighteenth Amendment never, of course, achieved the same level of public support as the Harrison Act. This lack of public support forced its repeal on December 5, 1933. With the repeal of federal prohibition, the states assumed responsibility to regulate the distribution and sale of alcohol. In most states, these regulatory units are referred to as alcoholic beverage control (ABC) agencies. They control the manufacture, distribution, and sale of alcoholic beverages.

Vendors are required to obtain licenses from the ABC. In 1991, there were over 500,000 retail licenses issued nationally. In 39 states, local communities regulate where and when alcohol can be sold. Although the National Minimum Drinking Age Act of 1984 required all states to raise their minimum alcohol purchase and possession age to 21, many state laws contain numerous loopholes.

POST-HARRISON ACT (1920–1929)

During the 1920s, enforcement of prohibition of alcohol surpassed that of narcotics by the Harrison Act. However, despite disparate resources, the smaller Narcotic Division successfully closed 44 opiate-dispensing clinics by 1923. This hard-line attitude reflected the prevailing public mood of the day that narcotic maintenance served only to contribute to or create a menacing personality. Not much has changed in contemporary society.

The Harrison Narcotic Act, as enforced by the *Narcotic Division of the Prohibition Unit*, had, therefore, become the first significant drug policy in this country, emphasizing a prohibitionist perspective while denying the concept of addiction as a disease. However, the prospect of a nation with 1 million narcotic addicts (contemporary estimates) in withdrawal was a sobering thought for the government. Therefore, temporary supply of drugs was discretely provided at carefully selected clinics.

Fortunately, the number of addicts estimated at the time appears to have been exaggerated. In New York City, for example, only 7500 addicts had been registered in city clinics, before they were closed in early 1920. Previous estimates for the city had been in the 100,000–200,000 range. Nevertheless, critics alleged that narcotic clinics did nothing more than providing a destabilizing influence by sanctioning the indefinite maintenance of addiction.

Although the *Narcotic Division was considerably smaller than the Alcohol Division of the Prohibition Unit*, it was quite effective. By the end of 1923, the population of addicts in the New York state penitentiary at Sing Sing had risen from 1 to 9%. By mid-1928, one-third of all male and female inmates in federal prisons were there by virtue of violating the Harrison Act.

Of the violators in federal prison, the majority were addicts and, therefore, presented a medical condition to wardens who did not wish to care for addicts. As a result of this situation, the *Porter Narcotic Farm* (as the facilities were originally known) bill was enacted on January 19, 1929, establishing the Lexington farm (opened in 1935) and the Ft. Worth farm (opened in 1938). These hospitals, as they were eventually referred to, were institutions that provided additional prison space (complete with iron bars) and segregation of the addicts from the general prison population. It was not until the late 1960s that the bars were removed from the Lexington facility and the cells converted into rooms.

FEDERAL MARIJUANA TAX ACT (1930–1937)

In 1930, the Narcotics Division became a separate entity (Federal Bureau of Narcotics[FBN]) within the Treasury Department. Harry J. Anslinger, then Assistant Commissioner of the Prohibition Bureau, became Acting Commissioner of Narcotics on July 1 and was appointed Commissioner on September 25 (a position he held for 32 years).

Anslinger was free of any of the prior scandals associated with the Alcohol Division (during prohibition) and was considered to have desirable diplomatic skills developed during his years in the foreign service. He had, however, only sporadic experience with narcotic control. Anslinger's tenure in office was characterized by his belief that the most effective strategy of achieving public compliance with a law regulating a dangerous drug was a policy of harsh fines and severe mandatory prison sentences for first convictions (sound familiar?). Anslinger had developed these proposals in the context of enforcing the Volstead Act (prohibition) but would refine them during the mid-1930s, with President Roosevelt's endorsement, in his attempt to enforce marijuana regulations.

The history of marijuana in the United States is not clear. However, it appears that hemp, hashish, and smokable marijuana were discovered at different times and were used in different contexts. The pilgrims, for example, brought hemp with them to Jamestown in 1611 and cultivated it for its fiber. The cultivation of hemp became so economically important that during the 1700s some states imposed penalties on those who did not produce it. In 1764, King George III offered American colonists a bounty of £8 for every bale of raw hemp delivered to London, to which Ben Franklin's reply was, "We have not yet enough for our own consumption."

In 1788, the Viceroy of Mexico ordered the mission at Monterey to plant hemp, thus starting hemp cultivation in California. The hemp industry remained important up to the Civil War. Following the war, production declined as cheaper imported hemp became available, and cotton and wool became less expensive alternatives.

Marijuana was first mentioned as a medicine in an American medical text in 1843 and in 1854 was listed in the U.S. Dispensatory. The latter year also marked the first written description by Bayard Taylor in The Atlantic Monthly of cannabis intoxication. In the 1850s, recommended medical uses for marijuana included the treatment of gout, rheumatism, tetanus, opiate and alcohol withdrawal, loss of appetite, dysmenorrhea, convulsions, depression, insanity, and asthma.

Although its suggested uses were widespread, marijuana never actually achieved popular use in the medical community. The reasons for this include variations in potency of commercial preparations, variability in patient's responses, slow onset of oral action, and lack of solubility preventing administration by injection. However, the drug was included in many patent medicine preparations and was officially recognized as a medicine in the *U.S. Pharmacopoeia* until 1937. In 1937, there were 28 pharmaceuticals that contained cannabis.

By 1906, the Pure Food and Drug Act required that the quantity of cannabis be clearly indicated on the label of any drug or food sold to the public. However, cannabis routinely escaped federal regulations including the Harrison Act. It was generally utilized in benign medical situations, and its use was not considered a significant problem. For example, in 1894, the Indian Hemp Commission, appointed by the British Parliament, concluded that moderate use of cannabis was not injurious to the majority of users. In fact, cannabis was defended by the *National Wholesale Druggists' Association* and a pharmaceutical company (Lehn and Fink) during Congressional hearings in 1911, dealing with a federal antinarcotic law.

Testimony by their respective representatives described cannabis as not being habit-forming and without attraction to narcotic addicts as an alternative. Conflicting testimony was provided by Charles B. Towns, dedicated antiaddiction crusader and formulator of Town's cure for addiction (1 part fluid extract of prickly ash bark, 1 part fluid extract of hyoscyamus, and 2 parts 15% tincture of belladonna; a tincture by definition contains alcohol).

Despite early passive views on cannabis use in America, however, a gradual accumulation of momentum in opposition to marijuana developed after World War I. Much of the antipathy was based on cultural fears relating to cannabis use by Syrians in New York, East Indians in California, and, principally, Mexicans in the Southwest. Much of the pressure for federal legislation regulating marijuana arose, not from the FBN, but from local law enforcement agencies in the South and Southwest who saw it as a link to violent crime presumably committed by Mexican immigrants.

In response to the international aspect of marijuana's intrusion into America, the United States succeeded at the *Second Geneva Convention in 1925* in obtaining an agreement that international traffic in cannabis should be regulated. Although domestic fear of marijuana was minimal during the 1920s, the federal government's view was different. For example, in 1929, habitual cannabis users were deemed eligible for treatment in the newly approved narcotic "farms."

Continuing bad press occurred during the early 1930s describing marijuana as a "menace," "developer of criminals," with the capacity to cause "intoxication" and facilitate prison "uprisings." Regardless of the extent of the marijuana "problem," the FBN believed, during its early years, that control should rest with state governments (particularly those with substantial Latin American populations). In fact, in their 1932 report, the Bureau comments that the use of marijuana had been exaggerated in the press (the Hearst newspapers were particularly active in this regard) and that its use was not inordinately large. As late as 1937, the Bureau still advocated that controlling the distribution of marijuana lay in adoption of uniform *state* narcotic laws.

Despite the Bureau of Narcotics file on marijuana being less than 2 in. thick in 1931, all 48 states had, by the early 1930s, similar laws regulating the illegal use, sale, and/or possession of marijuana under the *Uniform [state] Narcotic Drug Act*. As mentioned above, the Bureau was still reluctant to seek a federal law directed at marijuana. Commissioner Anslinger felt it would be difficult to enforce, would probably be unconstitutional, and felt that the Bureau was better advised to concentrate on heroin. However, the enactment in 1934 of a *"transfer tax"* on firearms, and the subsequent finding of its constitutionality in 1937, provided a legal precedent that the Treasury Department felt could be applicable to marijuana. Therefore, in response to increasing pressure from local police forces *the Bureau somewhat reluctantly agreed to pursue a federal antimarijuana transfer tax statute.*

Regardless of the ambiguous view that existed within the Bureau at that time, the Treasury Department opted to present a solid front before Congress. In the process, objectivity was not emphasized but, rather, bureaucratic excess supported the Tax Act, the goal being total prohibition. The only witness opposing the proposal to appear before the House Committee was an AMA spokesperson. He pleaded that the health professions did not need the burden of the bill's restrictions and that the evidence against marijuana was incomplete.

The AMA's legislative activities committee did write to protest the impending legislation. Their solicitation read in part, "There is positively no evidence to indicate the abuse of cannabis as a medicinal agent or to show that its medicinal use is leading to the development of cannabis addiction. Cannabis at the present time is slightly used for medicinal purposes, but it would seem worthwhile to maintain its status as a medicinal agent.... There is a possibility that a restudy of the drug by modern means may show other advantages to be derived from its medicinal use." Despite these protestations, the Federal Marijuana Tax Act was passed by Congress during a period of intolerance and came into effect on October 1, 1937.

The Marijuana Tax Act followed the regulation-by-taxation precedent set by the 1842 law, taxing opium importation. In essence, the law stipulated that nonmedical use of marijuana as well as the possession or sale of untaxed (i.e., unlicensed) marijuana was illegal. The courts were willing to accept the premise that it really was a tax violation when people got arrested for drugs. *The fact that the government would not issue any licenses (stamps) was not a defense.* Furthermore, a *legal* "*fiction*" was created that whatever a person puts into their bodies must have come as a result of some form of interstate commerce. Because this form of enterprise is regulated by the Federal Government, in the form of taxes and licenses, the Federal Government should be allowed to regulate what anyone puts into their own bodies.

Physicians and dentists, growers, and importer/manufacturers were required to pay $15, $25, and $50, respectively, in annual taxes. This was virtually impossible in practice since, as mentioned above, the government rarely issued the required stamps. An interesting amendment to the act allowed the use of sterilized marijuana seeds in birdseed. From 1937 to 1971, the federal government referred to marijuana as a narcotic.

The marijuana tax act of 1937 remained in effect until it was overturned by the Supreme Court in 1967. This was largely the result of Timothy Leary who led a movement pointing out the absurdity of a law that induced the public to break the law (i.e., obtain marijuana before applying for a fictitious license from the government). The government had the last say, however, when they passed the *Comprehensive Drug Act* in 1970 classifying marijuana as a Schedule I drug—no legal use.

Controversy continues to surround *Cannabis sativa* as to whether marijuana laws should be changed. Proponents argue that marijuana is less harmful than tobacco while opponents site undesirable behavioral effects. The dichotomy of viewpoints and legal status is illustrated by the conflict between state and federal officials regarding the medical use of marijuana. Despite the fact that voters in Arizona, Alaska, California, Colorado, Maine, Nevada, Oregon, and Washington have all approved ballot initiatives allowing the use of medical marijuana (Hawaii did so via legislative action), the U.S. Supreme Court in their wisdom concluded in 2001 that it is illegal to distribute marijuana for medical purposes.

In February 2002, agents of the DEA raided a medical pot club in San Francisco. Some 630 marijuana plants were seized and four arrests were made. If convicted, the sentences can range from *40 years to life in prison*. An outspoken group in favor of changing marijuana laws is the National Organization for the Reform of Marijuana Laws (NORML).

POST–WORLD WAR II (1945–1969)

It was once a patriotic duty for an American farmer to grow marijuana (hemp). In 1942, a film called *Hemp for Victory* was produced and distributed by the U.S. Department of Agriculture to encourage American farmers to grow cannabis for much-needed hemp products, particularly rope. During World War II, narcotic drug use reached its twentieth-century low point in the United States. This was due to a continual decline in use as well as diminished supply due to disrupted international transportation.

Between 1945 and 1970, a transition occurred from the application of strict legal sanctions to narcotic drug use during the 1950s to more medically based treatment during the 1960s. For example, under the tutelage of Representative Hale Boggs, the Uniform Narcotic Drug Act was significantly empowered in 1951 to impose mandatory minimum sentences of 2 years for *first*-time narcotic offenders. However, even this was not deemed sufficiently severe. The high water mark in punitive federal statutes against narcotics was reached in 1956. The Narcotic Control Act of that year (Little Boggs Act) authorized court verdicts to impose the *death penalty on anyone over the age of 18 who sold heroin to anyone under the age of 18*. The severity of these rather draconian sanctions ultimately elicited the opposition of the American Bar Association as well as the AMA.

Now that the respectable institutions of law and medicine were beginning to question the merits of narcotic regulations, the FBN began to go on the defensive. It took umbrage, for example, at a Joint ABA–AMA Committee Report in 1958 advocating a lessening of criminal penalties and, significantly, the reestablishment of an experimental clinic. The Bureau attempted to discredit the report. However, the document's reasoned views began to permeate a more receptive Congress and initiated the transfer of narcotic control from the FBN to mental health professionals.

With the coincidental retirement in 1962 of Commissioner Anslinger and the Supreme Court's decision that addiction was a disease, as well as the arrival of President Kennedy's New Frontier, the Bureau's approach was becoming anachronistic. The prevailing mood of the day encouraged reduced penalties, more medical treatment, possible development of maintenance clinics, and a reevaluation of drug laws. In 1962, a White House Panel on Narcotic and Drug Abuse reported that "*It is the opinion of the Panel that the hazards of marijuana per se have been exaggerated and that long criminal sentences imposed on an occasional user or possessor of the drug are in poor social perspective.*"

In 1963, the Presidential Commission on Narcotic and Drug Abuse recommended relaxation of mandatory minimum sentences, increased appropriations for research, and the dismantling of the FBN. The Drug Abuse Control Amendments of 1965 further diminished the role of the FBN by establishing the Bureau of Drug Abuse Control within the HEW (Department of Health, Education, and Welfare). The Act also shifted the basis for drug control from taxation to interstate commerce regulation. One of the most significant results of the more liberal view of the time was *the establishment of methadone maintenance clinics in the mid-1960s*. This program is, of course, by its very nature the direct antithesis of earlier federal prohibition policy outlawing addiction maintenance (Supreme Court decision of 1919), since one addiction is substituted for another.

In 1968, the FBN was transferred to the Justice Department, fused with the Bureau of Drug Abuse Control of HEW, to become the Bureau of Narcotics and Dangerous Drugs. By this time, the budget for the National Institutes of Mental Health was 40 times that of the FBN. This funding reflected the successful persuasiveness of the mental health establishment in convincing Washington that addiction was a disease and, as such, should be treated by the medical profession. In addition to the reorganization of federal agencies concerned with regulation of narcotic drugs, an amalgamation of the vast number of regulations in effect at that time was also undertaken. They were repealed, replaced, or updated.

In 1969, the U.S. Supreme Court ruled in the case of Timothy Leary that the Marijuana Tax Act could no longer be enforced because, had Dr. Leary tried to pay the tax on cannabis required by federal law, he would have broken Texas law prohibiting possession of marijuana. This meant that federal drug laws had to be rewritten. The result was the framing of the Comprehensive Drug Abuse Prevention and Control Act (Controlled Substances Act [CSA]) of 1970.

The CSA centralized federal regulations into one statute and separated marijuana from addicting drugs. At the federal level, both simple possession and nonprofit distribution of small amounts of marijuana were changed from *felonies to misdemeanors*. In addition, first-time offenders could have their criminal records expunged. Many states copied these federal efforts, and within a few years all but Nevada had reduced simple possession of marijuana to a misdemeanor.

THE CONTROLLED SUBSTANCES ACT (CSA-1970)

The CSA was an attempt by the government to rank drugs into categories, called *schedules*, according to their level of dangerousness (i.e., potential for abuse and dependency). The final decision about which schedule a drug was put in was made *not* by medical experts *but by the* Justice

Department and the Bureau of Narcotics and Dangerous Drugs, later named the *Drug Enforcement Administration* (DEA).

Schedule I includes drugs deemed to have no *accepted* medical use in the United States and cannot be prescribed (e.g., heroin, the hallucinogens dimethyltryptamine and psilocybin, *and marijuana*). The presence of marijuana in Schedule I is, of course, interesting because its inclusion is neither consistent with pharmacological data nor reflects the view of most qualified professionals in the medical field. This reality is dramatized by the DEA's own administrative law judge who ruled on September 6, 1988 that, *"The evidence in this record clearly shows that marijuana has been accepted as capable of relieving the distress of great numbers of very ill people, and doing so with safety under medical supervision. It would be unreasonable, arbitrary and capricious for DEA to continue to stand between those sufferers and the benefits of this substance..."*

Schedule II contains dangerous prescribed drugs (e.g., morphine, cocaine, amphetamines, certain barbiturates, and methylphenidate); Schedule III contains drugs that have potential for abuse less than those in Schedules I and II (e.g., most barbiturates); Schedule IV drugs produce only limited physical and psychological dependence (e.g., chloral hydrate and meprobamate); and Schedule V drugs contain moderate quantities of certain opioid drugs (e.g., antitussives and antidiarrheals) that may be obtained without a prescription. In order to avoid innocent violations of the law, medical practitioners may obtain a manual of guidelines from the Drug Enforcement Administration, Registration Unit, P.O. Box 28083, Central Station, Washington, DC 2005.

To some degree, the CSA was based on the British Pharmacy Act of 1868 that attempted to accomplish a similar goal (though not related to abuse or dependency). The CSA was originally presented to Congress focusing on rehabilitation, research, and education. However, because of conflicting philosophies of the day (treatment/tolerance versus Nixon's war on drugs), the act contained substantial law and order sentiment when passed. Nevertheless, this law has been viewed as a transition between reliance on law enforcement with severe penalties and a therapeutic approach. Significantly, it also *de facto* decriminalized marijuana to a certain extent by allowing first offenders possessing small amounts to be placed on probation for 1 year rather than mandatory incarceration. In the era from 1970 to 1980, law enforcement became more narrowly targeted on drug dealers.

THE 1970s

After the enactment of the CSA, there followed a period of uncertainty as the use of illicit drugs increased. Because of conflicts between the philosophy of enforcement and that of treatment or toleration, a presidential Commission on Marijuana and Drug Abuse (NCMDA) was established in 1972. Its task was to report within a year on marijuana, its highest priority, and within 2 years on drug abuse in general. The committee's first report recommended that possession of small amounts of marijuana should be decriminalized (i.e., a finable offense not subject to incarceration). The final report appeared in March 1973 and reconfirmed its original recommendation. *Despite these recommendations, President Nixon remained opposed to decriminalization.*

Nixon's successor, Gerald Ford, was less strident than Nixon on the question of recreational drug use. This is reflected in the *White Paper on Drug Abuse* prepared by the President's Domestic Council Drug Abuse Task Force and published in September 1975. The document acknowledged that elimination of drug abuse is unlikely but government can contain the problem. Importantly, it also stated that all drugs are not equally dangerous and that priority should be given to reducing supply and demand for those drugs that pose a greater risk (e.g., heroin, amphetamines, and certain barbiturates). This softened position toward marijuana reflected the more relaxed attitude of the country as evidenced by the decriminalization of marijuana by Oregon in 1973.

The election of Jimmy Carter in 1976 ensured a continuation of tolerance to drug use, particularly marijuana. In March 1977, the Special Assistant for Health Issues to the President, and high officials from DEA, the State Department, NIDA, NIMH, the Customs Service, and the Justice Department appeared before the House Select Committee on Narcotics Abuse and Control to argue for the decriminalization of marijuana. The President himself repeated a similar theme before Congress later that year.

In 1977, publications of the DEA de-emphasized the importance of the marijuana problem and argued that enforcement was a matter best left to the states. By 1978, eleven states, with one-third of the American population, had decriminalized marijuana use. Thirty others had provisions for conditional discharge (charges dropped or no penalty attached), and twelve allowed for the expungement of the record for first-possession offenders.

The year 1978 probably became a *watershed* in America's relaxed view toward drug use. The decriminalization of marijuana possession was significant because approximately 90% of arrests during this period were for possession (360,000 per year); this brief era of relaxed federal and states' attitude toward marijuana was about to change, however, as data emerged indicating a steep rise in marijuana and cocaine use, particularly among young people.

THE 1980s AND 1990s

By 1980, the DEA had reversed its position and now portrayed marijuana as the most serious *drug problem facing the United States*. The White House, now occupied by Ronald Reagan, also shifted its stance to more of an uncompromising Nixonian position. The average penalty for convicted marijuana *users* in federal courts rose from approximately 30 months in 1975 to over 50 months in 1982 (thus approaching the 1961 average of 70 months). The impact of the late-seventies/early-eighties backlash in societal opinion is also reflected in the fact that since 1977 no additional states have decriminalized marijuana. To the contrary, states have been reinstituting criminal penalties (including Alaska and Oregon, which were the most permissive).

In 1985, a new smokable form of cocaine ("crack") began to appear in certain parts of the United States. This new form of cocaine was cheap, highly effective, had a quick onset of action, did not require needle injection, and was less dangerous to manufacture than "freebase" cocaine. The violence and crime associated with this new, highly popular, and profitable drug had a significant impact on Americans. Because of the furor created, an Anti-Drug Abuse Act was signed into law in the autumn of 1986. This act authorized nearly $4 billion for an intensified battle against drugs. While most of the funding was destined for law enforcement, the law also provided some additional support for drug abuse research via the National Institute of Drug Abuse (NIDA).

In 1986, President Reagan also signed Executive Order Number 12564, the *Drug Free Federal Workplace Act*. This act initiated drug-testing programs for *federal employees* in safety-sensitive jobs. It also suggested procedures for drug-testing programs and plans for employee assistance programs to provide counseling and rehabilitation for workers with drug problems. In 1988, the drug-free policy act was extended to include all federal grantees and most federal contractors.

Drug use in the workplace is also a potential problem in nonfederal entities. According to an article in the *Houston Business Journal* in 2000, a recent survey by the *American Management Association's annual Survey on Workplace Drug Testing and Drug Abuse Policies*, workplace drug testing has increased more than 1200% since 1987. Virtually all companies that employ drug testing show steady decreases in drug use. Conversely, the number of employees trying to cheat, or adulterate their tests, is increasing. A quick search of the Internet reveals dozens of antidrug testing websites where so-called "cleansing" aids are sold for the sole purpose of helping drug users produce a clean urine drug screen (e.g., http://www.testclean.com). Drug users can even purchase freeze-dried urine, or human urine that is purported to be "clean."

Laws pertaining to workplace drug testing in the United States are always changing, with courts, legislatures, and regulatory agencies at both the federal and state levels continually modifying their approach. Employers must keep abreast of these changes and regularly reevaluate their drug policies. An employer's right to implement drug and alcohol testing depends on several factors, including whether the employer is in the public or private sector, the employees are contract or "at will," and whether the company is covered by the U.S. Department of Transportation regulations. Collective bargaining agreements may also enter into the mix.

In addition to narcotics and marijuana, the nonmedical use of anabolic steroids became increasingly popular during the eighties. This was particularly true for athletes seeking to increase skeletal muscle mass and performance, as discussed previously. The *Omnibus Anti-Substance Abuse Act of 1988* made the unlawful distribution of anabolic steroids across state lines a felony under federal law, punishable by 1–3 years in prison and a fine of up to $250,000. State laws governing the possession and distribution of anabolic drugs vary, but a conviction in most states carries a stiff fine and imprisonment.

The subsequent *Omnibus Crime Control Act (OCCA) of 1990* added certain anabolic–androgenic steroid substances to Schedule III of the Controlled Substance Act of 1970, which places them under the aegis of the DEA. Therefore, provisions for registration, reporting, record keeping, prescribing, as well as investigation of and penalties for misuse, now apply to these drugs. Only registered clinicians can issue prescriptions for these drugs, which can be refilled a maximum of 5 times within 6 months. The OCCA also regulates human growth hormone distribution for nonmedical purposes, since this drug was being turned to as an alternative for anabolic steroids. Possession and distribution of steroids without a prescription is a federal crime punishable by up to a year in prison and a fine of at least $1000.

According to the Office of National Drug Control Policy (ONDCP), federal spending on drug control programs has increased from $1.5 billion in fiscal year 1981 to $18.1 billion (enacted) in fiscal year 2001 (a 12-fold increase). The budget is divided into three main categories: domestic enforcement (the largest), international/border control, and demand reduction. The *1993 National Summit on U.S. Drug Policy* has made five recommendations to modify future policy: (1) reduce spending on international interdiction and eradication with corresponding increases for treatment and prevention; (2) fund only effective programs for drug dependence; (3) coerce hard-core users to get treatment; (4) continue strict law enforcement; and (5) avoid counterproductive prison terms for first-time offenders. A more specific breakdown of the federal budget for fiscal year 2000 and 2001 is shown in Table AI.1. Table AI.2 shows state spending for substance abuse in 1998. According to Bureau of Justice Statistics for 1990, U.S. law enforcement agencies now arrest more than 1.3 million citizens each year for the possession, distribution, and sale of prohibited drugs. More than a quarter of a million people are now incarcerated for drug offenses.

When he took office as the country's Drug Czar in 1996, Barry McCaffrey insisted there was not a shred of scientific evidence that smoking marijuana was useful or necessary. Nevertheless, McCaffrey commissioned yet another report to evaluate the scientific validity of marijuana for patients. *The National Academy of Sciences' Institute of Medicine* undertook an 18-month study

TABLE AI.1

Fiscal Year 2000 and 2001 Federal Drug Control Budget by Function

Function	2000 (in Millions)	2001 (in Millions)
Total	$17,940.3	$18,053.1
Drug treatment	$2,915.2	$3,168.3
Drug prevention	2,338.6	2,515.1
Criminal justice system	8,429.0	9,357.7
International	1,892.9	609.7
Interdiction	1,965.9	1,950.4
Research	89.6	106.1
Intelligence	309.1	345.2
International (U Support for Plan Colombia & the Andean Region)	954.4	

Source: ONDCP FY2002 National Drug Control Budget April 2001.

TABLE A1.2
State Spending for Substance Abuse in 1998

Function	FYI 998 (in Billions)
Total	$77.9
Justice	$30.7
Education	16.5
Health	15.2
Child/family assistance	7.7

Source: National Center on Addiction and Substance Abuse at Columbia University, "Shoveling Up: The Impact of Substance Abuse on State Budgets," January 2001, press release. Lesser amounts were budgeted for developmental disabilities (5.9) and public safety (1.5).

---

of all available scientific evidence on medical marijuana. The 1999 report's authors found that the active components in marijuana appear to be helpful in treating pain, nausea, and AIDS-related weight loss and muscle spasms in multiple sclerosis. While there is currently no legal source for marijuana, patients can get access to a synthetic THC pill. In 1986, the FDA approved Marinol®.

THE NEXT MILLENNIUM

Unlike cocaine and opium, tobacco and its primary psychoactive ingredient, nicotine, are products of the New World: two species being in cultivation at the time of Columbus. The sale of tobacco by the United States to France helped finance much of our Revolutionary War expenses. Thus, together with hemp, tobacco contributed to the young countries positive cash flow. Between the late-eighteenth and early-twentieth centuries, the primary forms of tobacco use in America were snuff and chewing. By 1911, smoking tobacco became the dominant form.

The government of the United States has supported these very important industries by various means for centuries. This support continues to this day even though tobacco contributes to approximately 400,000 deaths annually. A study published in 2004 indicated that the overall cancer death rate for African–American males alone would drop by nearly two-thirds (without any other intervention) if their exposure to tobacco smoke was eliminated.

"African–American men have had the highest cancer burden of any group in this country for decades," the author stated. Smoke exposure appears responsible for African–American males' high overall cancer mortality rates, not just their lung cancers. Research has linked their smoking to cancers of the colon, pancreas, and prostate. U.S. black male smoke exposures and nonlung cancer death rates have moved in near-perfect lockstep; the associations are very strong and have been consistent year-by-year for over 30 years. According to recent figures from the U.S. Centers for Disease Control and Prevention, the overall age-adjusted cancer death rate for African–American men is 330.9 deaths per 100,000 individuals, compared to 239.2 for white men.

Beginning in the late 1980, however, there were signs that the sacrosanct status of tobacco (i.e., nicotine) would be challenged. The warning shots were fired in 1988 when, then Surgeon General, C. Everett Koop testified before the Congress that *nicotine should be listed as an addictive drug and should be regulated by the FDA.*

In June of 1988, the tobacco industry lost its first court case involving liability in the death of a smoker after heavy, chronic cigarette use. Although the decision was subsequently reversed in 1990, it represents a significant application of tort law. The question of addiction liability was the core of a landmark *class action* case against the tobacco industry in federal court in New Orleans. (*Castano versus The American Tobacco Co.*) This case was settled as part of the general settlement.

Tobacco companies have always denied that nicotine is addictive. However, there may be evidence that tobacco firms knew as long ago as 30 years that the opposite was true and went to great lengths to control the levels of nicotine. In any event, an advisory panel to the FDA found nicotine to be addictive, comparing it to cocaine and heroin. Then FDA Commissioner Kessler indicated that the FDA would not back off from efforts to regulate tobacco (tobacco is not currently regulated by the FDA), labeling nicotine addiction a "pediatric disease" and that cigarettes are, in fact, nicotine delivery devices and thus under the purview of the FDA. The Centers for Disease Control estimate that 3000 American teenagers start to smoke each day. Tobacco firms' *intent* may be the key to federal control if the FDA is correct in alleging that the tobacco companies deliberately alter nicotine levels (e.g., the development of a high-nicotine tobacco plant) in order to achieve dependency.

It is the long-standing denial of addiction by the tobacco industry that may render them more susceptible to recent court challenges. Alcohol manufacturers, on the other hand, have long acknowledged alcohol's potential for addiction. Thus, they have shielded themselves from claims now confronting the tobacco industry, such as fraud and intentional concealment. The industry's denial that nicotine is addictive was becoming more and more scrutinized.

Some states began taking a more proactive position regarding smoking liability, independent of the government. In February of 1995, in a state court in Indianapolis, five of six jurors rejected four tobacco companies' defense in a product defect claim that a man's smoking was wholly voluntary. The case ended in a mistrial. As reported in the April 16, 1995 edition of the *New York Times*, the Massachusetts House may ban all products containing nicotine. However, cigarette makers scored two big victories in West Virginia and Florida. In the West Virginia case, the judge struck down eight of the ten counts in the attorney general's suit. In Florida, massive lobbying resulted in the repeal of a new law allowing the state to litigate against third parties responsible for Medicaid costs.

Despite those victories, there was evidence of possible erosion of the tobacco industry's position. In a December 8, 1995 decision by the *Labor Department*, regarding liability for secondhand smoke, a claimant's position was vindicated. In the first workers compensation case in the nation linking secondhand smoke to a cancer death, the Department of Veterans Affairs was ordered to pay the widower of a nurse $21,500 a year until his death. The decision was based on his wife's 18-year exposure to secondhand smoke at a veteran's hospital and expert testimony regarding causality. Although the workers compensation ruling is not admissible in court, it may impact cigarette smoking by rendering employers susceptible to future claims.

Most significantly, in December of 1995, Massachusetts became the fifth state to file a lawsuit against the tobacco industry (six major tobacco companies). The state was seeking more than $1 billion in damages to repay taxpayers for the money the state spent to fund medical care for poor people with tobacco-related maladies. The lawsuit alleged, "cigarette manufacturers and their trade associations have engaged in a conspiracy to mislead, deceive and confuse" the state and its citizens about "the overwhelming evidence that cigarette smoking causes fatal disease."

In August of 1996, Massachusetts passed a rigorous new cigarette disclosure law. If upheld, the bill will force tobacco companies to reveal additives in each brand, in descending order of weight, including ammonia-based compounds that critics say boost nicotine delivery and make cigarettes more potent. The tobacco industry responded by saying that "they wouldn't ask Coke, Pepsi or the Colonel to divulge their soft-drunk or chicken recipe, so why should we be deprived of trade-secret privileges?"

By March of 1996, the first real crack in the unified tobacco industry front became evident. Liggett group, the smallest of the nation's five major tobacco companies, and five states (Florida, Massachusetts, Mississippi, West Virginia, and Louisiana) *reached a settlement* of the lawsuits seeking to recover the public health care cost of treating illnesses linked to smoking; thus presaging the Master Settlement Agreement by two and a half years; see below. Simply getting a tobacco company to agree to pay plaintiffs anything is a watershed development in the 40-year history of tobacco litigation. Ligget *became the first cigarette company ever to settle smoking-related lawsuits.*

Liggett agreed to pay the five states $5 million over 10 years to defray the taxpayer costs of treating state Medicaid patients with smoking-related illnesses. If Liggett merges with RJR or another tobacco company, the settlement provides $160 million for all five states. The settlement also included annual payments of between 2 and 7% of Leggett's pretax profits for 24 years. At profit levels of the time, that amounts to approximately $250,000 per year for Liggett alone or $30 million annually if Liggett combines with RJR. The states estimated that together they spent in excess of $900 million on smoking-related health care costs. Significantly, Liggett also agreed to drop its opposition to the FDA proposal to regulate tobacco as a drug and to refrain from using various marketing and promotional gimmicks aimed at children.

The woes of the tobacco industry continued into the summer of 1996 when, on August 9, a Florida jury awarded a plaintiff and his wife $750,000 in their suit against Brown & Williamson Tobacco Corp. One document that was persuasive in the case was a 1963 memo from a former top counsel of the company. In that correspondence, the executive stated that "Nicotine is addictive. We are, then, in the business of selling nicotine, an addictive drug effective in the release of stress mechanisms."

One of the national health objectives for 2010 is to reduce the prevalence of cigarette smoking among adults. To assess progress toward this objective, the Centers for Disease Control and Prevention analyzed self-reported data from the 2002 National Health Interview Survey sample adult core questionnaire. This report summarizes the results of that analysis, which indicated that in 2002, approximately 22.5% of adults were current smokers. Although this prevalence was slightly lower than the 22.8% among adults in 2001 and 24.1% in 1998, the rate of decline has not been at a sufficient pace to achieve the 2010 objective.

SALES TO MINORS

It was also in August 1996 that a "final" rule on tobacco was published in the Federal Register. It identified the FDA as being in charge of regulating the sale and distribution of cigarettes and smokeless tobacco to children and adolescents. The action resulted from the agency's assertion of jurisdiction over tobacco products. This was based on an extensive FDA investigation of the tobacco industry, tobacco use, and its health consequences. The rule prohibits the sale of cigarettes and smokeless tobacco to those under 18 while leaving them on the market for adults.

Specifically, the rule made the sale of cigarettes and smokeless tobacco to children and adolescents, anyone younger than 18 years of age, a *federal violation*. In addition, the rule required manufacturers, distributors, and retailers to comply with certain conditions regarding the sale, distribution, and promotion of tobacco products. It prohibited all free samples and limits retail sales in most circumstances to face-to-face transactions. As a result, vending machines and self-service displays were prohibited, except in facilities where the retailer or operator ensures that no person younger than 18 is present or is permitted to enter at any time.

The rule limited advertising generally to a black-and-white, text only format to ensure that advertising was not used to create demand for these products among young people and thus undermine the restrictions on access. Billboards and other outdoor advertising were prohibited within 1000 ft of schools and public playgrounds. The sale and distribution of nontobacco items, such as hats and tee shirts that carry cigarette logos, such as Joe Camel, were prohibited, and sponsorship of sporting and other events was limited to the corporate name only.

The FDA's authority, in its opinion, to carry out its mission to protect public health derives *primarily* from the Federal Food, Drug, and Cosmetic Act of 1906. This statute provides the agency authority to regulate a wide variety of consumer products, including *drugs and devices*. FDA asserted that cigarettes were, in fact, combination products containing both an addictive drug (nicotine) and a delivery system (processed tobacco, ventilation system, and filters). As an historical aside, it is interesting to note that at the beginning of the twentieth century, an atropine-like drug (stramonium) was put in cigarettes to be delivered by smoking to asthmatics. The FDA determined that tobacco products are most appropriately regulated under the device provisions of the act and, thus, under its purview. The tobacco industry, of course, appealed. On August 14, 1998, the Fourth Circuit Court of Appeals ruled in the industry's favor stating that *Congress had never intended to give the FDA the regulatory to regulate tobacco* (2 to 1 decision) and overruled a lower court decision favoring the FDA.

As fate would have it, however, the tobacco industry had seen the writing on the wall and had been independently negotiating with a team of eight Attorneys General to reach a substantial settlement. On November 23, 1998, a *Master Settlement Agreement* (MSA) was signed with the Attorneys General of 46 states. The Attorneys General said, "This is litigation, not legislation. Congress should pass legislation to provide essential reforms—including full Food and Drug Administration authority over tobacco..."

The settlement, like the FDA proposal, has numerous provisions primarily aimed at protecting children. Under the settlement proposal, the tobacco industry would contribute $1.5 billion over the next 5 years for a national public education fund that would carry out a massive education and advertising campaign. It would also pay $250 million for a foundation dedicated to reducing teen smoking. Like the FDA proposal, the settlement would ban cartoon characters in tobacco advertising, prohibit the industry from targeting youth in ads and marketing, prohibit billboards and transit advertising, and ban the sale and distribution of apparel, backpacks, and other merchandise that bear brand name logos and become, in effect, walking billboards.

Under the settlement, tobacco companies would pay the states more than $9 billion a year, beginning in the year 2008. The industry will pay the states $12 billion in "up-front" money over 5 years. Total payments through the year 2025 would be approximately $206 billion. This does not include settlements already reached with four other states (Florida, Mississippi, Minnesota, and Texas) totaling over $40 billion in the same period. To ensure the industry lives up to the agreement, the settlement would be enforceable through consent decrees that will be entered in each state court. In addition, the industry will provide $50 million for an enforcement fund, which states could use to pursue violations of the settlement. To cover the cost of this settlement manufacturers raised prices; between January 1998 and January 2000, the average U.S. wholesale price of cigarettes climbed from $1.31 per pack to $2.35, a 79% increase in 2 years.

The effect of the settlement directives may already have been manifested in 1999. In 1999, the five "leading" cigarette companies reported that they sold 47.2 billion fewer cigarettes than in 1998. This encouraging news suggests that perhaps the first substantive steps have been taken to arrest the single greatest preventable disease factor in the United States. The 400,000 lives claimed each year in the United States matches the number of Americans who died in World War II. Comparable figures in the United Kingdom are 120,000 fatalities per year. Yet, incredibly, a 2001 survey in the United Kingdom reveals that 54% of smokers and 61% of nonsmokers believe that smoking cigarettes is not dangerous to their health.

The Master Settlement Agreement assumed that a large portion of the money would pay for tobacco-use prevention programs. However, a 2001 report by the National Conference of State Legislatures found that the 46 states that joined in the settlement, plus the four that reached separate deals with the tobacco companies, had used only 5% of the money for smoking prevention and cessation programs. (The General Accounting Office has found similar data.) Many states appear to be using the money for other needs, such as public schools, elderly care, and balancing their budgets.

In conclusion, lest we be too harsh on the tobacco industry, we should be cognizant of a study on the financial cost of smoking carried out by the research company Arthur D. Little International commissioned by Philip Morris. Researchers looked at the Czech Republic and concluded that the *government **saved** $30 million in 1999 because it did not have to support, house and care for smokers who **died prematurely** from tobacco-related illness.* The study also indicated that there were "indirect positive effects" of early deaths such as savings on health care, pensions, welfare, and housing for the elderly. The government's net gain from the tobacco industry was calculated to be $146 million. This reasoning was also actually argued at pretrial hearings in the Mississippi case in 1997. Citing a legal text on equity jurisprudence, the defendants wrote

A court of equity is a court of **conscience** (emphasis mine); it seeks to do justice and equity between all parties; it seeks to strike a balance of convenience as between all litigants; and it looks to the whole situation…. Here, the Court's duty to look at the 'whole situation' requires the Court to look at the full economic impact of the sale of cigarettes on the State.

The plaintiff's countered by characterizing the defendant's assertion as "ghoulish." Specifically, they wrote "Seeking a credit for a purported economic benefit from early death is akin to robbing the graves of Mississippi smokers who died from tobacco-related illness. No court of law or equity should entertain such a defense or counterclaim. It is offensive to human decency, an affront to justice, uncharacteristic of civilized society, and unquestionably contrary to public policy."

SELECTED BIBLIOGRAPHY

Baskys, A. and Remington, G. (Eds.) (1996) *Brain Mechanisms and Psychotropic Drugs*, Boca Raton, FL: CRC Press.

Bayer, R. and Oppenheimer, G. (Eds.) (1993) *Drug Policy: Illicit Drugs in a Free Society*, New York: Cambridge University Press.

Goldberg, R. (1994) *Drugs Across the Spectrum*, Minneapolis, MN: West Publishing Co.

Goldstein, A. (1994) *Addiction from Biology to Drug Policy*, New York: W.H. Freeman and Co.

Hardman, J.G., Limbird, L.L., and Gilman, A.G. (Eds.) (2001) *Goodman and Gillman's: The Pharmacological Basis of Therapeutics*, 10th ed., New York: McGraw-Hill.

Karch, S. (1993) *The Pathology of Drug Abuse*, Boca Raton, FL: CRC Press.

Lidow, M.S., (Eds.) (2000) *Neurotransmitter Receptors in Actions of Antipsychotic Medications*, Boca Raton, FL: CRC Press.

Moody, E. and Skolnich, P. (Eds.) (2001) *Molecular Basis of Anesthesia*, Boca Raton, FL: CRC Press.

Musto, D.F. (1987) *The American Disease*, 2nd ed., New York: Oxford University Press.

Niesink, R.J.M., Jaspers, R.M.A., Kornet, L.M.W., and van Ree, J.M. (Eds.) (1999), *Drugs of Abuse and Addiction: Neurobehavioral Toxicology*, Boca Raton, FL: CRC Press.

Orey, M. (1999) *Assuming the Risk: The Maverisks, the Lawyers, and the Whistle-Blowers Who Beat Big Tobacco*, Boston: Little, Brown and Co.

Pinger, R.R., Payne, W.A., Hahn, D.B. and Hahn, E.J. (1995) *Drugs: Issues for Today*, 2nd ed., St. Louis, MO: Mosby Publishing Co.

Ray, O. and Ksir, C. (1993) *Drugs, Society, and Human Behavior*, 6th ed., St. Louis, MO: Mosby Publishing Co.

Redda, K., Walker, C., and Barnett, G. (1989) *Cocaine, Marijuana, Designer Drugs: Chemistry, Pharmacology, and Behavior*, Boca Raton, FL: CRC Press.

Snyder, S. (1996) *Drugs and the Brain*, New York: Scientific American Library.

Snyder, S.H. and Pasternak, G.W. (2003) Historical review: Opioid receptors, *Trends in Pharmacol. Sci.*, 24: 198–206.

Weil, A. and Rosen, W. (1993) *From Chocolate to Morphine*, Boston, MA: Houghton Miflen Co.

Weisheit, R.A. (1992) *Domestic Marijuana: A Neglected Industry*, New York: Greenwood Press.

Zernig, G., Saria, A., Kurz, M., and O'Malley, S.S. (Eds.) (2000) *Handbook of Alcoholism*, Boca Raton, FL: CRC Press.

QUESTIONS

1. Drug companies have been required to demonstrate both safety and efficacy of their compounds since which year?
   a. 1906
   b. 1926
   c. 1933
   d. 1962
   e. 1970

2. The FDA was created by legislation in which year?
   a. 1906
   b. 1910

    c. 1947
    d. 1958
    e. 1976

3. The Opium Exclusion Act was enacted in which year?
    a. 1906
    b. 1909
    c. 1919
    d. 1933
    e. 1940

4. Isolation of pure cocaine occurred in which year?
    a. 1809
    b. 1812
    c. 1859
    d. 1861
    e. 1906

5. The Harrison Narcotics Act was passed in which year?
    a. 1906
    b. 1911
    c. 1914
    d. 1915
    e. 1919

6. Prohibition (The Volstead Act) was ratified in which year?
    a. 1906
    b. 1911
    c. 1914
    d. 1915
    e. 1919

7. The Federal Marijuana Tax Act came into effect in which year?
    a. 1906
    b. 1911
    c. 1919
    d. 1937
    e. 1938

8. Which of the following years was probably the "watershed" in terms of America's relaxed view toward illicit drug use?
    a. 1933
    b. 1952
    c. 1962
    d. 1978
    e. 1980

9. The Master Settlement Agreement between the tobacco industry and 46 states was signed in which year?
    a. 1989
    b. 1991
    c. 1993
    d. 1996
    e. 1998

Appendix II: Molecular Structure of Nucleic Acids

Here is James Watson and Francis Crick's historic paper on the structure of DNA, which ushered in a new era with the celebrated understatement near the end. It is of such a seminal nature that students interested in biology should be obliged to make its acquaintance.

Originally published in Nature, 171: 737, 1953.

We wish to suggest a structure for the salt of deoxyribose nucleic acid (DNA). This structure has novel features that are of considerable biological interest.

A structure for nucleic acid has already been proposed by Pauling and Corey.[1] They kindly made their manuscript available to us in advance of publication. Their model consists of three intertwined chains, with the phosphates near the fiber (sic) axis, and the bases on the outside. In our opinion, this structure is unsatisfactory for two reasons: (1) We believe that the material that gives the x-ray diagrams is the salt, not the free acid. Without the acidic hydrogen atoms it is not clear what forces would hold the structure together, especially as the negatively charged phosphates near the axis will repel each other and (2) Some of the van der Waals distances appear to be too small.

Another three-chain structure has also been suggested by Fraser (in the press). In this model, the phosphates are on the outside and the bases on the inside, linked together by hydrogen bonds. This structure as described is rather ill-defined, and for this reason we shall not comment on it.

We wish to put forward a radically different structure for the salt of DNA. This structure has two helical chains each coiled round the same axis (author note: diagram of an α-helix was displayed at this point in the text). We have made the usual chemical assumptions, namely, that each chain consists of phosphate diester groups joining β-D-deoxyribofuranose residues with 3', 5' linkages. The two chains (but not their bases) are related by a dyad perpendicular to the fiber axis. Both chains follow right-handed helices, but owing to the dyad the sequences of the atoms in the two chains run in opposite directions. Each chain loosely resembles Furberg's model No.1, that is, the bases are on the inside of the helix and the phosphates on the outside. The configuration of the sugar and the atoms near it is close to Furberg's "standard configuration," the sugar being roughly perpendicular to the attached base.[2] There is a residue on each chain every 34 Å in the z-direction. We have assumed an angle of 36° between adjacent residues in the same chain so that the structure repeats after 10 residues on each chain, that is, after 34 Å. The distance of a phosphorus atom from the fiber axis is 10 Å; as the phosphates are on the outside, cations have easy access to them.

The structure is an open one, and its water content is rather high. At lower water contents, we would expect the bases to tilt so that the structure could become more compact.

The novel feature of the structure is the manner in which the two chains are held together by the purine and pyrimidine bases. The planes of the bases are perpendicular to the fiber axis. They are joined together in pairs, a single base from one chain being hydrogen-bonded to a single base from the other chain, so that the two lie side by side with identical z-coordinates. One of the pair must be a purine and the other a pyrimidine for bonding to occur. The hydrogen bonds are made as follows: purine position 1 to pyrimidine position 1; purine position 6 to pyrimidine position 6.

If it is assumed that the bases only occur in the structure in the most plausible tautomeric forms (i.e., with the keto rather than the enol confifigurations), it is found that only specific pairs of bases can bond together. These pairs are as follows: adenine (purine) with thymine (pyrimidine), and guanine (purine) with cytosine (pyrimidine).

In other words, if an adenine forms one member of a pair, on either chain, then on these assumptions the other member must be thymine; similarly for guanine and cytosine. The sequence of bases on a single chain does not appear to be restricted in any way. However, if only specific pairs of bases can be formed, it follows that if the sequence of bases on one chain is given, then the sequence on the other side is automatically determined.

It has been found experimentally [3,4] that the ratio of the amounts of adenine to thymine and the ratio of guanine to cytosine are always very close to unity for DNA.

It is probably impossible to build this structure with a ribose sugar in place of the deoxyribose, as the extra oxygen atom would make too close a van der Waals contact.

The previously published x-ray data [5,6] on DNA are insufficient for a rigorous test of our structure. So far as we can tell, it is roughly compatible with the experimental data, but it must be regarded as unproved until it has been checked against more exact results. Some of these are given in the following communications. We were not aware of the details of the results presented there when we devised our structure, which rests mainly though not entirely on published experimental data and stereochemical arguments.

It has not escaped our notice that the specific pairing we have postulated immediately suggests a possible copying mechanism for the genetic material. (Italics mine.)

Full details of the structure, including the conditions assumed in building it, together with a set of coordinates for the atoms, will be published elsewhere.

We are much indebted to Dr. Jerry Donohue for constant advice and criticism, especially on interatomic distances. We have also been stimulated by a knowledge of the general nature of the unpublished experimental results and ideas of Dr. M.H.F. Wilkins and Dr. R.E. Franklin and their coworkers at King's College, London. One of us (J.D.W.) has been aided by a fellowship from the National Foundation for Infantile Paralysis.

J.D. Watson
F.H.C. Crick
Medical Unit Research Council for the
Study of the Molecular Structure of
Biological Systems,
Cavendish Laboratory, Cambridge

SELECTED BIBLIOGRAPHY

1. Pauling, L., and Corey, R.B. (1953) Structure of the Nucleic Acids, *Nature*, 171: 346 (1953), A Proposed Structure for the Nucleic Acids, *Proc. U.S. Nat. Acad. Sci.*, 39: 84.
2. Furberg, S. (1952) Genetical implications of the Structure of Deoxyribonucleic Acid, *Acta Chem. Scand.*, 6: 634.
3. Chargaff, E. (1952) for references see Zamenhof, S., Brawerman, G., and Chargaff, E., Separation of Calf Thymus Deoxyribonucleic Acid into Fractions of Different Composition, *Biochim. et Biophys. Acta*, 9: 402.
4. Wyatt, G.R. (1952) Molecular Structure of Nucleic Acids: A Structure for Deoxyribose Nucleic Acid, *J. Gen. Physiol.*, 36: 201.
5. Astbury, W.T. (1952) Molecular Structure of Nucleic Acids: A Structure for Deoxyribose Nucleic Acid, *Symp. Soc. Exp. Biol.* 1, Nucleic Acid, 66 (Camb. Univ. Press, 1947).
6. Wilkins, M.H.F., and Randall, J.T. (1953) Crystallinity in Sperm Heads: Molecular Structure of Nucleoprotein *in vivo*, *Biochim. et Biophys. Acta*, 10: 192.

Appendix III: Glossary

"When I use a word, it means just what I chose it to mean – neither more nor less."

Humpty Dumpty

Abbreviated New Drug Application, or ANDA: A simplified submission permitted for a duplicate of an already approved drug. ANDAs are for products with the same or very closely related active ingredients, dosage form, strength, administration route, use, and labeling as a product that has already been shown to be safe and effective. An ANDA includes all the information on chemistry and manufacturing controls found in an NDA, but does not have to include data from studies in animals and humans. It must, however, contain evidence that the duplicate drug is bioequivalent to the previously approved drug.

Accelerated approval: A highly specialized mechanism intended to speed approval of drugs promising significant benefit over existing therapy for serious or life-threatening illnesses. It incorporates elements aimed at making sure that rapid review and approval is balanced by safeguards to protect both the public health and the integrity of the regulatory process. This mechanism may be used when approval can be reliably based on evidence of a drug's effect on a "surrogate endpoint" (see "Surrogate Endpoint), or when the FDA determines an effective drug can be used safely only under restricted distribution or use. Usually, such a surrogate can be assessed much sooner than such an endpoint as survival. In accelerated approval, FDA approves the drug on condition that the sponsor studies the actual clinical benefit of the drug.

Acetylcholine: A chemical neurotransmitter released by nerve endings. Its effects include cardiac inhibition, increase in blood vessel diameter, and constricted pupils.

Acidosis/alkalosis: The condition when the pH of the blood falls/rises outside the normal acceptable limits.

Action letter: An official communication from the FDA to an NDA sponsor that informs of a decision by the agency. An approval letter allows commercial marketing of the product. An approval letter lists minor issues to be resolved before approval can be given. A not approvable letter describes important deficiencies that preclude approval unless corrected.

Active transport: Movement of materials across cell membranes, which requires direct expenditure of metabolic energy.

Acute: Short-term exposure or response.

Acute toxicity: The short-term effects of onetime exposure to a chemical substance.

Additive: When the therapeutic or toxic effect of several xenobiotics is equal to the sum of the individual components.

Adduct: Covalent binding of an exogenous chemical to a cellular macromolecule.

Adolescence: The period from puberty to maturity.

Adrenergic: Nerves responding to the neurotransmitter norepinephrine.

Adverse effect: A biochemical change, functional impairment, or pathological lesion that either singly or in combination deleteriously affects the performance of the whole organism, or reduces an organism's ability to respond to an additional environmental challenge.

Advisory committee: A panel of outside experts convened periodically to advise the FDA on safety and efficacy issues about drugs and other FDA-related products. FDA is not bound to make committee recommendations, but usually does.

Aerosol: A colloidal system with a gas as the dispersion medium (such as fog or mist of droplets or particles).

Agonist: A drug that both binds to receptors and has intrinsic activity.

Albumin: Protein component of blood, abnormal component of urine.

Alcohol: See ethanol.

Allergen: An antigenic substance capable of eliciting an allergic response.

Allergic reaction: A reaction to a foreign agent giving rise to a hypersensitive state, mediated via an immunological mechanism and resulting in a particular series of responses.

Allosteric modulator: A compound without inherent agonist or antagonist activity, but with the ability to modulate positively or negatively their effect on cells (e.g., alteration of receptor protein conformation resulting in alteration of function—noncompetitive receptor inhibition).

Amendment to an NDA: A submission to change or add information to an NDA or supplement not yet approved.

Amino acid: A component of every protein, in which up to 20 different amino acids are strung together into polymer chains.

Amphiphatic: A molecule possessing both polar and non-polar moieties.

Analgesic: Pain-relieving substance.

Anaphylactic reaction: A type I immunological response involving histamine and other mediator release.

Androgen: Any substance that produces masculinization, such as testosterone.

Anemia: Reduction of red blood cells or hemoglobin.

Aneurysm: Ballooning of a blood vessel (e.g., of the aorta), formed by weakness in the wall of a blood vessel.

Angina pectoris: Attack of chest pain caused by diminished blood supply to the heart muscle.

Anoxia: Absence of oxygen in the tissues.

Antagonism: When the therapeutic effect of a drug is reduced in either a competitive or noncompetitive manner.

Antagonist: A drug that impedes the action of another drug (may be competitive or noncompetitive).

Anterior: Situated in the front part of the organ or body.

Antibiotics: These are anti-infection drugs that inhibit the growth of or destroy microorganisms and are used extensively in treating bacteria-mediated disease.

Antibody: A protein produced by B-lymphocytes in response to, and specific for, a foreign substance or antigen.

Anticholinergic: An action by substances that block the parasympathetic system.

Anticoagulant: A substance that inhibits the normal process of blood clotting. An agent that prevents coagulation of blood (e.g., heparin or coumarin).

Anticonvulsant: A drug that counteracts or prevents convulsions caused by brain diseases, electric shock, and certain chemicals.

Antidote: A substance that specifically blocks or reduces the toxic action of a drug or poison.

Antihistamine: These drugs block the effects of histamine usually by competitive antagonism at the site. They can relieve symptoms such as sneezing, watery eyes, runny nose, and itching of the nose and throat.

Antihypertensive: A drug used for lowering blood pressure.

Antimetabolite: A chemical of a structure related to but not identical with normal metabolite. If it counteracts the effects of the metabolite, it may be useful as drug.

Antigen: A protein or other macromolecule that is recognized as foreign by the immune system in an animal.

Antitussive: A drug that prevents coughing.

Apoptosis: Programmed cell death.

Area under the curve (AUC):   For example, a measure of how much drug reaches the blood stream in a set period of time, usually 24 h. AUC is calculated by plotting drug blood concentration at various times during a 24-h or longer period and then measuring the area under the curve.

Arrhythmia: Irregularities in heart rate.

Arteriosclerosis: Common disease of old age; thickening of the artery walls and narrowing of arteries resulting in a variety of dysfunctions of different organs, especially the brain and heart.

Astrocyte: Cells found in the central nervous system.

Ataxia: Inability to coordinate balance.

Atherosclerosis: Common form of arteriosclerosis with deposits of yellow plaques containing cholesterol, lipid material within the intima and inner media of arteries.

Atopic: Pertaining to genetic predisposition toward developing immediate hypersensitivity reactions to antigenic substances.

Atrial fibrillation: Rapid, irregular contractions of the atrial chambers of the heart.

Atrophy: Reduction in size of a structure or organ resulting from lack of nourishment or functional activity, death and reabsorption of cells, diminished cellular proliferation, and ischemia or hormone changes.

Attention deficit hyperactivity disorder (ADHD):   A common disorder of unknown etiology that occurs primarily in children, characterized by marked restlessness and inability to concentrate.

AUC: Area under the curve when the plasma (blood) concentration of a substance is plotted against time.

Autoimmune disease: Immune response in which antibodies are directed against the organism itself.

Autosomal: Pertaining to the ordinary paired chromosomes that can be distinguished from the sex chromosomes.

Axon: The process of a neuron that conducts impulses traveling away from the cell body.

Axoplasm: Cytoplasm of an axon.

Bactericidal: A drug that kills bacteria.

Bacteriostatic: A drug that slows or prevents the multiplication of bacteria.

β-receptor: An autonomic receptor of which there are three types.

Basal ganglia: Deep areas of the brain regulating motility and vegetative functions.

Base pair: Unit of length for DNA work. Usually expressed as kb (Kilobase pairs). In the double-stranded molecule Guanosine pairs with cytidine and adenosine with thymidine (or uridine in RNA).

Bioaccumulation: The accumulation of a substance in a biological organism, usually due to its lipophilicity.

Bioactivation: Metabolism of a xenobiotic to a chemically more reactive metabolite.

Bioavailability: A measure of the degree to which a dose of a substance becomes physiologically available to body tissues based on blood levels. The standard of comparison is the intravenous dose.

Bioequivalence: Scientific basis on which generic and brand-name drugs are compared. To be considered bioequivalent, the bioavailability of two products must not differ significantly when the two products are given in studies at the same dosage under similar conditions. Some drugs, however, are intended to have a different absorption rate. FDA may consider a product bioequivalent to a second product with a different rate of absorption if the difference is noted in the labeling and does not affect the drug's safety or effectiveness or change the drug's effects in any medically significant way.

Biotransformation: An enzymatic chemical alteration of a substance within the body that generally leads to a more excretable metabolite, sometimes producing a more toxic form of the xenobiotic.

Blood–brain barrier: The combination of tight endothelial junctions in cerebral capillaries together with their covering of astrocytes.

Blood pressure, diastolic: Measurement of blood pressure at dilation of the heart.

Blood pressure, systolic: Measurement of blood pressure at contraction of the heart.

Bolus: A single dose.

Bradycardia: Slowing of the heart rate usually below 60 beats per minute.

Bronchiole: Smaller diameter, more distal branches of the bronchiole tree.

Bronchoconstriction: Constriction of the smooth muscle in airways in the lungs due to exposure to irritant chemicals or to an immunological reaction involving release of inflammatory mediators.

Bruxism: Involuntary grinding of the teeth.

Buccal: Pertaining to the cheek.

Carcinogen/carcinogenic: A substance/property of a substance that causes cancer when administered to an organism.

Cardiac arrythmias: Abnormal beating rhythms in the heart.

Cardiac output: The volume of blood pumped by the heart in one cycle.

Cardiomyopathy: Pathological changes to heart tissue.

Catabolized: Metabolically broken down.

Cathartic: A chemical that stimulates intestinal peristalsis and relieves constipation.

cDNA: A double-stranded copy of an RNA molecule that contains only the coding and flanking regions of the gene.

Cell culture: Growth of living cells or microorganisms in a controlled, artificial environment.

Centrilobular: The region of the liver lobule surrounding the central vein.

Cerebral vascular accident (CVA):   Destruction of brain tissue caused by a blood clot or gradual occlusion of the artery supplying blood.

Chelation: Binding of an inorganic ion (e.g., heavy metal) by an organic molecule.

Chemical proteomics: Is devoted to the parallel characterization of ligand interactions with all the proteins encoded by a genome.

Child: Covers the age range from birth to puberty.

Chiral: The presence of asymmetry in a molecule giving rise to isomers.

Cholestasis: Cessation of bile flow.

Cholinergic stimulation: Stimulation of the nerve fibers utilizing acetylcholine as the neurotransmitter.

Chromosome: A cellular structure comprised of a long, folded DNA molecule and protein.

Chronic: Long-term exposure to a xenobiotic.

Cirrhosis: Liver disease characterized by loss of the normal microscopic lobular structure with fibrosis (collagen deposition).Usually the result of chronic exposure to a noxious agent such as ethanol.

Clearance: The volume of plasma cleared of a drug in unit time.

Clinical trials: Divided into three phases involving pharmacokinetc studies of the drug as well as studies designed to assess efficacy. Such studies conducted in this country must be under an approved IND.

Cloning: The insertion of foreign DNA into host plasmids or genomes.

CNS: Central nervous system.

Coating, enteric: Encapsulating a biologically active chemical in a layer such as wax or biodegradable plastic that delays and regulates the rate of release of a drug into tissues.

Cocaine: An alkaloid obtained from the dried leaves of the coca shrub. It is a schedule I regulated drug with high addiction potential.

Codon: A group of three base pairs that code for a specific amino acid.

Cognitive: Brain functions related to sense perception or understanding.

Collagen: A fibrous protein.

Complement: A series of proteins found in extracellular fluids and involved in certain immunological reactions.

Cortex, cerebral: The outer layer (gray matter) of the brain.

Cremasteric reflex: Normal reflex elicited by stroking the skin of the upper leg near the scrotum, resulting in upward movement of the scrotum; absence may indicate lesions of the lower spine.

Cyanosis: The pathological condition where there is an excessive concentration of reduced hemoglobin in the blood.

Cytochrome P-448 and P-450: Isozymes that are important in the detoxification by biotransformation of many xenobiotics. These enzymes are found primarily in the liver and, to a lesser extent, in the lungs and other tissues.

Cytosol: The internal part of the cell excluding the organelles.

Dalton: Unit of molecular weight (e.g., hydrogen has a molecular weight of 1).

Database: A computerized collection of information

Deacetylation: Removal of an acetyl group.

Dealkylation: Removal of an alkyl group.

Deaminate: Removal of an amine group.

Dechlorination: Removal of a chlorine group.

Deethylation: Removal of an ethyl group.

Dehalogenation: Removal of a halogen group.

Delaney Amendment: Amendment to the Food, Drug, and Cosmetic Act of the Food and Drug Administration of the United States. The amendment states that food additives that cause cancer in humans or animals at any level shall not be considered safe and are, therefore, prohibited.

Demethylation: Removal of a methyl group.

Dendrites: Neuronal projections that usually convey impulses to the cell body.

Denervated: A tissue deprived of its nerve supply.

Dermatitis: Inflammation of the skin.

Desensitization: Loss of functional response. Can be short term (seconds or minutes) or long term (hours).

Detoxification: Reduction of a chemical's toxic properties by means of biotransformation processes, to form a more readily excreted, or a less toxic chemical than the parent compound.

Developmental toxicity: Adverse effects on the developing organism. Adverse developmental effects may be detected at any point in the life span of the organism. Major manifestations of developmental toxicity include death of the developing embryo, induction of structural abnormalities (teratogenicity), altered growth, and functional deficiency.

Diabetes insipidus: Disease due to lack of antidiuretic hormone.

Diabetes mellitus: Disease with enhanced blood glucose levels due to lack of insulin.

Dimer: Subunit of a macromolecule (e.g., certain proteins exist as dimers).

Distal: Remote from the point of reference.

Diuretic: A drug that increases the flow of urine. Some diuretics also lower blood pressure.

DNA: Deoxyribonucleic acid, the substance within cells that carries the "recipe" for the organism and is inherited from parents. A normally double-stranded molecule made up of Deoxyadenosine, Deoxycytidine, Deoxyguanosine, and Deoxythymidine, which follows Watson–Crick complementary rules.

Dopaminergic: Receptors responsive to dopamine.

Dorsal: Pertaining to the back.

Dose–response relationship: The relationship between (1) the dose, actually based on "administered dose" (i.e., exposure) rather than actual absorbed dose and (2) the extent of therapeutic or toxic effect produced by the xenobiotic.

Downregulation: Loss of total receptor number due to agonist-induced endocytosis and subsequent degradation. Can become significant after an hour or more of agonist treatment.

Drug insert: The paper in a drug package that contains a description of the drug, its main effects, toxicity, dosage form, and names.

Drug product: The finished dosage form (tablet, capsule, etc.) that contains a drug substance— generally, but not necessarily, in association with other active or inactive ingredients.

Drug substance: The active ingredient intended to diagnose, treat, cure, or prevent disease or affect the structure or function of the body, excluding other inactive substances used in the drug product.

Drugs, chiral: Drugs with unsymmetrical molecular structure. Chiral drugs exist as enantiomers.

Duodenum: First portion of the intestine between the pylorus and jejunum.

Dyspepsia: Gastrointestinal symptoms (heartburn) without demonstrable organic pathology.

EC$_{50}$ (effective concentration 50):   The concentration of agonist causing 50% of the maximal response, determined from an agonist dose–response curve.

ED$_{50}$:   The dose of a drug that is pharmacologically effective for 50% of the population exposed to the drug or a 50% response in a biological system that is exposed to the drug.

Edema: Abnormal accumulation of fluid in cells, tissues, or body cavities resulting in swelling.

Effectiveness: The desired measure of a drug's influence on a disease condition. Effectiveness must be proven by substantial evidence consisting of adequate and well-controlled investigations, including human studies by qualified experts, that prove the drug will have the effect claimed in its labeling.

Elderly: The *Census Bureau* defines "elderly" as 65+ years of age.

Electrophile: A chemical that is attracted to react with an electron-rich center in another molecule.

Elimination half-life: The time it takes the body to eliminate or breakdown half the dose of a xenobiotic.

Elixir: A solution, often an alcoholic tincture, of drugs.

Embolism: Sudden blocking of an artery with a blood clot or foreign material.

Embryo: In mammals, the stage in the developing organism at which organs and organ systems are developing. For humans, this involves the stage of development between the second through the eighth weeks of conception.

Emetic: To induce vomiting.

Endocytosis: Uptake or removal of a substance from a cell by a process of invagination of membrane and formation of a vesicle. Movement of receptor or ligand from the cell surface to an internal compartment. Usually occurs within minutes of agonist treatment. In the case of receptors there is a basal rate of endocytosis (usually slow, occurs without agonist ligand and is therefore constitutive) and an agonist-stimulating rate.

Endogenous: Part of the internal environment of a living organism.

Endoplasmic reticulum (ER):   May be divided into rough ER with attendant ribosomes involved with protein synthesis and smooth ER where cytochrome P-450 and many other drug metabolizing enzymes are located.

Endothelium: The layer of endothelial cells lining the interior of blood vessels.

Endpoint: Refers to the point in an animal experiment when no more information can be obtained and the experiment is stopped.

Enteral: Refers to the gut.

Enterohepatic circulation: The recycling of a drug from the blood into the liver, then into the bile and gastrointestinal tract. This is followed by reuptake into the bloodstream from the gastrointestinal tract possibly after chemical or enzymatic breakdown.

Eosinophile: A type of white blood cell.

Epidemiology: The study of diseases in populations.

Epidural: Outside or directly above the dura mater covering the brain and spinal cord.

Epigenetic: Nongenetically mediated.

Epinephrine: Adrenaline.

Ethanol (alcohol):   The world's most popular drug, legally used in most countries. Ethanol is produced through the fermentation of fruits, vegetables, and grains.

Etiology: The study of the cause and/or origin of a disease.

Euphoria: A feeling of well-being. It can be induced by certain drugs.

Excretion: Elimination of chemicals from the body. Chemicals may be excreted through feces, urine, exhaled breath, and so forth.

Exocytosis: Cellular discharge of material; opposite of endocytosis.

Expression: Transcription and translation of a gene to protein.

Extrapolation: An estimate of response or quantity at a point outside the range of the experimental data. Also refers to the estimate of a measured response in a different species or by a different route than that used in the experimental study of interest (i.e., species-to-species, route-to-route, acute-to-chronic, etc.).

Extrapyramidal symptoms: Facial rigidity, tremors, and drooling.

Extrasystole: Premature heart contraction.

Feedback inhibition: Mechanism that maintains constant secretion of a product by exerting inhibitory control.

Fenestrations: Perforations.

Fetus: The postembryonic stage of the developing young. In humans, from the end of the second month of pregnancy up to birth.

Fibrillation, cardiac: Heart flutter and irregular beats.

Fibroblast: Connective tissue cell capable of producing collagen.

Fibrosis: The formation of fibrous tissue that may be a response of tissue to injury resulting in increased deposition of collagen fibers.

Fick's Law: At constant temperature the rate of diffusion of a substance across a cell membrane is proportional to the concentration gradient and the surface area.

First-order process: The rate of the process is proportional to the present concentration of the substance.

First-pass metabolism: Metabolism of a drug or other xenobiotic during the absorption process. Typically occurs in the liver or gastrointestinal tract after oral dosing.

Forced diuresis: Induced increased urine formation.

Free radical: An atom or molecule that has an unpaired electron. They may be uncharged or charged depending on the number of electrons. Free radicals are usually chemically very reactive.

Ganglion: A group of nerve cell bodies located in the peripheral nervous system.

Gastric lavage: Washing or rinsing the stomach.

Gene: The simplest complete functional unit in a DNA molecule. A linear sequence of nucleotides in DNA, which is needed to synthesize a single protein and/or regulate cell function. A mutation in one or more of the nucleotides in a gene may lead to abnormalities in the structure of the gene product or in the amount of gene product synthesized. The gene is made up of coding regions (Exons) and noncoding regions (Introns).

Genetic code: The information contained in DNA molecules that scientists describe on the basis of a four-letter alphabet (A, C, G, and T).

Genetic engineering: The process of transferring DNA from one organism into another, which results in a genetic modification; the production of a transgenic organism.

Genomics: Complete set of hereditary factors found on chromosomes, all the genes of one organism, the study of genes and their function.

Genotoxic: Toxic to the genetic material of an organism.

Glial cells: Support cells located adjacent to neurons in the central nervous system; may be a component of the blood–brain barrier.

Glomerulonephritis: Inflammation of the capillary loops in the glomerulus.

Glomerulus: A functional unit of the mammalian kidney consisting of a small bunch of capillaries projecting into a capsule (Bowmans capsule) that serves to collect the filtrate from the blood of those capillaries and direct it into the kidney tubule.

Glucuronidation: Addition of glucuronic acid to form a more water-soluble conjugate.

Glycosuria: The presence of glucose in the urine.

Good laboratory practice (GLP): A system of protocols (standard operating procedures) recommended to be followed so as to avoid the production of unreliable and erroneous data. Accurate record keeping and careful forethought in the design of the study are important aspects of GLP.

Granuloma: Aggregation of Norman and abnormal white blood cells and epithelial cells in tissues forming nodes.

Gray baby syndrome: Cyanosis of the newborn due to inadequate capacity for glucuronidation of chloramphenicol.

GSH: Reduced glutathione (the tripeptide glutamyl-cysteinyl-glycine). Found in most tissues, particularly the liver; plays a major role in detoxification of electrophiles and cellular protection against oxidative damage.

GSSG: Oxidized glutathione.

Half-life: The time taken for the concentration of a xenobiotic in a body fluid to decrease by half.

Hapten: A molecule (e.g., a drug metabolite) that becomes attached to an endogenous protein or other tissue macromolecule and so renders it antigenic.

Hashish: Cannabis preparation more concentrated than marijuana. It comes from the resinous secretions of the marijuana plant's flowering tops.

Hemi-paresis: Paralysis of one-half of the body.

Hemodialysis: The process by which a drug is removed from the blood of a poisoned patient by allowing it to diffuse across a semipermeable membrane, while the blood is pumped through a dialysis machine.

Hemoglobin: Pigment in red blood cells that transports oxygen.

Hemolysis: Destruction of erythrocytes with the release of hemoglobin.

Hemolytic anemia: The pathological condition where red blood cells undergo uncontrolled destruction.

Hemoperfusion: The process by which a drug is removed from the blood of a poisoned patient by allowing it to be absorbed by activated charcoal or a resin, while the blood is pumped through a special machine.

Henderson-Hasselbach equation: $pH = pKa + \log A/HA$.

Heparin: Endogenous compound that prevents blood clotting.

Hepatocellular: Relating to hepatocytes.

Hepatomegally: Increase in liver size.

Heroin: Acetylated morphine.

Hill slope: The slope of the dose–response curve at the EC_{50} point.

Histamine: A mediator of inflammatory reactions in the body, which may be part of an allergic reaction. Present in preformed granules in mast cells and basophils.

Homeostasis: Maintenance of normal, internal stability in an organism by coordinated responses of the organ systems, particularly the endocrine.

Homogenate: The mixture resulting from the homogenization of tissue.

Hormone: A chemical (usually peptide, amino acid derivative, or steroid) produced by an endocrine gland that effects the function of target cells.

Hydrophobic/hydrophilic: A substance that repels/attracts water.

Hyper: Prefix indicating an increase.

Hyperkinesis: Hyperactivity.

Hyperplasia: An abnormal increase in the number of cells in a tissue.

Hypnotic: Generic term for a drug producing or facilitating sleep.

Hypo: Prefix indicating a decrease.

Hypoglycemia: The physiological state where there is a low blood glucose concentration.

Hypothalamus: The region of the brain lying immediately above the pituitary gland and responsible for coordinating and controlling the autonomic nervous system.

Hypoxia: The physiological state where there is a low oxygen concentration.

IC_{50} (inhibitory concentration 50): The concentration of antagonist causing 50% of the maximal inhibition; determined from an antagonist dose–response curve.

Icterus: Jaundice.

Idiopathic: Of unknown origin or cause.

Idiosyncrasy: In pharmacology, this is an adverse reaction to a drug that occurs in small numbers of individuals in a distinct frequency distribution as a result of a genetic abnormality.

Immune complex: A complex of antibody(ies) and antigen(s) that may lead to pathological consequences such as inflammation or blockage of a vessel (i.e., a type III reaction).

Immunoglobin (Ig):   One of five classes of antibody protein involved in immune responses (i.e., IgA, IgD, IgE, IgG, and IgM).

Infant: A more formal term for a baby, the youngest category of child. A child is no longer considered an infant when able to walk and talk, which, in most cases, is at about 1 year.

Infarction: Death of tissue (necrosis) caused by insufficient blood supply (a myocardial infarction is necrosis of the heart muscle).

Inflammation: A protective tissue response to injury that serves to destroy, dilute, or wall off both the injurious agent and the injured tissue. It is characterized by symptoms such as pain, heat, and redness and is the result of the combined effects of numerous inflammatory mediators (e.g., prostaglandins, histamine, cytokines, etc.).

Interferon: A protein produced by the body in response to a stimulus such as an infection.

Internalization: Loss of surface receptor number determined by a combination of the effects of endocytosis and recycling.

Interstitial: Between cells in tissue.

Intima: Innermost layer of a blood vessel.

Intraperitoneal/i.p.:   A route of drug administration for a drug to an animal by direct injection into the peritoneal cavity.

Investigational New Drug Application, or IND: An application that a drug sponsor must submit to the FDA before beginning tests of a new drug on humans. The IND contains the plan for the study and is supposed to give a complete picture of the drug, including its structural formula, animal test results, and manufacturing information.

***In vitro*:**   From the Latin meaning in glass; in an artificial environment such as a test tube.

***In vivo*:**   Tests conducted within the whole living body.

Ischemia: The condition where there is reduced or blocked blood flow to a tissue, which will lead to ischemic tissue damage.

Isoenzyme: One of several forms of an enzyme where the different forms usually catalyze similar but different reactions.

Isotonic: Having the same osmotic pressure and salt concentration as blood.

Kernicterus: Central neuropathy associated with high bilirubin levels and characterized by yellow staining of the basal ganglia.

Latency: The period of time between exposure to an injurious agent and the manifestation of a response (e.g., sensitization period following initial exposure to an antigen).

LD_{50}:   The lethal dose of a compound for 50% of the animals exposed.

L-DOPA: Dihydroxyphenylalanine, a drug used to treat Parkinson's disease.

Ligand: A substance that binds specifically to a receptor.

Ligation: The rejoining of restriction-digested DNA fragments using the enzyme T4 DNA Ligase.

Lipid peroxidation: Oxidative breakdown of lipids usually involving a free radical mechanism or active oxygen species and giving rise to reactive products that may be responsible for cellular damage.

Lipid solubility: See lipophilicity.

Lipophilicity: A term used to describe the ability of a substance to dissolve in, or associate with, fat and therefore living tissue. This usually applies to compounds that are nonionized or nonpolar or have a nonpolar portion. Therefore, high lipid solubility usually implies low water solubility.

Local toxicity: Toxicity that affects only the site of application or exposure.

LSD-d-lysergic acid diethylamide: This chemical was synthesized from ergot in 1938 by Albert Hoffman the Sandoz Laboratories, in Switzerland. It is a potent hallucinogen in the microgram range.

Lupus erythematosus: Autoimmune disease characterized by inflammation and localized skin discoloration.

Lymphocyte: Type of white blood cell produced in the thymus and bone marrow. Two types, T and B.

Lysis: Breakdown of a tissue or macromolecule.

Macrophage: Large phagocytic cells that are components of the reticuloendothelial system.

Mast cell: A granulated cell containing numerous preformed and formed mediators of inflammation. Distributed within the body but particularly concentrated in the lungs.

Messenger RNA (mRNA): Is the transcription-pertinent RNA; represents about 1–5% of total RNA.

Metastasis: Migration and relocation of malignant cancer cells.

Microflora: Microorganisms such as bacteria that normally inhabit the gastrointestinal tract.

Microsomes/microsomal: The subcellular fraction containing the fragments of the smooth endoplasmic reticulum (ER) after ultracentrifugation of a cellular homogenate.

Mitochondria: The intracellular organelle in which respiration and other important metabolic reactions take place.

Monooxygenase: Enzyme system (such as cytochrome P-450) involved in the oxidation of xenobiotics.

Monorchism: Absence of one testicle in the scrotal sac.

Mucosa: Membrane containing mucus secreting cells.

Muscarinic receptors: Receptors for acetylcholine found in smooth muscle, heart, and exocrine glands. Named after the substance muscarine that was used in the early experiments.

Mutagen/mutagenic: A substance/property of a substance that causes some type of mutation in the genetic material of an organism exposed to it.

Mutation: A change of one of the "letters" in the DNA "recipe" caused by chemicals, ultraviolet light, x-rays, or natural processes; a heritable change in DNA sequence; the rawmaterial for natural selection; and the driving force for the generation of biological diversity and evolutionary change.

Mydriasis: Dilation of the pupil of the eye.

Myesthenia gravis: Progressive disease with skeletal muscle weakness associated with neuromuscular junction cholinergic receptor autoantibodies.

Myocardial infarction: Damage to the heart muscle caused by obstruction of the blood flow in the coronary arteries.

Myocardium: The middle and thickest layer of cardiac muscle in the heart wall.

NADH: The coenzyme nicotinamide adenine dinucleotide.

NADPH: The coenzyme reduced nicotinamide adenine dinucleotide phosphate.

Necrosis: The process of cell death within a living organism and the end result of irreversible changes following cellular injury.

Neonate: Refers to a baby from birth to 4 weeks. Another word for neonate is "newborn."

Neoplasia: The pathologic process that results in the formation and growth of a tumor.

Nephritis: Inflammation of the kidney.

Nephron: The functional unit of the kidney that produces urine. It consists of a long tubule divided into sections in which reabsorption into the blood stream of certain solutes filtered by the glomerulus from the blood takes place.

Nephropathy: Pathological damage to the nephrons of the kidney.

Neuronal: Relating to nerve cells.

Neurotransmission: Passage of nerve impulses between neurons mediated by chemical neurotransmitters (e.g., norepinephrine and acetylcholine).

Neutrophil: A phagocytic white blood cell that plays an important role in the inflammatory process.

New Drug Application, or NDA: An application requesting FDA approval to market a new drug for human use in interstate commerce. The application must contain, among other things, data from specific technical viewpoints for FDA review—including chemistry, pharmacology, medical, biopharmaceutics, statistics, and, for anti-infectives, microbiology.

Nodes of Ranvier: Areas in peripheral nerves between myelin sheaths occurring at regular intervals of approximately 1 mm.

Nonsteroidal anti-inflammatory drug: A drug useful in arthritis and other inflammatory conditions, such as salicylates, indomethacin, and ibuprofen.

Occlusion: Constriction or blockage as can occur in a blood vessel.

Older: The Census Bureau defines "older" people as 55+ years of age.

Opiates: Compounds derived from, or similar in action to, potent analgesic opium alkaloids.

Organelle: A subcellular structure such as the mitochondrion or nucleus of a cell.

Organogenesis: The development of specific body structures or organs from undifferentiated tissue. In humans, this corresponds to weeks 2 through 8 postconception.

Orphan drug: A drug for which the target population is limited or for which the disease it treats occurs only rarely.

pA2 value: A value indicating the potency of a competitive antagonist independent of the agonist concentration. Calculated from the Schild analysis.

Parallel track mechanism: A U.S. Public Health Service policy that makes promising investigational drugs for AIDS and other HIV-related diseases more widely available under "parallel track" protocols, while the controlled clinical trials essential to establish the safety and effectiveness of new drugs are carried out. The system established by this policy is designed to make drugs more widely available to patients with these illnesses who have no therapeutic alternatives and who cannot participate in the controlled clinical trials.

Parathesias: Abnormal sensations such as tingling.

Parenteral: Routes of drug administration other than via the gastrointestinal tract.

Parkinson's disease: Neurological disorder accompanied by dopamine deficiency. Patients exhibit extrapyramidal symptoms.

PCR: The Polymerase Chain Reaction that utilizes a thermostable DNA polymerase to make many copies of the same piece of DNA. This allows specific amplification of rare pieces of DNA.

Pediatrics: Deals with the care of infants and children.

Percutaneous: Through the skin.

Peripheral neuropathy: Damage to nerves of the peripheral, rather than central nervous system.

Peroxidases: Enzymes that catalyze oxidation utilizing hydrogen peroxide. Found in many tissues including certain types of white blood cells (e.g., neutrophils).

Pesticide: An agent used to exterminate pests of various types (includes insecticides, herbicides, and fungicides).

Phago/pinocytosis: The uptake of a solid substance (phago) or solution (pino) into a cell by invagination of the cell membrane, eventually forming a vesicle inside the cell.

Pharmacodynamic: Relating to the effects of drugs on living systems.

Pharmacokinetics: The field of study concerned with defining, through measurement or modeling, the absorption, distribution, metabolism, and excretion of drugs or other xenobiotics in a biological system as a function of time.

Pharmacopoeia: An official compendium listing medicinal drugs, their properties, standards of purity, and other useful information.

Phase I: The term applied to the first stage of drug metabolism, commonly involving either oxidation, reduction, or hydrolysis of the molecule.

Phase II: The term applied to the second stage of drug metabolism, usually involving conjugation of a functional group with a moiety available endogenously and conferring water solubility on the molecule.

Phenotype: The expression of the genotype or genetic makeup of an organism.

Phocomelia: The syndrome of having shortened arms and legs due to an adverse effect on the embryo such as caused by thalidomide.

Phospholipid: A lipid in which one of the hydroxyl groups of glycerol or sphingosine is esterified with a phosphorylated alcohol.

Phosphorylation: The process of adding phosphate groups to a compound. Particularly important in the transduction processes of G-protein receptors.

pH partition theory: This states that a foreign compound in the nonionized state will pass across a cell membrane by passive diffusion down a concentration gradient.

Pill (the contraceptive): A mixture of synthetic estrogen and progestin that controls menstrual cycles and produces a state of pseudopregnancy.

Placebo: An inactive compound having no physiological effects; an inert substance identical in appearance to the treatment drug used in clinical studies.

Plasma: Blood from which the cells have been removed by centrifugation, but distinct from serum in which the blood is first allowed to clot.

Plasmid: An extrachromosomal circle of DNA found in bacteria and yeast, which can confer antibiotic resistance to a bacterial host and can be transferred from one cell to another. Capable of self-replicating and can exist in multicopy numbers within a cell. Used as the main vector for gene cloning.

Pneumonitis: Inflammation of the lungs.

Polar: A term used to describe a molecule that is charged or has a tendency to become polarized.

Polydipsia: Excessive thirst.

Polymer: A molecule formed by the joining of many smaller molecules; a protein, for example, is a polymer of amino acids.

Polymerase: An enzyme that forms long chain polymers from simple molecular components; DNA polymerase, for example, forms DNA strands from nucleotides.

Polypeptide: A chain of amino acids joined by peptide bonds.

Population variability: The concept of differences in susceptibility of individuals within a population to drugs or toxicants due to genetic variations in metabolism, for example, or differences in biological responses.

Portal: The term applied to the venous circulation draining the tissues of the gastrointestinal tract into the liver.

Postmarketing surveillance: FDA's ongoing safety monitoring of marketed drugs.

Potency: A comparative expression of drug activity measured in terms of the relationship between the intensity or incidence of a particular effect and the administered dose. Is most appropriately used when comparing drugs that interact with the same population of receptors.

Potentiation: When an effect due to two drugs with different modes of action is greater than expected from the effects of the individual drugs.

PPM: A measure of concentration of a substance in which the units of the substance are one millionth of the solvent (e.g., μg per g).

Preclinical studies: Studies that test a drug on animals and other nonhuman test systems. They must comply with FDA's good laboratory practices. Data about a drug's activities and effects in animals help establish boundaries for safe use of the drug in subsequent human testing (clinical studies). Also, because animals have a much shorter life span than humans, valuable information can be gained about a drug's possible toxic effects over an animal's life cycle and on offspring.

Prodrugs: Inactive drugs that undergo metabolic activation.

Promoter: Region of DNA close to the 5' end of the gene where transcription factors bind and help the binding of RNA polymerase at the *start* of transcription.

Prospective, randomized, double-blind trial: A clinical trial in which the method for analyzing data has been specified in the protocol before the study has begun (prospective), the patients have been randomly assigned to receive either the study drug or alternative treatment, and in which neither the patient nor physician conducting the study know which treatment is being given the patient.

Prostaglandins: Endogenous chemical mediators involved in inflammation derived from the cellular membrane unsaturated fatty acid, arachidonic acid.

Proteinuria: Presence of protein in the urine above normal limits.

Proteomics: Devoted to the study of the entire complement of proteins at once, rather than the tradional one-at-a-time strategy.

Psychoactive drugs: Drugs that produce behavioral changes.

Psychotomimetic: A chemical that produces symptoms similar to pathologic psychoses, such as amphetamine, LSD, and mescaline.

Quantal response: A response that is all-or-none rather than graded.

Racemate: A mixture of stereoisomers.

Raw data: Researcher's records of patients, such as patient charts, hospital records, x-rays, and attending physician notes. These records may or may not accompany an NDA, but must be kept in the researcher's file. FDA may request their submission or may audit them at the researcher's office.

Receptor cycling: Continual agonist-stimulated endocytosis and constitutive recycling of receptors.

Recombinant DNA: DNA formed by joining pieces of DNA from two or more organisms.

Recycling: Movement of receptor or ligand from an internal compartment to the cell surface. Recycling is assumed to be constitutive.

Renal elimination: Excretion of a substance via the kidneys.

Resensitization: Recovery of functional response after desensitization.

Restriction enzyme: An enzyme that cuts DNA at a specific sequence leaving a complimentary "sticky end."

Retrovirus: A type of virus whose genetic material consists of RNA rather than DNA.

Reverse transcriptase: A retro-viral enzyme that copies RNA into DNA.

Rhinitis: Inflammation of the mucous membranes of the nose.

Ribosomes: The intracellular organelles attached to the rough endoplasmic reticulum, which are involved with protein synthesis.

RNA: A single stranded copy of DNA consisting of Adenosine, Cytidine, Guanosine, and Uridine. Most commonly found as Messenger RNA (mRNA), Transfer RNA (tRNA), or Ribosomal RNA (rRNA).

RNA processing: The removal of the introns from the coding (exon) sequence to give the mRNA.

Safety: No drug is completely safe or without the potential for side effects. Before a drug may be approved for marketing, the law requires the submission of results of tests adequate to show the drug is safe under the conditions of use in the proposed labeling. Thus "safety" is determined case by case and reflects the drug's risk-versus-benefit relationship.

Safety update reports: Reports that an NDA sponsor must submit to FDA about new safety information that may affect the use for which the drug will be approved, or draft labeling statements about contraindications, warnings, precautions, and adverse reactions. Safety update reports are required 4 months after application is submitted, after the applicant receives an approval letter, and at other times on FDA request.

Schild analysis: Consists of a series of agonist dose–response curves obtained in the presence of increasing concentrations of antagonist. Allows the determination of antagonist potency independent of the agonist concentration.

Schwann cells: Large nucleated cells that wrap around myelinated peripheral neurons to form the myelin sheath.

Sequencing: The determination of the nucleotide sequence of a DNA fragment.

Sequestration: Synonymous with internalization.

Sensitization: A term used in reference to the period following exposure to an antigen when the body begins to produce antigens.

Sinsemilla: There are male and female marijuana plants. The flowers of the female plant contain the highest concentration of THC. Growers have learned that if the female plants are not allowed to be pollinated, the flowers cluster and excrete greater quantities of resin. Marijuana grown in this fashion is called Sinsemilla that means "no seeds."

Splanchnic: Pertaining to the internal organs.

St. Anthony's fire: Ergotism or toxicity from ingesting ergot alkaloids with cerebrospinal symptoms, spasms, cramps, and gangrene in the extremities.

Structure–activity relationship: Relationships of pharmacological activity or toxicity of a xenobiotic to its chemical structure.

Subchronic: An exposure of duration intermediate between acute and chronic (e.g., 28 or 90 days) or approximately 10% of the lifetime of an organism.

Subcutaneous: Below the skin.

Sublingual: Below the tongue.

Superoxide: The oxygen molecule with an extra unpaired electron. It is thus a charged free radical and is highly reactive.

Supplement: A marketing application submitted for changes in a product that already has an approved NDA. FDA must approve all important NDA changes (in packaging or ingredients, for example) to ensure that the conditions originally set for the product are not adversely affected.

Surrogate endpoint: A laboratory finding or physical sign that may not, in itself, be a direct measurement of how a patient feels, functions, or survives, but nevertheless is considered likely to predict therapeutic benefit. An example would be CD4 cell counts, used to measure the strength of the immune system in AIDS.

Synergism/synergistic: When effects of two or more drugs are greater than the sum of their individual effects.

Synovial: Relating to the lubricating fluid in joints.

Synovitis: Inflammation of the joints, arthritis.

Systemic toxicity: Toxicity that affects a system in the organism other than and probably distant from the site of application or exposure.

Tachycardia: Excess rapid heart rate.

Tachyphylaxis: Rapid decrease in physiological response to a drug after administration of a few doses (i.e., acute tolerance).

TD$_{50}$: The dose that is toxic to 50% of the population exposed to the substance or a 50% toxic response in a biological system exposed to the substance (i.e., nausea).

Teratogen/teratogenicity: A substance/property of a substance causing abnormalities in the embryo or fetus when administered to the maternal organism.

Therapeutic index: The ratio of LD$_{50}$ to ED$_{50}$.

Thiol: SH or sulfhydryl group.

Thromboembolism: Obstruction of a blood vessel by a broken thrombus (blood clot) that was transported to the occluded vessel from another site of formation.

Thrombosis: Formation of blood clots causing vascular obstruction.

Tinnitus: A "ringing" in the ears.

Tolerance: When repeated administration of or dosing with a drug leads to a decrease in the potency in the biological activity of that drug. May have a metabolic or cellular basis. Acute tolerance is referred to as tachyphylaxis.

Toxic effect: Any change in an organism that results in impairment of functional capacity of the organism (as determined by anatomical, physiological, biochemical, or behavioral parameters); causes decrements in the organism's ability to maintain its normal function; or enhances the susceptibility of the organism to the deleterious effects of other environmental influences.

Toxicology: The multidisciplinary study of toxicants, their harmful effects on biological systems, and the conditions under which these harmful effects occur. The mechanisms of action, detection, and treatment of the conditions produced by toxicants are studied.

Transcription: The process of copying DNA to RNA, performed by RNA polymerases.

Transdermal: Through the skin.

Transfection: Introduction of a foreign gene into a cell's genome.

Transgenic: An organism that has been modified by genetic engineering to contain DNA from an external source.

Transgenic animals: Animals in which a gene from a different species has been inserted.

Translation: The process of copying mRNA into protein, performed by ribosomal RNA.

Treatment IND: A mechanism that allows promising investigational drugs to be used in "expanded access" protocols—relatively unrestricted studies in which the intent is both to learn more about the drugs, especially their safety, and to provide treatment for people with immediately life-threatening or otherwise serious diseases for which there is no real alternative. But these expanded protocols also require researchers to formally investigate the drugs in well-controlled studies and to supply some evidence that the drugs are likely to be helpful. The drugs cannot expose patients to unreasonable risk.

Trimodal: Frequency distribution that divides into three groups.

Ultrafiltrate: The fluid formed in the renal tubule from blood passing through the glomerulus/ Bowman's capsule in the kidney.

Urticaria: A vascular reaction of the skin marked by the appearance of wheals, which may be caused by direct or indirect exposure to a toxic substance. Also known as hives.

User fees: Charges to drug firms for certain NDAs, drug products, and manufacturing establishments. FDA uses these fees to hire more application reviewers and to accelerate reviews through the use of computer technology.

Vasculitis: Inflammation of a blood vessel.

Vasoconstriction: Constriction of blood vessels.

Vasodilatation/vascular dilatation: Dilation of blood vessels.

Vector: Any DNA structure that is used to transfer DNA into an organism; most commonly used are plasmid DNA vectors or viruses.

Vivissection: Originally the surgical cutting of a living animal in scientific research; often used today as a synonym for any type of animal research.

Volume of distribution (Vd):   The volume of body fluid in which a xenobiotic is apparently distributed when administered to an animal.

Wheals: Raised patches on the skin; usually an immunological response.

Xenobiotic: A chemical foreign to the body.

Zero-order process: The rate of the process is independent of the concentration of the substance (e.g., liver metabolism of ethyl alcohol).

Appendix IV: Top 10 Drugs in History

A list of top 10 of anything is obviously arguable. This is my selection, which I have gleaned from WebMD. I think it is perfectly reasonable, and can stimulate the student to develop his or her own.

1. As the first antibiotic, penicillin led the way toward the treatment of microbial disease. As pointed out in this book, it is a unique drug in that it can actually cure a disease. Without penicillin, 75% of the people now alive would not be alive because their parents or grandparents would have died owing to infections. The effects of penicillin on mankind cannot be overestimated.

2. Insulin: The first widely used hormone. Its use in type 1 diabetes changed a death sentence to being able to live a long life. An untreated patient with type 1 diabetes will eventually succumb to blindness, peripheral vascular disease, or kidney failure. Fortunately, through the collaboration between industry and academic researchers, patients now have access to human insulin produced by recombinant technology.

3. Smallpox is by nearly universal acclaim foremost among the most dreadful scourges of humanity. One need only see the face and body of an afflicted poor soul to imagine what it must be like to suffer from this horrible malady. This makes its possible use as a bioterror weapon all the more terrible to contemplate. Thanks to vaccination, smallpox is the first disease wiped from the face of the earth. One can only hope that cultures that still exist in laboratories remain controlled.

4. Ether: imagine going to the dentist without aid of an anesthetic; imagine having a limb amputated or, a baby for that matter. The amount of pain that people have endured throughout history is incalculable. Ether made it possible to have an agent that can depress a person's brain so major operations can be carried out.

5. Despite the problem of narcotic addiction, a world without morphine would have had more suffering, not less. Without morphine, untold numbers of people would have spent their lives in great pain. It is the forerunner of several generations of pain-alleviating drugs—one of the great drugs of all time.

6. Aspirin was the first drug to demonstrate you can treat simple pain. Most people in the world have some kind of peripheral pain, muscle pain, or headache, or arthritis. For these people, morphine would be inappropriate; as an analgesic, aspirin can fill the bill.

7. Salvarsan is mentioned in this book and makes the list. It was Paul Ehrlich's magic bullet number 606 developed for the treatment of syphilis. It worked because the arsenic-based compound is a bit more poisonous to syphilis bacteria than it is to humans. Salvarsan was the first chemotherapeutic agent. Like anticancer drugs today, salvarsan made people dreadfully ill but didn't kill them, which syphilis would eventually do.

8. Insane asylums of the past were built to contain people suffering from severe psychiatric diseases known as psychoses. The advent of modern psychiatric drugs in the 1950s changed everything. Drugs such as Thorazine helped to control psychoses and manage the disorder on an out-patient basis. It was the first drug for modern psychopharmacology.

9. Oral contraceptives changed the world. By giving women control over their reproductive system, these drugs have had far-reaching medical and social impact.

10. One of the first loop diuretics was furosemide (Lasix). As such it found efficacy in the treatment of hypertension and heart failure. Despite the availability of newer drugs to treat congestive heart failure today, many patients can still be treated with inexpensive diuretics.

Appendix V: Answers to Self-Assessment Questions

Chapter 1	Chapter 2	Chapter 3	Chapter 4
1-c	1-d	1-a	1-c
2-b	2-a	2-e	2-e
3-d	3-c	3-e	3-e
4-e	4-b	4-e	4-d
5-e	5-a	5-c	5-e
6-e	6-c	6-d	6-d
7-d	7-c	7-e	7-c
8-b	8-d	8-e	8-b
9-d	9-a	9-a	9-a
10-e	10-a	10-d	10-e

Chapter 5	Chapter 6	Chapter 7	Chapter 8
1-c	1-b	1-d	1-a
2-e	2-c	2-a	2-e
3-e	3-c	3-c	3-d
4-e	4-c	4-e	4-e
5-e	5-e	5-b	5-e
6-d	6-e	6-d	6-e
7-d	7-d	7-c	7-e
8-e	8-e	8-a	8-c
9-b	9-e	9-c	9-c
10-d	10-c	10-e	10-e

Chapter 9	Chapter 10	Chapter 11	Chapter 12
1-e	1-e	1-e	1-d
2-d	2-c	2-e	2-a
3-e	3-b	3-e	3-b
4-d	4-b	4-c	4-c
5-c	5-d	5-e	5-c
6-e	6-d	6-d	6-e
7-e	7-e	7-c	7-d
8-e	8-e	8-d	8-d
9-c	9-e	9-d	9-e
10-b	10-e	10-d	10-c

Chapter 13	Chapter 14	Chapter 15	Chapter 16
1-a	1-e	1-d	1-e
2-d	2-e	2-e	2-c
3-c	3-a	3-e	3-d
4-d	4-c	4-e	4-c
5-d	5-d	5-c	5-a
6-e	6-d	6-e	6-a
7-b	7-e	7-e	7-e
8-e	8-b	8-b	8-e
9-e	9-d	9-e	9-c
10-e	10-b	10-b	10-e

Chapter 17	Chapter 18
1-c	1-e
2-c	2-b
3-d	3-e
4-c	4-a
5-e	5-c
6-b	6-a
7-c	7-e
8-e	8-e
9-e	9-c
10-b	10-c

Index

G